A Textbook of
Practical Physiology

A Textbook of Practical Physiology

Seventh Edition

CL Ghai MBBS MD

Formerly

Professor and Head, Department of Physiology
Government Medical College, Amritsar

Professor and Head, Department of Physiology
Government Medical College, Patiala

Professor and Head, Department of Physiology
GGS Medical College, Faridkot

Professor and Head, Department of Physiology
DAV (C) Dental College, Yamunanagar

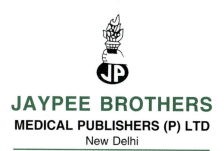

JAYPEE BROTHERS
MEDICAL PUBLISHERS (P) LTD
New Delhi

Published by

Jitendar P Vij
Jaypee Brothers Medical Publishers (P) Ltd
B-3 EMCA House, 23/23B Ansari Road, Daryaganj
New Delhi 110 002, India
Phones: +91-11-23272143, +91-11-23272703, +91-11-23282021, +91-11-23245672, Rel: 32558559
Fax: +91-11-23276490, +91-11-23245683,   e-mail: jaypee@jaypeebrothers.com
Visit our website: www.jaypeebrothers.com

Branches

- ❏ 2/B, Akruti Society, Jodhpur Gam Road Satellite
  Ahmedabad 380 015
  Phones: +91-079-26926233, Rel: +91-079-32988717, Fax: +91-079-26927094
  e-mail: ahmedabad@jaypeebrothers.com

- ❏ 202 Batavia Chambers, 8 Kumara Krupa Road, Kumara Park East
  Bengaluru 560 001
  Phones: +91-80-22285971, +91-80-22382956, Rel: +91-80-32714073, Fax: +91-80-22281761
  e-mail: bangalore@jaypeebrothers.com

- ❏ 282 IIIrd Floor, Khaleel Shirazi Estate, Fountain Plaza, Pantheon Road
  Chennai 600 008 Phones: +91-44-28193265, +91-44-28194897, Rel: +91-44-32972089
  Fax: +91-44-28193231   e-mail: chennai@jaypeebrothers.com

- ❏ 4-2-1067/1-3, 1st Floor, Balaji Building, Ramkote Cross Road
  Hyderabad 500 095, Phones: +91-40-66610020, +91-40-24758498, Rel:+91-40-32940929
  Fax:+91-40-24758499, e-mail: hyderabad@jaypeebrothers.com

- ❏ No. 41/3098, B & B1, Kuruvi Building, St. Vincent Road
  Kochi 682 018, Kerala, Phones: 0484-4036109, +91-0484 2395739, +91-0484 2395740
  e-mail: kochi@jaypeebrothers.com

- ❏ 1-A Indian Mirror Street, Wellington Square
  Kolkata 700 013, Phones: +91-33-22451926, +91-33-22276404, +91-33-22276415
  Rel: +91-33-32901926   Fax: +91-33-22456075, e-mail: kolkata@jaypeebrothers.com

- ❏ 106 Amit Industrial Estate, 61 Dr SS Rao Road
  Near MGM Hospital, Parel
  Mumbai 400 012
  Phones: +91-22-24124863, +91-22-24104532, Rel: +91-22-32926896
  Fax: +91-22-24160828,   e-mail: mumbai@jaypeebrothers.com

- ❏ "KAMALPUSHPA" 38, Reshimbag, Opp. Mohota Science College, Umred Road
  Nagpur 440 009 (MS)
  Phones: Rel: 3245220, Fax: 0712-2704275,   e-mail: nagpur@jaypeebrothers.com

A Textbook of Practical Physiology
© 2007, CL Ghai

First Edition :   1983
Second Edition: 1985
Third Edition: 1987
Fourth Edition: 1990
Fifth Edition: 1999
Sixth Edition: 2005
Reprint: 2006

Seventh Edition : **2007**

ISBN 81-8448-141-1

Typeset at   JPBMP typesetting unit
Printed at   Ajanta Offset & Packagings Ltd., New Delhi

To
Prem
Shobhit, Seema
and
Mehak and Akshay

PREFACE TO THE SEVENTH EDITION

The first edition of this book was published nearly 25 years ago. This is a long enough time for the evolution of a book and for assessing its value to the students.

During this period, the evolution of the book has been a continuous process depending, largely as it does, on the feedback received from various medical teachers and students. They have been generous in their appreciation as well as in their constructive criticism and suggestions for the further improvement of the book. I am confident that I shall continue to receive such help in the future as well.

The general organization and format of the book has been retained for the Seventh edition. The section on Hematology has been thoroughly revised. As per the new curriculum policy of the Medical and Dental Councils of India, the section on Human Experiments has been reorganized and expanded with the addition of new experiments, figures and diagrams. Other sections have also been appropriately revised to bring the book in conformity with modern concepts in the subject. A few experiments and other material that were not found beneficial to the students have been excluded.

The format of Questions/Answers introduced in the last edition has been particularly appreciated by the students and junior teachers. This material is not meant to replace the standard textbooks on physiology, but merely to act as a bridge between the theory and practical work.

A new feature is the introduction of **Student Objectives** at the beginning of most practicals. It gives an outline of what a student is expected to learn from that experiment and the clinical application of that knowledge. However, this has not been done at the cost of the fundamentals of physiological knowledge.

Every effort has been made to make the book easily readable and understandable by our students, some of whom find it difficult to overcome the language barrier. They have continuously demanded simplicity, directness, and clarity of expression that is within their grasp. I hope I have succeeded in this effort.

During the course of the evolution of the book I have received valuable help and guidance from many sources. Though it is not possible to thank everyone, I am particularly grateful to Dr Ashok Kumar, Dr OP Tandon, Dr SK Manchanda, Dr (Mrs) B K Maini, Dr RS Sidhu, Dr (Mrs) P Khetarpal, Dr Ram Sarup Sharma, Dr NK Mishra and Dr (Mrs) Usha Nagpal.

I particularly wish to express my thanks to Dr DK Soni and Dr AK Garg who were ever ready to extend suggestions as well as criticism for the improvement of the book.

I am indebted to Shri JP Vij, Chairman and Managing Director, Jaypee Brothers Medical Publishers (P) Ltd. and his team for their enthusiasm in bringing out the new edition. He and his team have done an excellent job.

I would be remiss if I do not express my gratitude to my students who have, over a period extending over 40 years, inspired me towards greater efforts to achieve excellence in this book.

C L Ghai

Panchkula , Haryana

PREFACE TO THE FIRST EDITION

The material included within the covers of this book conforms to the syllabi and courses of practical physiology laid down by the Medical Council of India, and followed by all the medical colleges. The book is divided into three main sections—amphibian, mammalian and human experiments. There is a separate section on electronic recorders and stimulators. If our students are not to be left behind the rapidly advancing field of medical electronics, they have to be introduced at the earliest to the use of some of these modern devices. The book also supplements the cyclostyled material provided by some physiology departments to their students.

In essence, each experiment begins with the **PRINCIPLE** on which it is based, and the **APPARATUS** required for it. Then follow the step by step **PROCEDURES** in which the working instructions are so framed that an average student will find no difficulty in tackling any experiment. Next come the **OBSERVATIONS, RESULTS,** and **CONCLUSIONS**. The relevant theoretical aspects of each experiment that are needed for immediate reference, including deviations from the normal, are then described under the heading of **DISCUSSION**. This is intended to obviate the necessity for the student to refer to the textbooks again and again. Finally, the **QUESTIONS** generally asked from the students are grouped at the end of the experiment. A student should be able to assess his/her comprehension of the relevant material in trying to answer these questions. The **APPENDIX** contains the units and measures employed in physiology, and the equivalents of metric, United States, and English (Imperial) measures. This is followed by some important reference values of clinical importance. These will certainly prove useful to the hurried and harried medical student for quick reference.

There is continuing controversy and divergence of opinion regarding the necessity of including amphibian experiments in the medical curriculum. Often, these experiments may appear to be time wasting and irrelevant to clinical medicine. However, they have to be included in a book meant primarily for the Indian medical student till such time the courses are revised by the MCI. In any case, they do serve a very useful purpose. They train the students to work with their hands in devising and setting up an experiment, making careful observations, critically analyzing the results and then drawing appropriate conclusions. These are the qualities that the students will depend on later in their clinical work. In fact, the ability to solve problems is the ultimate skill of the physician, and this ability will be honed if the above-mentioned qualities are suitably developed. A compromise can, however, be arrived at; the number of amphibian experiments to be done by the students themselves may be reduced while the rest are demonstrated to them in small groups by their tutors.

The chief aim of the book is to help the students in coping with the problems arising from the handling of various apparatuses during the practical work. If a student has a hazy notion of the purpose of an experiment and the correct technique of carrying it out, he/she will easily be disheartened and frustrated. We hope to help with a clear idea of what he/she is expected to do and a more definite plan of doing it.

It is a pleasure to acknowledge the valuable suggestions received from many friends and colleagues, especially Dr. (Mrs.) P. Khetarpal, Dr. (Mrs.) Usha Nagpal, Dr. Kanta Kumari, Dr. R. S. Sidhu, Dr. R. S. Sharma, Dr. Ashok Kumar, Dr. Parveen Gupta, Dr. O. P. Mahajan, Dr. S. Mookerjee, Dr. (Mrs.) B. K. Maini, Dr. S. K. Manchanda, Dr. O. P. Tandon, Dr. G. M. Shah, and Dr. M. Sayeed.

I must express my gratitude to my wife, Mrs. Prem Ghai, for her understanding and unstinted support during the long months of collecting the material and the writing of the book.

I fail to find adequate words to thank my students who prompted and encouraged me in the first instance to write this book. We physiologists recognise the importance of the feedback systems of the body, and so too, is feedback essential for the development of a book. Criticism and suggestions from teachers and students for the further improvement of the book will be thankfully received and acknowledged.

I am indebted to Mr. Jitendar P. Vij, my publisher, and his dedicated team for their continued cooperation, enthusiasm and their excellent work in bringing out this book.

May this book act as an effective stimulus for the students to gain first-hand knowledge of experimental physiology, and ease their journey through a complex but fascinating science. As they gather experience, the path will become easier. The discipline of work will then become the most exciting and rewarding experience in their lives.

As they say, "When the going gets tough, the tough get going".

C L Ghai

Amritsar
October 1983

CONTENTS

Section One
HEMATOLOGY

Section Two
HUMAN EXPERIMENTS

Section Three

CLINICAL EXAMINATION

Section Four

EXPERIMENTAL PHYSIOLOGY
(AMPHIBIAN AND MAMMALIAN EXPERIMENTS)

Section Five

CHARTS

Section Six

CALCULATIONS

The term "physiology" is derived from a Greek root with a Latin equivalent "physiologia", originally meaning "natural knowledge" (Physic- = nature; -logy = study of). Though first used by Jean Fernel, a French physician, in 1542, the word "physiology" did not come into common use till the 19th century. The subject of "physiology" now refers to the origin, development and progression of living organisms - from bacteria to vertebrates to trees. Thus, there are many branches of physiology. However, we are primarily concerned with "Human Physiology", i.e. the functional characteristics of the human body.

It is said that medicine is as old as man, and the growth of our knowledge of physiology is closely linked to the growth of medicine— the mother of all branches of natural science. Chemistry, physics, botany, zoology, pathology, pharmacology, microbiology and their branches have all evolved from the study of the art of healing. And they have, in turn, contributed tremendously to the advancement of medical science. Man is always in search of new and better means of maintenance of health and cure of diseases. This has resulted in new lines of thought and newer methods of investigations from time to time, thus creating new sciences.

It is interesting to note that many of the outstanding physiologists have been well known physicians. We are now aware of the tremendous body of physiological knowledge that has its origin in the study of disease. In turn, the exciting progress in physiology during the last two centuries has greatly enriched our knowledge of disease and put medicine on a scientific footing. The student must, therefore, never lose sight of the fact that the knowledge she gains from physiology will form the solid basis of all branches of medicine that she will be studying later— pharmacology, pathology, internal medicine, surgery, gynecology etc.

Over a century ago, William Osler, the famous physician said, "The study of physiology (and pathology) within the past half century has done more to emancipate medicine from the routine and thralldom of authority than all the work of all the physicians from the days of Hippocrates to Jenner, and we are as yet on the threshold."

THE INTERNAL ENVIRONMENT OF THE BODY

Life is believed to have originated in warm seas, which, therefore, formed the external environment of the early forms of life. While these unicellular and few-celled organisms could exchange oxygen and other nutrients, as well as their waste products, directly with the external (or general) environment (i.e., sea water), this process could not operate in multicellular organisms in which most of the cells were located deep within the body. But if these cells could not reach the sea, the sea would have to be brought to them within the body. Each cell in the depths of the body would then be bathed by a fluid with which it could enter into exchanges. This is exactly what is believed to have happened. As evolution proceeded, the external environment was 'internalized' and the sea became the tissue fluid (interstitial fluid), which, along with blood plasma, constitutes extracellular fluid (ECF). The evolution of ECF from the sea water is evident from its composition— it has more sodium, chloride, and bicarbonate as compared to intracellular fluid (ICF; the fluid within the cells), which has more potassium, magnesium, and proteins. The plasma membranes (cell membranes) of the cells, because of their selective permeability, keep the two chemical worlds separated from each other.

The adult human body consists of nearly 100 trillion cells (25 trillion of which are red cells), most of which live in an "internal sea" of ECF, as

xviii A Textbook of Practical Physiology

described above. Since these cells live within 20-30 μm of blood capillaries, materials can easily pass from the blood into the tissue fluid and thence into the cells, as well as in the opposite direction.

Claude Bernard, a French physician and a great experimental physiologist, employed the term "milieu interior" (internal environment), in the mid 19th century, for the very thin layer of tissue fluid that lies immediately outside each cell. Though the tissue fluid lies outside the cells, it is called the " internal environment" of the body because it has no direct communication with the external or general environment that surrounds the body of an organism.

HOMEOSTASIS – THE BASIC THEME OR PHILOSOPHY OF THE BODY

A necessary condition for the survival of each living cell (and the body as a whole) is that the physical and chemical composition of its immediate surrounding (i.e., interstitial fluid) must not change beyond a certain narrow range, although the external or general environment may show wide changes. For example, the temperature of external environment may vary between –60°C and +60°C, the temperature of the tissue fluid will not change by more than a few degrees.

Though the huge varieties of body cells are organized in tissues, organs and organ systems, they do not function in isolation. Rather they act in such a way that the body as a whole reacts as a unit to any change in the environment. Thus, all the specialized systems of the body—blood, circulatory, respiratory, digestive, and locomotor etc. – have one and only one aim in common, i.e. maintenance of a nearly constant condition of equilibrium or balance in the internal environment of the body. Walter Canon, in 1897, introduced the term **"homeostasis"** (homeo- = sameness; -stasis = standing still) to refer to the dynamic state of relative stability of the tissue fluid— in terms of its temperature, chemical composition, gas pressures etc – the so-called *"controlled conditions"*.

The ***nervous system*** and the ***endocrine (hormonal) system*** are the two major communication and control systems that coordinate the activities of all the other systems of the body. The nervous system is a "quick-reaction" system that is concerned with the immediate "*short-term*" maintenance of homeostasis. The endocrine system, on the other hand, maintains "*long-term*" homeostasis. In both cases, homeostasis is achieved through a "non-stop" interplay of feedback mechanisms (feedback loops) – some of which function at the macro level (e.g. regulation of body temperature, blood pressure, gas pressures, blood glucose, etc), while others operate at the micro level, i.e. within the cells. In fact, most of physiology deals with homeostatic mechanisms.

Many factors, within and outside the body, tend to disturb the body's state of equilibrium. If the disturbance is mild, the feedback systems help to quickly restore homeostasis required for health and life. However, if the imbalance is moderate, a disorder or disease may result. If, on the other hand, the imbalance is severe or prolonged, death may occur.

EXPERIMENTATION AND OBSERVATION

Experimentation

Science is the study of the world around us; rather it is an organized language for describing the world. An experimentation forms the core concept, and a time-honored procedure, in the process of learning about any science.

1. An experiment consists in making an event occur under certain known conditions, care being taken to exclude as many extraneous factors as possible. Only then observations can be made and proper conclusions drawn.

2. It is very important for the student to understand the workings of various instruments and apparatuses that she/he will be using. There is a definite protocol or procedure for conducting every experiment. Careful attention given to apparently minor and seemingly

unimportant, yet troublesome, points and the precautions to be taken, usually determine the outcome of an experiment. It is an important axiom of science that "mistakes in technique can lead to misleading results".

3. The fundamental idea in experimentation is that "*you learn by doing*". It is an opportunity provided to the student to gain first-hand knowledge about various aspects of the functioning of one's own body.

4. Laboratory work in Physiology is meant to inculcate in the students the habit of carrying out certain procedures in an orderly manner, make careful observations, and draw appropriate conclusions. This will help them in developing scientific skills that will aid them when they approach a problem in clinical setting.

5. Practical work and theory always complement each other. Therefore, the student must read up as much as possible about the practical and theoretical aspects of an experiment beforehand. Francis Bacon, a great philosopher of science, said, "Read not to contradict, nor to believe and take for granted... but to weigh and consider." So, read critically and reflectively, with an open mind.

Observation

1. Relations between phenomena can only be revealed if proper observations have been made. Observations should not be passive. Active and effective observation involves noticing something and giving it significance by correlating it with something else noticed or already known.

2. The student must keep an open mind, forget for the time being, her preconceived notions and be on the lookout for the unusual. "Look out for the unexpected" is a good maxim for the medical student.

New knowledge very often has its origin in some quite unexpected observation or chance occurrence arising during an experiment.

Alfred North Whitehead, the famous philosopher says, "First-hand knowledge is the ultimate basis of intellectual life. The peculiar merit of scientific education is that it bases thought upon first-hand observation; and the corresponding merit of a technical education is that it follows our deep natural instinct to transfer thought into manual skill, and manual activity into thought. The thought which science evokes is logical thought."

REPORTING THE RESULTS

1. Students have a common tendency to report their observations and results similar to those described in the books. One should always remember that the result of an experiment is, strictly speaking, valid only for the precise conditions under which the experiment was conducted.

2. It is well known that the accuracy with which an experiment is conducted varies from person to person. Therefore, if your results are at variance with those expected, some unrecognized factor or factors might be operating. Such occurrences must always be welcomed, because the search for the unknown factor may lead to an interesting discovery. It is when experiments go wrong that we find things out.

INSTRUCTIONS TO THE STUDENTS

1. Check the laboratory schedule a day earlier and read up the relevant material in the practical physiology book. This will help you to plan and organize each experiment.

2. Pay due attention to the practical demonstration given by your teacher before each experiment.

3. Always bring your practical physiology book as well as your practical work-book (file) to the laboratory.

4. Check out the apparatus being issued to you by the lab technician at the distribution table, and see that it is in proper working condition. This will avoid frustration and wastage of time

once you start your work. You will be required to sign for the apparatus and return it after completing your work. If there is any breakage or damage to the apparatus, it must be reported to the teacher-in-charge.

5. As you may be working in groups of two, you should not expect nor depend entirely on the efforts of your work-partner to do most of the work. Each student is expected to be able to independently carry out each experiment.

6. As you and your partner will be acting as the 'subject' in human experiments and clinical examination, try to be gentle and considerate. You will need these qualities later when you handle patients.

Important

As you start each practical, be certain to go through the **"Student objectives"** at the start of each experiment. This will help you to focus on what is important and what is expected from you.

LABORATORY DISCIPLINE

1. Wear a clean overall, as it constitutes an essential part of laboratory discipline.
2. The working area on the worktable must be kept clean and the equipment placed in proper and convenient locations. Avoid clutter.
3. Do not throw any used cotton/ gauze, pieces of paper etc. into the sink.
4. Do not indulge in idle gossip. However, discussions with your work partner and other students will be of tremendous help.
5. Guidance from your teacher is always available and should be actively sought and welcomed.
6. **Equipment.** The department will provide most of the equipment needed by you. However, you must bring your own colored pencils (blue, heliotrope, black lead, etc.) ruler, rubber, clean piece of cloth, etc. You will be told about other instruments (e.g. stethoscope, percussion hammer, etc.) required for

"Human Experiments", "Clinical Examination," and "Amphibian Experiments."

WRITING RECORDS

1. The practical notebook should be of good quality paper, blank (unruled) on the left side for diagrams, and ruled on the right side for description of the practical work.
2. Every student must keep a record of the demonstrations attended and experiments conducted. Get every experiment signed from your teacher regularly. Make an index of your work in your notebook, and get each entry initialed by your teacher.
3. Remember that **Relevance**, the **Principle** on which the experiment is based, **Observations** and **Results**, **Conclusions** and the **Precautions** taken constitute an important part of your training in basic scientific work. Enter all this material in your notebook.
4. Observations and results should be properly entered, and diagrams, graphs and tables prepared as and when needed.
5. Variations under normal and abnormal conditions form an important part of a medical experiment. These should also be recorded.

SUGGESTIONS FOR TUTORS/ JUNIOR TEACHERS

1. Teachers are managers of the learning process of the students. Every student needs help and guidance in her/his learning process and teachers are meant to fulfill this need.
2. Teachers have great responsibility of inculcating discipline and work culture in their students.
3. They must ensure that the students do not indulge in idle gossip. However, they should be easily accessible to the students in need of guidance.
4. Students are generally afraid to seek help and ask questions out of fear of the teacher, or out of a fear of exposing their ignorance of the subject and cutting a sorry figure in front

of other students. They need to be assured that it is all right to ask questions (and even make mistakes in the process). In these days of knowledge explosion, nobody can even hope to know everything even about a limited part of knowledge available.

5. Junior teachers should acquaint themselves thoroughly with the subject so that they can help students effectively.

Objective Assessment of Students' Practical Skills

The assessment of students in practical work during class tests and university examinations has been more or less a subjective process. Usually the student has finished her/his practical by the time the examiner comes to assess the students' work. Questions are asked about the practical and its theoretical aspects and what is then assessed is the students' knowledge rather than the practical skills. Depending on the experience of the examiner, the method has stood the test of time to quite a satisfactory extent.

However, the trend has changed at many colleges. The examiner asks the students to carry out the given practical exercise, say, preparation of a blood film and staining it for differential leukocyte count. Each step is checked against a previously-prepared 'checklist'. Questions may be asked and awards are then given accordingly. This **objective method** of assessment of practical skills is, of course, time-consuming and requires detailed planning and cooperation of the teaching staff.

Hematology

Hematology (Gr. Hema- = Blood; - logy = Study of). Hematology is the branch of medical science that deals with the study of blood. *Blood*, along with the *cardiovascular system* constitutes the *Circulatory system* and performs the following functions:

1. **Transport.** Blood provides a pickup and delivery system for the transport of gases, nutrients, hormones, waste products, etc over a route of some 1,12,000 km of blood vessels, with 60-70 trillion customers (cells).

2. **Regulation.** It regulates the body temperature by transporting heat from the tissues (mainly liver and muscles) to the skin from where it can be lost. Its buffers regulate pH of the body fluids, while its osmotic pressure regulates water content of cells through the actions of its dissolved proteins and ions.

3. **Protection.** The blood protects the body against diseases caused by harmful organisms by transporting leucocytes and antibodies against more than a million foreign invaders.

It also protects the body against loss of blood after injury by the process of blood clotting.

Physical features. The blood is denser and more viscous than water, slightly alkaline, sticky to touch, and salty in taste. It clots on standing, leaving behind serum. The normal total circulating blood volume amounts to 8 % of the body weight, i.e., 5-6 liters in an average adult male weighing 70 kg, and 4-5 liters in a female. The interplay of various hormones that control salt and water excretion in the urine keep the blood volume remarkably constant.

Composition. Blood consists of 55 % of watery liquid plasma that contains various proteins and other solutes dissolved in it. The rest 45 % is the formed elements— mainly the red blood cells (RBCs) but also white blood cells (WBCs), and platelets (cell fragments). The RBCs are the most numerous (4.5-5.5 million/mm^3) and are medium sized (7-8 µm). Next in number are platelets (2.5-4.5 lacs/mm^3) and are the smallest (2-4 µm) in size. The WBCs number 4000-11000/mm^3 and vary in size from 8 to 20 µm. The percentage of whole blood that is red cells is called *hematocrit*, its value being 45.

Hematological tests. The experiments described in this section are carried out as routine hemato-logical tests in hospitals and clinical laboratories for aiding in the diagnosis and prognosis of disease. Some tests (e.g., hemoglobin, cell counts etc) are simple enough, while others require some degree of practice and understanding.

The use of microscope, diluting pipettes counting chamber, collection of blood samples are described in details in the first few experiments. This will avoid repetition later on. The student can refer to them later on as required.

Electronic hematology analyzers. Automatic electronic analyzers under various trade names are now available (Eg; Nihon Kohdon, model MEK-6318 K). Though costly, they are easy to operate and highly accurate.

The measured parameters include: TLC, WBC population percentages. Hb concentration, HcT, absolute corpuscular values (MCV, MCH, MCHC, etc), platelet count and volume, etc. The detection methods include: electrical resistance detection, spectrophotometry, histogram calculations, etc.

The volumes of blood samples required are small and may be venous (50 µl) or capillary (10 µl). Once the sample is aspirated through the sampling nozzle, all other operations, such as dilution or adding hemolysing agent, are carried out automatically. There is an LCD screen that displays calibration and error messages, numerical data and histograms for individual samples. Printouts can be obtained and data stored for recall.

There is a provision for automatic cleaning and waste fluid treatment.

CAUTION

The patient's blood, as that of a volunteer, must be regarded as a possible source of communicable infections, particularly immunodeficiency virus (HIV), hepatitis B, and recurrent venereal disease. Always handle blood specimens as potential hazards capable of transmitting infection.

Do not touch blood other than your own.

Every student should bring his/her own disposable blood lancet for finger pricks.

1-1

The Compound Microscope

"Come here! Hurry! There are little animals in this rain water. They swim! They play around! They are a thousand times smaller than any creature we can see with our eyes alone. Look! See what I have discovered"

Antony Leeuwenhoek (1632-1723), a Dutch store keeper and an amateur microscopist, to his daughter, Maria, on seeing microbes for the first time, in rain water, in about 1685.

STUDENT OBJECTIVES

After completing this experiment, you should be able to:
1. Name the different parts of the microscope and explain the functions of each.
2. Explain the physical basis of microscopy and define the terms magnification, resolution, and numerical aperture.
3. Describe the mechanism of image formation and the type of image seen.
4. Explain how to get different magnifications.
5. Describe the procedure (protocol) that must be followed every time you use a microscope.
6. Explain why cedar wood oil is used with oil immersion lens.
7. Name the precautions that must be observed during and after using the microscope.
8. Solve the common problems that may arise during microscopy.
9. Explain the basic working of other types of microscopes.

Introduction

It was known at the time of Galileo (1584-1642) that when one looked through a system of suitably arranged lenses; one could not only magnify distant objects but also nearby objects that were invisible to the naked eye. However, even after the invention of the microscope and telescope in 1609, it was over half a century later that Malpighii discovered capillaries in the frog's lung in 1661, and independently by Leewenhoek in 1676 in the tail of a fish (thus completing the circuit of blood circulation discovered by William Harvey in 1628).

Perhaps one of the greatest microscopists of his time was Anton von Leeuwenhoek, a town clerk and owner of a dry goods store in the city of Delft. He constructed hundreds of microscopes (grinding his own lenses and melting the metals he needed) and confirmed and extended the studies of others. He examined everything he could get his hands on— from insect wings to semen, blood, rainwater to the food stuck between his teeth. In fact, he put microscopy on a solid footing.

The compound microscope is called so because, in contrast to a single magnifying convex lens, it has two such lenses— the *objective* and the *eyepiece*. It magnifies the image of an object that is not visible to the naked eye to an extent where it can be seen clearly.

The microscope is one of the most commonly used instruments in the medical and life sciences colleges, and in clinical laboratories. Students of Physiology use it in the study of morphology of blood cells and in counting their numbers. They will use it in histology, histopathology and microbiology and later in various clinical disciplines.

- Before using a microscope, the students must familiarize themselves with its different parts and how to use it and take its care. It will be discussed under the following heads:

1. Parts of the Microscope.
   A. The support system.
   B. The focusing system.
   C. The optical (magnifying) system.
   D. The illumination system.
      i. Source of light.
      ii. Mirror.
      iii. Condenser.
2. Physical Basis of Microscopy.
   A. Visual acuity.
   B. Resolving power.
   C. Magnification.
   D. Numerical aperture.
   E. Image formation
   F. Working distance.
   G. Calculation of total magnification.
3. Protocol (Procedure) for the Use of Microscope
   A. Focusing under low power (100 x).
   B. Focusing under high power (450 x).
   C. Focusing under oil immersion (1000 x).
   D. "Racking" the microscope.

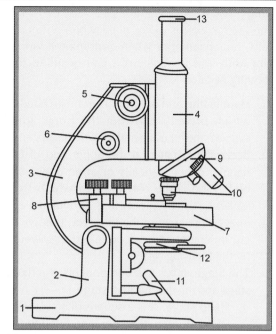

Figure 1-1. Compound microscope: (1) Base, (2) Pillars, (3) Handle, (4) Body tube, (5) Coarse adjustment screw, (6) Fine adjustment screw, (7) Fixed stage, (8) Mechanical stage, (9) Fixed and revolving nose pieces, (10) Objective lenses, (11) Mirror, (12) Condenser, and (13) Eye-piece.

4. Common difficulties faced by students.
5. Precautions and routine care.
6. Other types of microscopes.
7. Questions/Answers

1. PARTS OF THE MICROSCOPE

A. The Support System.

The support system functions as a framework to which various functional units are attached:

i. Base. It is a heavy metallic, U- or horseshoe-shaped base or foot, which supports the micro-scope on the worktable to provide maximum stability.

ii. Pillars. Two upright pillars project up from the base (**Figure 1-1**) and are attached to the C-shaped handle. The hinge joint allows the microscope to be tilted at a suitable angle for comfortable viewing.

Note

The microscope is never tilted when counting cells in a chamber or when examining a blood film under oil immersion. It can be tilted for viewing histology slides.

iii. **Handle (the arm or limb).** The curved handle, which projects up from the hinge joint supports the focusing and magnifying systems.

iv. **Body Tube.** Fitted at the upper end of the handle, either vertically or at an angle, the body tube is the part through which light passes to the eyepiece, thus conducting the image to the eye of the observer. It is 16-17 cm in length, and can be raised or lowered by the focusing system.

v. **The Stage.** It has two components: the **fixed stage** and the **mechanical stage.**

   a. **Fixed stage.** It is a square platform with an aperture in its center, and fitted to the limb below the objective lenses. The slide is placed on it and centered over the aperture for viewing. The converging cone of light emerging from the condenser passes through the slide and the objective into the body tube.

   b. **Mechanical stage.** It is a calibrated metal frame fitted on the right edge of the fixed stage. There is a spring-mounted clip to hold the slide or counting chamber in position while two screw-heads move it from side to side and forwards and backwards. The vernier scale on the frame indicates the degree of movement. In some microscopes the screw-heads are mounted on a common spindle under the fixed stage.

Note

In some sophisticated and binocular microscopes, the entire stage, fixed and mechanical, can be raised or lowered (the aim in all microscopes is to bring the material under study and an objective lens at the proper working distance).

B. The Focusing System

The focusing system consists of **coarse** and **fine** adjustment screw-heads. It is employed for raising or lowering the optical system with reference to the slide under study till it comes into focus. Thus, the adjustments place an objective lens at its optimal working distance, i.e., its focal length.

There are two coarse and two fine adjustment screws working on a double-sided micrometer mechanism, one pair (one coarse and one fine) on either side. If one coarse (or fine) adjustment is turned, its partner on the other side also rotates at the same time. It is, therefore, not sensible to use both hands on the coarse or the fine screws simultaneously.

The **coarse adjustment** moves the optical system up or down rapidly through a large distance via a rack and pinion arrangement. The fine adjustment works in the same way but several rotations of the screw-head are required to move the tube through a small distance; e.g., one rotation moves the tube by 0.1 mm or less. The **fine adjustment** is usually graduated in l/50ths, where each division corresponds to a movement of 0.002 mm of the tube. It is employed for accurate focusing.

Important

The left hand is used both, for coarse and for fine focusing, while the right hand is used for the mechanical stage to move the slide in various directions. The student is advised to get into the habit of using the hands simultaneously for different purposes.

C. The Optical (Magnifying) System

The optical system consists of the body tube, the eyepiece, and the nosepiece that carries the objectives. It can be raised or lowered as desired.

i. **The body tube.** The distance between the upper ends of the objectives and the eyepiece is called the tube length, which is 16-17 cm. The distance between the upper focal point of the eyepiece and the lower focal point of the objective is called *the optical tube length*, which is about 25 cm (A x10 lens will produce an image 10 times the diameter of the object as it naturally appears when held at 25 cm from the eye).

ii. The eyepiece. The eyepiece fits into the top of the body tube. Most microscopes are provided with 5 x, 8 x, and 10 x eyepieces, though 6 × and 15 × are also available. Each eyepiece has two lenses—one mounted at the top, the **'eye lens'**, and the other, the **'field lens'** is fitted at the bottom. The field lens collects the divergent rays of the primary image (see below) and passes these to the eye-lens, which further magnifies the image.

Note
The height of the eyepiece, when taken out of the body tube, is also variable. The 5 x eyepiece is tallest, while 10 x is shortest. A 'pointer' eyepiece has a small pin mounted in it which is used to point out a particular cell or object in a field. A 'demonstration' eyepiece, in which a teacher and a student can look through separate eyepieces mounted on a horizontal barrel, is a useful device (A short piece of hair gummed on the inside next to the eye-lens can serve as a pointer).

iii. The nosepiece. It is fitted at the lower end of the body tube and has two parts: the **fixed** nosepiece, and the **revolving** nosepiece. The latter carries interchangeable objective lenses. Any lens can be rotated into position when desired, its correct position being indicated by a 'click'.

iv. Objective lenses (also called objectives, or; simply 'lenses'). Three spring-loaded objectives of varying magnifying powers are usually provided with the student microscope. In some cases, there is a place provided for a 'scanning' lens as well. Each objective has a cover glass which forms its outer covering and protects it. Though each lens can be unscrewed for cleaning, the students are not supposed to remove them.

The magnifying power of each lens and its numerical aperture (NA) rather than its focal length, are etched on each.

Note
Sign of multiplication. The magnifying power of each objective, as that of the eyepiece, is etched on it. The sign 'x' is not the capital letter (upper-case letter) X but the sign of multiplication.

The objective lenses are
a. Low-power (LP) Objective (10 x; NA= 0.25; focal length =16 mm) The LP objective in common use magnifies 10 times. It is used for initial focusing and viewing a large area of the specimen slide. The numerical aperture (NA) of this lens is always less than that of the condenser in most microscopes. In order to achieve focus, therefore, the NA has got to be closely matched by reducing the light reaching the specimen under study. This is achieved by lowering the condenser and partially closing the iris diaphragm. (See below).

b. High-power (HP) Objective (45 x; NA=0.65; focal length= 4 mm) This lens magnifies the image 45 times. Because of its higher magnification, it is used for more detailed study of the material before switching to oil immersion lens. The NA of HP lens is almost equal to, or slightly less than that of commonly used condenser. Therefore the latter has to be slightly raised and the iris diaphragm opened to get more light and maximum clarity in focusing.

c. Oil-immersion (OI) Objective (100 x; NA= 1.30; focal length=2mm) The OI lens magnifies the image 100 times. Since the lens almost touches the slide it has to be immersed in a special medium (most commonly cedar wood oil), a drop of which is first placed on the slide. The oil is used to increase the NA and thus the resolving power of the objective. Since the NA of OI objective is always greater than that of the condenser, the latter has to be raised to its highest position and iris diaphragm fully opened. As this lens gives (with an eyepiece of 10 x) a total magnification of 1000 times, it is employed for detailed study of the morphology of blood cells and tissues.

d. Scanning Objective (3 x; NA= 0.10; focal length= 40 mm). This objective, a very low power lens, magnifies the image 3 times. It is used for scanning (or viewing) a much larger area on the slide.

Parfocal system. The objectives these days are so constructed that when one lens (LP, for example) is in focus, the others are more or less in focus. Thus switching from one lens to another (e.g., from LP to HP) requires only a little turn of fine adjustment to bring the image into sharp focus. This arrangement of lenses is called "parfocal system."

D. The Illumination System

No microscope can function optimally unless proper illumination (lighting) is provided. All the light that will reach the eye should come from the specimen under study. Light from any other part of the slide will tend to obscure the details. Such extra (extraneous) light is called glare. The illumination system must, therefore, provide uniform, soft, and bright illumination of the entire field of view. Two factors are involved in providing such uniform illumination:

   i. The construction and position of the condenser.

   ii. The size of the iris diaphragm.

Types of Illumination. The compound microscopes work on six types of illumination: **'Bright-field' or 'light' microscope**. This is the usual student microscope that uses white light, either external or internal, as the source of illumination. Seen under this light, the objects look darkish or colored, contrasted against a lighted background. The **other types** of illumination systems include: *Dark-field microscope, Phase-contrast microscope. Fluorescent microscope, Polarizing microscope,* and *Interference-contrast microscope.* (See below for their brief descriptions).

The **illumination system** of the bright-field microscope consists of: a source of light, and a mechanism to condense the light and direct it into the specimen under study.

i. Source of light. The light source may be outside the microscope or within the microscope.

External light source. It may be the diffuse, natural daylight (sunlight) reflected and scattered by the atmosphere and its dust particles and reflected from the buildings. On bright, sunny days, the north daylight, which is a distant light source, is ideal for routine student work.

If daylight is not available, or is not sufficient, an artificial source of light— a fluorescent tube, or an electric lamp housed in a lamp box with a frosted glass window, fitted on the worktable can provide enough light.

Internal light source. In most microscopes, there is a provision to remove the mirror and fit an electric microscope lamp in its place. This unit has frosted tungsten lamp to provide uniform white light.

ii. The mirror. A double-sided mirror, in fact two mirrors, one flat or plane and the other concave, fitted back to back in a metal frame is located below the condenser; it can be rotated in all directions. The plane mirror is used with a distant source of light (natural, or daylight). The parallel rays of light are reflected parallel into the condenser. The concave mirror, on the other hand, is employed when the light source is near the microscope. The divergent rays of light are reflected as parallel rays and directed into the condenser.

iii. The condenser ('Substage' or 'substage condenser'). The condenser is a system of lenses fitted in a short cylinder that is mounted below the stage. It can be raised or lowered by a rack and pinion, and focuses the light rays into a solid cone of light onto the material under study. It also helps in resolving the image.

   a. The lens system. The commonly used substage is Abbe-type condenser. It is composed of two lenses which should be corrected for spherical and chromatic aberrations.

     Since the condenser is a lens system, it has a fixed NA, which should be equal or less than that of the objective being used. Raising or lowering the condenser can vary its NA. And with the axes of the two being the same, all the light passing through the condenser is collected by the objective, thus allowing maximum clarity.

Note

It is clear from the above that the position of the condenser must always be adjusted with each objective to get best focus of light and resolving power of the microscope.

b. **The iris diaphragm.** It is fitted within the condenser. A small lever on the side can adjust the size of the aperture of the diaphragm, thus allowing more or less light falling on the material under study. Reducing the size of the field of view (i.e., by narrowing the aperture) decreases the NA of the condenser. Thus, proper illumination includes a combination of position of light source, regulation of light intensity, position of condenser, and regulation of the size of field of view.

c. **Filter.** A metal ring can accommodate a pale blue or green filter since monochromatic light is ideal for microscopy.

   • Generally, when viewing clear preparations under low power, we need less light, but more illumination is required when studying stained preparations under oil-immersion lens.

2. PHYSICAL BASIS OF MICROSCOPY

A. Visual Acuity

The term visual acuity (VA) refers to the ability of the eye to resolve or recognize two very closely situated points of light or lines, which are not touching, as separate from each other rather than one. If the distance between the two points is less than a certain value, the two points are not resolved but appear as one. (See Expt (Chart) 5-11 for details).

B. Resolving Power (Resolution)

The utility of a microscope depends not only on its magnifying power but also on its power of resolution, i.e. its ability to show closely located structures as separate and distinct from each other.

This translates into the ability to improve the details of structures within a cell.

Generally the resolving power of the unaided human eye is said to be between 0.15 mm and 0.25 mm. The resolving power of a lens depends on its NA as well as the wavelength of light. With the light microscope and OI lens of 100x, and NA of 1.30, its resolving power is about 0.25 μm (2500 Angstroms) with white light, and about 0.19 μm with monochromatic green light (shortest wavelength: 5.5×10^{-5} cm). The electron microscope, however, gives very high magnifications and can separate dots that are about 0.5 nm apart or even less.

The resolving power of a microscope is expressed in terms of *limit of resolution (LR)*, or the minimum separable distance. If this distance is less than LR, the two points appear as one. The formula for determining LR is: LR = 0.61 × W/NA, where W= wavelength of light being used, and NA= the numerical aperture of the objective in use.

C. Magnification

In order to see clearly and distinctly the details and contours of closely- located structures (say in a cell), their image has to be magnified many times. How this is achieved is explained below.

D. Numerical Aperture (NA)

A powerful lens is made of glass of high refractive index, has a short focal length, and a small diameter. The small diameter allows only the central cone of light to pass through without getting too much refracted, while the peripheral rays that would be refracted more, are cut off.

The value "n sine alpha" – where 'n' is the refractive index of glass, and 'alpha' the angle subtended by it at the object is called the numerical aperture, as shown in **Figure 1-2**. Thus, the NA of a lens, which is an index of its power of resolution, is the ratio of its diameter to its focal length. As the NA increases, the resolving power of the lens increases.

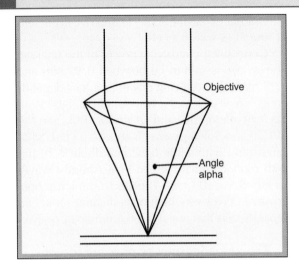

Figure 1-2. Diagram to explain the numerical aperture. The angle alpha is shown.

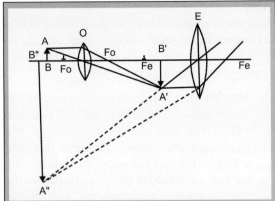

Figure 1-3. The ray diagram of a compound microscope. AB = object; A' B' = real, inverted, magnified image; A" B" = Virtual, inverted, magnified image. O = objective lens, E = Eye-piece; Fo = Focus of objective; Fe = Focus of eye-piece.

The NA is also an index of light gathering power of a lens, i.e., the amount of light entering the objective. The NA can be decreased by decreasing the amount of light passing through the lens. Thus, as shown below, the illumination has to increase as the objectives are changed from LP to HP to OI.

E. Image Formation in the Compound Microscope

It is the objective that starts the process of magnification. It forms a real, inverted, and enlarged image (primary image: A' – B' (**Figure 1-3**) in the upper part of the body tube. (A real image is that which can be received on screen). The field lens of the eyepiece collects the divergent rays of light of the primary image and passes these through the eye lens, which therefore the image seen by the eye is virtual, inverted, and magnified, and appears to be further magnifies the image. The light rays reaching the observer's eye are divergent and about 25 cm in front of the eye. **Figure 1-3** shows the ray diagram of a compound microscope.

F. Working Distance

The working distance is the distance between the objective and the slide under study. This distance

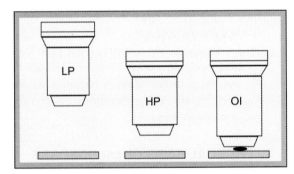

Figure 1-4. Diagram to show the working distances of LP, HP and OI lenses

decreases with increasing magnification. It is 8-13 mm in LP, 1-3 mm in HP, and 0.5-1.5 mm in OI lenses respectively. **Figure 1-4** shows the approximate working distances for each lens. Note that the OI lens has to be immersed in a drop of oil.

G. Calculation of Total Magnification

Since the objective and eyepiece both magnify the image, it is easy to calculate the total magnification of any combination of objective lens and eyepiece. For example, with an eyepiece of 10X, the magnifications with the three objectives will be:-
Scanning objective (3 x or 4 x) = 3 or 4 × 10 = 30 or 40 times.

Low power objective (10 x) = 10 × 10 = 100 times.
High power objective (45 x) = 45 × 10 = 450 times.
Oil immersion objective (100 x) = 100 × 10
= 1000 times.

3. PROTOCOL (PROCEDURES) FOR THE USE OF MICROSCOPE

Principle

A focused beam of light passes through the material under study into the microscope. Parts of the specimen that are optically dense and having a high refractive index or are colored with a stain (dye), cast a potential shadow which is magnified in 2 main stages as it passes into the observer's eye.

Procedures

The student must avoid the bad habit of using objective lenses in a haphazard manner, starting with any lens at random and then switching over to another. A brief protocol (procedure) for using a microscope is given below:

Important
The first rule in examining any slide/blood film/specimen is always to examine it with the naked (unaided) eye. This important step which is often ignored by the student, can help in identifying some histology slides (e.g., a section of spinal cord, cerebellum etc.) and assessment of a blood smear. This will also confirm whether a stained slide is worth proceeding further.

- After this step, the slide is viewed under low magnification to get a general view all over. One can then choose an area of interest for viewing it under higher magnifications.

A. Focusing Under Low Power (100 x)

a. Place the microscope on your work-table in an upright position, and raise the body tube 7-8 cm above the stage. Put the slide on the stage and, using the mechanical stage, bring the specimen over the central aperture.

b. Select and adjust the mirror (plane or concave) so that the light shines on the specimen. Rack the condenser well down (low position), and partly close the diaphragm to cut down excess light.

c. Looking from the side, and using the coarse adjustment, bring the body tube down so that the LP lens is about 1 cm above the slide. Now look into the eyepiece and gently raise the tube till the specimen comes into focus. But if it does not, i.e., if you have missed the focusing position, repeat the whole procedure. When the image comes into focus, scan the entire field, racking the fine adjustment all the time.

CAUTION
Do not bring the body tube down from any height while looking into the microscope. You might miss the focusing position and continue moving it down thereby breaking the slide or permanently scratching the objective lens.
- In some microscopes the body tube can be pre-locked in any position below which it will not go unless it is unlocked first.
- If with low-power lens, you use plane mirror and the condenser is 'up', you will see the image of the window frame/wire gauze which will interfere with microscopy. The image will disappear when the condenser is moved down.

B. Focusing Under High Power (450 x)

a. For focusing under high magnification, simply rotate the nosepiece so that the HP lens clicks into position. Raise the condenser to mid-position and open the diaphragm to admit enough light. Use fine adjustment as required.

b. If the lens system is not parfocal, look from the side and bring the lens down to about 1-2 mm above the slide. Now look into the microscope and raise the tube slowly and gently till the image comes into focus.

C. Focusing Under Oil-immersion (1000 x)

This objective is the most frequently used in hematology because of its high magnification and resolution. (It can also be used for mounted histology and pathology slides).

The two features of this objective are: its very small aperture through which light enters it, and its deep focusing position that is about 1 mm from the slide.

The reason why this lens is immersed in oil and not the LP or HP lenses is the thin layer of air between this objective and the glass slide when the lens is in focus. (Without the oil the image can be seen but it is very faint and blurred).

We know that when light passes from a denser medium (glass of the slide) into a rarer medium (the thin layer of air), they are refracted away from the normal. As a result, when light rays emerge from the slide, many of them are refracted away from the aperture of the objective and very few enter it, and a faint image results. Cedar wood oil, which has the same refractive index as that of glass, i.e., 1.55 (air=1.00; water= 1.33), removes this layer of air so that the glass of the slide and the objective lens become a continuous column (thus avoiding refraction) and allow enough light to enter the objective. Other mediums that can be used are glycerin and paraffin, their refractive index being 1.35-1.40. However, cedar wood oil, though costly, gives best results.

Raise the body tube so that the O.I. lens is about 8-10 cm above the slide. Place a drop of cedar wood oil on the slide, and looking from the side, slowly bring the objective down till it just enters the oil drop. The oil will spread out in the capillary space between the slide and the lens (thus effectively removing the thin layer of air).

While looking into the eyepiece, slowly and very carefully raise the objective with coarse adjustment (without taking it out of the oil) till the cells come into view, (if no cells are seen, repeat the whole process). Use the fine adjustment for fine tuning. When you move the slide, the oil will move with it. It is therefore, a bad habit to cover the entire slide with oil to begin with.

Important

A proper illumination of the specimen slide is very essential. However, the students often forget about its importance. The broad rule about illumination is as follows:

Objective	Condenser - position	Iris- diaphragm
Low power (10x)	Low	Partly open
High power (45x)	Midway	Half open
Oil-immersion	High	Fully open

This rule is not rigidly fixed. Depending on the source and strength of light, the condenser position and diaphragm size have to be combined to get optimal illumination.

"Racking the Microscope"

The cells and their constituents are 3-dimensional structures and lie at different levels. Therefore, it is important not to keep a fixed focus but to continuously "rack" the microscope by using fine adjustment after the specimen has been brought under focus under any magnification. By turning the fine adjustment screw this way and that, various structures come into and go out of focus alternately. A good microscopist will always have his/her left hand on the fine adjustment (and the right hand on the mechanical stage) and "rack" it continuously while looking into the microscope.

Important

Whenever you are asked by your teacher to look into the microscope to identify or describe something—the very first thing you should do is to put your left hand on the fine adjustment screw and rack it. You may change the field if permitted by the teacher. Illumination may, however, be adjusted as required.

Note

Although you will be using one eye with the monocular microscope, do not close the other eye as this will cause lot of strain on that eye. Practice keeping both the eyes open and, with practice, you will be able to ignore the unwanted image, and continue working for long hours.

4. COMMON DIFFICULTIES ENCOUNTERED BY STUDENTS

The beginner is likely to face some difficulties when starting to use the microscope for the first time, but these can be minimized if the procedures are strictly followed and proper precautions taken. Some common problems are:

A. The material cannot be focused or the image is very faint.

i. The slide may not be near the focus of the objective, or there may be no visible material under it (e.g., part of the blood film may be missing from this area). Check this out and start with coarse adjustment once again.

ii. The slide bearing the material may have been placed upside down on the stage, a common mistake made by the students with a blood film. The thickness of the glass slide does not allow the OI lens to reach down to its working distance. Reversing the slide will solve the problem.

iii. If focusing is achieved with LP and HP lenses but not with OI lens despite all efforts, the lens may have been damaged earlier. Seek the help of your tutor.

B. There may be a dark shadow or smudge in the field. If the shadow rotates when the eyepiece is rotated, remove it and clean it. Or there may be an air bubble in the cedar wood oil.

C. The field of view appears oval instead of round. This problem arises when the objective has not been properly "clicked" into position.

D. The illumination of the image is poor. Check the source of light, angle of the mirror, the position of the condenser, and iris diaphragm.

E. The image does not come into focus even when the objective is in the lowest position and the fine adjustment cannot move down any further.

i. This happens when the fine adjustment screw reaches the end of its thread (turn) before the image is brought to its focus. To overcome this problem, turn the adjustment screw in the opposite direction for several turns and then use the coarse adjustment screw to regain the focus once again. (It is therefore;

best to keep the fine adjustment screw near the middle of its turning range).

ii. The problem may also arise if the body tube has been kept in the 'locked' position, and so cannot be taken down to focus the slide.

5. PRECAUTIONS AND ROUTINE CARE

1. Select a stool or chair of suitable height so that your eyes are at a level slightly above the eyepiece. This will ensure comfortable working for long periods.

2. Ensure that all the lenses are clean and free from dust and smudges. Do not touch them with your fingers, nor blow on them to remove dust.

3. Check the position of the objective, condenser, and diaphragm, to ensure optimal illumination.

4. Never lower any objective from any height while looking into the microscope.

5. If the objectives are not parfocal, check the working distance of each objective separately by using fine focusing.

6. Once a specimen has been focused, continuously "rack" the microscope.

7. *Cleaning the microscope.* Never leave cedar wood oil on the OI lens, because it may seep into the body of the objective and damage the lens permanently. Dried oil is difficult to remove. Remove oil with lens paper, then xylene to clean the lens.

6. OTHER TYPES OF MICROSCOPES

Various types of microscopes have been specially introduced for particular purposes over the past many decades. They differ from the compound "bright-field" microscope in fundamental ways by employing different illumination and image-formation systems. Some of these are:

1. **Binocular Microscope.** It is a compound bright-field microscope but having two eyepieces instead of one so that both eyes are used simultaneously. This prevents eyestrain.

2. **Dissection Microscope.** It is a binocular microscope used for micro dissection under magnification.

3. **"Dark-field" Microscope.** It employs a special condenser that causes light waves to cross on the material under study rather than passing through it. As a result the field of view appears dark (hence called "dark-field" in contrast to "bright-field" microscopy) against which the object appears bright. It is used in microbiology to study spirochetes.

4. **Phase-contrast Microscope.** Since the living cells are mostly transparent, they must be stained with vital stains, or they must be first fixed in alcohol and then stained with acid or basic dyes before they can be viewed under the microscope. In this microscope, a special phase plate is inserted into the condenser, which can retard the speed of some light waves. Since the tissue cells and organisms have different refractive indices, this microscope uses these differences to produce an image with good contrast of light and shade. Thus, unstained wet preparations can be studied (e.g., platelets). The interference microscope is based on similar principle.

5. **Interference-contrast Microscope.** A special prism that can split a beam of light is added to the condenser. The two split beams are then polarized, but only one resultant beam passes through the specimen under study while the other (reference beam) does not. The 2 beams are then recombined to produce a three-dimensional image.

6. **Polarizing Microscope.** It has a polarizer (filter), which is usually placed between the light source and the specimen, and an analyzer, which is, located between the objective and the eyepiece. Such a system is used to study tissues that have the property of birefringence (e.g., muscle fibers).

7. **Fluorescence Microscope.** A fluorescent dye is used to stain tissues which are then studied under this microscope.

8. **Transmission Electron Microscope (TEM).** Invented by Knoll and Ruska in 1940, the TEM uses a strong beam of electrons instead of light and electromagnetic fields in place of glass lenses. The electrons produce a wavelength of about 0.05 Å, and provide a practical resolution of about 5 Å (theoretically possible resolution is about 1 Å). The magnified image, which is visible on a fluorescent screen, can be recorded on a photographic film, and the negative further enlarged 6 to 8 times. Thus, the total magnification obtained can vary from one to several hundred thousand times.

9. **Scanning electron microscope (SEM).** This microscope, which achieves a resolution of about 30 Å, has been developed for three-dimensional study of surface topography of cells and object. Though similar to TEM, the SEM employs a different technique.

QUESTIONS

Q. 1 Why is your microscope called a compound microscope? What type of image is produced by it?

A single convex lens works like a simple microscope. In the student microscope, there are two lens systems—the objective and the eyepiece which take part in the formation of the image—hence the term compound in contrast to simple. The image seen by the eye is a virtual, inverted and magnified image produced by the eyepiece from the real, inverted and magnified image (primary image) produced by the objective lens.

Q. 2 When is plane mirror used and when concave?

See page 6.

Q. 3 What is the total magnification you are getting now (at the time of viva)?

The total magnification obtained at any time depends on the combination of the objective and the eyepiece being used (see page 8 for details).

Q. 4 What is meant by the term numerical aperture? What is its significance?

See page 7.

Q. 5 How will you identify oil-immersion objective lens ? Why is cedar wood oil used with this lens and not with others?
See page 10.

Q. 6 Will you see any image with the oil-immersion lens without the cedar wood oil?
The image will be visible but will be very faint because of the layer of air present between the slide and the lens. Removal of this air by the cedar wood oil clarifies the image.

Q. 7 Why does the oil-immersion lens have pin-hole sized aperture?
The aperture being very small, it allows only the central cone of light to pass through and form the image. Had the diameter been large, excessive refraction would have caused spherical and chromatic aberrations, thus making the image indistinct.

Q. 8 Why should the position of the condenser be low with the LP lens and highest with oil-immersion lens?
Since the aperture of the LP lens is wide, a high condenser would allow too much light to enter the microscope and cause glare. The position of the condenser with the oil-immersion lens has to be highest to allow enough light to enter it through its pin-hole aperture.

Q. 9 Why are different degrees of illumination required when using a microscope and why?
The clarity of an image depends on an optimal (ideal) amount of light available. The illumination (the process of providing light) can be altered by raising or lowering the condenser and opening or closing the diaphragm. A proper combination of the two has to be selected under different conditions. In general, we require less illumination when viewing a clear, unstained object, and greater illumination when viewing a stained preparation.

Q. 10 What is meant by racking the microscope and what is its importance?
Since the cells and their components are 3-dimensional entities, and situated at different levels, the focus has to be constantly changed to see all these structures.

Q. 11 What are the other types of microscopes?
See page 11.

1-2

The Study of Common Objects

The purpose of this experiment is to familiarize the student with the proper use of the microscope and how to take its care. As the student gets used to handling the microscope in this and later experiments, she/he will realize that common objects of interest in microscopy such as, dust particles, cotton/wool/silk/synthetic and other fibers, air bubbles, stain precipitate, etc are the usual artifacts which may cause confusion to a beginner.

STUDENT OBJECTIVES
After completing this experiment, you should be able to: 1. Explain the functions of each part of the microscope. 2. Name some common objects, which may cause confusion. 3. Focus and identify an object under different magnifications. 4. Take care of the microscope during and after use. 5. Answer all the questions relating to the use of microscope in Experiment 1-1.

PREPARATION OF SLIDES

About 8 to 10 clean, grease-free, standard microscopy glass slides (75 mm × 25 mm) and cover-slips will be required. Once cleaned, do not touch their surfaces but hold them from their edges.

Place one drop of water in the middle of each slide. Then add a pinch of dust, starch powder, a few well-teased (dissected, separated) cotton, wool, and other fibers, drop of milk, and a few hairs to each drop of water separately. Then holding a cover-slip by its edges, place its edge in the edge of the water drop, and using a pencil point to support it, gently lower it on to the water drop. This avoids trapping of air under the cover-slip. The various objects are now ready for examination under low and high magnifications of the microscope.

1. **Dust particles.** The usual house and garden dust contains inorganic, and organic matter—including silica, graphite, mica, carbon, calcium carbonate (from white washing, chalk etc.), iron oxide (iron is the most common metal in the earth's crust), cellulose, natural and synthetic fibers, keratin and epithelial cells shed off from the skin and so on. The particulate matter is of different sizes (usually larger than 8-10 μm), angular or irregularly polygonal; with sharp edges, and unevenly light or dark brown, black, or yellow in color. A few cotton or other fibers or hairs may be seen.

2. **Starch granules.** These granules are oval or pear-shaped and usually have a hilum at their narrow ends. Concentric rings (lines) are seen, especially when stained blue with dilute iodine solution added to a watery suspension of starch powder.

3. **Hairs.** Hairs are the growths of epidermis, and composed of dead, keratinized cells. The human hairs (pili) are long, filamentous and cylindrical and cover most of the skin surfaces except palms and soles. Each hair has 3 layers: the inner medulla consists of cells containing pigment granules and air spaces. The next

layer, cortex, which forms the major part of the shaft, consists of cells which contain pigment granules (melanin, or its variants which have different colors) in dark hair but mostly air in gray hair. The outermost layer, the cuticle, is a single layer of heavily keratinized thin, flat cells arranged like the tiles of a roof, with their free edges appearing as minute projections.

The medulla appears dark and the cortex light in deep focusing position. If the focus is changed (as it always is during racking) the darker medulla appears lighter and the cortex appears darker.

4. **Cotton fibers.** Undyed cotton fibers appear as long, ribbon-like, semi-transparent filaments which are spirally twisted at intervals. Two faint lines appear to enclose a light central zone throughout the twisted fiber. Unlike hair, there is no medulla or cortex.

5. **Woollen fibers.** These are the body hairs of sheep, rabbit, or other animals. They appear as long, filamentous structures showing a cortex and medulla. Minute hairlets may be seen projecting from the surface.

6. **Stain granules.** Place a drop of Leishman's stain on a slide, spread it out thickly with another slide, and allow it to dry at room temperature. Examine it under LP and HP lenses. Then put a drop of cedar wood oil and examine it under OI lens. The stain precipitate appears as round, uniformly dark blue-violet granules of uniform size (about 2 μm). The granules usually lie singly and do not form aggregates or clusters (this is how you will see the granules on a blood smear when the stain dries up during staining, as mentioned in Expt 1-12. These granules have to be distinguished from platelets which form clusters of 2 to 12, and show a central darker and a peripheral lighter zone.

7. **Fat globules.** A drop of diluted milk shows fat globules, most of which are round and of uniform size. A few may be found in clumps

like a bunch of grapes. (The fat in milk is neutral fat, or triglycerides, TGs, the storage form of fat in adipose tissue of the body).

8. **Air bubbles.** Drop a cover-slip over a drop of water taken on a slide. This usually traps air bubbles of various sizes. They are usually round or oval due to surface tension of water around them. They appear as darkish rings with a clear area in the centre, an appearance that changes when the focus is changed.

1-3

Collection of Blood Samples

STUDENT OBJECTIVES
After completing this experiment, you should be able to:
1. Explain what a blood sample is, what are its sources, and what are its main constituents.
2. Describe the purpose of collecting a blood sample.
3. Indicate how to attain and maintain asepsis when collecting a blood sample.
4. Collect capillary blood from a finger-prick, heel-prick, and earlobe prick, and precautions to be taken during a skin-prick.
5. Indicate the steps for obtaining a blood sample by venepuncture.
6. Name the various anticoagulants employed in hematological studies and their mode of action.
7. Provide samples of plasma and serum.

Since blood is confined within the cardio-vascular system, the skin has to be punctured before blood can be obtained. There are two common sources of blood for routine laboratory tests: *blood from a superficial vein* by puncturing it with a needle and syringe, or *from skin capillaries* by skin-prick. Arterial blood and blood from cardiac chambers may be required for special tests.

None of these samples can be called a representative sample because there are minor variations in their composition. But for routine hematological tests, however, these differences can safely be ignored.

1. **Asepsis.**
   A. Sterilization of equipment.

B. Cleaning/sterilizing of skin.
   C. Prevention of contamination.
2. **The blood sample.**
   A. Sources and amount of blood.
   B. Containers for blood samples.
   C. Differences between venous and capillary blood.
3. **Commonly used anticoagulants.**
4. **Collection of venous blood.**
5. **Collection of capillary blood.**
   A. Selection of site.
   B. Apparatus.
   C. Procedure.
6. **Precautions.**
7. **Questions/Answers.**

1. ASEPSIS

The term asepsis refers to the condition of being free from septic or infectious material—bacteria, viruses, etc. The skin is a formidable barrier to the entry of foreign invaders and the first line of defence against bacteria and other disease-causing microorganisms which are present in abundance on the skin and in the air. Therefore, puncturing the skin always poses the danger of infection

In order to achieve asepsis, the following aspects need to be kept in mind:

A. Sterilization of Equipment

All the instruments to be used for collecting blood—syringes, needles, lancets, and cotton and gauze swabs—should preferably be sterilized in an autoclave. The old practice of boiling glass syringes and needles in tap water is now obsolete. Irradiated and sealed, single-use syringes, needles, lancets and blades are now freely available and are in common use.

B. Cleaning/Sterilization of Skin

Though it is impossible to completely sterilize the selected site for skin puncture, every aseptic precaution must be exercised. The selected area need not be washed and scrubbed unless grossly dirty. If washed, the area should be allowed to dry before applying the antiseptics because these agents do not act well on wet skin. At least 2-3 sterile cotton/gauze swabs soaked in 70% alcohol, methylated spirit, or ether should be used to clean and scrub the area. Cotton swabs are likely to leave fibers sticking to the skin and provide an undesirable contact, or they may appear as artifacts in a blood film. But if they are used, the final cleaning should be done with gauze swab.

Note
After cleaning the skin, allow the alcohol to dry by evaporation (do not blow on it), because sterilization with alcohol is effective only after it has dried.

C. Prevention of Contamination

Any material used for skin puncture, or the operator's hands may cause contamination. Therefore, once the site has been cleaned and dried, it should not be touched again. Care must be taken to prevent contamination until the puncture wound has effectively closed/healed.

2. THE BLOOD SAMPLE

The term "blood sample" refers to the small amount of blood—a few drops or a few milliliters—obtained from a person for the purpose of testing or investigations. These tests are carried out for aiding in diagnosis and/or prognosis of the disease or disorder.

A. Sources and Amount of Blood Sample

i. **Capillary blood.** The skin and other tissues are richly supplied with capillaries, so when a drop or a few drops of blood are required, as for estimation of Hb, cell counts, BT and CT, blood films, micro chemical tests, etc, blood from a skin puncture (skin-prick) with a lancet or needle is adequate.

ii. **Venous blood.** When larger amounts (say, a few ml that cannot be obtained from a skin puncture) are needed as for complete hematological and biochemical investigations, venous blood is obtained with a syringe and needle by puncturing a superficial vein. In infants, venous blood may have to be taken from the femoral vein, or the frontal venous sinus.

Note
Venous blood is always preferred for clinical tests.

iii. **Arterial blood.** When arterial blood is needed for special tests such as blood pH, gas levels, etc, an artery such as radial or femoral is punctured with a syringe and needle. This, however, is not a routine procedure.

iv. **Cardiac catheterization.** Blood from a heart chamber, taken through a cardiac catheter, may be required for special tests.

B. Containers for Blood Sample

A container is a receptacle into which blood is transferred from the syringe before sending it to the laboratory. Clean and dry 10 ml glass test tubes, collection bottles such as clean and dry 10 ml discarded medicine vials, glass bulbs, etc are the usual ones in use.

A container may or may not contain an anticoagulant depending on whether a sample of blood/plasma, or serum is required.

For a sample of whole blood or plasma. The blood is transferred to a container containing a suitable anticoagulant. This is to prevent clotting of blood.

For a sample of serum. No anticoagulant is used. The blood is allowed to clot in the container and serum is collected as described later.

Obviously, capillary blood does not require a container or anticoagulant.

C. Differences Between Venous and Capillary Blood

The differences between these two sources of blood are given in Table 1.1.

3. COMMONLY USED ANTICOAGULANTS

Anticoagulants are substances employed to delay, suppress, or prevent clotting of blood. They are classified into 2 groups: the *in vitro* (outside the body) anticoagulants, and the *in vivo* (in the body) anticoagulants.

The commonly used *in vitro anticoagulants* include: EDTA, trisodium citrate, double oxalate, sodium fluoride, heparin, and ACD and CPD-A mixtures. The use of fluoride and heparin is limited to pH, blood glucose and gas analysis. *The in vivo anticoagulants* include: heparin and dicoumarol derivatives (warfarin, dicoumarin). Thus, heparin is both an *in vivo* and an *in vitro* anticoagulant.

A. In vitro Anticoagulants

1. Ethylene Diamine Tetra-acetic Acid (EDTA). EDTA is also known as *sequestrene* or *versene*, and both its potassium and sodium salts are strong anticoagulants. The dry (anhydrous) dipotassium salt of EDTA, being more readily soluble than the sodium salt, is the anticoagulant of choice for most of the hematological tests, except coagulation studies. The tripotassium salt of EDTA causes some shrinkage of RBCs that results in 2-3 % decrease in packed cell volume.

Mode of action. EDTA prevents clotting by removing ionic calcium (which is an essential clotting factor) from the blood sample by chelation. The platelets appear clear and are neither aggregated nor destroyed.

Effective concentration. EDTA is used in a concentration of 1 mg/ml of blood. 0.2 ml of 2.5% solution of the salt placed in a container and dried in gentle heat in an oven is sufficient for 5 ml of blood. This provides 1 mg of EDTA/ml of blood. (A number of containers can be prepared from the stock solution at a time).

TABLE 1.1

Sources and differences between Venous blood and Capillary blood	
Venous blood	*Capillary blood*
1. It is obtained from a superficial vein by venepuncture.	1. It is obtained from a skin puncture, usually over a finger, ear lobe/or the heal of a foot.
2. A clean venepuncture provides blood without any contamination with tissue fluid.	2. Blood from a skin prick comes from punctured capillaries and from smallest arterioles and venules.
3. There is less risk of contamination since sterile syringe and needle are used.	3. There is greater risk of contamination and transmission of disease as one may be careless about sterilization since skin prick is considered a harmless procedure.
4. Cell counts, Hb, and PCV values are generally higher.	4. These values are likely to be on the lower side since some tissue fluid is bound to dilute the blood even when it is free-flowing.
5. Venous blood is preferable when normal blood standards are to be established, or when two samples from the same person are to be compared at different times.	5. Capillary blood is not suitable for these purposes.

Note

Excess of EDTA (more than 2 mg/ml blood) affects all blood cells. Red cells shrink, thus reducing PCV, while WBCs show degenerative changes. Platelets break up into large enough fragments to be counted as normal platelets. Care should, therefore, be taken to use correct amount of EDTA, and blood should be thoroughly mixed with the anticoagulant.

2. Trisodium Citrate ($Na_3 C_6 H_5 O_2 . 2 H_2O$). Trisodium citrate is the anticoagulant of choice in blood tests for disorders of coagulation. A 3.8 % solution is prepared in distilled water and then sterilized.

Mode of action. Any substance that deionizes the blood calcium will prevent clotting. The negatively charged citrate ion is particularly useful for this purpose, usually in the form of sodium, ammonium, and potassium citrate. The citrate ion combines with calcium in the blood to form an unionized calcium compound.

Citrated blood, citrate and blood in the ratio of 1:9, is used for coagulation studies, and for ESR test by the Westergren method in the ratio of 1:3. Along with other components, sodium citrate is used for storing donated blood in blood banks (see Expt. 1-18), since it can be safely given intra-venously. Oxalates are toxic and cannot be given intravenously.

3. Double Oxalate mixture. A mixture of ammonium oxalate and potassium oxalate in the ratio of 3:2 is an effective anticoagulant. A large number of containers can be prepared at a time by placing 0.2 ml of oxalate mixture (3.0 gm of ammonium oxalate and 2.0 gm of potassium oxalate in 100 ml of distilled water) in each container and drying in gentle heat in an oven. This amount is sufficient for 8-10 ml of blood. Too much oxalate is hypertonic and damages all blood cells, while too little will not prevent clotting.

Though each oxalate by itself (also sodium and lithium oxalate) can prevent clotting, a mixture is used since the ammonium salt increases cell

volume while potassium salt shrinks them. Sodium oxalate should not be used since it causes crenation of red cells. Ammonium salt should not be used in urea and non-protein nitrogen tests. *Oxalates prevent clotting* by forming insoluble calcium salts, thus removing ionic calcium.

4. Sodium Fluoride. A mixture of 10 mg of sodium fluoride and 1 mg thymol is an anticoagulant as well as a preservative when a blood sample has to be stored for a few days. Since fluoride inhibits glycolytic enzymes (thus preventing loss of glucose), it is employed when plasma glucose is to be estimated.

5. Heparin. Heparin, a highly charged mixture of sulphated polysaccharides, and related to chondroitin, has a molecular weight ranging from 15000-18000 and is a naturally occurring powerful anticoagulant. It is normally secreted by mast cells that are present in many tissues, especially immediately outside many of the capillaries in the body. Both mast cells and basophils release heparin directly into blood. Heparin is also a cofactor for the lipoprotein lipase – the clearing factor.

Commercial heparin is extracted from many different tissues and is available in almost pure form (It was first extracted from the liver—hence the name 'heparin'). Low m.w. fragments (m.w. 5000) have been produced from unfractionated heparin and are being used clinically since they have a longer half-life and produce more predictable results.

Mode of action and uses. Heparin by itself has no anticoagulant activity. However, when it combines with antithrombin III, the ability of the latter to remove thrombin (as soon as it is formed) increases hundreds of times. The complex of these two substances removes many other activated clotting factors- such as IX, X, XI, and XII.

Theoretically, heparin is an ideal anticoagulant since no foreign substance is introduced into the blood. The required amount of stock solution is taken in a number of containers and dried at low heat. At a concentration of 10-20 IU /ml blood, it does not change red cell size and their osmotic fragility. It is, however, inferior to EDTA for general use. It should not be used for leucocyte counts, as these cells tend to clump. It also imparts a blue tinge to the background of blood films. Clinically, it is used to prevent intravascular clotting of blood.

6. Dicoumarol and warfarin. The coumarin derivatives are vitamin K antagonists and thus inhibit the action of this vitamin that is essential as a cofactor for the synthesis of six glutamic acid-containing proteins—namely, factors II (prothrombin), VII, IX, and X, protein C, and protein S. The action of this anticoagulant is, however, slower than that of heparin.

7. ACD and CPD-A. Acid-citrate-dextrose (ACD) and citrate-phosphate-dextrose-adenine (CPD-A) are the anticoagulants of choice for storing donated blood in blood banks (See Expt. 1-18). The CPD-A mixture is preferred as it preserves 2-3 DPG better.

B. In Vivo Anticoagulants and Their Clinical Use

The two *in vivo* anticoagulants are heparin and coumarins. Patients at increased risk of forming blood clots in their blood vessels, e.g, leg veins during prolonged confinement to bed, or during long flights, are sometimes put on these drugs (e.g, warfarin) to prevent thromboembolism. Their BT, CT, and PT are checked from time to time to adjust the dosage of the drug.

Heparin is particularly used during open-heart surgery in which the blood has to be passed through a heart-lung machine; or the dialysis machine during hemodialysis in kidney failure, and then back into the patient.

Important
Anticoagulant therapy should not be confused with thrombolytic agents employed for dissolving blood clots (see Q/A 22, Expt 1-19).

4. COLLECTION OF VENOUS BLOOD

CAUTION
The blood sample from a vein must be collected by a medically qualified staff member who should screen the volunteer for any communicable diseases/especially viral hepatitis, and AIDS. *Do not touch blood other than your own.*

Puncturing a vein and withdrawing blood from it will be demonstrated to you because it requires some degree of skill and confidence. It needs assistance and complete aseptic precautions. (In due course of time, you will also learn to do venepuncture).

Note
Two types of blood samples are not suitable for hematological tests:
1. *Clotted samples.* Even tiny clots in the anticoagulated blood can negate the results.
2. *Hemolysed samples.* The red cells may be damaged and ruptured during collection or handling of blood. The released Hb tinges the plasma or serum red, rendering the sample unfit for tests.

For a Sample of Whole Blood or Plasma. (Plasma= Blood minus all the blood cells). Draw blood from a vein as described below and transfer it from the syringe to a container containing a suitable anticoagulant. Mix the contents well without frothing. A sample of whole blood is now ready for tests.

If plasma is desired, centrifuge the anticoagulated blood for 20-30 minutes at 2500 rpm, as described later. Collect the supernatant plasma with a pipette and transfer it to another container. (The packed RBCs will be left behind).

For a Sample of Serum. (Serum= Plasma minus fibrinogen and all the clotting factors). Transfer the blood from the syringe to a container *without any anticoagulant in it,* and keep it undisturbed. After the blood has clotted in an hour or two and the clot shrunk in size, the serum will be expressed.

Remove the supernatant serum with a pipette and transfer it to a centrifuge tube. Centrifuge it to remove whatever red cells may be present. Clear serum can now be collected with another pipette.

APPARATUS AND MATERIALS

Keep the following equipment ready before venepuncture:

1. Disposable gloves. These should always be worn before venepuncture.
2. Sterile, disposable, one-time use, 10 ml syringe with side nozzle. Two 22-gauge needles with short bevels (the flattened puncturing points).
3. 10 ml test tubes, or vials, with or without anticoagulant.
4. Sterile gauze pieces moist with 70 % alcohol/methylated spirit.
5. Tourniquet. A 2-3 cm wide elastic bandage with Velcro strips to keep it securely in place. (It will be used to obstruct the venous return and make the veins prominent just before venepuncture). Alternately, a blood pressure cuff attached to its apparatus, or a 'twisted' handkerchief can serve the purpose.

PROCEDURES

1. Seat the subject comfortably on a chair with an arm rest, or near a table. The subject, if nervous, may lie down on a bed. Reassure the subject by your approach and conversation.
2. Examine both arms in front of the elbows to locate a suitable vein. Ask your assistant to compress the upper arm with his hands to make the veins prominent. The antecubital (medial basilic) vein is embedded in subcutaneous fat and is usually sufficiently large to take a wide-bore needle. It also runs straight for about 3 cm, and is usually palpable—even in obese subjects. If the vein is neither visible nor palpable, try the other arm. (You should avoid superficial veins because they are notoriously slippery. Veins above the ankle or on the back of the hand may have to be used).
3. Once a suitable vein has been selected, support the subject's arm over the edge of the table. Wash your hands with soap and water, dry them on a sterile towel, and put on the gloves. Ask your assistant to open the syringe pack. Take out the syringe and attach the needle (it is attached/detached with a little twist), with its bevel facing you.
4. Ask your assistant to apply the tourniquet about 2-3 cm above the elbow to obstruct the venous return. The subject may open and close her fist to increase the venous return and make the veins engorged (filled) with blood. If the vein is still not sufficiently prominent, a few 'slaps' with your fingers over the region may do so.

   Clean the skin over the selected vein with gauze and alcohol and allow it to dry. With the fingers of your left hand supporting and steadying the elbow from behind, stretch the skin over the vein downward with your left thumb placed about 4 cm below the vein. This traction fixes the vein and prevents its slipping when it is punctured.
5. With the piston pushed in, the side nozzle towards the subject's arm, and the bevel of the needle facing you, hold the syringe between your fingers and thumb of the right hand.
6. With the first finger placed near the butt of the needle, puncture the skin and push in the needle under the skin with a firm and smooth thrust, at an angle of 15-20° to the skin.
7. Slightly pull the plunger back with your thumb and little finger to produce a little negative pressure in the syringe. Advance the needle gently along the vein and puncture it from the side, a few mm ahead of the skin puncture. This prevents counterpuncture of the far wall of the vein and formation of a hematoma (local leakage of blood).

8. As the vein is punctured, all resistance will suddenly cease and blood will start to enter the syringe. With the needle still in the vein, and supporting the syringe with your left hand, gently pull the plunger back with the thumb and fingers of your right hand. Do not withdraw blood faster than the punctured veins is filling as too much pressure applied to the plunger is likely to cause mechanical injury and hemolysis of red cells. The subject may open and close the fist to enhance venous return.

9. When enough blood has been collected, release the tourniquet and press a fresh swab over the skin puncture. Withdraw the needle gently but keep the swab in position. Ask the subject to flex the arm and keep it so to maintain pressure on the puncture site till the bleeding stops. The arm may be raised above the head for a minute or so if required.

10. Hold the syringe vertical with the plunger supported, and remove the needle with a slight twist. Expel the blood gently into the container; do not apply force as it may cause mechanical injury to red cells. Gently shake, or swirl the container between your palms so that the anticoagulant (if used) mixes well with the blood without frothing.

Note
If an autoclaved glass syringe has been used and is required to be used again, wash it under tap water, passing a syringeful of water forcefully through the needle. This will clean the needle from inside.

Important
The entire process of withdrawing blood should be completed within two minutes of applying the tourniquet because, stagnation of blood in the vein is likely to alter its composition—the cell counts usually increasing.

PRECAUTIONS

1. All aseptic precautions must be observed and disposable gloves, syringe and needles must be used.

2. The tourniquet (or the BP cuff) must be removed before taking the needle out of the vein to avoid formation of hematoma.

3. The blood from the syringe should be transferred to the container without delay to prevent clotting.

4. Ask the subject to keep the swab in position till the bleeding from the puncture site stops.

5. COLLECTION OF CAPILLARY BLOOD (SKIN-PRICK METHOD)

In most medical colleges and clinical laboratories, trained laboratory technicians give the skin prick because an anxious student may only make a superficial prick on her or his partner's finger. This will force her to squeeze the finger that will expel tissue fluid along with blood to come out of the puncture site. The dilution of blood will, thus, nullify the results. *Hence for clinical work, venous blood is always preferred.* Skin-prick may be used on the bedside of a patient, or in an emergency when it is not convenient to take a venous sample. With a little practice, and confidence, the students should be able to give skin pricks to their work-partners with confidence.

Note
Remember that one deep puncture, which will give you free-flowing blood, is less painful than 3 or 4 superficial stabs.

• *Capillary blood* is also called *"peripheral blood"* as it comes out of the peripheral vessels (capillaries) in contrast to venous blood.

Selection of Site for Skin Prick

In adults and older children, capillary blood is generally obtained from a skin puncture made on the tip of the middle or ring finger, or on the lobe of the ear. In infants and young children in whom the fingers are too small for a prick, the medial or lateral side of the pad of the big toe or heel is used.

The site for skin-prick should be clean and free from edema, infection, skin disease, callus, or circulatory defects.

Important

The thumb and little finger are never pricked because the underlying palmar fasciae (venous bursae) from these digits are continuous with those of the forearms. Any accidental injury to these fasciae may cause the infection to spread into the forearm.

APPARATUS

Note

Since our aim is to get free-flowing blood drops with only a single prick, without squeezing the skin around the puncture, choosing a suitable instrument is very important, whether a blood lancet, an injection needle, or a pricking gun. Your teacher will guide you accordingly.

1. **Blood Lancet/Pricking needle.** Disposable, sterile, one-time use, blood lancets (flat, thin metal pieces with 3-4 mm deep penetrating sharp points) are commercially available and should be preferred. Lancets with 3-sided cutting points and mounted in plastic are also suitable. However, lancets with thin and shallow points are not satisfactory.

   Ordinary, narrow-bore **injection needles** are useless since they only make shallow cuts rather than deep punctures. However, wide-bore (22 gauge) needles may be used in an emergency or if blood lancets are not available.

   A **cutting needle** with 3-sided cutting point (used by surgeons) can serve the purpose well.

   Pricking gun. A spring-loaded pricking gun that has a disposable, 3-sided sharp point, and a loading and releasing mechanism, is ideal because the depth of the puncture can be preselected. After pulling back the release lever, and thus "loading" the gun, it is placed on the ball of the finger and the release lever pressed. The subject does not see the sharp point and the pain is thus minimized.

2. Sterile gauze/cotton, moist with 70 % alcohol/methylated spirit.

3. Glass slides, pipettes, etc, according to requirements.

Note

The students should bring their own lancets. These may be reused 2-3 times, if required, after passing their points through a flame. Too much heating, however, is likely to blunt the pricking points.

PROCEDURES

All aseptic precautions must be taken. The person giving the prick should wash his/her hands with soap and water, and wear gloves if possible.

Note

Keep all the equipment ready before getting a prick. If the finger to be pricked appears cold and bloodless, especially in winter, immerse it in warm water for 2-3 minutes.

1. Clean and vigorously rub the ball of the finger with the spirit swab, followed by a final cleaning with dry gauze. (Scrubbing increases local blood flow).
   Allow the alcohol to dry by evaporation for the following reasons:
   i. Sterilization with alcohol/spirit is effective only after it has dried by evaporation.
   ii. The thin film of alcohol can cause the blood drop to spread sideways along with alcohol so that it will not form a satisfactory round drop.
   iii. The alcohol may cause hemolysis of blood.
2. Steadying the finger to be pricked in your left hand, apply a gentle pressure on the sides of the ball of the finger with your thumb and forefinger to raise a thick, broad ridge of skin. (Do not touch the pricking area).
3. Hold the lancet between the thumb and fingers of your right hand, and keeping it directed along the axis of the finger, but slightly "off" center so as to miss the tip of the phalanx (i.e., not too far down or too far near the top of the nail bed), prick the skin with a

sharp and quick vertical stab to a depth of 3-4 mm and release the pressure. The blood should start to flow slowly, spontaneously and freely (without any squeezing) — if a good prick has been given.

Important
Do not squeeze or press the finger as the tissue fluid squeezed out will dilute the blood and give false low values. The squeeze also tends to close the wound edges. You may exert a slight tension on either side of the puncture with your thumbs in order to open up the wound more widely (a plug of epithelial cells tends to block the puncture especially if the wound is shallow, as often happens if a narrow-bore injection needle is used). The forearm or the hand may be squeezed or milked towards the fingers to facilitate blood flow. If all efforts fail, a fresh prick may be required.

4. Wipe away the first 2 drops of blood with dry, sterile gauze as it may be contaminated not only with tissue fluid, but also with epithelial and endothelial cells which will appear as artifacts in the blood film.
5. Allow a fresh drop of blood of sufficiently large size (about 3-4 mm diameter) to well up from the wound, and make a blood smear, or fill a pipette as the case may be.
6. Clean the area of the prick with a fresh swab and ask the subject to keep the swab pressed on the wound with his/her thumb till the bleeding stops, which occurs in a minute or so.

Ear-lobe Prick

1. After selecting the site, rub the lobe of the ear between your thumb and finger until warm. Clean the skin with alcohol and give a 2 mm deep prick. (The skin here is usually thinner than at the fingertip). Wipe away the first drop and allow a new one to form).
2. Alternately, a nick may be given with the corner edge of a sterile blade to obtain blood.

(The BT and CT tests give better results here than at the finger-prick).

Pricking the Heel

In infants and young children, blood can be collected from the cleaned and warmed medial or lateral areas of the heel. The central plantar and the posterior curvature areas of the heel should be avoided as the prick may cause injury to the underlying tarsal bones which lie near the surface.

PRECAUTIONS

1. Keep the equipment for the test ready before getting/giving a finger prick.
2. The selected site should be clean, free from infection, edema, or skin disease.
3. The site should be vigorously cleaned and scrubbed with sterile gauze and alcohol. Scrubbing increases local blood flow.
4. The lancet/needle should be sterile, and if it is to be refused, it should be passed through a flame.
5. The puncture should be deep enough to give free-flowing blood but not so very deep that it takes inordinately long time for the bleeding to stop.
6. Do not press or squeeze the finger to increase the blood flow from the skin-prick, though the arm or the hand may be milked towards the fingers.

QUESTIONS

Q. 1 What measures are taken to prevent infection during venepuncture and skin-pricking?
The instruments to be used should be properly sterilized . The site selected for puncturing should be clean and free from any disease. The area should be properly sterilized. The person withdrawing blood should wash his/her hands.

Q. 2 What are the sources and main differences between venous blood and capillary blood? Why is capillary blood called peripheral blood?
See page 17.

Q. 3 What is the difference between plasma and serum? How will you get a sample of each?
See page 19.

Q. 4 What precautions will you observe to prevent hemolysis of venous blood sample?
The syringe, needle and the container should be clean and dry. The needle should be of wide bore, and the blood should be drawn slowly and without frothing. The needle should be removed from the syringe and blood should be expelled slowly into the container.

Q. 5 What are anticoagulants? What is meant by *in vivo* and *in vitro* anticoagulants?
See page 17.

Q. 6 Why are the thumb and little finger not pricked for blood?
See page 22.

Q. 7 What are the sites for collecting capillary blood in infants?
See page 23.

Q. 8 Why should the pricked finger not be squeezed? What is meant by free-flowing blood and why should it be preferred over squeezed blood?
Squeezing or pressing the finger contaminates blood with tissue fluid, (thus diluting the blood and giving low values), and epithelial and/or endothelial cells. Free-flowing blood is that which comes out of the wound without pressing or squeezing.

1-4

Hemocytometry (Cell Counting) The Diluting Pipettes

STUDENT OBJECTIVES
After completing this experiment, you should be able to:
1. Describe the principle underlying hemocytometry.
2. Identify the RBC and WBC pipettes, name their parts, and the differences between them.
3. Name the precautions to be observed during dilution of blood in a pipette.
4. Calculate the dilution obtained with each pipette.
5. Describe the possible sources of error during dilution of blood.

Hemocytometry	Diluting pipettes
Principle.	Parts of a diluting pipette.
Units for reporting	Principle underlying their use.
Sources of error.	Differences between RBC and WBC pipettes.

Steps in hemocytometry	Filling the pipette with blood and diluting it.
Hemocytometer	Calculation of dilution apparatus obtained.
Diluting pipettes	Precautions.
Counting chamber	Questions

HEMOCYTOMETRY

Hemocytometry is the procedure of counting the number of cells in a sample of blood, the red cells, the white cells, and the platelets being counted separately. It is assumed that the cells are homogenously mixed (suspended) in the plasma in all regions of the body. However, even under physiological conditions, there are slight differences (e.g., higher red cell counts in venous and capillary blood than in arterial blood) which, though minor, are accentuated by muscular exercise, changes in posture, meals etc. Nevertheless, important clinical information can be obtained if cell counts are done carefully on a venous blood sample.

Principle

Since the number of blood cells is very high, it is difficult to count them even under the microscope. This difficulty is partly overcome by diluting the blood to a known degree with suitable diluting fluids and then counting them.

The sample of blood is diluted in a special pipette and is then placed in a capillary space of known capacity (volume) between a specially ruled glass slide (counting chamber) and a coverslip. The cells spread out in a single layer which makes their counting easy. Knowing the dilution employed, the number of cells in undiluted blood can then easily be calculated.

Units for Reporting

The result of cell counting is usually expressed as "so many cells per cubic millimeter (c.mm; mm^3;μl) of blood". For example, RBC count = 5.0 million/c.mm. The SI unit, however, is ......cells per liter of blood.
1 mm^3 = 1 μl = 10^{-6} liter.
1 μl x 10^6 = 1 liter.

Significance of Counting the Cells in a Chamber

How much important information can be obtained from this method? Does counting the cells in this traditional manner give useful clinical information as compared to counting them in electronic counters?

Automatic Electronic Cell Counters

The electronic cell counter uses volumetric impedence method. An electrolyte solution (diluent) containing suspended blood cells is aspirated through the aperture. Two electrodes are located close to the aperture and a constant current

flows between them. When a blood cell passes through the aperture, the resistance between the electrodes momentarily increases and a very small voltage change occur corresponding to the resistance. The voltage signal is amplified and sent to the electronic circuit. The data is then corrected by the CPU and displayed on the screen.

RBC Counting

The counting of red cells in a chamber is a time-consuming and tedious procedure and difficult to perform accurately even in the hands of experts. Therefore, RBC counting, because of their great number and high dilution employed, has not much of clinical value. (However, it is needed in the calculation of some blood standards). By the time changes occur in their number, the diagnosis is already clear to the clinician.

WBC Counting

The white cell counting is comparatively simpler to carry out and also more reliable.

Sources of Error in Cell Counting

Three important sources of error, pipette error, chamber error, and field error (see Expt 1-8 for details) can produce a variation of as much as 10-15%, or even more in the hands of a student. On the other hand, hemoglobin and packed cell volume are easy to determine and give enough information about the blood picture.

Steps in Hemocytometry

The whole process of cell counting involves the following steps:
1. Keeping all the equipment ready.
2. Getting a sample of blood.
3. **Pipetting,** i.e., filling the pipette with blood and diluting it.
4. **Charging**, i.e., filling the counting chamber with diluted blood.
5. Counting the cells and reporting the results.

Hemocytometer

The hemocytometer set consists of the following:

1. **The diluting pipettes** Two different glass capillary pipettes, each having a bulb, are provided for counting RBCs and WBCs. (These pipettes are sometimes called "cell pipettes" or blood pipettes. The third pipette that the students will be using is the hemoglobin pipette, which does not have a bulb).

2. **The counting chamber** It is a thick glass slide, appropriately ruled with a counting grid, i.e., squares of varying dimensions.

3. **Coverslips** Special coverslips having an optically plane and uniform surface should be preferred over ordinary coverslips.

4. **RBC and WBC** diluting fluids.

5. **Watch glasses** • Spirit swabs, • Blood lancet/needle, etc.

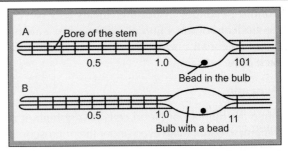

Figure 1-5. The diluting pipettes (blood pipettes) (A) RBC pipette: it has 3 markings—0.5, 1.0, and 101, (B) WBC pipette: it has 3 markings—0.5, 1.0, and 11 (see text for dilutions obtained)

> ### Note
> In this experiment we shall study the diluting pipettes, while the counting chamber will be studied in the next experiment.

For practice. Since this and the next experiment are study/practice exercises, the whole class may use anticoagulated blood obtained from a student volunteer. Or a spare anticoagulated blood sample obtained from the clinical laboratory may be used (Of course with all precautions about handling blood from an unknown person). Alternatively, and more conveniently, you may place a drop of washable red ink on your or your partner's fingertip, or on a glass slide, and then practice pipetting.

STUDY OF THE DILUTING PIPETTES

Figure 1-5 shows the two glass capillary pipettes used for diluting the blood. Each pipette has a long narrow stem (for measuring the blood), which widens into a bulb (for diluting the blood/ which in turn, leads to a short stem.

Parts of a Diluting Pipette

The stem. The long narrow stem has a capillary bore and a well-grounded conical tip. It is divided into 10 equal parts (graduations) but has only two

numbers etched on it—0.5 in the middle of the stem, and 1.0 (or 1) at the junction of stem and the bulb. The pipette, has a glossy white surface behind the graduations to facilitate their reading. (Note that some pipettes have only two graduations- 0.5 and 1.0).

The bulb. The stem widens into a bulb which contains a free-rolling bead—red in the RBC pipette, and white in the WBC pipette. The bead helps in mixing the blood and the diluent and also helps in quick identification at a glance.

Rubber tube and mouthpiece. The bulb narrows again into a short stem to which a long, narrow, soft-rubber tube bearing a mouthpiece (often red in RBC pipette, and white in WBC pipette) is attached. The rubber tube should be at least 25-30 cm long to facilitate filling of the pipette by gentle suction. It also allows the pipette to be held horizontally so that one can comfortably watch the blood or diluting fluid entering the pipette.

Just beyond the bulb, the number 101 is etched on the RBC, and 11 on the WBC pipettes.

Principle Underlying the Use of Diluting Pipettes

It is important to understand that the numbers marked on the pipettes—0.5, 1.0 and 101 on the RBC pipette and 0.5, 1.0 and 11 on the WBC pipette—do not indicate absolute or definite amounts (or volumes) in terms of so many cubic millimeters (or µl), a mistake commonly made by the students. These figures only indicate relative volumes (parts)/or relative volumes in relation to each other. That is, half volume (from tip to mark 0.5), one volume (from the tip to mark 1.0) in both pipettes; and eleven volumes (from tip to mark 11 above the bulb in WBC pipette), and hundred one volumes (from tip to mark 101 in RBC pipette). Of course, all these volumes will have certain definite volumes in terms of cmm, but we are not concerned with these but only the relative volumes or parts in relation to each other. It can be seen that the capillary bore in WBC pipette is wider than that in RBC pipette, and therefore, will hold more blood though the volume of the stem in both cases is 1.0 (one).

Differences Between the Two Pipettes

The differences between the two pipettes are given below:

RBC pipette	WBC pipette
1. Calibrations are 0.5 and 1.0 below the bulb, and 101 above the bulb.	1. Calibrations are 0.5 and 1.0 below the bulb and 11 above it.
2. The capillary bore is narrow, thus it is a slow-speed pipette.	2. The capillary bore is wider, hence it is a fast-speed pipette.
3. Bulb is larger and has a red bead.	3. Bulb is smaller and has a white bead.
4. The volume of the bulb is 100 times the volume contained in stem.	4. The volume of the bulb is 10 times the volume of the stem.
5. The dilution can be 1 in 100 or 1 in 200.	5. The dilution can be 1 in 10 or 1 in 20.

• Note that though the dilution obtained with the RBC pipette is 10 times that obtained with WBC pipette, its bulb is not 10 times bigger. The reason is the much finer bore in the red cell pipette.

Filling the Pipette

1. Place a drop of anticoagulated blood on a glass slid, or a drop of red ink on your fingertip, or get a finger-prick under aseptic conditions.
2. Holding the mouthpiece of the pipette between your lips and keeping the pipette

(with its graduations facing you) at an angle of about 40° to the horizontal, place its tip within the edge of the drop. Gently suck on the mouthpiece and draw blood until it is just above the mark 0.5 (capillary action cannot fill the pipette at this angle).

• The blood drop should be of adequate size (say 3-4 mm in diameter). If it is too small or if the tip is lifted out of the drop, air will enter the pipette along with blood. If the tip presses against the skin, the bore at the tip will get blocked and no blood will enter the stem even if you suck hard at the mouthpiece.
• Alternately, the pipette (after removing the rubber tube) may be filled with blood (without sucking/by lowering its bulb end below the horizontal and allowing the blood to flow down the stem by gravity.
3. Remove the pipette from the blood drop and clean its outer surface with a cotton swab by wiping it toward the tip. Do not touch the bore at the tip otherwise some blood will be pulled out.
4. Keeping the pipette horizontal all the time, bring the blood in the stem to the exact mark 0.5 by wiping the tip on your palm (or on a paper) a couple of times till the blood recedes to the exact mark.

Note

Do not use filter paper for this purpose as it will absorb a large amount of blood, and neither should you try to blow out the extra blood.

5. Holding the pipette nearly vertical, immerse its tip in the diluting fluid taken in a watch glass, and suck the diluent to the mark 11 (WBC) or 101 (RBC). As the fluid is sucked up, the blood is swept before it into the bulb of 10 volumes (WBC) or 100 volumes (RBC pipette).

• The sucking up of diluting fluid should not be done very quickly because blood being viscous, if a sufficient time is not allowed, a thick film of blood will remain sticking to the inside of the capillary bore, thus introducing a significant error.

- The dilution of blood should not be delayed otherwise it is likely to clot in the stem.
- Once the diluent has been taken to the appropriate mark, keep the pipette horizontal so that the fluid does not run out by gravity.
- Do not place the pipette on the table, or delay the mixing because it becomes impossible to dislodge the cells from the walls of the bulb once they settle down.

6. **Mixing the Blood with the Diluting Fluid.** Once the diluting fluid has been sucked up, remove the rubber tube. Holding the short stem above the bulb between your thumb and first two fingers, and pressing the tip of the pipette against the palm of the other hand, rotate it to and fro for 3-4 minutes so that the blood and diluent get thoroughly mixed.

   - Alternately, remove the rubber tube, close the pipette ends with thumb and forefinger of your right hand, and shake it vigorously with a figure of eight motion.
   - Do not shake the pipette with an end-wise motion as this will force the cells out of the bulb into the stem. A pipette shaker, if available, may be used.

7. **Charging the Chamber.** Once the blood and the diluent have been mixed well, 'charge' the chamber as described in the next experiment.

8. **Cleaning the Pipette.** Pipette should be cleaned as soon as possible after the experiment is over. Rinse it in running water, sucking and expelling water with maximum force, a few times. Remove water by sucking and expelling alcohol a couple of times. Finally, rinse it with ether or acetone to remove alcohol.

Calculation of Dilution Obtained (Dilution Factor)

When blood is sucked up to the mark 0.5 (half part or volume) and is followed by the diluting fluid, the blood enters the bulb first and is followed by the diluent to the mark 101 (RBC pipette), or mark 11 (WBC pipette). The stem in both pipettes contains only the diluent. Thus, *the dilution of the blood occurs in the bulb only.*

RBC pipette. Since the volume of the bulb is 100 (101-1.0 = 100), it means that 100 volumes (or parts) of diluted blood contain 0.5 (half) part of blood and 99.5 (100-0.5 = 99.5) parts or volumes of diluent. This gives a dilution of 0.5 in 100 (half in hundred), or 1 in 200 (one in two hundred); i.e., 1 part blood, and 199 parts of diluent, or 200 times. This figure of 200 is called **the dilution factor.**

- If blood is taken to the mark 1.0 in the stem and followed by diluent to the mark 101, the dilution obtained would be 1 in 100, or 100 times; the dilution factor being 100.

WBC Pipette. In this case the volume of the bulb is 10 (11-1= 10). When blood is taken to the mark 0.5 (half part or volume) followed by diluent to the mark 11, the volume of the diluted blood is now 10, which contains 0.5 part blood and 9.5 parts or volumes of the diluting fluid. This gives a dilution of 0.5 in 10 (half in ten), or 1 in 20 (one in twenty), the dilution factor being 20 (the blood will be diluted 20 times). Similarly, if blood is taken to the mark 1.0 followed by diluted to mark 11, the dilution now would be 1 in 10.

Example
A simple example will make the calculation of dilution clear. We have one cup of milk and it is to be diluted 10 times or 1 in 10, taking this one cup of milk and adding 9 cups (1 cup milk and 9 cups of water), giving us a dilution of 1 in 10 or 10 times.

If we have ½ cup of milk and want a dilution of 1 in 10, we will add 4½ cups of water to it, making it 5 cups of diluted milk. This gives a dilution of ½ in 5 or 1 in 10. Again, if we want 50 times dilution, we will add 49 cups of water to 1 cup of milk, thus making a total of 50 cups of diluted milk, the dilution factor being 50.

PRECAUTIONS

1. The pipette should be clean and dry and the bead should roll freely.

2. The pipette should not be lifted out of the blood drop while filling it with blood, otherwise air will enter it.
3. The drawing up of diluent, after blood has been taken in the stem, should not be delayed, otherwise it will clot in it.
4. The pipette should be cleaned soon after the experiment is over.

QUESTIONS

Q. 1 How will you identify a red cell pipette and a white cell pipette?
See page 27.

Q. 2 What is the function of the bead in the bulb?
The bead helps to mix the blood with its diluent. It tells whether the pipette is dry or not. (It rolls freely if it is dry.) It also helps to identify the pipette by just glancing at it.

Q. 3 What are the units of markings on the pipettes?
There are no absolute units of volume marked on the pipette. They only denote relative volumes or parts in relation to each other.

Q. 4 What is the function of the bulb in a diluting pipette?
The dilution of the blood occurs in the bulb only, and since the volume of the bulb is known, it is possible to dilute the blood with a diluent in accurately known proportions.

Q. 5 Why is it important to discard the first two drops of diluted blood from the pipette before charging the counting chamber?
After the blood has been diluted in the pipette, the stem contains only the cell-free diluent. This fluid has, therefore, to be discarded before the chamber can be filled.

Q. 6 How will you clean a pipette when blood has clotted in the stem?
The pipette is kept in strong nitric acid for 24 hours. A flexible suitably thick metal wire is used to clean the capillary bore after washing the pipette in running water. The process may have to be repeated.

Q. 7 What is the significance of the tenth graduations on the stem?
Instead of taking 0.5 or 1.0 volume of blood we can take smaller volumes, say 0.2 or 0.3 to get higher dilutions.

Q. 8 Can a pipette be used for any other purpose than cell counting?
The RBC pipette can be used for counting platelets, WBCs (when their number is very high, as in some leukemias) or spermatozoa in the semen.

1-5

Hemocytometry (Cell Counting) The Counting Chamber

STUDENT OBJECTIVES	
After completing this experiment you should be able to: 1. Describe the counting chamber, and the dimensions of different squares on the counting grid. 2. Name the diluting fluids and their composition.	3. Name the precautions observed during charging the chamber. 4. Focus the counting grid for RBC and WBC counting under low and high magnifications. 5. Explain the possible sources of error for cell counting.

Improved Neubauer Chamber

The Counting Grid.	Charging the Chamber.
For RBC counting.	High-speed pipette.
For WBC counting.	Slow-speed pipette.
Focusing the Counting	Ideally charged
Grid.	chamber.
	Precautions
	Questions.

The counting chamber was introduced by Crammer in 1805. Its modification by Thoma, and later by Neubauer remained in use for a long time. Improved Neubauer chamber is in current use.

Note

Since this is a practice experiment, anticoagulated blood from a student, capillary blood from a skin-prick, or washable red ink may be used.

Improved Neubauer Chamber (Counting Chamber)

The counting chamber (**Figure 1-6**) is a single, solid, heavy glass slide. Extending across its middle third are 3 parallel platforms (pillars, or flanges) separated from each other by shallow trenches (moats, gutters, or troughs). The central platform or "floorpiece" (sometimes also called the plateau) is wider, and exactly 0.1 mm (one-tenth of a mm) lower than the two lateral pillars. The floorpiece is divided into two equal parts by a short transverse trench in its middle as shown in **Figure 1-6**. Thus, there is an H-shaped trench or trough enclosing the two floorpieces.

The two lateral platforms can support a coverslip which, when in position, will span the trenches and provide a capillary space 0.1 mm deep between the under surface of the coverslip and the upper surface of the floorpieces.

Identically ruled areas, called "counting grids", consisting of squares of different sizes, are etched on each floorpiece. The two counting grids allow RBC and WBC counts to be made simultaneously if needed, or duplicate samples can be run.

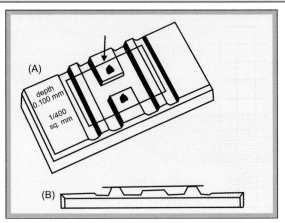

Figure 1-6. Hemocytometer, or counting chamber with improved Neubauer's ruling (A) Surface view, with the cover slip in position. The locations of the counting grids on the two platforms ("Floor pieces") are indicated. The arrow indicates the place where the tip of the pipette should be placed for "charging" the chamber, (B) Side view with the coverslip in position. The space between the underside of the coverslip and the surface of the platform is 0.100 mm in depth. The depth and the area of the smallest square are etched on the surface of the chamber

Note

Hemocytometers with silver-coated floor-pieces show the grids beautifully, which makes them easier to use by the students.

The Counting Grid

The ruled area on each floorpiece, the counting grid, has the following dimensions:

- Each counting grid (**Figure 1-7**) measures 9 mm^2 (3 mm × 3 mm). It is divided into 9 large squares, each 1 mm^2 (1 mm ×1 mm).
- Of these 9 squares, the 4 large corner squares are lightly etched, and each is divided by single lines into 16 medium-sized squares each of which has a side of 1/4 mm, and an area of 1/16 mm^2 (1/4 mm × 1/4 mm). These 4 large corner squares are employed for counting leucocytes and are, therefore, called WBC squares (**Figure 1-7**).

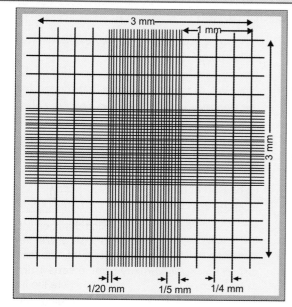

Figure 1-7. The counting grid of improved Neubauer's ruling. The four corner groups of 16 squares (side = 0.25 mm) are used for counting WBCs. The RBCs are counted in 5 groups of 16 smallest squares each (side = 0.05 mm). The grid also provides a convenient scale for measuring the size of small objects like parasite eggs

- The central densely etched large square (1 mm × 1 mm), called the RBC square, is divided into 25 medium-sized squares, each of which has a side of 1/5 mm.
- Each of these medium squares is set off (separated) from its neighbors by very closely placed double lines (tram lines) or triple lines. These double or triple lines extend in all directions beyond the boundaries of the 9 mm² ruling i.e., in between all the WBC squares around the central RBC square.
- Each of the 25 medium squares (side= 1/5 mm), bounded by double lines (which are 0.01 mm apart) or triple lines, is further divided into 16 smallest squares by single lines. Thus, each smallest square has a side of 1/5 × 1/4 = 1/20 mm, and an area of 1/4000 mm².

Note

Since each group of 16 smallest squares is demarcated from its neighbors by double or triple lines, the dimensions of the RBC square (largest central square) must be slightly larger than 1 mm × 1 mm, as indeed they are (the exact dimensions of the smallest squares (1/400 mm²) are etched on the chamber surface.

For RBC Counting

The red cells are counted in 4 corner groups and one central group of medium squares, each of which has 16 smallest squares, i.e., in a total of 80 smallest squares.

Area of smallest square = 1/20 mm × 1/20 mm
= 1/400 mm²

Since the depth of the chamber is 1/10 mm, the Volume of the smallest square = 1/400 ×1/10
= 1/4000 mm³.

For WBC (Total Leucocyte) Counting

This count is done in the 4 corner groups of large squares, each of which has 16 medium squares.

Area of one medium square = 1/4 mm × 1/4 mm = 1/16 mm².

Volume of this square = 1/16 mm² × 1/10 mm = 1/160 mm³.

Thoma's Chamber. In this counting chamber, not used now, the central depressed platform is circular. The grid is only 1 mm², consisting of 25 groups of 16 smallest squares each. The dimensions of the smallest squares are the same, i.e., 1/20 mm × 1/20 mm. The 1 mm squares at the corners are absent.

Old Neubauer Chamber. There are nine 1 mm squares. The 4 corner groups of 16 squares each are for WBC counting, while the central 1 mm² area has 16 groups of 16 squares each for RBC counting (rather than 25 groups of 16 smallest squares as in improved Neubauer chamber). The medium squares are separated by triple lines.

Focusing the Counting Grid

Examine the grid on each floorpiece, without the coverslip, under low and high magnifications. Rack the condenser up and down, closing/adjusting the diaphragm at the same time. Find out the best combination of these two that shows the grid lines and squares clearly. When properly focused, the rulings (lines) appear as translucent darkish lines.

- With low magnification of 100 times, one large square, 1 mm × 1 mm is visible in one field, i.e. a group of 16 medium squares (for WBC counting), or a groups of 25 medium squares (for RBC counting).
- Examine the squares under high magnification. Compare what you see with the diagram of **Figure 1-6** and identify, understand, and draw the dimensions of various squares in your workbook.

Charging the Counting Chamber

Charging the chamber requires patience, practice, and understanding of how to correctly judge the size of the drop, the angle at which the pipette should be held on the floorpiece and the time needed for filling (charging) the chamber. This is called the **"speed of the pipette"**. Obviously, it varies with the size of the capillary bore in the stem of the pipette.

- **High-speed pipette.** Since the bore of the WBC pipette is wider, a drop will form more quickly at its tip, and it will be larger, as compared to the RBC pipette. This requires that this pipette should be held more horizontally—say, at an angle of 10-20° and for a shorter time.
- **Slow-speed pipette.** The bore of the RBC pipette being narrow, it will take a longer time for a suitable drop to form. It should, therefore, be held at a steeper angle—say, 60-70°.

It is for this reason that the students should first practice charging a chamber with the RBC pipette and then with the WBC pipette.

PROCEDURES

1. Assuming that the blood and the diluent have been properly mixed, the next step is to charge the chamber. Place a coverslip on the chamber so that it spans the floorpieces and the trenches around them—a process called "centering" the coverslip.
2. Roll the pipette once more between your palms to mix the contents of the bulb. If this precaution is not taken the counts are bound to be unreliable.
3. Keeping your finger over the top of the pipette and releasing it in a controlled manner, allow the first 2 drops to drain the gravity. This fluid contains cell-free diluting fluid in the stem which has not taken any part in the dilution of blood.
4. Hold the pipette at an appropriate angle (depending on the speed of the pipette) and watching carefully, allow a drop of diluted blood to form at its tip. Then quickly place the tip of the pipette on the floorpiece in gentle contact with the edge of the coverslip. As the surface of the drop touches the coverslip, the fluid will run under it by capillarity and form a uniform film. Lift the pipette as soon as the floorpiece is covered with diluted blood.
   - The chamber should be charged at one go and not in parts. For this, one needs a drop of proper size. Try to achieve an ideally-charged chamber.
     Ideally-charged chamber
     An ideally-charged chamber is completely filled with diluted blood. If any blood flows into the trenches, it is called **"overcharging"**. If the fluid is insufficient to cover the floorpiece, or if there are air bubbles, it is called **"undercharging"**, (air bubbles are formed if the coverslip or the floorpiece is dirty with grease or is moist).
   - If there is over or under-charging, wash the chamber and coverslip in soap and water, dry them and recharge the chamber.

5. Once the chamber has been properly charged, move it to the microscope. Wait for 2-3 minutes so that the cells settle down. Counting cannot be started when the cells are moving and changing places due to currents in the fluid.

   Counting the cells. Focus the appropriate squares under the required magnification and start counting as described in Expts 1-8 (RBC) and 1-11 (WBC).

PRECAUTIONS

1. Ensure that the counting chamber and the coverslip are absolutely clean, grease-free, and dry.
2. While charging the chamber ensure that it is neither under nor over-charged.

3. Never bring the objective lens down while looking into the microscope as the chamber is likely to be scratched or broken.

QUESTIONS

Q. 1 What is the principle underlying the use of a counting chamber?
See page 25.

Q. 2 What are the dimensions of WBC and RBC squares?
See page 31.

Q. 3 What are the features of an ideally-charged chamber?
See page 32.

Q. 4 How does the improved Neubauer chamber differ from the older variety of Neubauer chamber?
See page 31.

1-6

Examination of Fresh Blood:
A. Drop Preparation
B. Preparing a Peripheral Blood Film

A. DROP PRESENTATION

The first and obvious way to study the cells of the blood is to examine fresh blood under the microscope in the form of a drop preparation and in a thin blood film or smear made on a glass slide.

In this experiment, the students will examine some features of blood cells and record their observations. They will also practice making (preparing) blood films and examine them without staining. In later experiments, they will prepare and stain blood smears and identify and count various blood cells, reticulocytes, and platelets.

- Anticoagulated blood obtained from a student volunteer, or spare blood obtained from the clinical laboratory may be provided to the students to avoid skin pricks at this time (a drop of blood can be put on the slide without touching it). Students may also use their own blood from skin pricks.

APPARATUS AND MATERIALS

1. Disposable, sterile blood lancet/pricking needle.
   - Sterile cotton/gauze swabs.
   - 70% alcohol/methylated spirit.

2. 8-10 thin, absolutely transparent, grease-free standard glass slides (75 mm × 25 mm).
   - Vaseline.
   - Toothpicks.

Important
Once cleaned, do not touch the surfaces of the glass slides and cover slips.

PROCEDURES

While you prepare the drop preparation, your work-partner can make blood films from the same finger-prick blood.

1. Get a finger-prick under aseptic conditions. Discard the first 2 drops and allow a good drop to form. Holding a coverslip by its edges between your thumb and finger, touch its centre to the blood drop, thus forming a bead.
2. Invert and carefully drop the coverslip (along with the blood drop under it) in the centre of a glass slide. Do not press. The blood drop will spread into a thick film by the weight of the coverslip.
3. Using a toothpick, apply a little vaseline all around the edges of the coverslip to seal the capillary space under it. This will prevent evaporation of water and drying up of the preparation.
4. Examine the preparation under low and high magnifications and record your observations.

OBSERVATIONS

Note the degree of separation of cells. Do they lie in a single layer or in 2, 3 or more layers? The red cells are non-nucleated, flat biconcave discs, round, oval or pear-shaped, thinner in the centre and appear as colorless, or pale pink structures. (When stained with Leishman's stain, they appear dull orange-pink). Note if there is any rouleaux formation (cells lying on top of each other like a pile of coins) and the number of cells in a rouleaux. Observe if any leucocytes are seen, and their types if possible. Do they show any ameboid movement?

Do you see any platelets—in clumps, or showing disintegration? After a time you may see fibrin threads when clotting starts.

B. PREPARATION OF A BLOOD FILM (BLOOD SMEAR)

Blood films can be made from anticoagulated, or finger-prick blood.

PROCEDURES

1. Place 3 or 4 slides on a white sheet of paper on your work-table, the surface of which should be even and smooth.
2. Allow a medium-sized drop of blood to form on the finger-tip.
3. Steady the pricked finger of your partner with your left hand. Lift a slide from the table, holding it along its long edges. Then touch its centre, about 1 cm from the narrow end, to the blood drop. (If anti-coagulated blood is being used place a drop of blood in a similar position with a dropper).
   - Do not apply the blood drop at the finger to the slide placed on the table. One cannot see the amount of blood placed on the slide.
4. Place the slide flat on the table, with the blood drop to the right side (neither your fingers, nor the skin of the subject's finger should touch the surface of the slide).
5. Support the left end of the slide with your thumb and fingers of your left hand. Now grasp the long edges of a second slide, the "spreader" between thumb and fingers of your right hand, so that its free left end extends downwards and to the left at an angle of about 40° to the horizontal.
6. Place the narrow edge of the spreader on the first slide, at an angle of 40°, just in front of the blood drop (**step 1, Figure 1-8**). Pull the spreader back gently so that it touches the front of the blood drop. Hold it there, (or move it a little from side to side) till the blood,

moving along the junction of the two slides by capillarity, almost reaches the ends of the spreader, except the last 2 mm on each side, thus distributing the blood evenly across its width. (If the blood drop is too big, you may start to spread the smear before the whole of the blood spreads along the slide).

7. Steady the first slide with your left hand, and maintaining a light but even pressure and 40° angle (**step 2, Figure 1-8**), move the spreader forwards to the left in a single, smooth, fairly fast gliding motion, pulling the blood behind it in the form of a thin smear.
   - The smear should be spread in about half a second. Any hesitation will result in striations in the film.

8. Make as many trials as possible to get acceptable films, keeping in mind the features of an ideal blood smear, as described below. Dry the film by waving the slide in the air (Do not try to blot-dry the film).

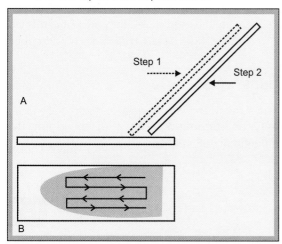

Figure 1-8. (A) Method of spreading a blood film. Step 1: The spreader is placed in front of the blood drop and pulled back till it touches the blood Step 2: Spreader is pushed forwards to spread the film. (B) The appearance of a well-prepared film, showing the movement of the objective over it

OBSERVATIONS

Examine the slides against diffuse light, with naked eye. What is the color of the smear? Does it appear thick, thin, or granular? Are there any striations— longitudinal or transverse? Are there any vacant places in the film? Is it uniformly distributed in the middle two-thirds of the slide? Is its head—the starting point, straight and about 1 cm from the end? Are its edges about 2 mm from the long sides of the slide? Is there a tail? Try to answer all these questions.

Examine the slides under low and high magnification. Describe what you see about the various cells and compare with what you saw in the drop preparation.

Features of an Ideal Blood Film

1. The blood film should occupy the middle two-thirds (about 5 cm) of the slide, with a clear margin of about 2 mm on either side.
2. It should be tongue-shaped, i.e., broad at the head (starting point), and taper towards the other end, but without any 'tails'.
3. It should be translucent, uniformly thick throughout, with no vacant areas, striations (longitudinal or transverse), or 'granular' areas.
4. It should be neither very thick nor very thin (this can be learned only with practice). A thin film looks faintly pink against a white surface, while a thick smear appears red. An ideal film appears 'buff' colored.
5. The red cells, as seen under the microscope, should lie separately from each other, just touching here and there, but without any crowding, or rouleaux formation.

Note
A thick blood film results from taking too large a drop of blood, a faster movement, and a smaller angle of the spreader.

PRECAUTIONS

1. The slides should be absolutely free from dust and grease, because blood will not stick to areas where oils from your fingers have been left. New slides should be preferred. But if

old ones are to be used, they should be properly cleaned, as described below.

2. The edge of the spreader should be smooth and not chipped, otherwise the slide would leave striations along or across the smear. Leucocytes may also be caught in chipped places and be carried towards the tail.

3. When applying the slide to the blood drop from a finger-prick, do not touch the skin with the slide, but only the periphery (top) of the blood drop. This is to avoid taking up epidermal squamous or sweat.

4. The blood should be spread immediately after taking it on the slide. Any delay will cause clumping of cells due to partial coagulation. This will give a 'granular' appearance to the blood film, which is visible to the naked eye.

5. The angle of the spreader should be 35° to 40°. The more the angle of the spreader approaches the vertical, the thinner the film, and the lesser the angle, the thicker the film.

6. The pressure of the spreader on the slide should be slight and even and the pushing should be fairly quick while maintaining a uniform pressure throughout.

7. The film should be dried by waving it in the air immediately after spreading it. A delay can cause not only clumping, but also crenation and distortion of red cells in a damp atmosphere (if water is allowed to slowly evaporate from the blood plasma on the slide, crenation occurs due to gradual increase in the concentration of salts).

8. By turning the spreader over, you can use it to make 4 blood films.

Cleaning the Slides

Prepare acid-dichromate solution by mixing 1 part of concentrated sulfuric or nitric acid with 9 parts of 2-3% potassium dichromate solution.

1. Wash the slides and coverslips with soap and water and rinse in running water. Then soak them overnight in the acid-dichromate solution. Follow this with a wash in running water, then in distilled water.

2. Dip the slides in 90-95% alcohol and dry with a clean, lint-free cloth.
   - Another method is to use a good detergent for overnight soak in place of acid-dichromate solution.
   - The acid-dichromate solution is best kept in a 1-2 litre, wide-mouth jar. After washing the used slides, they are put in this jar. The slides can then be treated as described above.

QUESTIONS

The Questions/Answers are listed with Expt 1-12 on staining a blood film and doing the differential cell counts.

Estimation of Hemoglobin

Student Objectives	
After completing this experiment you should be able to: 1. Indicate the relevance of this estimation. 2. Which characteristics of hemoglobin can be used to estimate its concentration?	3. Explain the absolute and relative Hb scales. 4. Determine the Hb level by the Sahli's acid hematin method. 5. List the sources and degree of error in this method. 6. Name the advantages and disadvantages of his method.

7. Name other methods of estimation of Hb.
8. Indicate normal levels of Hb in different age groups and sexes.
9. Describe the structure, synthesis, and functions of Hb.
10. Name the varieties and derivatives of Hb.
11. Name the common causes of increased and decreased levels of Hb.
12. Classify anemias, and mention the commonest type of anemia in India.

Relevance.

Hemoglobinometry
  Basis.
  Absolute and relative Hb scales.

Principle.

Apparatus and Materials.
Procedures.

Sources and degree of error.
Observations and results.
Normal values.
Advantages and disadvantages of Sahli's method.
Other methods of Hb estimation.
Precautions.
Questions.

Relevance

The hemoglobin concentration is always estimated as part of routine tests in outpatients department and also as a bedside test in indoor patients. It is indicated as part of complete hematological studies in all diseases of blood, especially all types of anemias, leukemias, and in chronic diseases such as tuberculosis, chronic infections, malignancies, renal failure, etc.

Hemoglobinometry

The term refers to measurement of the concentration (amount) of Hb in the blood. For this purpose, advantage is taken of the following characteristics of Hb:
1. Ability to combine with oxygen.
2. Presence of known amount of iron in each gram of Hb.
3. Ability of a solution of a derivative of Hb to refract specific wavelengths of light, thus giving typical absorption bands.

Based on these features of Hb, the various methods can be grouped into the following categories:

I. **Gasometric method.** The Hb is fully saturated with oxygen and its amount is then measured with van Slyke apparatus. Though very accurate, the method is time-consuming and tedious.

II. **Visual color comparison.** This group includes Sahli, Haldane, and Tallqvist methods. The Sahli method is the most acceptable since the golden brown color of acid hematin is much easier to match with the standard than the red color of oxyHb.

III. **Spectrophotometric methods.** The Hb is converted to other compounds (e.g., cyanmetHb, carboxyHb, alkaline hematin), and by using definite wavelengths of light; each of the derivatives can be measured.

IV. **Electronic Hematology Analyzer.** The electronic analyzer, along with cell counts, can also provide Hb concentration automatically. A hemolysing agent is added to the diluted blood to release the Hb, which reacts with potassium ferricyanide and potassium cyanide in the solution to produce cyanmetHb. The cyanmetHb is then measured by specytrophotometry.

V. **Other methods.** These include: estimation of iron content of blood, and the copper sulphated specific gravity method.

Note
Since many of the above methods are unsuitable for routine use, indirect methods based on color comparison are used. However, a standard solution of a derivative (e.g., acid hematin) cannot be used, as its color will fade with time. Also there are personal errors in preparing standard solutions. To overcome these drawbacks, permanent colored glass rods, exactly matching the color of standard solution, are provided with the apparatus. Though these glass rods or strips maintain their color for a long time, they can be got tested from the National Standards Institute.

Absolute and Relative Hemoglobin Scales

In the past, when deciding the color density of the standard solutions in different methods, the same amount of blood was not taken. And since the earlier Hb tubes were calibrated only in percentage of normal, one had to know how much Hb was represented by 100 percent in each case. For example, a sample of blood containing 14.5 g/dl Hb would report 87% Hb by Sahli, 108% by Haldane, and 100% by Wintrobe methods, and so on. The values for 100% Hb by these methods are given below:

Sahli   = 17.0 %   Sahli-Adams = 14.8 %
Haldane = 13.8 %   Dare   = 16.0 %
Wintrobe = 14.5 %

To avoid this confusion, the practice of expressing Hb in "percentage" has been discarded and the Hb tubes are now graduated directly in **g percent**. However, most manufacturers needlessly continue to indicate percentages in addition to readings in grams percent on the Hb tubes.

PRINCIPLE

The Hb present in a measured amount of blood is converted by dilute hydrochloric acid into acid hematin, which in dilution is golden brown in color. The intensity of color depends on the concentration of acid hematin which, in turn, depends on the concentration of Hb. The color of the solution (i.e., its hue and depth), after dilution with water, is matched against golden-brown tinted glass rods by direct vision. The readings are obtained in g%.

APPARATUS AND MATERIALS

A. Sahli (Sahli-Adams) Hemoglobinometer (Hemometer). The set consists of:

1. **Comparator.** It is a rectangular plastic box with a slot in the middle which accommo-dates the calibrated Hb tube. Non-fading, standardized, golden-brown glass rods are fitted on each side of the slot for matching the color. An opaque white glass (or plastic)

is fitted behind the slot to provide uniform illumination during direct visual color matching.

2. **Hemoglobin tube.** The square or round glass tube is calibrated in g Hb % (2-24 g%) in yellow color on one side, and in percentage Hb (20-140%) in red color on the other side. There is a brush to clean the tube (**Figure 1-9**).

3. **Hemoglobin pipette.** It is a glass capillary pipette with only a single calibration mark-0.02 ml (20 cmm, cubic millimeters; or 20 ml, micro liters). There is no bulb in this

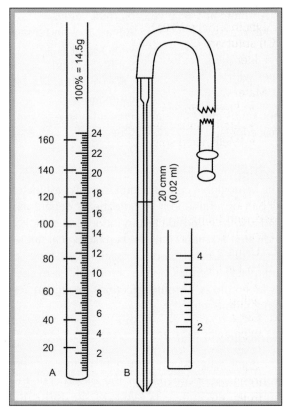

Figure 1-9. (A) Sahli-Adam's hemoglobin tube: It has graduations in g% on one side, and in percentage on the other. In this tube, 100% is equal to 14.5 g Hb per 100 ml blood. (B) Hemoglobin pipette: It has only one marking, indicating 20 cmm (0.02 ml, or 20 μl). There is no bulb (Inset: Each division represents 0.2 g of Hb)

pipette (as compared to cell pipettes) as no dilution of blood is done. **Figure 1-9B** shows the Hb pipette.

Note The calibration mark 20 cmm indicates a definite, measured volume and not an arbitrary volume, as is the case with diluting pipettes.

4. **Stirrer.** It is a thin glass rod with a flattened end which is used for stirring and mixing the blood and dilute acid.

5. **Pasteur pipette.** It is a 8-10 inch glass tube drawn to a long thin nozzle, and has a rubber teat. Ordinary glass dropper with a rubber teat also serves the purpose.

6. **Distilled water.**

B. **Decinormal (N/10) hydrochloric acid (0.1 N HCl) solution.** Mixing 36 g HCl in distilled water to 1 liter gives 'Normal' HCl; and diluting it 10 times will give N/10 HCl solution.

C. **Materials for skin prick.**
- Sterile lancet/needle.
- Sterile gauze and cotton swabs.
- Methylated spirit/70% alcohol.

PROCEDURES

Review the instructions for obtaining skin-prick blood, and filling a pipette as described in Expts 1-3 and 1-4.

1. Using a dropper, place 8-10 drops of N/10 HCl in the Hb tube, or up to the mark 20% or 3 g, or a little more till the tip of the pipette will submerge, and set it aside.

2. Get a finger prick under aseptic conditions, wipe away the first 2 drops of blood. When a large drop of free-flowing blood has formed again, draw blood up to the 20 cmm mark (0.02 ml). Carefully wipe the blood sticking to the tip of the pipette with a cotton swab, but avoid touching the bore or else blood will be drawn out by capillarity.

Note
If any blood remains sticking to the outside of the pipette, it will be that much extra blood in addition to 20 cmm.

3. Without any waiting, immerse the tip of the pipette to the bottom of the acid solution and expel the blood gently. Rinse the pipette 3-4 times by drawing up and blowing out the clear upper part of the acid solution till all the blood has been washed out from it. Avoid frothing of the mixture. Note the time.

4. Withdraw the pipette from the tube, touching it to the side of the tube, thus ensuring that no mixture is carried out of the tube. Mix the blood with the acid solution with the flat end of the stirrer by rotating and gently moving it up and down.

5. Put the Hb tube back in the comparator and let it stand for 6-8 minutes (or as advised by the manufacturer). During this time, the acid ruptures the red cells, releasing their Hb into the solution (hemolysis). The acid acts on the Hb and converts it into acid hematin which is deep golden brown in color.

- The color of acid hematin does not develop fully immediately, but its intensity increases with time, reaching a maximum, after which it starts to decrease. An adequate time, usually 6-8 minutes, must be allowed before its dilution is started. Too little time and all Hb may not be converted into acid hematin. And, waiting too long, may result in fading of color. In either case, the result will be falsely a low.

6. **Diluting and matching the color.** The next step is to dilute the acid hematin solution with distilled water (preferably buffered water, if available) till its color matches the color of the standard tinted glass rods in the comparator.

Note
Each time you compare the color, lift and hold the glass stirrer against the side of the Hb tube above the solution (rather than taking it out completely) thus allowing it to drain fully back into the tube. (If the stirrer is left in the solution when comparing the color, the solution will appear lighter).

7. Take the Hb tube out of the comparator and add distilled water drop by drop (or larger amounts depending on the experience), stirring the mixture each time and comparing the color with the standard.

8. Hold the comparator at eye level, away from your face, against bright but diffused light. Read the lower meniscus (lower meniscus is read in colored transparent solutions).

Sources and Degree of Error

False results with this method may be due to:

i. *Technical error.* It may be due to: not taking exactly 20 c.mm blood, or not giving enough time for formation of acid hematin, or using an old comparator that has faded glass rods.

ii. *Personal error.* Generally, it is not difficult to match color but since it is a visual method, color matching may vary from person to person. For example, you may think that the color is matching, while your work-partner may consider it lighter or darker than the standard.

The *Degree of Error* may be as high as 10 to 15 %. However, it can be reduced to about 5 % by taking 3 readings on the same test solution as described below.

OBSERVATIONS AND RESULTS

Compare your color matching with that of your work-partner and record the observations in your workbook. Take the average of 3 readings as shown below, and report your result as: Hb = ...g/dl.

1st reading, when the color is slightly darker than the standard:.................g/dl.

2nd reading, when, after adding a few drops of distilled water, the color exactly matches the standard: .... g/dl.

3rd reading, when, after adding some more drops, the color becomes a little lighter than the standard:................. g/dl.

For report. Express your result as: Hb= ....g/dl.

• **Oxygen carrying capacity:** Knowing your Hb concentration, and that 1.0 g of Hb can carry 1.34 ml of O_2 calculate its oxygen-carrying capacity as ....ml O_2/dl.

• **100 % Saturation.** When blood is equilibrated with pure (100 %) oxygen at a PO_2 of 120 mm Hg, the Hb gets 100 % saturated, i.e.; it picks up as much O_2 as it possibly can.

For report:
• Oxygen carrying capacity.
• 100% saturation.

Normal Values

The levels of Hb in normal Indian adults, especially in the economically deprived population, are on the lower side of those reported from affluent countries. The reason may be the poor intake of grade 1 proteins and other nutrients. The average levels and their ranges are as follows:
Males: 14.5 g/dl (13.5-18 g/dl).
Females: 12.5 g/dl (11.5-16 g/dl).

Advantages of Sahli Method

The method is simple, fairly quick, and accurate. It does not require any costly apparatus, since it needs only direct color matching. Its running cost is minimal and can, therefore, be used in mass surveys.

Disadvantages of Sahli Method

Since the acid hematin is not in true solution, some turbidity may occur. The method estimates only the oxyHb and reduced Hb, other forms-such as carboxyHb and metHb are not estimated. Also the degree of error may be high if proper precautions are not taken.

OTHER METHODS OF ESTIMATING HEMOGLOBIN

A. **Spectrophotometric methods.** In these methods, a photoelectric colorimeter is employed to measure the amount of light absorbed by a derivative of Hb.

1. *Cyanmethemoglobin method.* All forms of Hb normally present in blood (i.e., oxyHb, reduced Hb, carboxyHb, and metHb) are converted into a stable compound—*cyanmetHb*. The sample of blood is treated with modified Drabkin's reagent (it contains potassium cyanide, potassium ferricyanide, and potassium phosphate—the last replacing sodium bicarbonate of Drabkin's reagent). The modified reagent speeds up the conversion, reduces turbidity, and enhances RBC lysis. The amount of light absorbed with yellow-green filters (peak at 450 nm) is compared with a standard solution in a photoelectric colorimeter. This method is the most accurate method of estimating Hb.

2. *Wu's Alkaline Hematin Method.* The blood is treated with N/10 NaOH, which converts all forms of Hb into alkaline hematin, which is in true solution. These are two methods: the standard method and the acid-alkaline method.

3. *Haldane's CarboxyHb Method.* The red cells are Hemolysed in distilled water to release Hb. Carbon monoxide is then passed through the solution to form carboxyHb that is bright red in color. The color is then compared with that of the standard.

4. *OxyHb Method.* The blood is treated with ammonium hydroxide or sodium carbonate. The red cells are hemolysed and the Hb is converted immediately and quickly into oxyHb. The solution is then compared with a standard gray screen in photoelectric colorimeter.

B. **Tallqvist method.** A drop of blood, absorbed on a white filter paper is allowed to spread over the paper to form an even spot. As soon as the blood spot loses its shine (gloss), but before it dries, it is matched against a scale of increasingly dark red-colored round spots printed on a card. The method, though quick is rather inaccurate due to personal error. It is sometimes used in mass surveys for anemia.

C. **Iron content**. The iron in blood is separated with sulphuric acid, and its amount measured. Since 1 g of Hb contains 3.35 mg iron, the amount of Hb can be calculated.

D. **Copper sulphate falling drop method.** It is a rapid method for estimating the approximate level of Hb, and is used in large surveys. It was used extensively during World War II where an indication of the necessity for blood transfusion was immediately required (see Expt 1-21).

PRECAUTIONS

1. All precautions mentioned for collecting finger-prick blood, and filling the pipette must be observed.
2. The finger should not be squeezed, and there should not be any blood sticking to the outside of the pipette tip.
3. Only the recommended time should be allowed for the formation of acid hematin by the action of acid on Hb.
4. When diluting the color of acid hematin solution, avoid over-dilution because the color cannot be concentrated.
5. When matching the color, the solution should be uniformly golden brown throughout the solution. Dark color near the bottom of the tube indicates poor mixing.
6. During color matching, 3 readings should be taken to reduce the personal error.

QUESTIONS

Q. 1 What is the principle on which the Sahli method is based?
See page 38.

Q. 2 Why is Sahli method most frequently employed as a routine test?
See page 40.

Q. 3 What is meant by the term 'normality' of a solution? What is N/10 HCl and how will you prepare it?

The normality (N) of a solution is the number of gram equivalents in 1 litre of water. A 1 N solution of HCl contains 1 + 35 = 36 g of HCl in water made to 1 litre. Diluting this solution 10 times will give N/10 HCl.

Q. 4 Can strong acids (such as nitric, sulphuric, and hydrochloric acids) or alkalis be used in place of decinormal HCl?

The strong acids, which are very strong oxidizing agents, and alkalis will cause disruption of Hb and thus cannot be used. Only N/10 HCl is used because standardization has been done for acid hematin.

Q. 5 How would estimation of Hb be affected if less or more than 8-10 drops of N/10 HCl is taken in the Hb tube?

If less (3-4 drops) acid is taken, the blood may not mix well and/or may clot. All the Hb will not be converted into acid hematin. This will result in false low value. If much more acid is taken (say, up to the level of 10 g), the final color developed in a case of anemia (Hb 6-8 g%) would be much lighter than the standard. Color matching will then not be possible, because the color of the solution cannot be concentrated.

Q. 6 Can tap water be used for diluting and color matching?

No, it cannot be used because its salt content may cause turbidity which will interfere with color matching.

Q. 7 Can N/10 HCl be used (if distilled water is not available) for diluting and color matching?

Yes, it can be used because it being transparent, it cannot further deepen the color once all the Hb has been converted into acid hematin.

Q. 8 Why is it necessary to wait for 6-8 minutes after adding blood to N/10 HCl solution?

See page 38.

Q. 9 While matching the color, why is it important to lift the stirrer above the solution and not leave it there or take it out?

If the stirrer is left in the solution, it will lighten the color (since it is translucent) and thus matching will occur earlier. This will give a false low value. If, however, it is taken out every time the color is matched, it is bound to take away some of the solution out of the tube, thus, again giving a low value.

Q. 10 Which of the two scales given on the Hb tube is preferred over the other and why?

The scale which gives the Hb concentration in a blood sample directly in grams percent is used, as this is what is required. The scale in percentages is of no value, except academic interest.

Q. 11 What are the normal levels and ranges of Hb at different ages?

   i. Newborns   : 18-22 g/dl.
   ii. At 3 months : 14-16 g/dl.
   iii. 3 months-1 yr : 13-15 g/dl.
   iv. Adult males : 14.5 g/dl (13.5-17 g/dl).
   v. Adult females : 12.5 g/dl (11.5-15.5 g/dl).
- There may be some decrease after age 60 years.

Q. 12 Compared to males, why are the hemoglobin levels lower in females?

All other factors (age, body mass, etc.) being equal, the levels are lower in healthy females not because of menstrual loss of blood (20-30 ml). It is the estrogens in the females which have an inhibitory effect on the secretion of erythropoietin (EP) which is the main stimulant of red cell production. Also, the androgens (mainly testosterone) have a stimulatory effect on EP secretion. Both these factors tend to keep the red cell count higher in males.

Q. 13 Why is the hemoglobin level high in the newborns?

The Hb may be as high as 20-22 g/dl at the time of birth due to the high red cell count (>6 million/mm^3). The newborn has been living in state of relative hypoxia, which is a very potent stimulus for the secretion of EP. As age advances the Hb levels decrease, and adult levels are reached in a few years.

Q.14 What would happen if Hb were present freely in the plasma instead of in the red cells?

Normally, only a very small amount is present in the plasma—about 3 mg/dl, most of it being confined to red cells. If it were present in the plasma, it would increase the viscosity (thus raising blood pressure), and the osmotic pressure of blood (thus affecting fluid exchanges). It would also be excreted in the urine, besides being taken up and rapidly destroyed by the reticuloendothelial system.

Q.15 What are the common causes of increased and decreased Hb readings?

Hb readings (apparent levels) may show an increase or decrease due to experimental error, or increase or decrease of red cell count.

A. Increased level of Hb may be due to:
  1. Experimental Error.
    i. Blood taken more than 20 cmm or blood sticking to the outside of the pipette tip.
    ii. Fading of colored glass standards (rods).
  2. High Red Cell Count.
    i. Physiological: males, newborns, high altitude, etc.
    ii. Pathological: polycythemia/hypoxia due to heart or lung diseases.
B. Decreased level of Hb may be due to:
  1. Experimental error.
    i. Blood sample diluted with tissue fluid.
    ii. Blood taken is less than 20 cmm.
    iii. Color of acid hematin not allowed to develop fully.
  2. Decreased red cell count.
    i. Physiological: females during pregnancy (hemodilution).
    ii. All cases of anemia.

Q.16 What is the structure of hemoglobin, where is it synthesized, and what are the materials required for its synthesis?

Hemoglobin (mw 64,450) is a chromoprotein present in the red cells, and gives red color to the whole blood. It constitutes 95% of dry weight and 32-34% wet weight of red cells. It is a globular molecule consisting of 4 subunits. Each subunit consists of heme conjugated to a polypeptide chain. Two subunits contain alpha (α) chains (141 amino acid residues), while the other two contain beta (β) chains (146 amino acid residues). The four polypeptide chains taken together make up the protein part called globin. (Globin constitutes 96% of the molecular mass of Hb). The heme is an iron containing porphyrin pigment, called iron proto-porphyrin IX. The porphyrin nucleus has 4 pyrrole rings synthesized from acetyl CoA and glycine.

The synthesis of Hb begins in the proery-throblast, though it appears first in the intermediate normoblast, and continues till the reticulocyte stage. The materials required for Hb synthesis include: grade 1 proteins, metals such as iron, copper, nickel, cobalt, and vitamins such as vitamin C, pyridoxin, riboflavin, nicotinic acid.

Q.17 Name some derivatives of hemoglobin.

  1. *Oxyhemoglobin.* There is a loose and reversible binding of oxygen with one of the coordination bonds of the iron atom. Since Hb contains 4 iron atoms, each molecule of Hb carries 4 molecules of oxygen.
  2. *Reduced hemoglobin.* It results from release of O_2 from oxyHb.
  3. *Carbaminohemoglobin.* In this, CO_2 is attached to the globin part of Hb. The affinity of Hb for CO_2 is about 20 times that for oxygen.
  4. *Carboxyhemoglobin.* Carbon monoxide is attached to Hb where O_2 is normally attached. The affinity of Hb for CO is 200-300 times that for O_2. It is normally present in small amounts, but in large amount in smokers in whom it impairs O_2 transport.
  5. *Methemoglobin.* When blood is exposed to some drugs, or oxidizing agents *in vitro* or *in vivo*, the ferrous iron of Hb is conver-ted into ferric iron, forming metHb, which is dark in color. When present in large amounts, it gives a dusky appearance to the skin. Small amounts of metHb are

formed normally but an enzyme system converts it back to Hb.

6. *Sulfhemoglobin.* It is formed by the action of some drugs and chemicals (e.g., sulphonamides), the reaction being irreversible.

7. *Cyanmethemoglobin (hemiglobincyanide).* It is formed by the action of cyanide on Hb. (Hemiglobin is metHb).

Q. 18 What are the different varieties of hemoglobin and what is their significance?

The amino acid sequences of the polypeptide chains are determined by the globin genes. Slight variations in their composition can alter the properties of Hb.

i. HbA ($\alpha_2 \beta_2$): About 95% of Hb in a normal adult is HbA.

ii. HbA$_2$ ($\alpha_2 \delta_2$): About 2-5% of Hb in an adult is HbA$_2$.

iii. HbF (α_2, γ_2): During fetal life HbF predominates, in which 2 gamma chains replace the 2 beta chains. The gamma chains also contain 146 amino acid residues but have 37 that differ from those in beta chains. Since Hb has less affinity to 2-3 BPG, it can accept greater amounts of O_2 from mother's blood at low PO_2.

Diffusion of CO_2 from fetal blood into mother's blood causes alkalinity of fetal blood and acidity of mother's blood. This causes increase in the affinity of fetal Hb for O_2, and release of O_2 from mother's Hb—this has been called *double Bohr effect.*

In young embryos, there are in addition 2 zeta (ζ_2) and 2 epsilon (ε_2) chains, forming Gower 1 Hb ($\zeta_2 \varepsilon_2$) and Gower 2 Hb, that contains 2 alpha and 2 epsilon chains ($\alpha_2 \varepsilon_2$).

iv. HbA$_{1c}$ is characterized by α_2 and β_2 globin chains. Hb$_{1c}$ is formed by the covalent binding of glucose to HbA. The levels of HbA1c increase in poorly controlled diabetes mellitus.

Abnormal Hemoglobins

Sometimes, abnormal polypeptide chains are synthesized due to mutant genes. These defects are widespread and over 1000 abnormal hemoglobins have been described in humans. They are usually identified by letters.

In **HbS** (sickle cell anemia), the alpha chains are normal but in each beta chain, one glutamic acid residue has been replaced by a valine residue. HbS polymerizes at low O_2 tensions and forms elongated crystals (often 15 μm long) inside the RBCs, which assume sickle shapes. They pass through small capillaries with difficulty, and the spiked ends of the crystals cause rupture of these cells resulting in anemia.

In **HbC,** there are 2 alpha and 2 beta chains. The glutamate of beta chains in 6th position is replaced by lysine residue. HbC disease occurs in black population. **HbD** has also 2 alpha and 2 beta chains. However, glutamine replaces glutamate in 12th position of beta chains. **Hb E, I, J, H, Barts,** etc are other abnormal hemoglobins. Many of these are harmless while some have abnormal O_2 equilibriums and cause anemia.

The abnormal hemoglobins are associated with two types of inherited anemias:

i. *Hemoglobinopathies.* These are due to abnormal chains.

ii. *Thalassemias.* The chains are normal, but are less in amount or even absent. The α and β thalassemias are defined by decreased or even absent α and β polypeptides. The defects in the genes are in their regulatory proteins.

Q. 19 How does adult Hb differ from fetal Hb?

The differences between the two hemoglobins are:

Adult hemoglobin	Fetal hemoglobin
1. Contains 4 polypeptide chains (2 alpha and 2 beta).	1. The 2 beta chains replaced by gamma chains.
2. Appears in red cells of the fetus in 5th month. At birth 20% of total Hb is HbA.	2. HbF at birth makes up 80% of total Hb. Disappears by 5th month after birth.
3. Life span long—120 days.	3. Life span short— about 2 weeks.
4. It has the usual affinity for oxygen.	4. It has greater affinity for oxygen as it binds 2, 3 BGP less avidly.
5. Percentage saturation at PO_2 of 20 mmHg = 30-35%	5. Percentage saturation at a PO_2 of 20 mmHg = 70%.

Q. 20 What is the fate of hemoglobin?

Old and effete red cells, and their fragments in the blood are ingested by the tissue macrophages, largely in the spleen and liver. Here iron and globin are split apart and stored in their respective pools for reuse. The protoporphyrins from the breakdown of heme (this is the only reaction in the body where carbon monoxide is formed) are converted into biliverdin and bilirubin (the bile pigments) which are excreted in bile and then into urine and feces.

Q. 21 What are the functions of hemoglobin?

1. **Carriage of oxygen**. It carries O_2 from the lungs to all the tissues. Each iron atom loosely binds one molecule of O_2 at the 6th covalent or coordination bond. Each gram of Hb, when fully saturated, carries 1.34 ml of O_2 (1.39 ml by pure Hb). The affinity of Hb for O_2 is affected by pH, H^+, temperature, and 2-3 BPG.

2. **Carriage of CO_2.** Hb carries about 23 % of the total CO_2 carried by the blood from the tissues to the lungs. The CO_2 reacts with the amino radicals of the goblin to form carbaminoHb—a reversible reaction that occurs with a loose bond.

3. **Homeostasis of pH (buffer action of Hb)** Buffer systems convert strong acids and bases (which ionize easily and contribute H^+ or OH^-) into weak acids and bases that do not ionize as much to contribute H^+ or OH^-. As H^+ or OH^- are formed in red cells, or enter them, they are readily accepted by Hb (Hb + H = HbH) that gives up its oxygen. Hb is an excellent buffer and is responsible for 75% of the buffering power of blood. In fact all proteins act as buffers because of the terminal carboxyl and amino groups.

4. **Stabilization of Tissue PO_2.** Hb is mainly responsible for stabilizing PO_2 in the tissues because sufficient amounts of O_2 are delivered between a PO_2 of 20 and 40 mmHg.

5. **Regulation of Blood Flow and Blood Pressure.** In addition to the key role of Hb in carriage of O_2 and CO_2, Hb also plays a role in the regulation of *local blood flow* and *blood pressure.*

The iron ions of Hb have a strong affinity for *nitric oxide (NO)*, a local vasodilator gas produced on demand by the vascular endothelium (NO was formerly called "endothelium derived relaxing factor (EDRF)". The action of NO is immediate but very brief.

In the tissues, the reduced Hb, in addition to picking up CO_2 also picks up and removes excess of NO. The lack or removal of NO tends to cause vasoconstriction due to contraction of vascular smooth muscle. The result is decrease in blood flow and rise of blood pressure. In the lungs the CO_2 is exhaled, and NO being a highly reactive free radical, combines with O_2 and water to form inactive nitrates and nitrites. The Hb now picks another form of NO (along with fresh O_2) called *super nitric oxide* (SNO) formed in the lungs. In the tissues, Hb gives up O_2, while SNO causes vasodilatation of resistance vessels. (The Hb also picks up excess NO here). Thus, by transporting NO and SNO throughout the body, Hb helps to regulate peripheral resistance and, thus, bloods flow and pressure.

Note

Blocking the synthesis of NO in experimental animals causes a prompt rise in blood pressure. This suggests that a tonic release of NO is essential for maintaining normal blood pressure. (Being a hormone and a neurotransmitter, NO has been shown to have a variety of other physiological functions.

Q. 22 What is anemia and how is it graded according to Hb concentration? What are its common causes in India?

Anemia is a condition in which the oxygen carrying capacity of blood is reduced. There are many kinds of anemia, and in all anemias there is a decreased concentration of Hb, usually below 11-12 g/dl as a result of decrease in red cell mass (RBC count below 4-4.5 million/mm^3).

Depending on Hb concentration, anemia may be:

Mild: Hb   = 10-12 g/dl
Moderate: Hb = 7 - 9 g/dl
Severe: Hb   = Below 6 g/dl

The common causes of anemia in India are
   i. *Chronic loss of blood.*
   ii. *Deficiency of nutrients.*

Q. 23 What are the common causes of anemia and how will you classify it ?

Normally, about 1% of RBCs are destroyed daily (cells present in about 50 ml of blood) and equal numbers (about 3 million/per second) enter the circulation. Anemia may be caused when more cells are lost, or when less cells are produced, or both. Anemia will develop if:

   i. red cell production is normal but loss is increased.
   ii. red cell production is decreased but loss remains normal.
   iii. red cell production is decreased and loss is also increased.

Classification of anemia. The anemia may be classified on the basis of morphology of red cells, or the etiology (causes) of anemia:

A. Depending on the size and saturation of red cells with Hb, anemia may be **microcytic, normocytic,** or **macrocytic,** and each type may be **hypochromic,** or **normochromic.** For example, iron deficiency anemia is usually microcytic hypochromic. B_{12} and folic acid deficiency anemia is macrocytic normochromic (there can be no hyperchromic anemia because the saturation of red cells with Hb cannot exceed the normal upper limit of 36%).

B. Depending on the etiology (causation) of Anemia. Depending on the cause, the anemia may be grouped into:

   a. Anemias due to excessive RBC loss or destruction.
   b. Anemias due to inadequate RBC production.
   c. Anemias due to excessive loss and decreased production of RBCs.

1. Blood Loss (hemorrhagic) Anemia. The loss of blood (i.e., RBCs) through bleeding may be mild or severe, internal or external, and acute or chronic (prolonged). The anemia is usually normocytic. The common causes include: large wounds, bleeding piles, peptic ulcer, hookworm infestation, malarial parasites, or heavy menstruation. Enough iron cannot be absorbed to make up for the loss.

2. Hemolytic anemias. The red cell plasma membranes (cell membranes) rupture prematurely and pour their Hb into the plasma (hemolysis).

It may be inherited or acquired:

   a. Inherited. Structural abnormalities (spherocytosis, sickle cells, etc.), enzyme deficiencies (glutathione reductase). Thalassemia is a group of hereditary anemias associated with deficient synthesis of Hb. The RBCs are microcytic and short-lived.

   b. Acquired. The hemolysis of red cells may result from parasites (malaria), bacterial toxins, snake venom, adverse drug reactions (aspirin), autoimmunity, etc.

3. Nutritional (deficiency) anemias. These are due to lack of essential nutrients such as iron, vitamin B_{12}, folic acid, etc.

   a. Iron deficiency anemia. This is the most common type of anemia. It may be caused by insufficient intake, inadequate absorption from GI tract, increased iron requirements, or excessive loss of iron. Women are more likely to get it because of menstrual blood losses and increased iron demands of growing fetus during pregnancy.

   b. Deficiency of vitamins B_{12} and folic acid (folate). Both of these vitamins are required for normal erythropoiesis. Deficiency of either causes anemia. There is a derangement of DNA synthesis (DNA is required by dividing cells). As a result, large immature, nucleated red cell precursors (megaloblasts) appear in the circulating blood; their life span is also short—

about 40 days (red cell production cannot keep pace with their destruction, hence anemia). The large mature red cells (macrocytes) are fully saturated with Hb.

Deficiency of B_{12} may be due to: (1) inadequate intake, as in pure vegetarians ('vegans') because vegetables and fruits contain very little or no B_{12}; (2) lack of intrinsic factor (IF), which is a glycoprotein produced by gastric parietal cells that helps in the absorption of B_{12}. The IF binds with B_{12} in food (in this bound state, B_{12} is protected from being digested by GIT enzymes) and both are absorbed together in distal ileum. B_{12} then gets freed from the IF and is released into portal blood. The basic abnormality is the destruction of parietal cells by autoimmune antibodies in the disease called **atrophic gastritis** (total gastrectomy can also lead to B_{12} deficiency). The result is that the patient develops a type of anemia called **pernicious anemia,** or **Addison's anemia.** Nervous lesions occur ultimately.

Deficiency of folic acid is a nutritional disease and is more common than B_{12} deficiency. Like B_{12} deficiency, folic acid deficiency is characterised by macrocytic anemia. Production of IF and HCl is normal. In patients with intestinal malabsorption (e.g., sprue) there is a serious difficulty in absorbing folic acid (and B_{12}).

4. Aplastic anemia. There is suppression or destruction of red bone marrow due to overexposure to ionizing radiations (gamma rays, X-rays); adverse drug reactions that inhibit enzymes needed for erythropoiesis (drugs such as chloramphenicol, sulphonamides, and cytotoxic drugs used in treatment of cancers may cause this anemia). Certain poisons and severe infection may also produce aplastic anemia. The anemia is usually nomocytic.

5. Anemias due to Chronic diseases. Tuberculosis, chronic infections, cancers, lung diseases, etc. frequently cause anemia. The mechanism of causation is complex. The tissue macrophages are believed to become activated so that red cells are removed from the blood faster than they can be produced by the bone marrow.

This type of anemia is diagnosed by determining various blood indices and absolute corpuscular values, as described in the next experiment. Estimation of levels of iron, vitamins, intrinsic factor, etc. are also done.

Q. 24 What are the signs and symptoms of anemia?

Symptoms (They are what the patient complains or experiences). The person complains of fatigue and cannot tolerate cold; both of these symptoms are due to lack of oxygen that is needed for production of ATP and heat. Other symptoms are breathlessness (dyspnea) on exertion, or even at rest, palpitation (unpleasant awareness of heart beat), loss of appetite, and bowel disturbances.

Signs are what can be seen by the doctor on examination of the patient. The signs of anemia include paleness of skin and mucous membranes (the paleness of these tissues is due to low red-colored Hb in their capillaries), especially the inside of cheeks, gums, underside of tongue. (These are the sites where one looks for anemia during the clinical examination of a person. The nail-beds, and the surface of the tongue—which may be red due to glossitis are not the ideal sites for this purpose). In chronic cases of anemia, there may be spoon-shaped nails and even retinal hemorrhages. Some cases may show cardiac enlargement and heart failure.

Q. 25 Name some other methods for the estimation of hemoglobin.
See page 40.

1-8

The Red Cell Count

STUDENT OBJECTIVES

After completing this experiment, you should be able to:
1. Describe the relevance of doing red cell count.
2. Identify the RBC pipette; fill it with blood and diluent.
3. Charge the counting chamber and count the red cells.
4. Describe the composition of diluting fluid and the function of each.
5. Give the normal RBC count in different age groups.
6. Describe the site and stages of erythropoiesis, and factors that regulate it.
7. Explain the causes of anemia and polycythemia.

Relevance

Principle	Calculation of dilution
Apparatus and materials	obtained.
Principle.	Calculation of volume of fluid examined.
Procedures.	Degree and sources of error.
Filling the pipette with blood and diluting it.	• Pipette error. • Field error.
Charging the chamber.	• Chamber error.
Counting the cells.	• Experimental error. Normal red cell count.
Rules for counting.	Precautions. Questions.

Relevance

Since there is likely to be a high degree of error in RBC counting by the manual method, this count by itself may not be of much clinical significance. Estimation of Hb, being less time-consuming and more accurate, can give the required information in a patient. Nevertheless, RBC count, if done carefully and as part of full blood count (FBC), is required for the calculation of absolute corpuscular values and indices in anemia. Of course, automatic cell counters are available.

PRINCIPLE

The blood is diluted 200 times in a red cell pipette and the cells are counted in the counting chamber. Knowing the dilution employed, their number in undiluted blood can easily be calculated.

APPARATUS AND MATERIALS

1. **RBC pipette.** Consult Expt 1-4 and **Figures 1-5** and 1-10 for its discription. It should be clean and dry and the bead should roll freely.
2. **Improved Neubauer chamber with coverslip.** These should be clean and dust free.
3. **Microscope with LP and HP objectives and 10 x eyepiece.**
4. **Disposable blood lancet/pricking needle.**
   • Sterile cotton/gauze swabs.
   • 70% alcohol/methylated spirit.
5. **Hayem's fluid (RBC diluting fluid).** The ideal fluid for diluting the blood should be isotonic and neither cause hemolysis nor crenation of red cells. It should have a fixative to preserve the shape of RBCs and also prevent their autolysis so that they could be counted even several hours after diluting the blood if necessary. It should prevent agglutination and not get spoiled on keeping. All these properties are found in Hayem's fluid.
   Composition of Hayem's fluid. The diluting fluid contains the following:

Sodium chloride (NaCl)	0.50 g
Sodium sulphate (Na_2SO_4)	2.50 g
Mercuric chloride ($Hg\ Cl_2$)	0.25 g
Distilled water	100 ml

Dissolve all these chemical in distilled water and filter several times through the same filter paper. Discard the solution if a precipitate forms.

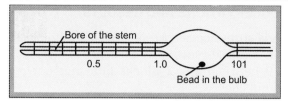

Figure 1-10. The RBC pipette. It has 3 markings—0.5, 1.0, and 101

- Sodium chloride and sodium sulphate provide isotonicity so that the red cells remain suspended in diluted blood without changing their shape and size. Sodium sulphate also acts as an anticoagulant, and as a fixative to preserve their shape and to prevent rouleaux formation (piling together of red cells).
- Mercuric chloride acts as an antifungal and antimicrobial agent and prevents contamination and growth of microorganisms.

PROCEDURES

- Consult Expt 1-3 for obtaining a sample of capillary blood, Expt 1-4 on filling a pipette with blood and diluting it, and Expt 1-5 on charging a counting chamber.
1. Place about 2 ml of Hayem's fluid in a watch glass.
2. Examine the chamber, with the coverslip 'centred' on it, under low magnification. Adjust the illumination and focus the central 1 mm square (RBC square on the counting grid) containing 25 groups of 16 smallest squares each. All these squares will be visible in one field. Do not change the focus or the field.
- Admitting too much light is a common cause of the inability to see the grid lines and squares clearly.
3. Move the chamber to your work-table for charging it with diluted blood. (It can be charged while on the stage, but it is more convenient to charge it on the table).
4. **Filling the pipette with blood and diluting it.** Get a finger-prick. Wipe the first 2 drops of blood and fill the pipette from a fresh drop of blood up to the mark 0.5. Suck Hayem's fluid to the mark 101 and mix the contents of the bulb for 3-4 minutes as described earlier.
5. **Charging the chamber.** Observing all the precautions, fill the chamber with diluted blood.
- Since the RBC pipette is a slow-speed pipette, it will need to be kept at an angle of 70-80° while charging the chamber.
6. Move the chamber to the microscope and focus the grid once again to see the central 1 mm square with the red cells distributed all over.
- Wait for 3-4 minutes for the cells to settle down because they cannot be counted when they are moving and changing their positions due to currents in the fluid. During this time draw a diagram once again showing the RBC square. Then draw 5 groups of 16 squares each, showing their relative positions—the 4 corner groups and one central group for entering your counts.
7. **Counting the cells.** Switch over to high magnification (HP lens) and check the distribution of cells. If they are unevenly distributed, i.e., bunched at some places and scanty at others, the chamber has to be washed, dried, and re-charged.
8. Move the chamber carefully and bring the left upper corner block of 16 smallest squares in the field of view. (There are no smallest squares above and to its left).

Rules for Counting

Note that the immediate boundary of each smallest square is formed by the 4 lines forming the square (side: 1/20 mm; area: $1/400$ mm^2) the other lines of the tram or triple lines do not form part of the boundary of that square.

i. Cells lying within a square are to be counted with that square.
ii. Cells lying on or touching its upper horizontal and left vertical lines are to be counted with that particular square.

iii. Cells lying on or touching its lower horizontal and right vertical lines are to be omitted from that square because they will be counted with the adjacent squares. In this way you will avoid counting a cell twice. (You may omit cells lying on the upper horizontal and left vertical lines and count those lying on its lower and right lines. But whichever method is chosen, it is best to follow it for all cell counts).

• While counting the cells, continuously "rack", the fine adjustment up and down so that cells sticking to the underside of the coverslip are not missed.

• An occasional WBC (may be 1 in 600-700 RBCs) may be seen—appearing greyish and granular but it is not to be counted with the red cells.

9. We have already focused the upper left block of 16 smallest squares in the high power field. First count the cells in the upper 4 horizontal squares from left to right, then come down to the next row and count the cells in each square from right to left. Then count the cells in the 3rd row from left to right, and in the 4th row, from right to left. As the counts are made, enter your results in the appropriate squares drawn in your workbook, showing the count in each square.

• Count once more in these 16 squares and note the result in your work-book. The difference between the two counts should not be more than 10.

10. Move the chamber carefully till you reach the right upper corner block of 16 smallest squares (there are no smallest squares above and to the right of this group), and count the cells as before. Then move on to the right lower corner and then left lower corner groups, and finally count the cells in the central block of 16 smallest squares.

Thus, the counting will have been done in 80 smallest squares, i.e., in 5 blocks of 16 squares each.

OBSERVATIONS AND RESULTS

Add up the number of cells in each of the 5 blocks of 16 smallest squares. A difference of more than 20 between any 2 blocks indicates uneven distribution.

A. Calculation of dilution obtained (dilution factor).
Consult Expt 1-4 once again. Recall that the dilution with this pipette can be 1 in 100 or 1 in 200 depending on whether blood is taken to mark 1.0 or 0.5.

Thus, the dilution factor is
$$= \frac{\text{Final volume attained (100 parts)}}{\text{Volume of blood taken (0.5 part)}}$$

B. Calculation of volume of fluid examined. We know the count in 80 smallest squares which have a volume (space) of $1/50$ mm^3. We can also know the cell count in 1 smallest square, which has a volume (space) of $1/4000$ mm^3. We can now calculate the number of red cells in two ways as shown below:

C. Calculation of red cell count
i. Let x be the number of cells in $1/50$ mm^3 of diluted blood.
Cells in 1 mm^3 of diluted blood = x × 50
Dilution employed was = 1 in 200
∴ Number of cells in 1 mm^3 of undiluted blood will be = x × 50 × 200 = x × 10000
Thus, adding, 4 zeros in front of x will give the RBC count per 1 mm^3 of undiluted blood.

Example:
Number of cells in 80 smallest squares = 480
These cells are present in $1/50$ mm^3 of diluted blood.
Dilution employed is = 1 in 200
∴ Number of cells in 1 mm^3 of undiluted blood will be = 480 × 50 × 200
= 480 × 10,000
= 4800000, i.e., 4.8 million/mm^3.
ii. The other way to calculate is
Number of cells in 80 smallest squares = x

Number of cells in 1 smallest square = $\dfrac{\times}{80}$

$\dfrac{\times}{80}$ cells are present in $1/4000$ mm^3 of diluted blood.

Dilution employed = 1 in 200

∴ Number of cells in 1 mm^3 of undiluted blood

$\dfrac{\times}{80} \times 4000 \times 200 = x \times 50 \times 200 = x \times 10,000$

Example:

Number of cells in 80 smallest squares = 480

∴ Number of cells in 1 smallest square = 480/80 = 6

Volume of 1 smallest square $= 1/4000$ mm^3

Dilution employed $= 1$ in 200

∴ Number of cells in 1 mm^3 of undiluted blood

$= 4000 \times 6 \times 200 = 4800000 = 4.8$ million/mm^3.

Degree and Sources of Error

As mentioned in Expt 1-4, despite all precautions in the procedures the degree of error with this method is said to be about 15%. Thus, with a count of 5.0 million/mm^3, the technical error of a single count comes to about ± 0.75 million/mm^3. And in the hands of a student, this error can be as high as 20%.

The following factors are responsible for the error:

i. **Pipette error.** It may be due to inaccuracy of graduations, the method of filling with blood and diluent, or mixing.

ii. **Chamber error.** The counting grid and the depth of the chamber may not be accurate, or the process of charging it may introduce an error.

iii. **Field error.** The distribution of cells on the grid may not be uniform.

iv. **Experimental error.** Since the multiplication factor is 10,000, an error in counting of 5 cells in 80 smallest squares may cause a variation of 50,000/mm^3 of blood.

Note
- To be of any value, the test must be carried out as meticulously as possible.
- Repeated counts of a charged chamber do not give significantly better results. Counting the cells in more than 80 smallest squares has similar effect.
- Taking repeated samples of blood, counting the cells in each, and taking their mean value can eliminate pipette error. But this has hardly any practical value.

Normal Red Cell Count

Express your result as ..... million/mm^3

The average cell counts and their ranges are:

Males = 5.0 million/mm^3 (4.75-6.0 million/mm^3)

Females = 4.5 million/mm^3 (4.0-5.5 million/mm^3).

PRECAUTIONS

1. Observe all precautions described for getting a finger-prick, filling the pipette with blood and diluent, and charging the chamber.
2. Clean the chamber with a lint-free piece of cloth. Once cleaned, do not touch the central part. Any oils left from your fingers on the coverslip or the chamber are fatal to cell counting.
3. If there is over-charging or under-charging, wash, clean, dry, and refill the chamber.
4. Continuously rack the fine adjustment while counting the cells.

QUESTIONS

Q. 1 When blood is taken to the mark 0.5 and the diluent to mark 101, why is the dilution 1 in 200 and not 1 in 202?

Dilution of the blood occurs in the bulb, the volume of which is 101 − 1.0 = 100. Hence half volume in hundred gives a dilution of 1 in 200.

Q. 2 Why is blood diluted 200 times for red cell count?

A high dilution is needed because the number of RBCs is very high.

Q. 3 What is the function of the bead in the bulb?

The bead (red in this case) helps in mixing the contents of the bulb thoroughly. It helps in identifying the pipette at a distance. And, thirdly, it tells whether the bulb is dry or not (If it is not, the bead will not roll freely).

Q. 4 Would not the bead decrease the dilution of blood due to its own volume?

The volume of the bead is taken into consideration during manufacture of the pipette.

Q. 5 How will you clean the pipette and the chamber after your experiment is over?

See page 28.

Q. 6 How will you clean a pipette/blocked with clotted blood?

See page 22.

Q. 7 What are the units of markings on the pipette?

These markings (0.5, l.0, 101) do not represent any units but relative volumes or parts in relation to each other.

Q. 8 When drawing blood into the pipette, why do you take it to slightly, above 0.5 mark? And, why should the excess blood not be blown out or removed with cotton, gauze, or blotting paper?

The blood is taken slightly to above the mark because it is now easier to bring it to the exact mark. In trying to blow out the excess blood, more than the extra blood may be removed. Similarly, cotton swabs or filter paper should not be used because they are likely to remove more than the required blood. (The level is brought to the exact mark by wiping the tip against one's palm or finger-tip).

Q. 9 If Hayem's solution is not available, can you use any other?

  i. *Dacie's solution.* This diluting fluid is an alternative to Hayem's solution. It is simple to prepare and keeps for a long time. It contains 3.13 g of trisodium citrate, 1.0 ml of 37% formalin (commercial formaldehyde), and distilled water to 100 ml.

  ii. *Normal saline.* 0.9% sodium chloride solution can be used if Hayem's or Dacie's fluids are not available. However, the red cells have to be counted within an hour or so of filling the pipette. Also the RBCs are likely to form rouleaux. Further, a stock solution of normal saline cannot be kept for this purpose.

Q. 10 Why should you discard the first two drops from the pipette before charging the chamber?

Even after thorough mixing the blood and the diluent, the stem contains only the diluent which is cell-free.

Q. 11 What are the features of a properly charged chamber? How will over- or under-charging of the chamber affect the red cell count?

See page 32 for features of properly charged chamber.

   When the chamber is over charged, diluted blood flows into the trenches where the red cells being heavier, sink down. This gives a false low count. Under charging, due to less blood in the chamber will also give a low count.

Q. 12 What is the function of the coverslip?

Since the coverslip is absolutely flat and smooth, it ensures a uniformly deep capillary space between it and the floor-piece. Surface tension holds the diluted blood in place without its spilling into trenches unless the volume is more than the space available to it.

Q. 13 Why should a chipped coverslip not be used?

A chipped or broken coverslip will not cover the floor-piece properly, thus resulting in uneven distribution of cells.

Q. 14 Why should both sides of the chamber be charged?

Charging on one side may lift the coverslip unevenly on that side. Charging the two sides keeps them uniformly deep on both sides, Duplicate samples can be run or RBC and WBC counts can be done simultaneously.

Q. 15 Why is it difficult to see the grid lines and cells clearly at the same focus?

Since the grid lines, the cells lying on the floor-piece, and those sticking to the underside of the coverslip are located at different levels in the 0.1 mm space, all of them may not be seen clearly at one focusing position. It is for this reason that 'racking' of fine adjustment is required.

Q. 16 How will you differentiate red cells from dust particles?

Dust particles may be present on the objective, eyepiece, or in the diluent. They are angular, of different sizes and colors. (If they are on the eyepiece, they will rotate with the eyepiece.) Red cells, on the other hand, are round discs, of uniform size, light pink in color which is lighter in the centre.

Q. 17 Can the red cells be counted with the low power objective?

Though the cells can be seen clearly under low power and can be counted by an experienced person, it is best for the student to count them under high power.

Q. 18 Why is it necessary to follow the rules of counting?

The rules must be followed to avoid the error of missing some cells, and counting others more than once.

Q. 19 What are the sources of error in this experiment?

See page 41.

Q. 20 What is the fate of leucocytes in this experiment?

An occasional leucocyte may be seen. It is larger than a red cell, appears refractile (shiny) and granular, it also contains a nucleus. Since there is 1 WBC to 600-700 RBCs, one may come across a single WBC in a count of red cells in 80 smallest squares. But if it is counted with the red cells, it will increase the count by 10,000/mm^3 since the multiplication factor is 10,000 for cells in 80 smallest squares.

Q. 21 Since the mature red cells do not contain 'nuclei, are they dead cells?

The RBCs, though without nuclei, are not dead in the usual sense. Since there are no mitochondria (and other organelles), energy is not available from oxidative phosphorylation (Krebs cycle). However, they contain a number of enzymes which control important functions. The cells contain all enzymes necessary for energy supply from anaerobic glucose metabolism via the Embden-Meyerhof pathway (hexose monophosphate shunt). (Glucose enters RBCs by an active process which is insulin-independent). Energy is needed to maintain the shape, flexibility, and ionic composition of red cells. MetHb reductase converts metHb into its functional divalent form of Hb. ATPase keeps a high K$^+$ and a low Na$^+$ inside. Carbonic anhydrase promotes formation of carbonic acid from CO$_2$ and H$_2$O. Glutathione reductase helps to stabilize red cell membrane and in detoxifying (reducing) toxic oxygen metabolites.

Q.22 What is the site of formation of red cells during fetal life and after birth? Are they being formed in your body at this time?

During early fetal life, the primitive nucleated red cells are formed in the blood islands of yolk sac. (This is the only time when they are formed within blood vessels. Later they are formed extravascularly from where they enter the circulating blood). From 2 to 5 months, they are formed mainly in the liver, but also in spleen, thymus, and lymph glands. During the last trimester, they are formed only in the bone marrow. At birth, all marrow is red, but the adult pattern is reached by the age of 15 years.

The red cells are being continuously formed in and released from (my) red bone marrow at a rate of about 3.5 million per second which is equal to the rate of their destruction (About 1% of red cells, i.e., those present in about 50 ml of blood, are destroyed every day).

The red bone marrow is a highly vascularized connective tissue present in the minute spaces between the trabeculae of spongy bone confined to flat bones (pelvis, sternum, ribs, skull, vertebrae) and the proximal epiphysis of humerus and femur. The rest of the bone marrow, i.e., in the medullary (marrow) cavities of long bones, is the inactive yellow bone marrow – mainly fat cells and some blood vessels.

Q. 23 What is the life span and fate of red cells?

The average life span of red cells, as determined by radioactive and agglutination methods is about 120 days (about 40 days in macrocytic anemia and spherocytosis). During their life time, they circuit the cardiovascular system some 300,000 times. (Their elastic framework, formed by the protein spectrin, permits them to regain their biconcave shape as they emerge through the capillaries). As they squeeze through 5-6 μm capillaries again, they are subjected to severe mechanical stress and wear and tear of their plasma membranes. Since there is no nucleus and other organelles, the red cells cannot synthesize new components to replace the damaged ones. The plasma membranes become more and more fragile with age; they are now more likely to burst, particularly as they squeeze through' the narrow trabecular spaces of the spleen.

About 10% of the worn-out RBCs fragment in the circulating blood. These fragments and old cells are removed from the blood and destroyed by the fixed phagocytic macrophages in the spleen, liver etc. (The spleen has been called the graveyard of RBCs). The breakdown products, globin and iron of heme, are recycled for reuse by the body.

Q. 24 What is erythropoiesis? What are the stages of differentiation and maturation of red cells?

The term hemopoiesis (-poiesis= making), or hematopoiesis, refers to the formation of blood cells, while erythropoiesis refers to the formation of red cells. All the cells of the blood develop from *pluripotent (pluri- = many)* **hematopoietic stem cells (PHSCs; or hemocytoblasts),** that are derived from mesenchyme and constitute about 0.01—0.1% of bone marrow cells. They have the capacity to develop into many different types of cells (e.g., blood cells, macrophages, reticular cells (they form the stroma of bone marrow) mast cells, bone and

cartilage cells, fat cells etc). These PHSCs, or the common (uncommitted) stem cells, replenish themselves, proliferate and give rise to two main types of committed stem cells — *the myeloid stem cells*, and *the lymphoid stem cells* as shown in Figure 1-11.

The myeloid and lymphoid stem cells, which give rise to all the specific cell lines of blood, form 'colonies' in soft gel cultures and are, therefore, called *"colony forming units"* *(CFUs; the so-called progenitor cells).* Thus, the CFUs are separate pools of progenitor cells for megakaryocytes CFU-M, granulocytes and monocytes CFU-GM, and erythrocytes CFU-E).

The erythrocytes (RBCs) that develop from CFU-E pass through various stages: CFU-E———→ Proerythroblast———→(pronormoblast)———→ Normoblasts———-→ Reticulocyte———→ Mature red cells.

As these cells develop and mature, they become smaller, the cytoplasm changes color from blue to pink (in stained smears) their nucleus becomes condensed and is finally extruded. The cells that have developed outside the blood vessels so far now enter the blood stream through enlarged and leaky capillaries (sinusoids) that surround marrow cells and fibers at the non-nucleated stage of reticulocytes, the network disappearing within a day or so.

Except lymphocytes, the blood cells do not divide after they leave the bone marrow. The lymphoid stem cells *("bone marrow lymphocyte precursors")* begin their development in red bone marrow but complete it in lymphoid tissue to become T and B lymphocytes (see Expt. 1-12).

Q. 25 How is erythropoiesis regulated?

The proliferation and differentiation of various cells in the bone marrow is very accurately controlled by various hormones or factors (hemopoietic growth factors) that include: colony stimulating factors (CSFs), cytokines, interleukins (ILS), erythropoietin (EPO), etc.

Cytokines (small glycoprotein molecules) are secreted by marrow cells, lymphocytes, endothelial cells, and fibroblasts etc. Conventionally,

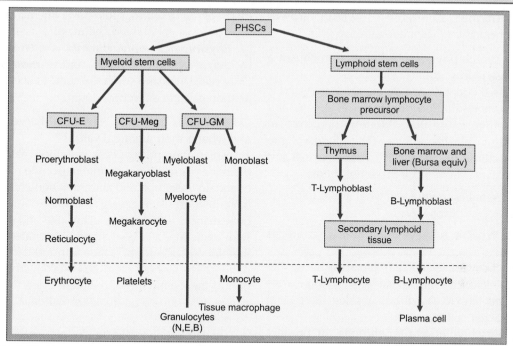

Figure 1-11. Hemopoiesis-Development of blood cells. Cells above dotted line: development and maturation in bone marrow. Cells below dotted line: cells present in blood. CFUs: Colony forming units are committed (progenitor) cells. PHSCs: Pluripotent hematopoietic stem cells

once the amino acid sequence is known, its earlier name is changed to **interleukin**. Interleukins 1, 3, and 6 and CSFs stimulate proliferation of different blast cells. Thus, cytokines function as local hormones (autocrine and paracrine). Cytokines also control phagocytosis and immune responses of lymphocytes.

Factors that Regulate Erythropoiesis.
1. *Erythropoietin (EPO).* The total red cell mass and therefore, the RBC count, is kept remarkably constant although there is a huge turnover of these cells in 24 hours.

This critical balance between RBC production and destruction is maintained by adjustments in the circulating levels of EPO.

EPO is a glycoprotein that contains 105 amino acid residues and 4 oligosaccharide chains. About 95% of EPO is secreted by the peritubular interstitial cells of the kidneys, and 15% from the perivenous hepatocytes of liver. Tissue oxygenation, i.e., the quantity of O_2 delivered to the tissues, is said to be the basic regulator of the basal secretion of EPO. Thus, hypoxia due to any cause—low blood volume, anemia, poor blood flow, and heart and lung diseases—increase EPO secretion. Transfusion of blood reduces EPO secretion. Recent evidence suggests that the O_2 sensor regulating EPO secretion is a heme protein that in deoxy form stimulates, and in oxy form inhibits formation of EPO mRNA. Cobalt salts and androgens also stimulate EPO secretion.

EPO has been produced by recombinant method and is available for clinical use in treating anemias of end-stage renal failure.

2. *Grade I proteins.* Proteins of animal origin, and soya beans, etc.

3. *Vitamins.* B_{12}, folic acid, pyridoxine, other B complex vitamins, and vitamin C are needed for red cell formation.

4. *Trace metals.* Iron, copper, zinc, and cobalt are required in trace amounts.

5. *Hormones*. Androgens, thyroxin, growth hormone and cortisol are required.

Q. 26 Which physiological condition causes a decrease in RBC count?

Decreased count is seen during pregnancy and is due to hemodilution. Increased estrogens and aldosterone cause fluid retention and thus an increase in plasma volume. (The blood volume may increase by about 25% above normal just before term. The red cell mass also increases.

Q. 27 What is anemia and what are its causes?
See Q/A 23 in Expt 1-7.

Q. 28 What is polycythemia and what are its causes?

Polycythemia. It refers to an increase in the number of red cells above the normal level. *Erythrocytosis* is a better term to describe an absolute increase in the total red cell mass.

1. Polycythemia vera (erythremia, or primary polycythemia). A gene abnormality in the early red cells causes them to form more and more cells. Erythropoietin production is not raised, but may be decreased.

2. Secondary polycythemia. Hypoxia due to lung diseases, congenital heart disease, cardiac failure increases the RBC count.

3. Polycythemia due to hemoconcentration. Fluid loss during severe vomiting and diarrhea; and loss of plasma in burns, cause polycythemia. There is no increase in total red cell mass.

Physiological polycythemia is seen during residence at high altitudes, and in newborns. Emotional stress and severe exercise may cause a temporary increase in RBC count.

Q.29 What is meant by "Stem cell harvesting" and what is their practical value?

Transplantation of stem cells (confined mainly to red bone marrow) from normal persons to patients of certain leukemias and abnormal bone marrow, have been in use for many years. The abnormal bone marrow is first destroyed by drugs and whole-body radiation, and bone marrow aspirated from the hipbone of a donor is then transfused into the patient. The normal stem cells (taken from the donor) then settle in the recipient bone marrow where they start to produce normal cells in due course of time.

The harvesting (collecting) of pluripotent stem cells (PHSCs) from the umbilical cord blood (where they are present in much larger numbers than in adult bone marrow) is now being employed. The PHSCs taken from the blastocysts of human embryos have been cultured and work on these cells may prove beneficial to currently incurable diseases like Parkinson's, Alzheimer's, diabetes mellitus, and repair of damaged heart muscle in coronary artery disease.

1-9

Determination of Hematocrit (HcT)
(Packed Cell Volume; PCV)

Relevance.

Principle.

Apparatus and materials.

Procedures

Observations and results.

Normal values.

True hematocrit.

Microhematocrit method.

Whole body hemato-crit.

Precautions.

Questions.

Relevance

Measurement of hematocrit (Hct) or packed cell volume (PCV) is the most accurate and simplest of all tests in clinical hematology for detecting the presence and degree of anemia or polycythemia. In comparison, hemoglobin estimation is less accurate, and RBC count far less accurate.

Also, if Hb, RBC count, and PCV are determined at the same time, various absolute corpuscular values (e.g., volume and Hb content of a single red cell) of a person can be determined. These values help in the laboratory diagnosis of the type of anemia in a person.

APPARATUS AND MATERIALS

1. **Equipment for venepuncture.**
   - Sterile swabs, alcohol, syringe and needle.
   - Container (penicillin vial or bulb) with anticoagulant (double oxalate or sequestrene).
2. **Wintrobe tube (hematocrit tube). Figure 1-13** shows a Wintrobe tube. It is 11 cm long, heavy, cylindrical glass tube, with a uniform bore diameter of 2 mm. Its lower end is closed and flat. The tube is calibrated in cm and mm from 0 to 10 cm from above downwards on one side of the scale (for ESR), and 10 to 0 cm on the other side (for PCV). The mouth of the tube can be covered with a rubber cap to prevent loss of fluid by evaporation. A Wintrobe stand is provided for holding the tube upright when doing ESR.
3. **Pasteur pipette.** It is a glass tubing drawn to a long thin nozzle about 14 cm long. A rubber teat is provided to suck blood into the pipette

by a slight pressure. It is used for filling the Wintrobe tube.

4. **Centrifuge machine.** It packs the red cells in the Hct tube by centrifugal force. The magnitude of force produced by rotation of the tube depends on:
   a. The radius, i.e., the distance between the center of the shaft and the bottom of the centrifuge tube when laid horizontally, and
   b. The number of revolutions per minute (rpm).

In terms of gravitational force (G), the value of this force should be 2260 units. This much force is created when the radius is 9 inches and the speed is 3000 rpm.

Note

Increasing the duration of centrifugation does not compensate for a low centrifugal force. For example, with decreased rpm and reduced force, the red cells do not get packed to their minimum volume (which is the purpose of centrifugation) even if centrifuged for hours. A proper machine that would create the required force is therefore, essential.

PROCEDURES

1. Draw 5 ml of venous blood and transfer it to a container (penicillin vial or bulb) of anticoagulant. Rotate the bulb between your palms, (i) to ensure proper mixing of cells and plasma (inaccurate results are likely if this precaution is not taken), and (ii) to oxygenate blood cells to remove CO_2 (red cells are larger when CO_2 is high, in venous blood).
2. Fill the Pasteur pipette with blood and take its nozzle to the bottom of the Wintrobe tube. Expel the blood gently by pressing the rubber teat, and fill the tube from below upwards while withdrawing the pipette but always keeping its tip below the level of blood. Ensure that there is no air bubble trapped in the blood.
   - Do not try to fill the tube from its top as blood will not flow down to its bottom because of air present in the tube.

3. Bring the blood column exactly to the mark 10 (or the mark 0 on the other side of the scale) at the top. There should not be any bubbles at the top of blood.
   - If less blood is available, note the level.

   For ESR. Before centrifuging the tube, ESR can be determined by placing the tube in its stand and taking the reading of clear plasma above the red cells, as described in Expt 1-16.

4. Close the mouth of the tube with its rubber cap and centrifuge it at 3000 rpm for 30 minutes (slower speed will not pack the red cells fully). Balance this tube with another tube filled with water, or another sample of blood placed in the opposite tube holder.

5. At the end of 30 minutes, take the reading of upper level of packed red cells on the side of the scale where zero is at the bottom. Replace the tube in the machine and centrifuge it again for 15 minutes. Read the packed cell height again; it should be the same as before. If the height is reduced, centrifuge it again for 5 minutes. To be reliable, at least 3 successive readings, at intervals of 5 minutes, should be the same.
   - Note that unnecessarily prolonged centri-fugation may cause mechanical hemolysis of red cells which must be avoided.

OBSERVATIONS AND RESULTS

Note that the blood has been separated into 3 layers:
   i. A tall upper layer of clear plasma—amber or straw-colored. It should not be pink or red which would indicate hemolysis of red cells in the sample or within the body (i.e., before withdrawal of venous blood) in hemolytic diseases. If there is hemolysis, the test must be repeated on a fresh sample.
   ii. A greyish-white, thin layer (about 1 mm thick) the so-called **"buffy layer"**, consisting of platelets above and leucocytes below it.
   iii. A tall bottom layer of red cells which have been closely packed together. A greyish red

line separates red cell layer from the layer of leucocytes above it. This line is due to the presence of reduced Hb in the red cells lying next to the leucocytes which reduce the oxyHb of the cells. The line marks the upper limit of the red cell layer.
   - The percentage of the volume of blood occupied by the red cells constitutes hematocrit or packed cell volume, i.e., the percentage of whole blood that is red cells

$$\text{Hematocrit (Hct)} = \frac{\text{Height of packed red cells (mm)}}{\text{Height of packed RBCs and plasma (i.e., height of blood column)}} \times 100$$

For example, if the height of packed red cells is 45 mm, then

$$= \frac{45}{100} \times 100 = 45 \text{ percent.}$$

   - It also means that out of 100 volumes (or parts) of blood 45 volumes (or parts) are red cells and 55 volumes (or parts) are plasma. Thus, out of 1 litre of blood, 450 ml are red cells and 550 ml are plasma.

Normal values. The average value of PCV is 42% when the RBC count is 5 million/mm^3 and their size and shape are normal.

Males: 44 percent (38-50 percent)
Females: 42 percent (36-45 percent)
The PCV for newborns is about 50 percent.

'True' hematocrit [true cell volume (TCV)]. Even under optimum conditions it is impossible to completely pack the red cells together, and about 2% plasma remains trapped in between the red cells. This percentage is more (i.e., more plasma) if the red cells are abnormal in shape (e.g. spherocytosis, sickle cells). To compensate for the trapped plasma, the 'true' cell volume (true hematocrit) can be obtained by multiplying the observed Hct value with 0.98.

The microhematocrit. Two heparinised glass capillary tubes, each about 6 cm long, are filled with blood and centrifuged at 12,000 rpm for 3 minutes. Readings of packed cells are taken from the scale on the tube holder. This method is very accurate and can be used on free-flowing capillary blood from a skin puncture in infants, or when the amount of blood available is very small, or in mass surveys for anemia.

Whole body hematocrit. Determination of total red cell mass by using chromium (^{51}Cr) has shown that the Hct of venous blood is higher than that of the blood in microcirculation vessels (metarterioles, arterioles, capillaries). In these small vessels, the red cells tend to move in the centre of the blood stream (axial flow). As a result, the blood along the sides of the vessels has a low Hct, and branches leaving at right angles may receive cell-poor blood. In capillaries, the effect is marked because the RBCs move in a single file in the middle of the stream. This phenomenon, called plasma skimming, may be responsible for the capillary blood hematocrit being about 20% lower than the whole body hematocrit.

Venous blood hematocrit. The Hct of venous blood is slightly higher than that of arterial blood, because as the pH changes from the arterial value of 7.41 to 7.37 in the venous blood, the red cells gain a little water.

PRECAUTIONS

1. Use the recommended amount of EDTA as the anticoagulant. There should be no clotting or hemolysis of the blood.
2. The test should be done within 6-8 hours of collection of the sample.
3. The Wintrobe tube should be filled from below upwards so that no air bubble is trapped in the tube.

QUESTIONS

Q. 1 What is the importance of determining hematocrit?

It is a simple but accurate test for determining the presence of anemia or polycythemia, as it is more accurate than the red cell count or Hb. It is also employed for determining various absolute, corpuscular values. Sometimes, it is used for screening for anemia.

Q. 2 Which cells make up the buffy layer? How thick is it and when can it increase in thickness?
The buffy layer consists of packed platelets and leucocytes. Platelets being less dense, settle in a separate layer above the leucocytes. The buffy layer is about 1 mm thick but the thickness increases in cases of severe leucocytosis, leukemia, and thrombocytosis, especially primary thrombocytosis where the count may exceed 800,000/mm^3.

Q. 3 What is the effect of a high hematocrit?
Increase in Hct increases the viscosity of blood which leads to an increase in peripheral resistance, and thus the blood pressure.

Q. 4 What is the difference between the PCV of arterial and venous bloods?
The PCV of venous blood is a little higher than that of arterial blood because the red cells gain a little water due to chloride shift.

Q. 5 Name the conditions where the PCV is increased and those where it is decreased?
Increased PCV is seen in:
 i. All cases of polycythemia (newborns, high altitude, hypoxia due to lung and heart diseases, etc.
 ii. Congestive heart failure, burns (loss of plasma), dehydration, after severe exercise, and emotional stress. In all these cases, there is a change in the plasma volume, or redistribution of red cells. (The spleen is not responsible for these changes in man because there is no smooth muscle in this organ).
Decreased PCV is seen in:
 i. All types of anemia
 ii. Pregnancy (due to hemodilution), and ingestion of large amounts of water.

Q. 6 What further information can be obtained from the buffy coat in a centrifuged tube of blood?
Studies on the buffy coat obtained after ultra-centrifugation of blood in special glass tubes (one for venous blood, another for capillary blood) have provided important information on certain parameters of complete blood count (CBC) or full blood count (FBC).

For example, the quantitative blood count (QBC) system which uses mechanical expansion and optical magnification of the buffy coat, augmented by supravital staining, yields the following information:

Hematocrit, platelet count, white blood cell count, granulocyte count (% and number), and lymphocyte-monocyte count (% and number). Counts of specific cell types of leucocytes are now possible.

1-10

Normal Blood Standards
(Absolute Corpuscular Values and Indices)

STUDENT OBJECTIVES
After completing this experiment, you should be able to:
1. Explain the clinical significance of calculating absolute corpuscular values.
2. Describe the normal corpuscular values and how to obtain them.
3. Describe the classification of anemia based on these standards.

Relevance

The basic values of Hb, RBC count, and PCV (Hct) do not give any information about the condition of an average red cell, such as its volume, Hb content, or its percentage saturation with Hb. Neither can this information, which is important in diagnosing the type of anemia in a patient, be obtained directly from any experimental method. However, this information, in the form of absolute corpuscular values, especially if these are done electronically. Can be calculated from 3 basic values of Hb, RBC count, and PCV.

Further, the basic values found in a patient/subject can be compared with arbitrarily set

"normal" values. This information, the red cell indices, have been discarded in favor of absolute corpuscular values.

Note
In addition to the indirect methods of calculating absolute corpuscular values from manually done Hb, HcT, and RBC, these values can be determined directly with automated electronic computers.

APPARATUS AND MATERIALS

The apparatus and materials required are those used for Hb, RBC count, and PCV.

PROCEDURES

1. Use your own values of Hb, RBC count and the value of PCV obtained during the demonstration experiment on a volunteer. This value of PCV, however, will not be strictly applicable to any person other than the volunteer.

- Your teacher may also provide each one of you with an arbitrary value of PCV from your Hb and RBC counts.
2. Calculate your absolute values for MCV, MCH, MCHC, and color index as shown below:

I. Mean Corpuscular Volume (MCV)

The MCV is the average or mean volume of a single red blood cell expressed in cubic micrometers (μm^3). It is calculated from the following two basic values:
  i. Red cell count in million/mm^3, and
  ii. Packed cell volume (PCV) in 100 ml blood.

Formula

$$\frac{PCV \times 10}{RBC \text{ count in million/mm}^3} \quad OR \quad \frac{PCV \text{ per liter}}{RBC \, (10^6/mm^3)}$$

For example
PCV = 45%   RBC count = 5.0 million/mm^3

$$MCV = \frac{45 \times 10}{5} = 90 \,\mu m^3$$

Normal range = 74-95 μm^3

Derivation of the formula. In order to know the volume of one red cell from this formula, we have to determine either of the following two:
  A. The packed volume of RBCs in 1 mm^3 of blood, since we know their number (i.e., 5 million), or
  B. The number of RBCs in 100 ml blood, since we know their packed volume (e.g., 45 ml) in the same volume of blood.
    The calculations according to both the methods are described below:
    [A] Since PCV is 45%, the volume of packed cells in 1 mm^3 of blood = 0.45 mm^3
    Number of red cells in the same volume of blood (i.e, 1 mm^3) = 5 million
    Thus, there are 5,000,000 red cells in 0.45 mm^3 of blood.

Therefore, the volume of 1 red cell $= \dfrac{0.45 \, mm^3}{5,000,000}$

Because 1 mm = 1000 micrometers, the MCV is:

$$MCV = \frac{0.45 \times 1000 \times 1000 \times 1000}{5,000,000} = \frac{0.45 \times 1000}{5} = 90 \mu m^3$$

[B] The PCV of RBCs in 100 ml blood = 45 ml
    Because 1 meter (100 cm) = 10^6 micrometers
              1 cm = 10^4 micrometers
For volume, 1 cubic cm $=10^4 \times 10^4 \times 10^4 = 10^{12}$ μm
[Since the density of water at 4°C is taken as 1, for practical purposes, the density at room temperature may also be taken as 1.]
    So, 1 cubic cm = 1 ml, and 1 ml = 10^{12} cubic micrometers (μm^3)
∴ 45 ml = 45 × 10^{12} cubic micrometers (μm^3)
    [We now have converted the volume of red cells (i.e., 45 ml) that are present in 100 ml blood into cubic microns (45 × 10^{12}), we now want to find out the number of RBCs in 100 ml blood, i.e., in 45 ml of packed red cells].
    Because 1 cm = 10 mm
    1 cubic cm = 10 × 10 × 10 = 10^3 mm^3
                                    (cmm)
∴ 1 ml   = 10^3 mm^3
And, 100 ml = $10^3 \times 10^2 = 10^5$ mm^3
Since 1 mm^3 blood contains = 5 × 10^6 red cells
100 ml will contain   = 5 × $10^6 \times 10^5$
                          = 5 × 10^{11} red cells
    Thus, the volume of 5 × 10^{11} RBCs in 100 ml blood = 45 × 10^{12} cubic micrometers (μm^3).

The volume of 1 red cell will be $= \dfrac{45 \times 10^{12}}{5 \times 10^{11}} = \dfrac{45 \times 10}{5} = 90 \, \mu m^3$

$$So, MCV = \frac{PCV \times 10}{RBC \text{ count in million/mm}^3}$$

II. Mean Corpuscular Hemoglobin (MCH)

The MCH, which is also determined indirectly, is the average hemoglobin content (weight of Hb) in a single red blood cell expressed in picograms (micro-microgram, μμg). It is calculated from the following basic values:

i. RBC count in million/mm^3, and
ii. Hb in g percent

Formula

$$\frac{Hb\ in\ g\% \times 10}{RBC\ count\ in\ million/mm^3}$$

For example   Hb   = 15 g%
                 RBC count   = 5 million/mm^3

$$MCH = \frac{15 \times 10}{5} = 30\ pg$$

Normal range = 27 – 32 pg

Derivation of the formula. The derivation of the formula is on the same lines as that for MCV. We want to convert the g Hb into picograms (pg).

Since 1 g = 10^{12} pg
       15 g = 15 × 10^{12} pg

Thus, the Hb content of 5 × 10^{11} RBCs in 100 ml blood = 15 × 10^{12} pg
The Hb content of 1 red cell will be

$$= \frac{15 \times 10^{12}}{5 \times 10^{11}} = \frac{15 \times 10}{5} = 30\ pg$$

(5 × 10^{11} red cells are present in 100 ml blood, as described earlier)

The formula can also be expressed as $= \dfrac{Hb\ in\ g\ per\ liter}{RBC\ count\ in\ million/mm^3}$

In macrocytic (large red cells) anemia, the MCH may be as high as 39 pg, because the cells are larger, but MCHC (see below) would be within normal range.

III. Mean Corpuscular Hemoglobin Concentration (MCHC)

The MCHC represents the relationship between the red cell volume and its degree or percentage saturation with hemoglobin, that is, how many

parts or volumes of a red cell are occupied by Hb. The MCHC does not take into consideration the RBC count, but represents *the actual Hb concentration in red cells only*, (i.e., not in whole blood)—expressed as saturation of these cells with Hb.

The Hb synthesizing machinery of red cells does not have the Hb concentrating capacity beyond a certain limit, i.e., RBCs cannot be, say 70% "filled" with Hb; this upper limit is only 36%. MCHC is calculated from the following formula:

$$MCHC = \frac{Hb\ in\ g\ per\ 100\ ml\ blood}{PCV\ per\ 100\ ml\ blood} \times 100$$

$$\left[\frac{Hb\ g\%}{PCV\%} \times 100 \right]$$

For example   Hb = 15 g%   PCV = 45%

$$MCHC = \frac{15}{45} \times 100 = 33.3\ percent$$

Normal range = 30 – 36%
If the MCHC is within the normal range, the cell is normochromic, if it is below the range, the cell is hypochromic. However, it cannot be hyperchromic for the reason mentioned above. A large cell may contain more Hb, but its percentage saturation will not be more than 36%.

Derivation of the formula. The derivation of the formula is as under:

45 volumes of red cells contain = 15 g of Hb

1 volume of red cells contain $= \dfrac{15}{45} g$

100 volumes of rec cells will contain $= \dfrac{15}{45} \times 100 \quad = 33.3\%$

Another way of expressing MCHC is as follows:

$$MCHC = \frac{MCH}{MCV} \times 100$$

(because MCH is Hb concentration in 1 red cell, and MCV is the volume of one red cell).

Taking MCH as 30 pg, and MCV as 90 cubic microns, MCHC

$$= \frac{30}{90} \times 100 = 33.3\%$$

IV. Mean Corpuscular Diameter (MCD)

The MCD is determined by direct micrometric measurements of the red cells in a stained film. The range is 6.9 to 8 micrometers, with an average of 7.5 μm. MCD can be used for measuring the mean corpuscular average thickness (MCAT).

V. Color Index (CI)

For the determination of CI, the results obtained in a particular case are compared with arbitrarily set "normal" values. The three traditional indices are: color index, volume index, and saturation index, which are the relative measures of Hb, cell size, and Hb concentration of red cells as compared to "normal" values. Only the color index is mentioned below.

To establish a relation between Hb concentration and the RBC count, they are expressed in the same unit, i.e., "percentage of normal", it being assumed that a normal person has 100% Hb, and 100% RBC count. Traditionally, the normal 100% RBC count is fixed at 5 million/mm^3, and the normal Hb at 15 g%, irrespective of age and sex.

For CI, we require the Hb concentration and the RBC count determined in an individual.

$$\text{Color index} = \frac{\text{Hb concentration (percentage of normal)}}{\text{RBC count (percentage of normal)}}$$

$$= \frac{100}{100} = 1.0$$

Normal range = 0.85 - 1.15

$$\text{Color index} = \frac{\dfrac{\text{g\% Hb found}}{\text{Normal Hb (15 g\%)}}}{\dfrac{\text{RBC count found}}{\text{Normal RBC count (5 mill./mm}^3)}}$$

The color index is low in iron deficiency anemia and high in macrocytic anemias. But since both RBC count and Hb may decrease simultaneously in a way the CI remains normal, the CI does not have much clinical value.

QUESTIONS

Q. 1 Consult and answer question numbers 4, 5, 6, and 7 in Section 6 on calculations.

Q. 2 Which absolute corpuscular value is most useful?

MCHC is the most reliable and useful value for the following two reasons:-
  i. It does not take RBC count into consideration for its calculation. MCH and MCV, on the other hand, both depend on the RBC count which has a high degree of error of ±15 percent.
  ii. MCHC tells us the actual Hb concentration in red cells only and not in whole blood.

Q. 3 Why cannot the MCHC exceed the saturation limit of 36?

The value of MCHC cannot exceed 36% because the Hb synthesizing and concentrating machinery does not have the capacity to saturate the cell beyond this limit. Thus, a cell can have more MCV and MCH but the saturation will not exceed 36%?

Q. 4 How will you classify anemias according to their causation?
See Expt. 1-7.

Q. 5 How will you classify anemias on the basis of MCV and MCHC?

The anemias can be classified on this basis as follows:

	Normochromic	*Hypochromic*
Normocytic	i. After acute hemorrhage. ii. Hemolytic anemias, except thalassemias. iii. Renal disease. iv. Aplastic anemia	After chronic blood loss.
Microcytic	Chronic infection.	i. Iron deficiency anemia. ii. Thalassemias (due to globin deficiency. iii. Hypoproteinemia.
Macrocytic	Deficiency of vitamins B_{12} and folic acid.	Secondary to liver disease.

1-11

The Total Leucocyte Count (TLC) White Cell Count (WCC)

Relevance.

Principle

Apparatus and materials

Procedures.

Filling the pipette.

Charging the chamber

Observations and results.

Dilution obtained.

Calculations.

Sources and degree of error.

Precautions.

Questions.

Relevance

The white blood corpuscles (WBCs; leucocytes) constitute the major defence system of the body against invasion by bacteria, viruses, fungi, toxins and other foreign invaders. Their number is kept remarkably constant in health, but it increases or decreases in many diseases, particularly acute and chronic infections. A clinician generally wants this test done, along with differential count, Hb etc. as part of "full blood count" (FBC or complete blood count, CBC) in cases of fever, especially if the cause of fever is not immediately apparent (pyrexia of unknown origin, PUO).

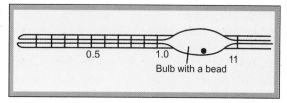

Figure 1-12. The WBC pipette. It has 3 markings—0.5, 1.0, and 11

PRINCIPLE

A sample of blood is diluted with a diluting fluid which destroys the red cells and stains the nuclei of the leucocytes. The cells are then counted in a counting chamber and their number in undiluted blood reported as leucocytes/mm^3.

APPARATUS AND MATERIALS

1. Microscope •Counting chamber with a heavy coverslip. •Blood lancet/pricking needle. •Sterile cotton/gauze swabs. •70% alcohol.
2. **WBC pipettes (Figures 1-5** and **1-12):** white bead in bulb, and markings 0.5, 1.0, and 11. Two such, clean and dry pipettes, with free-rolling beads are required.
3. **Turk's Fluid.** This fluid is used for diluting the blood.
   Glacial acetic acid = 1.5 ml (hemolyses RBCs without affecting WBCs).
   Gentian violet (1% solution) =1.5 ml (it stains the nuclei of leucocytes).
   Distilled water to 100 ml.

> **Note**
> It would be impossible to count WBCs unless the RBCs were first destroyed. This is achieved by acetic acid. (This concentration does not affect the cell membranes of WBCs.) The dye gentian violet stains only the nuclei of leucocytes without staining their cytoplasm.
> Go through Expt. 1-4 on filling the pipette, and Expt. 1-5 for charging the chamber.

PROCEDURES

1. Take 1 ml of Turk's fluid in a watch glass. Place the counting chamber on the microscope stage. Adjust the illumination, and focus the right upper group of 16 WBC squares. You will see all the squares in one field.
2. Observing all the aseptic precautions, get a finger-prick, discard the first 2 drops of blood, and let a good-sized drop to form.
3. **Filling the pipette.** Dip the tip of the pipette in the edge of the drop, draw blood to the mark 0.5 and suck Turk's fluid to the mark 11. Mix the contents of the bulb thoroughly for 3-4 minutes.
   • Your partner can draw blood up to the mark 1.0 in the second pipette, followed by Turk's fluid to mark 11. This will give a dilution of 1 in 10.
4. **Charging the chamber.** Discard the first 2 drops of fluid from the pipette and charge the chamber on both sides, 1 in 10 dilution on one side and 1 in 20 dilution on the other. The chamber should neither be over-charged nor under-charged.
5. Allow the cells to settle for 3-4 minutes, then carefully transfer the chamber to the microscope. Use the fine adjustment again and try to identify the WBCs.
   Under low magnification, the leucocytes appear as round, shiny (refractile), darkish dots, with a halo around them. These 'dots' represent the nuclei, which have been stained by gential violet. The cytoplasm is not stained.
   • Do not confuse with dust particles which have varying sizes and shapes, often angular. They are usually opaque, with no 'halo' around them. They may be brown, black or yellow in color.

Important

When examining cells or counting them, do not keep a fixed focus but continuously "rack" the microscope so that the cells and the lines come into and go out of focus. In this way you will not miss cells sticking to the undersurface of the cover-slip, or confuse dust particles for WBCs.

6. **Switch to High Magnification** and study the leucocytes. By racking the microscope, you should be able to make out the morphology, of these cells—their round shapes, the clear unstained cytoplasm, and the deep blue-violet nuclei which appear lobed in some cells and single in others. You will also see the remnants of the red cell membranes; these are called 'ghost' cells since they are faintly visible.

7. **Counting the cells.** The procedure for counting the WBCs is similar to that employed for red cells.
   • Count the cells under high power lens; once some practice is gained they can be counted under low power.
   • You may count the WBCs in 16 squares under low power and then under high power and compare the results.
   • Count the cells in the 4 groups of 16 squares each, i.e., in a total of 64 squares.
   • Draw appropriate squares in your work-book for entering the counts.

OBSERVATIONS AND RESULTS

Note that the deep brown color of the diluted blood is due to the formation of acid hematin by the action of acetic acid on the Hb released from the ruptured red cells. However, hemolysis and formation of acid hematin (the principle used for estimation of Hb by the Sahli method) does not interfere with the counting of leucocytes.

Calculations. The leucocytes were counted in 64 squares, the volume of one square being $1/160$ mm^3.

Volume of 64 squares = $1/160 \times 64 = 4/10$ mm^3.

Thus, the total volume of diluted blood in which WBCs were counted = $4/10$ mm^3.

Let the count in $4/10$ mm^3 be = x

Then 1 mm^3 of diluted blood will contain = x × 10/4 white cells.

Since the dilution employed is 20 times (10 times in the 2nd pipette) 1 mm^3 of undiluted blood

$$\text{will contain} = x \times 10/4 \times 20$$
$$= x \times 200/4$$
$$= x \times 50$$

(x × 10/4 × 10 in the 2nd pipette)

This means that multiplying the number of cells in 64 squares with 50 will give the total leucocyte count (multiply the number of cells in 64 squares with 25 in the 2nd pipette).

Compare the two counts. The difference between the two should not be more than 10 %. It will confirm the accuracy of your procedures in the two counting.

Sources and Degrees of Error

The sources of errors are the same as described for RBC counting and include: *pipette error, chamber error, field error, and experimental error.*

The degree of error, which may be 30% or more in RBC counting, is much less in TLC (about 5-10%) because of the low dilution employed (1 in 20) in this case. The error can be further reduced if counting is done on both platforms of the counting chamber. That the error in TLC counting is much less important than that in the RBC count is obvious from the following example: in a TLC of 8000/mm^3, even an error of 20% will give a count of 9600/mm^3, which is again well within the normal range.

PRECAUTIONS

1. Observe all precautions described for getting a finger-prick, filling the pipette, and charging the counting chamber.
2. Keep all equipment ready before getting a prick.
3. When mixing the blood with the Turk's fluid, give sufficient time for complete hemolysis

of red cells. However, ensure that the leucocytes are not centrifuged towards the ends of the pipette—which can be avoided by keeping the pipette horizontal while mixing the contents of the bulb.

4. Continuously "rack" the microscope while identifying and counting the cells for reasons described earlier.

5. Though the condition of a charged chamber may remain stable for 80-90 minutes, the count is usually stable for 30-40 minutes. After that the diluted blood starts receding due to drying and the count decreases. The counting of the cells should, therefore, not be delayed.

QUESTIONS

Q. 1 How will you differentiate a WBC pipette from a RBC pipette?
See page 27.

Q. 2 What do the three markings on the pipette indicate? How do you get a dilution of 1 in 20 and not 1 in 22?
See page 28.

Q. 3 What is the volume of the bulb in the WBC pipette? Why is its bulb smaller than that of the RBC pipette?
The volume of the fluid in the bulb is 10 times the volume of fluid in the stem, which can give a dilution of 1 in 10 or 1 in 20. In the RBC pipette, the volume of the bulb is 100 times the volume of the stem, which can give a dilution of 1 in 100 or 1 in 200. Since the count of leucocytes is in thousands/mm^3, the blood requires much less dilution as compared to red cell count which is in millions/mm^3.

Q. 4 What is the function of the bead in the bulb?
The bead serves 3 purposes:
  i. It aids mixing the blood with the diluent.
  ii. It helps in identifying the pipette by just looking at it.

iii. It tells whether the pipette is dry or not. In a dry pipette, the bead rolls freely without sticking to the inside of the bulb, which would happen if the bulb were wet.

Q. 5 What are the other uses of WBC pipette?
The WBC pipette can be used for diluting the blood much less for counting RBCs in cases of severe anemia, or for counting platelets. It can also be used for counting sperms, and bacteria.

Q. 6 What is the composition of Turk's fluid? What is the function of each constituent?
The diluting fluid for TLC contains glacial acetic acid, gentian violet and distilled water. The acid hemolyses the red cells, without affecting the WBCs at this concentration. The dye stains the nuclei of leucocytes.

Q. 7 What is meant by the term 'glacial'? Why should the acid in the 'Turk's fluid be glacial?
The term glacial means pure acetic acid. Only the glacial acid can give the typical 'shine' (halo) or clear refractility around the WBCs due to swelling of nuclei. This differentiates them from dust particles which are opaque and of different shapes. (It is called glacial because during its manufacture, it gives the appearance of a glacier at one stage).

Q. 8 Why are the red cells not seen when counting the leucocytes?
The red cells are not seen because they are hemolysed by the acid (they would, otherwise, not allow counting of leucocytes). The remnants of red cell membranes are faintly visible—the so-called ghost cells.

Q. 9 Can any other agent be used to hemolyse the red cells?
No. Any weak hemolytic agent would take an inordinately long time to lyse them. A strong agent, in addition to lysing the red cells, will also damage the leucocytes.

Q. 10 What is the normal total leucocyte count?
The normal count in adults ranges between 4000/mm^3 and 11,000/mm^3, with an average of 7000/mm^3. The count after birth may be as high

as 18,000 to 20,000/mm^3, the normal levels being reached in a few years. In the adults, about 55 to 75% of the WBCs are granulocytes, while in young children, lymphocytes dominate. The count may be high in some physiological conditions (see below) such as heavy exercise, stress, etc. This fact should be kept in mind while interpreting the results of cell counts.

Q. 11   What is the difference between differential leucocyte count and absolute leucocyte count?
In differential leucocyte count (DLC), the percentages of various types of WBCs are determined, while in absolute leucocyte count, the number of different WBCs per mm^3 are calculated. (This is done from TLC and DLC).

Q. 12   What are the various types of leucocytes and what are their functions?
The WBCs, unlike red cells, contain nuclei but no hemoglobin. Depending on the presence or absence of clearly visible and conspicuous, chemical filled granules (vesicles) in their cytoplasm (that are made visible by staining), they are grouped into 2 types: *granular* and *agranular.*
a. Granulocytes. There are 3 types of granulocytes that can be recognized under the compound microscope according to the coloration of their cytoplasmic granules: *neutrophils, eosinophils* (eosin loving) *and basophils* (basic loving).

Note
The neutrophils are often called polymorpho-nuclear leucocytes; PMNs; polymorphs, or simply "polys", because of many differently- shaped nuclear lobes connected by chromatin threads. The younger cells are often called 'bands' because their nuclei are more rod-shaped.

b. Agranulocytes (mononuclear cells). In contrast to granulocytes whose nuclei are lobed, the nuclei of agranulocytes are not lobed but appear as a single mass. Although the cytoplasm contains chemical filled granules, these are not visible under the light microscope due to their small size and poor staining with the usual dyes. The agranulo-cytes include: *monocytes,* and *lymphocytes.*

Chief Functions of Leucocytes
The skin and the mucous membranes of the body, which normally harbor harmful bacteria, and which are constantly exposed to disease-causing bacteria, viruses, fungi, parasites and their toxins, form a formidable barrier and the first line of defense against these foreign agents. Once these invaders succeed in breaking down this barrier, they enter the deeper tissues to cause damage, inflammation and disease.

The chief function of leucocytes is to provide immunity (protection) against these invaders and thus constitute an important mechanism of survival by preserving health and fending off disease. The immune system consists of task-specific cells that are in a constant state of vigilance and readiness—like the branches of armed forces. They recognize the invaders as "foreign" to the body and engage them in combat at the site of invasion.

The *tissue macrophages* (that develop from blood monocytes and act as the "sentinels"), and *neutrophils* (they act as the "infantry" and are transported by blood to the site of invasion), respond most quickly and destroy the invaders by phagocytosing them (both these cells move through the tissues by active ameboid movements and are attracted to the inflamed area). Thus, these two types of WBCs, along with antimicrobial proteins (interferons — alpha, beta, and gamma, and complement system and natural killer lympho-cytes, form the second line of defense.

The macrophages and various types of lymphocytes (see next Expt) are the major combatants in the immune responses against viruses, fungi, some bacteria, foreign cells and cancer cells (thus they act as the "artillery" of the body). The tissue macrophages finally come round to clean up the debris from the battlefield and carry away the results of carnage.

Q. 13   What is leucopoiesis? Where does it occur? Are leucocytes being formed in your body at this time?
Leucopoiesis, i.e., production of WBCs, occurs both in the bone marrow and in the lymphatic tissues. The two major lines of WBCs –the *myeloid*

and the *lymphoid* — arise from pluripotent (multipotent, or totipotent) hematopoietic stem cells (PHSCs) in the bone marrow (see Expt 1-8; Q. 24, and **Figure 1-11**) Once they become committed, the different types of WBCs pass through various stages of development before entering circulation.

The granulocytes, monocytes, and "*lymphocyte precursors*" are formed in the bone marrow (as are RBCs and platelets) while "*blood lymphocytes*" (those seen in blood films) are formed mainly in the "*peripheral (secondary) lymphoid tissue*" scattered throughout the body, such as lymph glands, tonsils, spleen, Pyer's patches of intestinal mucosa, and the "lymphoid nests in the bone marrow".

Lymphocytes. All lymphocytes come originally from "*bone marrow lymphocyte precursors*", most of which are released into circulation though some remain in the bone marrow. Those that enter blood are pre-processed (programmed, specialized) in either of the two *central (or primary) lymphoid tissues—thymus,* or *bursa equivalent,* as shown in **Figure 1-11.**

Those that take up residence in *thymus* are programmed by its environment into T- lymphocytes (T cells), while those that are processed *in bursa equivalent tissues (fetal liver and bone marrow*) become B lymphocytes (B cells). (In birds, the bursa of Fabricius, a lymphoid structure near cloaca, is the site of pre-programming of B-lymphocytes).

After pre-processing in the central (or primary) lymphoid tissue, both T and B cells take up residence in *peripheral (or secondary) lymphoid tissue*, as described above. From these locations, various types of lymphocytes continue to divide and re-divide and enter circulation throughout life via the lymphatic channels.

Thus, after birth, most lymphocytes are being formed in the peripheral lymphoid tissue, thymus and spleen, though some are formed in the bone marrow.

Granulocytes and *monocytes* are continuously formed in the red bone marrow to replace those

millions of cells that leave the blood and enter the tissues, or those that are destroyed. Similarly, lymphocytes are being formed continuously to replace those lost.

Note
With the exception of lymphocytes, the other cells of blood do not divide once they leave bone marrow.

Q.14 How is leucopoiesis regulated?
Over 70 billion WBCs pass from the blood into the tissues every day, and the same number enter the circulation from their sites of production. In spite of these huge numbers involved, the constancy of TLC suggests a very efficient feed-back mechanism that controls their production and release.

The substances which stimulate or inhibit this process appear to be many and varied. They include **colony stimulating factors. CSFs** (formed by monocytes and T lymphocytes); **interleukins** (formed by monocytes, macrophages, and endothelial cells); **prostaglandins** (formed by monocytes), **lactoferrin**, and possibly other agents. All these substances were collectively called **leucocyte promoting factor** (or **leucopoietin**). Thus, unlike RBCs, the products of dead and dying cells themselves control leucopoiesis. The CSF, a glycoprotein present in the body fluids appears to play an important role in the physiological regulation of leucopoiesis. During tissue injury and infection, the bacterial toxins, products of injury, etc. cause great increase in the rate of production and release of leucocytes.

Q.15 What are the kinetics, life-span and fate of leucocytes?
The 3 main varieties of WBCs—granulocytes, monocytes, and lymphocytes have different origin, kinetics (within the body), life-span, fate, and functional characteristics.

Granulocytes. These cells exist in 2 equal populations: the **"circulating pool"** and the **"marginal pool"** (those sticking to the endothelial cells of closed capillaries, venules, small veins, and sinusoids). However, there is a rapid exchange between the two pools (it has a physiological significance as described below). There are about 100 billion neutrophils in the blood and the entire population turns over each day (i.e., removed and renewed). For each mature cell in the blood, there are 50-100 such cells held in the bone marrow, which acts as a reservoir for a few days. The life-span of these cells after they enter circulation, is not fixed. They may remain there for 8-10 hours, or enter the tissues in thousands and millions by emigration (formerly called diapedesis; adhesion molecules, called **selectins** on endothelial cells and **integrins** on neutrophils, cause these cells to roll along the endothelium, slow down, and stick to it and then squeeze between endothelial cells), never to return again to the blood. In the tissues, they may live for a few more days before they die and are ingested by macrophages. A large number is also eliminated into the intestine (and out via feces), and into the respiratory passages. When there is infection, they are attracted to the site by bacterial toxins and products of inflammation (histamine, serotonin, bradykinin, prostaglandins, and reaction products of complement system and blood clotting). The neutrophils contain various enzymes which kill the bacteria (see below). Some enzymes escape from these cells, which liquefy dead tissues and form pus.

Eosinophils. Large numbers of these cells are present in the mucosa of lungs, GI tract and urinary tract where they provide **"mucosal immunity"**. They are weakly phagocytic.

Basophils. These cells along with tissue mast cells, play a role in allergic conditions.

Lymphocytes. The lymphocytes, along with lymph, are drained from the lymphoid tissue into the blood. After spending a few hours in blood, they pass back into the lymphoid tissue by emigration from the blood capillaries. They stay there for some days but re-enter the circulation via lymph once again. In this way they may circulate for months or even years.

Monocytes-Macrophages (Monocyte-macro-phage System, MMS). The blood monocytes, which are weakly phagocytic, enter tissues after 2-3 days. In the tissues, they increase in size from 15-20 μm to 90-100 μm, when they become actively phagocytic. They may remain motile and wander through tissues, or they may become fixed and become **tissue macrophages.** (It appears that they do not re-enter the blood.) The tissue macrophages (MMS), formerly called **"reticulo-endothelial system (RES)"**, are strategically located to guard all points of entry of microbes, etc. They constitute the body's 2nd line of defense, and include the following: histiocytes of skin and subcutaneous tissues, pulmonary alveolar macrophages (PAMs; or dust cells), the endothelial cells that line blood sinusoids in spleen, lymph glands; and bone marrow, cells lining the lymphatic paths in the lymphoid tissue including tonsils, the Kupffer cells of liver, osteoblasts of bone, and the microglia in the brain. Their life-span may be days, weeks, or 5-6 months.

Normally, the life-span of granulocytes and lymphocytes is quite different. Whereas the former may live for 8-10 hours or a few days, most lymphocytes re-circulate between blood and lymphoid tissues and may survive for months.

Q. 16 What is meant by the terms leucocytosis and granulocytosis? Name the physiological and pathological conditions which cause leucocytosis.
Leucocytosis. The term refers to an increase in the number of WBCs beyond 11000/mm^3 irrespective of the type of cells (granulocytes, monocytes, lymphocytes, etc.) that are involved in raising TLC. Thus, unless mentioned otherwise (e.g., lympho-cytosis, eosinophilia, etc.), the term refers to an increase in the number of neutrophils—the commonest cause of a raised TLC. The terms leucocytosis, granulocytosis, and neutrophilia, are more or less synonymous.

• Leucocytosis is a normal, protective response of the body to various types of stresses, such as infections, severe exercise, surgery, tissue injury, etc.
  The TLC may rise due to:

a. Redistribution within the blood: The WBCs from the "marginal" pool are mobilized and poured into the circulating blood.

b. Release from bone marrow reserve: This is another process by which the number of WBCs can be raised in a short time.

- These two processes raise the TLC without increasing their rate of production. There are no immature cells in the blood. (See "Cooke-Arneth" count in the next experiment).

c. Increased production and release from the bone marrow: The TLC rises as a result of suitable stimulation.

Physiological Leucocytosis

About 95% of the people have a TLC within the normal range. Physiological leucocytosis (i.e., in the absence of infection or tissue injury) has no clinical significance. There is no decrease or absence of eosinophils (eosinopenia), which is a feature of leucocytosis due to infection. Physiological leucocytosis is due to mobilization of WBCs from the marginal pool or bone marrow reserve ("Shift" leucocytosis). It is seen in the following conditions:

1. Normal infants: The count may be as high as 18-20,000/mm^3 but it returns to normal level within 1-2 years.

2. Food intake and digestion ("digestive leucocytosis"): There is a mild increase which returns to normal within an hour or so.

3. Physical exercise.

4. Mental stress.

5. Pregnancy: The count may be quite high, especially during the first pregnancy.

6. Parturition: The high TLC is possibly due to tissue injury, pain, physical stress, and hemorrhage.

7. Extremes of temperatures: Exposure to sun, or to very low temperature can increase the WBC count.

Pathological Leucocytosis

A rise in TLC in disease is seen in:

1. Acute infection with pyogenic (pus forming) bacteria: The infection (due to cocci bacteria—streptococcus, staphylococcus) may be:

a. localized, such as boils, abscess, tonsillitis, appendicitis, etc. or

b. generalized, such as in septicemia and pyemia, bronchitis, pneumonia, peritonitis, meningitis, etc.

2. Myocardial infarction: The rise in TLC due to tissue injury is not seen immediately after a heart attack but only after 4-5 days.

3. Acute hemorrhage: Maximum response occurs in 8-10 hours, the count returning to normal in 5-6 days.

4. Burns: Maximum response occurs in 5-15 hours, the count returning to normal in 2-3 days.

5. Amebic hepatitis.

6. Malignancies: High counts are seen in half the cases; secondary infection enhances the count.

7. Surgical operations: A postoperative rise is seen in all cases.

Q. 17 What is leucopenia? Name the physiological and pathological conditions causing it.

Leucopenia. The term refers to a decrease in the number of white cells (usually granulocytes; granulocytopenia) below the normal lower limit of 4000/mm^3.

Physiological Leucopenia

A decrease in TLC under normal physiological conditions is unusual and rare. Exposure to extreme cold, even under arctic conditions and in spite of acclimitization, may reduce the count to only slightly below the 4000/mm^3 level.

Pathological Leucopenia

Leucopenia due to disease, where TLC is abnormally low, is never beneficial to the body. In fact, it may endanger the life of the patient. The condition is almost always due to a decrease in neutrophils (neutropenia) and may be caused by various drugs used in treatment, radiation, or certain infections as described below?

1. Infection with non-pyogenic organisms: Typhoid and paratyphoid fevers, and sometimes in protozoal infection like, malaria.

2. Viral infections: Influenza, mumps, smallpox, AIDS (acquired immunodeficiency syndrome).

3. Drugs: Chloramphenicol, sulphonamides, aspirin, penicillins, cyclosporins, phenytoin, etc. Cytotoxic drugs used in treating malignancies may also cause leucopenis by depressing the bone marrow (other blood cells may also decrease).

4. Repeated exposures to X-rays and radium: These are used as radiotherapy in cancers, and cause bone marrow depression.

5. Chemical poisons that depress bone marrow: Arsenic, dinitrophenol, antimony and others.

6. Malnutrition: Deficiency of vitamin B_{12} and folate, general malnutrition, starvation, extreme weakness and debility.

7. Hypoplasia and aplasia: Partial or complete depression of bone marrow, i.e., failure of stem cells, may occur as a result of autoimmunity, and other factors.

8. Preleukemic stage of leukemias may show leucopenia.

> **Note**
> It is important to remember that leucopenia due to any cause makes a person more likely to get pyogenic and other infections. Prolonged leucopenia of more than 15 days increases the risk of many other infections. (Consult next experiment for neutropenia.)

Q. 18 What is leukemia and what are its major types?

Leukemias is a group of malignant (dangerous) neoplasms (new growths) of WBC forming organs—bone marrow and lymphoid tissue. There is an uncontrolled production and release of mature and immature WBCs into the circulation. The leukemias (commonly called blood cancers) may be myeloid (usually involving neutrophils) or lymphatic (involving lymphocytes), and acute or chronic.

In acute leukemia, there is accumulation of immature cells in the blood. (Acute lymphatic leukemia is the most common malignancy in children while acute myeloid leukemia is common in adults.) Chronic leukemia begins more slowly and may remain undetected for months. Mature cells accumulate in blood, because they do not die at the end of their normal life-span.

In most cases the cause is not known. However, genetic factors, viruses (e.g., human T cell leukemia, lymphoma virus-1; HTLV-1) chemical factors, and ionizing radiations (accidents in atomic power plants, atomic blasts, such as in Hiroshima and Nagasaki during World War II), are involved.

Q. 19 What is the difference between leucocytosis, leucostasis, leukemoid reaction and leukemia?

Leucocytosis is an increase in TLC count above $11,000/mm^3$, irrespective of the types of cells involved. It may be physiological or pathological. The pathological causes include infection and tissue injury. The count usually does not exceed $20\text{-}25,000/mm^3$ and there are no immature cells in the circulation.

Leucostasis. If the count is more than $100,000/mm^3$, white cell thrombi may form in the brain, lung, and heart—a condition called leucostasis. Transfusion of blood before TLC is reduced, increases blood viscosity, thus increasing the risk of leucostasis.

Leukemoid reaction. It is an extreme elevation of TLC above $50,000/mm^3$ as a result of the presence of mature and or immature neutrophils. The causes include: severe chronic infections, especially in children, severe hemolysis, malignant growths (cancer of breast, lung, kidney). It is not leukemia, and can be distinguished from chronic myelogenous leukemia (CML) by estimating the leucocyte alkaline phosphatase (LAP level which is elevated in leukemoid reaction, but depressed in CML.

Leukoerythroblastic reaction is similar to leukemoid reaction but with the addition of nucleated red cells (normoblasts) on blood smear. The causes include: marrow infiltration by malignancy, hypoxia, and severe anemia.

Leukemia. As descr-ibed above, leukemia is a cancerous growth of blood forming organs (bone marrow or lymphatic tissues). Due to uncontrolled production, both immature and mature WBCs are released into circulation. The TLC is generally above 40-50,000/mm^3 or even a few lacs. Even when the count is moderately high, it is not called leucocytosis. Most cells are, however, functionally incompetent.

The term aleukemic leukemia is sometimes used for the preleukemic stage when blood picture is normal but the bone marrow study points to leukemia.

Bone marrow study is always undertaken when there is a doubt about diagnosis.

Q. 20 Name a condition where the TLC may be markedly high or markedly low.

In leukemia, the count may be within the normal range, low or greatly increased.

Q. 21 What do you know about bone marrow transplantation? What are its indications?

Bone marrow transplantation is the intravenous transfusion of red bone marrow from a healthy donor (commonly taken from iliac crest) to a recipient. The purpose is to establish normal hemopoiesis and so, normal blood cell counts in the recipient. The procedure has been successfully used to treat certain types of leukemia, some cancers, severe combined immunodeficiency disease (SCID), some genetic disorders, hemolytic anemia and so on. The patient's defective red bone marrow must first be destroyed by whole body irradiation and high doses of chemotherapy. The donor's marrow must, of course, be closely matched with that of the recipient to avoid rejection. The stem cells from the donor's marrow settle down and start to grow in the recipient's bone marrow cavities, where they begin to produce healthy cells of various types.

1-12

Staining a Peripheral Blood Film
The Differential Leucocyte Count (DLC)

STUDENT OBJECTIVES

After completing this experiment, you should be able to:

1. Describe the relevance and special importance of preparing and staining a blood smear and doing the differential leucocyte count.

2. Name the components of Leishman's stain and explain the function of each.

3. Prepare satisfactory blood films, fix and stain them, and describe the features of a well-stained film.

4. Identify different blood cells in a film, and indicate the identifying features of each type of leucocyte.

5. Differentiate between neutrophils, eosinophils, and basophils and between a large lymphocyte and a monocyte.

6. Carry out the differential count and express your results in their percentages and absolute numbers.

7. Describe the functions of each type of leucocyte

8. List the conditions in which their numbers increase and decrease.

Relevance

Principle.

Special importance
of a blood smear

C. Assessment of stained
films.
Feature of a well-
stained film

D. Identification of
stained leucocytes
under OI.

E. Differentiation
between various

Apparatus and materials.

Steps in DLC Counting.

Procedures.

A. Preparing the blood film.

B. Fixing and staining the film.

Observations and results.

Leucocytes.

F. Differential counting of leucocytes.

G. Differential and absolute counts.

Precautions

Questions.

Relevance

Many hematological and other disorders can be diagnosed by a careful examination of a stained blood film. A physician may order a differential leucocyte count (always along with TLC) to detect infection or inflammation, determine the effects of possible poisoning by chemicals, drugs, chemotherapy, radiation, etc. DLC is also done to monitor blood diseases like leukemia, or to detect allergic and parasitic infections. The determination of each type of WBC helps in diagnosing the condition because a particular type may show an increase or decrease.

PRINCIPLE

A blood film is stained with Leishman's stain and scanned under oil immersion, from one end to the other. As each WBC is encountered, it is identified until 200 leucocytes have been examined. The percentage distribution of each type of WBC is then calculated. Knowing the TLC and the differential count, it is easy to determine the number of each type of cell per mm^3.

Special Importance of a Blood Smear

The special importance of a stained blood smear is that, unlike any other routine blood test, the smear can be retained and preserved as a permanent original record. The slide can be taken out and re-assessed whenever required after days, weeks, months or even years. The slide can also be conveniently sent to specialists for their opinion in doubtful cases.

The stained smears can also provide information about the morphology and count of red cells and platelets, and Hb status, besides detecting the presence of various parasites (e.g., malaria).

APPARATUS AND MATERIALS

1. Microscope. • 5-6 Clean glass slides. • Sterile lancet. • Cotton and gauze swabs. • 70% alcohol. • Glass dropper.
2. A drop bottle containing Leishman's stain.
3. A wash bottle of distilled water (or buffered water, is available). • Fluff-free blotting paper.

Leishman's stain. This stain is a simplification of Romanowsky group of stains. It is probably one of the simplest and most precise method of staining blood for diagnostic purposes. It contains a compound dye—eosinate of methylene-blue dissolved in acetone-free methyl alcohol.

i.   **Eosin.** It is an acidic dye (negatively charged) and stains basic (positive) particles—granules of eosinophils, and RBCs a pink color.

ii. **Methylene-blue.** It is a basic dye (positively charged) and stains acidic (negatively charged) granules in the cytoplasm, nuclei of leucocytes, especially the granules of basophils, a blue-violet color.

iii. **Acetone-free and water-free absolute methyl alcohol.** The methyl alcohol is a fixative and must be free from acetone and water. It serves two functions:

a. It fixes the blood smear to the glass slide. The alcohol precipitates the plasma proteins, which then act as a 'glue' which attaches (fixes) the blood cells to the slide so that they are not washed away during staining.

b. The alcohol preserves the morphology and chemical status of the cells.

   • The alcohol must be free from acetone because, acetone being a very strong lipid solvent, will, if present, cause crenation, shrinkage, or even destruction of cell membranes. This will make the identification of the cells difficult. (If acetone is present, the stain deteriorates quickly).

- The alcohol must be free from water since the latter may result in rouleaux formation and even hemolysis. The water may even wash away the blood film from the slide.

Steps in Differential Leucocyte Counting

1. Getting a blood sample from a finger-prick and making blood smears. If blood is obtained from a vein, place a drop of blood (through the needle) on each of the 4-5 slides and spread blood films.
2. Examining the blood smears under LP and HP and choosing the ideal films for staining.
3. Fixing and staining the blood films.
4. Identification and counting of various leucocytes.

PROCEDURES

A. Preparing the Blood Films

Prepare 4 or 5 blood films as described in Expt. 1-6. Air dry the slides immediately by waving them in the air. Examine them under low and then under high magnifications, and choose the best for staining.

Note
Aim for 'ideal' blood films as already described in Expt. 1-6 (shape, area covered, thickness, no striations or vacules etc.). Start the next step only if you are satisfied with the smears.

B. Fixing and Staining of Blood Films

While supravital staining is employed for living cells, the staining of blood films involves dead cells. **Fixation** is the process that makes the blood film and its cells adhere to the glass slide. It also preserves the shape and chemistry of blood cells as near living cells as possible. (See Q/A 8).

Staining is the process that stains (colors) the nuclei and cytoplasm of the cells. Both these purposes are achieved by the Leishman's stain.

Note
If it is not possible to stain a blood film within an hour or so, it should be fixed by immersing it in absolute methyl alcohol for 4-5 seconds and then air-dried.

- Since the timings for fixing and staining of the films with the Leishman's stain vary with different batches of the stain, check the timings with the laboratory assistant.

1. Fixing the Blood Films. Place the slides, smear side up, on a 'staining rack' assembled over a sink (two glass rods placed across the sink, with the ends fitted into short pieces of rubber tubing). Ensure that they are horizontal.

2. Pour 8-10 drops of the stain on each unfixed slide by dripping it from a drop bottle, or use a dropper. This amount of stain usually covers the entire surface and "stands up" from the edges of the slides without running off. Note the time.

3. Allow the stain to remain undisturbed for 1-2 minutes, as advised.

- During this time, watch the stain carefully, especially during hot weather, and see that it does not become syrupy (thick) due to evaporation of alcohol. If the stain dries, it will precipitate on the blood film and appear as round, blue granules. This can be prevented by pouring more stain on the slides as required.

4. Staining the blood film. After the fixing time is over, add an equal number of drops of distilled water (or buffered water, if available) to the stain. If the water is carefully dripped from a drop bottle or a dropper, the entire mixture will stand up from the edges of the slides (due to surface tension) without spilling over.

5. Mix the stain and water by gently blowing at different places on the slides through a dropper, without scratching the smear. A glossy greenish layer (scum) soon appears on the surface of the diluted stain. Allow the diluted stain to remain on the slide for 6-8 minutes, or as advised.

6. Flush off the diluted stain in a gentle stream of distilled water for about 30 seconds and leave the slides on the rack for about a minute with the last wash of water covering them. Drain the slides and put them in an inclined position against a support, stained sides facing downwards (to prevent dust particles settling on them) to drain and dry. The under sides of the slides may be blotted with filter paper.

- [You may also try the following method on an unfixed slide which gives very good results. Cover the smear with 10 drops of stain. After 30 seconds, add 20 drops of water, and leave for 15 minutes. Pick up the slide with forceps (to avoid purple fingers), and rinse in fast-flowing tap water for 1 second only. Dry as before].

OBSERVATIONS AND RESULTS

C. Assessment of Stained Blood Smears

Before starting the actual counting of WBCs, you should—

i. Take an assessment of all the blood films. Examine with naked eye first, and then under low and high magnifications. Choose the best stained films for cell counting.

ii. Make sure that you can identify all the leucocytes with certainty.

- Ensure that you are examining the blood smear side of the slide. Hold the slide in bright light and tilt it this way and that to see if there are any reflections. The clean side shows reflections, while the side which has the blood smear appears dull and does not show any reflections. (You may also scratch the margin of the smear with a pin).

Feature of a Well-stained Blood Smear

1. Naked eye appearance. The smear appears translucent and bluish-pink when seen against a white surface, its thickness being uniform throughout. (It is assumed that an ideal blood film has been stained).

2. Under low magnifications (100 x). The red cells appear as dots, uniformly spread-out in a single layer. The WBCs cannot be differentiated.

3. Under high magnification (450 x). The red cells are stained dull orange-pink and show a central pallor (due to biconcavity) which, if wide, may give the appearance of rings. The WBCs, with their nuclei deep blue-violet, lie unevenly here and there among the red cells. The platelets occur in small groups.

Staining Defects. The staining defects include: precipitation of stain particles, over staining, or under staining:

1. *Presence of stain granules.* Occasionally, round, solid-looking, deep blue-violet particles of stain get precipitated all over a blood film. They appear if the Leishman's stain is old, or if it has not been properly filtered, or if it was allowed to dry up on the slide during fixing. Finally, it may be due to insufficient washing of the greenish metallic scum that forms on the stain-water mixture during staining.

2. *Excessively blue appearance.* The RBCs appear deep blue or even bluish-black. The nuclei of WBCs are stained dark blue, with bluish cytoplasm in all cells; the PMNs cannot be differentiated. This appearance may be due to over-staining, over-fixing, insufficient washing or the use of alkaline stain or water. It can be corrected by reducing the fixing and staining times, and proper washing under running water.

3. *Excessively reddish appearance.* In this case the red cells appear pale pink. The WBCs show pale blue cytoplasm, while the nuclei typically appear lighter than the cytoplasm, or even colorless. This appearance may be due to under-staining, over- washing or the use of more acidic stain or water. The defect may be rectified by re-staining, if required.

4. *Faded appearance of blood cells.* This may result from the use of old stain, under-staining, or over-washing.

D. Identification of Leucocytes Under Oil-immersion

a. **Cells seen in a Blood Film.** The following cells can be identified:

1. **The red cells.** Stained orange-pink, the red cells appear as numerous, evenly spread out, non-nucleated, biconcave discs of uniform size of 7.2-7.8 µm. Normally, the central paleness occupies the middle third of the cells but is wider in anemias. There may be some overcrowding and overlapping, or even rouleaux formation in the head end of the blood film.

2. **The leucocytes.** Five main types of WBCs are commonly seen in blood films. They are all larger than the red cells, nucleated, and unevenly distributed here and there among the red cells. They include 3 types of granulocytes (polymorphonuclear leucocytes, PMNs; neutrophils being the most numerous), and 2 types of agranulocytes (monocytes and lymphocytes). A sixth type of leucocyte, the plasma cell, is occasionally seen in the blood films. The plasma cells are found in abundance in the lymphoid tissues. It is a specialized lymphocyte (B lymphocyte) that secretes antibodies. The chromatin of this cell gives a typical "cartwheel" appearance.

There are fewer and poorly-stained WBCs in the head end and the extreme tail; and some of these may be distorted. There appear to be more monocytes in the tail end, probably dragged there by the spreader because of their larger size. Plenty of leucocytes are found along the edges though they may be poorly stained.

Population-wise, neutrophils are the most numerous leucocytes, then come the lymphocytes, monocytes, eosinophils, and basophils, in that order.

3. **The Platelets.** They are membrane-bound round or oval bodies, with a diameter of 2-4 µm. They lie here and there in groups of 2-12, which is an *in vitro* effect, i.e., they do not form clumps in the circulating blood. They stain pink-purple, and being fragments of megakaryocytes, they do not possess nuclei.

b. **Identifying a Leucocyte.** A leucocyte is identified from its size, its nucleus, and the cytoplasm—its color, whether vesicles (granules) are visible or not, their color and size if visible, and the cytoplasm/nucleus ratio.

1. **Size.** The size of a WBC is assessed by comparing it with that of the surrounding red cells which have a uniform size of 7.2-7.8 µm. Try to assess whether 1½, 2, or 3 red cells will span across a leucocyte under study.

2. **The nucleus.** Note if the nucleus can be clearly seen through the cytoplasm and whether it is single or lobed. If single, note its

TABLE 1.2

Appearance of white blood corpuscles in a stained blood film				
Cell type	*Diameter (µm)*	*Nucleus*	*Cytoplasm*	*Cytoplasmic granules*
Granulocytes				
Neutrophils (40-70%)	10-14 (1.5-2X a RBC)	• Blue-violet. • 2-6 lobes, connected by chromatin threads. Seen clearly through cytoplasm.	• Slate-blue in color.	• Fine, closely-packed violet-pink. • Not seen separately. • Give ground-glass appearance. • Do not cover nucleus.
Eosinophils (1-6%)	10-15	• Blue-violet • 2-3 lobes, often bi-lobed, lobes connected by thick or thin chromatin band. • Seen clearly through cytoplasm.	• Eosinophilic. • Light pink-red. • Granular.	• Large, coarse. • Uniform-sized. • Brick-red to orange. • Seen separately. • Do not cover nucleus.
Basophils (0-1%)	10-15	• Blue-violet. • Irregular shape, may be S-shaped, rarely bilobed. • Not clearly seen, because overlaid with granules.	• Basophilic. • Bluish. • Granular.	• Large, very coarse. • Variable-sized. • Deep purple. • Seen separately. • Completely fill the cell, and cover the nucleus.
Agranulocytes				
Monocytes (5-10%)	12-20 (1.5-3 X a RBC)	• Pale blue-violet. • Large single. • May be indented horse-shoe, or kidney shaped (can appear oval or round, if seen from the side).	• Abundant. • 'Frosty'. • Slate-blue. • Amount may be larger than that of nucleus.	• No visible granules.
Small Lymphocyte (20-40%)	7-9	• Deep blue-violet. • Single, large, round, almost fills cell. • Condensed, lumpy chromatin, gives 'ink-spot' appearance.	• Hardly visible. • Thin crescent of clear, light blue cytoplasm.	• No visible granules.
Large lymphocyte (5-10½)	10-15	• Deep blue-violet. • Single, large, round or oval, almost fills cell. • May be central or eccentric.	• Large, crescent of clear, light blue cytoplasm. • Amount larger than in small lymphocyte.	• No visible granules.

location—central or eccentric, its shape—round, oval, or horse-shoe or kidney-shaped. Study its chromatin and whether condensed and lumpy or open and reticular. If lobed, count their number. Also note whether the lobes are connected by chromatin filaments or wider bands.

3. **The cytoplasm and cytoplasmic granules.** The cytoplasm may or may not show "visible" granules, or they may be very fine and not visible separately. Note the color of the cytoplasm and the granules, whether neutral color (light violet-pink taking up both acid and basic stains), or large and coarse—brick-red or red-orange (eosinophils) or deep blue-violet (basophils).

4. **Cytoplasm nucleus ratio.** Note the amount of cytoplasm in relation to the size of the cell and the nucleus.

Important

Whenever there is a doubt about a cell, try to draw its diagram exactly as you see it—its size (draw 2-3 RBCs alongside), nucleus (single or lobed, and how they are connected to each other), and the cytoplasm—its granules, their size and color, etc. In most cases, this will make the identification possible.

E. Differentiation Between Various Leucocytes

The students often find it difficult to differentiate between a neutrophil and an eosinophil, and a monocyte and a large lymphocyte.

Neutrophils, Eosinophils, and Basophils. All these cells are about the same size (10-14 μm) and have lobed nuclei. Neutrophils (polymorphonuclear leucocytes, PMNs, nuclei of many shapes) are the predominant WBCs. Their usual 3-5 lobed nucleus, and the fine, sand-like, sky-blue cytoplasmic granules identify them easily. The granules are not visible clearly and separately even with Leishman's stain, but give the cytoplasm a ground-glass

(translucent) appearance. Some difficulty may arise when its nucleus has 2 lobes (which may appear spectacle-shaped) and there appear to be visible granules in the cytoplasm. Such a cell is likely to be mistaken for an eosinophil or a basophil.

However, the presence of 15-20 round or ovoid, coarse, closely-packed, refractive (shining), even-sized, red-orange or brick-red acidophilic (= acid or eosin loving) granules; and the clearly-visible 2 lobes of the nucleus connected with a thick band of chromatin (spectacle-shaped nucleus) are typical of an eosinophil (the nucleus may sometimes be obscured by the granules).

The basophil (a rare cell of the blood) may be of the same size but is commonly smaller. The nucleus, which is bilobed or S-shaped, is usually obscured (covered, making it indistinct) by the deep blue-violet, basophilic (= basic loving) granules. These granules are round, variable-sized, coarse and closely packed.

Note

A degenerating neutrophil is occasionally confused for a basophil.

It is said that one should label a cell as basophil only when one is absolutely certain of its identification.

Small and large lymphocytes. Though small (7-9 μm) and large (10-15 μm) lymphocytes are commonly seen, a few intermediate cells also occur. The small lymphocyte, filled with a round or slightly indented and intensely blue-violet nucleus, and hardly containing any cytoplasm, is easy to differentiate from a large lymphocyte. It is about the size of a red cell, and its condensed chromatin gives it an ink-spot appearance. The bigger size of the large lymphocyte, with a round, oval, or indented nucleus, and larger amount of cytoplasm, which forms a small crescent on one side, help to identify it. However, the cytoplasm may form a thin rim around the nucleus in both cells. (The small lymphocyte is the more mature of the two cells).

- A plasma cell shows the typical "cartwheel" appearance of the chromatin of its nucleus.

Monocyte and large lymphocyte. The monocyte, which is the largest of the blood cells (12-20 µm) and 2-2½ times bigger than a red cell, can be identified by its pale-staining, oval, kidney or horseshoe-shaped nucleus, which is usually eccentric. The difficulty in differentiating it from a large lymphocyte may arise when the cell is seen from the side when it will appear oval or round. (The kidney shape of the nucleus cannot appear so from all directions). Then the much larger amount of pale-blue cytoplasm (about 1-2 times the size of the nucleus), as compared to a large lymphocyte (where it forms only a rim or crescent), and its frosty nature helps to identify it.

CAUTION
Occasionally, deep blue-violet, solid-looking granules of precipitated stain may appear on a blood film. These uniformly round artifacts, spread all over the film, should not be mistaken for cells, especially platelets.

F. Differential Counting of Leucocytes

1. Draw 200 squares in your workbook for recording various WBCs as they are encountered and identified one after another. Enter these cells by using the letters 'N' for neutrophils, 'M' for monocytes, 'LL' for large lymphocytes, 'SL' for small lymphocytes, 'E' for eosinophils, and 'B' for basophils.

- You can indicate these cells in a column (instead of the 200 squares), and as you identify a cell, put a short vertical stroke against that cell. In this way, you can place different types of cells in groups of 5, a horizontal stroke representing the 5th cell (e.g., Neutrophils = ⧍⧍ III, etc.)

2. Place a drop of cedar wood oil on the right upper corner of the film, a few mm away from the head end. Bring the oil immersion lens into position till it enters the oil drop. Adjust the focus.

- Do not flood the entire surface of the slide with oil; as you move the slide, the oil will move with the objective lens.

3. Move the slide slowly to the right (the image will move to the left) and as you encounter a leucocyte, identify it, and enter it in your workbook. As you approach the end of the smear, move 2 fields down and scan the film in the opposite direction. As you near the head, again move 2 fields down and scan the film towards the tail. Traverse the film in this to and fro fashion till you have examined 200 cells (count 400 cells for good results). This "battlement" procedure, as shown in **Figure 1-7**, ensures that you do not count a leucocyte more than once.

- The possibility of WBCs sticking to the edge of the spreader should be kept in mind.

4.   Recount. After you have, counted 200 (or 400) cells, count the leucocytes once more, starting from the lower left corner of the film, and going up in the "battlement" procedure.

Differential leucocyte count. When counting has been done, calculate the percentage of each type of cell in your count of 200 (or 400) white cells. The neutrophils are the prominent cells of the blood and constitute about 50-60% of the WBCs. The next predominant cells are lymphocytes (20-40%), which may be small or large. The third cell in the order of population is the monocyte which constitutes 8-10% of the WBCs.

Absolute leucocyte count. Use your value of TLC (though it should be done at the same time as DLC) obtained in the last experiment to express these percentages in terms of absolute values of each type of leucocyte per mm^3 of blood.

The absolute values are more significant than the DLC values alone. The reason is that the DLC may show only a relative increase or decrease of a particular type of cell with a corresponding change in the other cell types. For example, a neutrophil count of 85% may suggest neutrophilia, but if the TLC is, say, 8000/mm^3, then the absolute neutrophil count of 6800/mm^3 (8000 × 85/100 = 6800) would be within the normal range.

Normal values. The normal values for differential and absolute counts are given below:

Differential count	(per cent)	Absolute count (per mm³)
Neutrophils	40-75	2000-7500
Eosinophils	1-6	4-440
Basophils	0-1	0-100
Monocytes	2-10	500-800
Lymphocytes (both)	20-45	1300-3500

Spell out your results clearly, showing the percentage and absolute value of each type of leucocyte. Indicate whether your results lie within the normal range.

Note

When counting the cells in a blood film, you can make a rough estimate of the TLC depending on whether the cells appear more frequently, or are sparsely populated amongst the red cells.

Diagrams

While drawing the diagrams of the leucocytes in your workbook, keep in mind the size of the cells in relation to that of red cells. Use appropriate colors to represent the nuclei and the cytoplasm.

PRECAUTIONS

1. Observe all precautions described in Expt. 1-6 for making blood films.
2. Absolutely clean, grease- and dust-free slides must be used.
3. When taking blood on to the slide before spreading it, do not touch the skin with the slide but only the periphery (top) of the blood drop. This is to avoid taking up epidermal squamous cells or sweat. (Do not place the slide on the table and then touch the blood drop on to it. You will not be able to see how much blood has been taken).

4. Do not allow Leishman stain to become syrupy (thick) or dry up on the slide as this is likely to cause precipitation of the stain.
5. Avoid tap water for diluting the stain, and for washing off the diluted stain after 'staining', because methylene-blue components may not stain the cells properly.
6. The Leishman stain should be kept in well-stoppered bottles. After use, the stopper should always be turned so as to keep out air from the solution. (The stain can be kept for months provided it is kept in airtight bottles).
7. Avoid bringing the stained film in contact with alcohol. If you do this, the stain will be extracted in a few seconds.
8. When counting the cells, use the "battlement" method. This is to avoid counting a cell twice.
9. Avoid counting the leucocytes in the extreme ends of the head or tail, and along the edges of the blood film.

QUESTIONS

Q. 1 Name the methods employed for studying the blood cells. Which method is most commonly used?

Since the blood cells are suspended in fluid plasma, they can be studied in the form of a **"drop preparation"** (Expt 1-6), or a **"thin blood film"** spread on a glass slide (Expt 1-6). Also, a **"thick blood film"** can be made by taking a drop of blood on a glass slide and spreading it in a thick film with the corner of another slide. A thick film can also be made by placing a drop of blood between two coverslips and then pulling them in the opposite directions. It is employed in studying malarial parasite, etc. In **"centrifugal method"**, a drop of blood taken on a glass slide used to be centrifuged so that it spread across the slide in a thin layer.

The **"glass slide method"**, also called the **"wedge method"** (because the blood film resembles a wedge, wide at one end and tapering a the other), used in this experiment is the one that is most commonly used. A properly spread film is about 10-20 μm thick.

Q.2 How are the glass slides cleaned?
See Expt 1-6.

Q. 3 What precautions will you take while preparing blood films? Why are 4 or 5 (or more) slides prepared at a time?
A number of slides are prepared for 2 reasons: one, to get practice in the procedure, and two, the best-stained slide can be chosen for counting the cells.

Q. 4 Why should the blood film be dried quickly soon after spreading it?
See page 35.

Q. 5 What are the features of an ideal blood film?
See page 35.

Q. 6 What is the composition of Leishman's stain and what is the function of each component? Why should the stain be acetone free?
See page 74.

Q. 7 What is buffered water? Why should it be preferred over distilled water?
Buffered water is phosphate buffer in which the pH is adjusted at 6.8. At this pH, there is optimal ionization of the stain particles so that they can penetrate the cells better. The buffer is prepared by dissolving 3.7 g of disodium hydrogen phosphate and 2.1 g of potassium dihydrogen phosphate in distilled water made to 1000 ml. The pH is tested with a pH meter. If it is lower, the former is added; if it is higher than 6.8, the latter is added till the desired pH is reached.

Q. 8 Why is Leishman's stain diluted after 1-2 minutes? What happens to the blood film during this period?
During the fixation period of 1-2 minutes, the pure absolute alcohol serves two purposes: one, it precipitates the plasma proteins, which act as glue and attach (fix) the blood cells on to the glass slide, and two, it preserves the shape and chemistry of cells to as near the living state as possible.

The cells are not stained during this time, because the stain particles cannot enter the cells in their unionized state. Their ionization occurs

only when water is added to the salts in the undiluted stain. (If diluted stain were added to start with, the blood smear itself would be washed away. Diluted Leishman's stain can be used if the blood film is first fixed in absolute alcohol).

Note
The appearance of the glossy greenish scum (layer) floating on the surface of the diluted stain shows that the staining has been done properly. If the scum does not float, it means it has been deposited on the surface of the blood smear. The cells will now look hazy under the microscope.

Q. 9 Can tap water be used for diluting the stain after fixation?
Tap water should not be used because the methylene-blue components (methylene-blue plus methylene-azure formed from the former) may not stain the cells due to the unknown pH and salt content of this water. Also, tap water may contain impurities that may show up as artefact on the blood film.

Q.10 Can any other stain be used for blood films?
Yes. Giemsa's stain, like Leishman stain, is a mixture of methylene-blue methylene-azure, and eosin. Since it is an aqueous stain (i.e, containing water), the film is first fixed in absolute methyl or ethyl alcohol for 3-5 minutes. It is then stained in a staining-jar containing the diluted stain. The staining is very similar to Leishman's.

Wright's blood stain is still another stain commonly used in some laboratories

Q.11 What other information can be obtained from a blood film?
The other applications of blood film are:
1. Diagnosis of malaria, from malarial parasite seen in the red cells.
2. Diagnosis of leukemia from the type of blast cells.
3. Various parasitic infections, like filariasis, trypanosomiasis, etc.
4. Sex determination can be done from the presence of female sex chromatin which

appears as a "drum stick" (bar body) attached to a lobe of neutrophil nucleus.

5. Study of morphology of red cells in various types of anemias.

Q. 12 Why is cedar wood oil used with oil-immersion objective?

See Expt 1-1.

Q. 13 Which part of the blood film should be avoided for counting the cells? Which is the best part?

The 'head' (start) of the film and the extreme tail should be avoided because these areas contain fewer cells which are commonly distorted. They should also be avoided in the extreme edges. The area, in between these regions is the most suitable for counting leucocytes.

Q. 14 Which is the largest cell in the blood film? Which is the smallest ? How do you assess the size of a cell?

The monocyte is the largest cell in a blood film. Its diameter is usually 15-18 μm, though a few may be somewhat smaller and others a little larger than these. The diameter of small lymphocytes varies between 7-9 μm. So, a few may be slightly smaller than the red cells.

Normally, the size of the red cells is unchanging— being 7.2-7.8 μm. Therefore, the size of a WBC can be estimated by assessing how many RBCs will span across a given leucocyte.

Q. 15 What is a micrometer?

Micrometer is a measure of length in the SI system. The prefix 'micro' means a millionth (10^{-6}). Thus, a micrometer is one millionth of a meter. A millimeter is one thousandth of a meter (milli = one thousandth, 10^{-3}). A micrometer (μm) would be one thousandth of a millimeter. (It is difficult to imagine how much a μm would be, because rasing 10 to the power -6 does not tell us much. If it is remembered that a human hair is about 1/10 of a mm (100 μm) thick then one can imagine the diameter of a red cell, which will be about 1/13 of a hair thickness; i.e., about 13 red cells will span across the thickness of one hair).

Q. 16 Have you seen all the different leucocytes? Which WBC did you find difficult to identify?

(The student should be able to answer this question in the affirmative. Then one should describe one's experiences in identifying these cells).

Q. 17 How are leucocytes classified?

Consult Q/A 12 Expt 1-11.

Q. 18 Can the Leishman's stain be used for any other purpose than for staining a blood film?

Yes, the Leishman's stain is excellent for all body fluids containing cells.

Q. 19 What are the functions of various leucocytes?

Neutrophils

The neutrophils (along with tissue macrophages) are the first to arrive at the site of invasion by microbes. The toxins from the bacteria and kinins from damaged tissues, and some of the CSFs **attract** more and more of these cells by chemo-attraction (chemotaxis). The bacteria, which are made more 'tasty' by a coating of opsonins (IgG, and a CSF), are then phagocytosed by the neutrophils. Once the bacteria are ingested by a process of endocytosis, they get enclosed in membranous phagosomes within the neutrophils.

The neutrophil cytoplasmic granules contain various enzymes and chemicals that can kill bacteria and fungi within fractions of a second. These include 3 main groups of chemicals:

a. Lysozymes, proteases, and myeloperoxidases.
b. Proteins called **'defensins'** (α and β), form peptide "spears" that punch holes in bacterial membranes so that the resulting loss of cell contents kills the bacteria.
c. A group of strong oxidants, which kill the bacteria within fractions of a second, includes: superoxide (O^-_2, oxygen carrying an extra electron), hypochlorite (OCl^-), hydroxyl, halide, and hydrogen peroxide.

The neutrophil granules fuse with the phagosome and discharge the above-mentioned chemicals. In this way, each neutrophil can kill

8-10 bacteria before it itself is killed in the defence of the body.

The neutrophils also release leukotrienes, prostaglandins, thromboxanes, etc. that bring about the reactions of inflammation, like vasodilation and hyperemia, edema, redness, and pain. (All these are part of the body's defences).

Note
The myeloperoxidases catalyze conversion of Cl^-, Br^-, and I^- to the corresponding acids, which are potent oxidants.

Eosinophils
Large numbers of eosinophils are present in the mucosa of lungs, and gastrointestinal and urinary tracts, where they provide "mucosal immunity." They play the following roles:

1. **Antiallergic role.** These cells are believed to release enzymes such as histaminase, leucotriene C_4, aryl sulphatase, which neutralize the effects of histamine and other agents involved in allergic inflammation.

2. **Phagocytic function.** These cells are weakly phagocytic and so not of much use against the usual bacteria. However, they can ingest (phagocytose) and destroy antigen-antibody complexes; this prevents further spread of local allergic inflammation.

3. **Antiparasitic action.** The eosinophils are effective against certain parasites that are too big to be engulfed, e.g., larvae of trichinosis, (pork worm), schistosomiasis, etc. These cells attach themselves to these parasites and their granules release hydrolytic enzymes, reactive form of oxygen (superoxide), and the larvicidal agent called 'major basic protein' (MBP) which destroy the parasites.

Basophils
The basophils resemble mast cells which are found in large numbers around small and medium blood vessels and in the connective tissue under the epithelial surfaces. According to another view, some basophils leave the capillaries, enter the tissues, and become (develop into) mast cells. Like mast cells, the basophils liberate histamine, heparin and serotonin. Heparin prevents blood clotting and also removes fat particles from blood after a fatty meal.

Basophils collect where allergic reactions are taking place e.g., lung in asthma, and connective tissue in skin allergy. Here they release histamine, serotonin (5 HT), bradykinin, eosinophil chemotactic factor, slow-reacting substance (SRS), and other chemicals. These agents promote and intensify the inflammatory reactions and are involved in immediate hypersensitivity reactions.

Thus, though eosinophils and basophils appear to have opposite effects in allergy, they act in a balanced manner to control the harmful effects of the offending antigens.

Monocytes, (the monocyte-macrophage system, MMS; formerly called reticuloendothelial system, RES).
The monocytes, after spending a day or two in the circulation (here they are immature), enter the tissue where they increase in size and become actively-phagocytic tissue macrophages. They guard all the possible points of entry of foreign invaders. (Consult Q/A 15, Expt. 1-11) for details. They become activated by T lymphocytes.

The activated tissue macrophages migrate in response to chemotactic stimuli and engulf, and kill the bacteria by processes similar to those seen in neutrophils. Over 100 chemicals are secreted by these cells, including most of the bactericidal agents described for neutrophils. They also contain lipases which dissolve the lipid coating of bacteria like tuberculosis and leprosy. Each macrophage can kill up to 100 bacteria before it itself is killed.

The macrophages also play an important role in immunity. They pass (present) the partly-digested antigens of the organisms directly to T and B cells, thus activating them to perform their specific functions in immunity.

Lymphocytes
They play a fundamental role in immune responses of the body.

Types of Lymphocytes. There are 3 primary lymphocyte populations: T- lymphocytes,

B-lymphocytes, and third party or nil (non-T, non-B) lymphocytes. The function of 3rd party cells is not clear, and unlike T and B cells, they do not contain antigen receptors in their plasma membranes. *Innate or Inborn Immunity*. This immunity is present from birth and does not require first exposure to foreign agents (antigens). The cells involved include: neutrophils, macrophages, natural killer (NK) cells, and large lymphocytes that are cytotoxic.

Acquired Immunity. ("My" body contains a huge variety of chemical substances, especially proteins, which are part of me and constitute my "self" material. Material which is not part of me, such as another person's cells, or microbes, etc. which invade the body, is "nonself" material).

The key to acquired immunity is the inborn ability (without first exposure) of lymphocytes to recognize a billion or more non-self antigens. Before T cells and B cells leave thymus and bone marrow, they start to form a number of distinct proteins that are inserted into their plasma membranes. Many of them function as antigen receptors ("**T cell markers**" or "**T cell receptors**", **TCRs**) in T cells and "**surface antibody receptors**" in B cells). In addition to antigen receptors, they also contain other markers, which have been given CD (clusters of differentiation) numbers. Most cytotoxic T cells have glycoprotein CD8 and helper T cells have glycoprotein CD4. These proteins are closely associated with T cell receptors and may function as coreceptors.

Types of Acquired Immunity. There are 2 types of acquired immunity: *humoral* and *cellular*.

a. *Humoral Immunity*. It is mediated by circulating antibodies (immunoglobulins) that circulate in the gamma globulin fraction of plasma proteins. Activated B cells develop into plasma cells and each cell can secrete up to 2000 specific antibody molecules. Humoral immunity is the major defense against the common bacteria.

b. *Cellular ("cell mediated") Immunity*. There are 4 main types of T cells that take part in this type of immunity: helper/inducer (T4 cells), suppressor (Ts or T8) cells, cytotoxic (Tc, killer cells), and memory T cells. The cellular immunity is the major defense against viruses, fungi, some cancer cells, and foreign cells/tissues.

After an antigen (e.g., a microbe) is phagocytosed by tissue macrophages and other antigen presenting cells (APCs, such as dendritic and Langerhan cells of the skin) it is processed. Some of the partly digested products are presented to T and B cells which get activated.

Q.20 What is human immunodeficiency virus (HIV)? How does it affect immunity?

HIV is the causative agent of a very serious worldwide disease—AIDS in which there is a progressive destruction of the immune system. The disease was first described in patients receiving transfusions of blood or blood products. Its mode of spread is now well-known.

The HIV is a retrovirus whose genetic information is carried in RNA instead of DNA. The virus binds to CD4 and enters the host's T4 (helper/inducer) cells, where an enzyme reverse transcriptase (a part of HIV) makes millions of DNA copies of viral RNA. The loss of CD4 helper cells results in failure of proliferation of CD8 and B cells. For a few years, the body is able to replace these killed cells but then their number progressively decreases. The result is a variety of opportunistic infections that are the ultimate cause of death.

Q.21 How does the immune system respond to tissue and organ transplantation?

In organ and tissue transplantation, a diseased injured organ (e.g., heart, kidneys, lungs, liver, pancreas) is replaced with an organ donated by some other person. Generally, the proteins in the transplanted organ are recognised by the immune system as "**foreign**" or "**nonself**". The system reacts by both cell-mediated and antibody-mediated responses against the nonself material, which is destroyed. This phenomenon is called graft rejection. This is generally true even if donor and recipient are closely related. The only transplants that are not rejected are those from identical twin.

To reduce the chance of rejection, blood grouping and tissue typing is done to check incompatibility. The recipient also receives azathioprine (a purine antimetabolite) to kill T cells, glucocorticoids to inhibit cytotoxic T cells proliferation, and cyclosporine.

The cause of graft rejection is the mismatching between a special group of antigens called **"major histocompatibility complex (MHC)"** of the donor and those of the recipient. These antigens, which are glycoproteins, are also called **"human leucocyte associated (HLA)"** antigens, because they were first identified on WBCs. Thousands to many hundreds of thousands MCH molecules (which are unique to every person except in identical twins) are present on the surface of all body cells (except RBCs, which have blood group antigens). Though MHC antigens are involved in tissue rejection, their normal function is to help T cells to recognize that an antigen is foreign, not self, which is an essential first step in any immune response.

Q. 22 How would you differentiate between neutrophils, eosinophils, and basophils?
See pages 79, 80.

Q. 23 How will you differentiate between a small and a large lymphocyte?
See page 79.

Q. 24 How will you differentiate between a large lymphocyte and a monocyte?
See page 80.

Q. 25 What is the clinical importance of doing DLC?
The differential count is done to find out if there is an increase or decrease of a particular type of WBC. Knowing the TLC, the absolute number of each type can be calculated. This information is important in detecting infection or inflammation, allergic and parasitic infections, and effects of chemotherapy and radiation therapy.

Q.26 What is absolute leucocyte count and what is its importance?
See page 80.

Q.27 Can you get a rough idea of total leucocyte count while doing DLC?
See page 80.

Q. 28 How does the DLC of a child differ from that of an adult?
While granulocytes predominate in an adult where they form 50-70% of the TLC, the lymphocytes predominate in children where they form up to 40-50% of TLC.

Q. 29 Is it possible to know the sex of a person from the blood film?
Yes. It is possible to do so. In females, the chromatin of the sex chromosome is seen as a "drum-stick" (Barr body) extending from one lobe of the nucleus into the cytoplasm. However, it is not visible in all neutrophils.

Q. 30 What is meant by the terms neutrophilia and neutropenia, and what are their causes?
The suffix "-philia" means an increase in the number and the suffix "-penia" means a decrease in the number (of cells).

Neutrophilia. Increase in neutrophils in absolute and differential counts is called neutrophilia. (Leucocytosis or granulocytosis are a result of neutrophilia). It is the usual response to certain physiological and pathological stimuli. In the latter case, relatively younger cells appear in blood and cause "left shift" (see below). The causes include physiological and pathological. (See Q/A 16 Expt 1-11).

Physiological neutrophilia. It is seen in muscular exercise, physical and mental stress, after meals, and during pregnancy and after parturition. Neutrophils are mobilized from the "marginal" and "bone marrow" pools. There is no new formation of these cells.

Pathological neutrophilia (absolute count = >10,000/mm^3) can be due to
1. Acute infections, especially localized due to pus-forming bacteria (streptococci and staphylococci), such as superficial or deep

abscess, boils, tonsillitis, appendicitis, pneumonia, lung abscess.

2. Surgery, trauma, burns, acute hemorrhage, hemolysis.
3. Tissue necrosis (tissue death) myocardial, pulmonary, renal infarction amebic hepatitis, malignancies.
4. Drugs: Adrenaline, glucocorticoids (mobilization of marginal and "sequestered" cells in closed capillaries). No left shift.

Neutropenia (absolute count = < 2500/mm³). The terms leucopenia and granulocytopenia, usually mean neutropenia. Neutropenia is never beneficial. The major effect is a reduced ability of the patient to localize and confine infections (especially if the count is < 1000/mm³). The infection may spread to blood and cause septicemia, a serious emergency.

Infections with usual organisms, which rarely cause disease in normal persons (e.g., fungi, viruses like herpes simplex and herpes zoster), called **"opportunistic infections"**, may cause a serious condition if neutropenia is prolonged (>15 days).

Physiological neutropenia is unusual and rare.

Pathological neutropenia. The causes are:
1. Typhoid and paratyphoid infections, viral influenza, kala azar.
2. AIDS.
3. Depression of bone marrow due to drugs, chemicals, radiation, etc.
4. Autoimmune disease—the neutrophils are destroyed by neutrophil antibodies (The autoimmune diseases are due to immune responses against one's own "self " material, other examples are diabetes mellitus, rheumatoid arthritis, purpura, etc).
5. Severe overwhelming infection—the neutrophils are "used up"at a much faster rate than they are produced.

Q.31 Enumerate the conditions that cause eosinophilia and eosinopenia.
Eosinophilia (absolute count = > 500/mm³). The causes are:

1. Allergic conditions: Bronchial asthma, skin diseases like urticaria, eczema, and food sensitivity, etc.
2. Parasitic infections: Intestinal worms like hook-worms, tapeworms, round worms, especially those which invade tissues.

Eosinopenia (absolute count < 50/mm³). The causes include: acute stressful illness, Cushing's syndrome (excess steroids), ACTH, and glucosteroid treatment, and acute pyogenic infections.

Q.32 Name the conditions where basophils increase and decrease in number.
Basophilia (absolute number = > 100/mm³).
The condition is seen in viral infections (influenza), allergic diseases, smallpox, and chickenpox.
Basopenia. It is seen in acute pyogenic infections and during glucocorticoid treatment.

Q. 33 What is leukemoid reaction?
See Q/A 19, Expt. 1-11.

Q. 34 What are the causes of monocytosis and monocytopenia?
Monocytosis (Absolute count = > 800/mm³). It is seen in:
1. Infectious mononucleosis (IM). It is a contageous viral disease caused by Epstein-Barr virus (EBV) and occurs mainly in children. Signs and symptoms include fever, fatigue, dizziness, enlargement of lymph glands, high TLC, especially large number of lymphocytes. There is no cure but the disease runs its course in a few weeks.
2. Malaria, kala azar, subacute bacterial endocarditis, rheumatoid arthritis.
3. Leukemias, collagen diseases, malignancies.
Monocytopenia. It may be seen in bone marrow depression due to any cause.

Q. 35 What are the causes of lymphocytosis and lymphocytopenia?
Lymphocytosis (Absolute count= >5000/mm³). High counts are seen in:
1. Healthy infants and young children. DLC may be about 60% though the TLC may be normal.

This is sometimes called "relative lymphocytosis".

2. Viral infections: whooping-cough, chicken-pox, etc.; autoimmune disease.
3. Chronic infections like tuberculosis and hepatitis.
4. Chronic lymphocytic leukemia—this is the most common cause of lymphocyte count above 10,000/mm^3.

Lymphocytopenia. The causes of decrease include:
1. Patients on steroid therapy.
2. Acquired immunodeficiency syndrome (AIDS). The virus particularly attacks the helper/inducer (T4) cells.
3. Depression of bone marrow due to any cause.

Q. 36   What is Cooke-Arneth count and what is its importance?
Consult next Experiment (Expt 1-13).

Q.37 What is peroxidase reaction? Which types of leucocytes give a positive reaction?
Peroxidase Reaction (Peroxidase stain) for Leucocytes: This test is carried out as follows: A dry blood film is first treated with a solution of benzidine and sodium nitroprusside dissolved in ethyl alcohol and then with hydrogen peroxide. After a thorough wash with water, the film is counter-stained with Leishman's stain in the usual manner.

The peroxidase reaction detects the presence of oxidizing enzymes in the cytoplasm of myeloid series of WBCs. Oxidase granules are seen in myelocytes and myeloblasts. Eosinophils show deeper blue granules, while basophils show no granules. Lymphoid series of cells are peroxidase negative. This reaction helps in distinguishing immature cells of the myeloid series from lymphoid series in cases of leukemia (the two series of immature cells look similar with Leishman stain alone).

Demonstration Slides
Stained and mounted blood and bone marrow smears of leukemic patients (obtained from Pathology department) showing immature WBCs of myeloid and lymphoid series will be focused on the demonstration table. Note the descriptions listed on the cards besides the microscopes, and enter these in your workbooks.

1-13

The Cooke-Arneth Count (Arneth Count)

Relevance

Young neutrophils have fewer lobes as compared to older cells which have 5 or 6 lobes. A higher percentage of younger or older cells in a blood film can provide useful information about the functional status of the bone marrow.

APPARATUS AND MATERIALS

As for differential leucocyte count.

Procedures

1. Prepare and stain a fresh blood film in the usual manner. (You may use the film you employed for DLC if it is satisfactory).
2. Examine 100 (or 200) neutrophils, noting the number of lobes in each cell. Enter your observations in your workbook. Use the tally-bar method for this and calculate the percentages of each stage (for example: N_1 = IIII I = 6%).

Stage		Description	Normal count (%)
Stage I	(N_1)	• Nucleus is C- or U-shaped, the two limbs being connected by a thick band of chromatin.	5-10
Stage II	(N_2)	• The 2 lobes are connected by a narrow band of chromatin.	20-30
Stage III	(N_3)	• 3 lobes connected by chromatin filaments. (Actively motile and functionally most effective).	40-50
Stage IV	(N_4)	• 4 lobes connected by chromatin filaments.	10-15
Stage V	($N_{5,6}$)	• 5 lobes or more (N_6 = > 6 lobes). • Outline may be irregular. • Cytoplasmic granules poorly stained. • Functionally least motile and effective.	3-5

Note
Occasionally it is not possible to do the staging of some neutrophils accurately, especially when the lobes of the nuclei are folded. Two other factors may then be used:
  i. The cell size, which decreases with ageing.
  ii. The older cells contain fewer granules. In older cells (stages N 5,6) there may be no granules and the nucleus may show fragmentation).

PRECAUTIONS

1. Choose a stained slide that shows neutrophils to best advantage.
2. If the lobes cannot be seen, consider the size of the cell and the number of granules in the cytoplasm.
3. For good results, count 200 cells.

QUESTIONS

Q. 1 What is the relation between the number of lobes of the nucleus and the age of a neutrophil?
A newly formed neutrophil in the bone marrow is one-lobed and may be C- or U-shaped. Such cells are called 'stabs'. They enter blood mostly as bilobed cells. As their age increases, the number of lobes increase to 5 or 6 by the end of their short life-span of 8-10 hours.

Q. 2 Which stage is most effective and which stage least effective?
A 3-lobed neutrophil is the most motile and functionally the most efficient in killing the bacteria. A senile neutrophil is less motile and least effective. Shape may be irregular, and the granules fewer and poorly-staining. These cells commonly break up during the spreading of a blood film.

Q. 3 What is meant by the terms left shift and right shift? Is the Cooke-Arneth count of any clinical value?
The terms 'left shift" and "right shift" refer to the appearance of younger neutrophils (shift to the left), or more mature cells (shift to the right) in the blood.

"Left shift" ("Regenerative shift") =
  $N_1 + N_2 + N_3$ = > 80%
This indicates hyperactive bone marrow.

Right shift" ("Degenerative shift") =
  $N_4 + N_5 + N_6$ = > 20%
This indicates a hypoactive bone marrow.
  A shift of the count to one or the other side can provide important information about the functional status of bone marrow. It can tell us whether or

not the bone marrow is actively forming and releasing neutrophils into the circulation.

Q. 4 If Cooke-Arneth count can provide such useful information about the functioning of bone marrow, why is it not used as a routine?

There are two reasons for this test not being used as a routine:

1. Some physiological conditions cause shifting of neutrophils from various pools into the circulating blood. This is likely to cause confusion about left or right shift.

2. Better methods, e.g., bone marrow biopsy, are now available for assessing bone marrow function.

   Nevertheless, this count can provide some useful information from a blood film without bone marrow biopsy. It is also a good laboratory exercise.

Q. 5 Plot a graph of your own values with the neutrophil stages on the X-axis, and their percentage on the Y-axis. Draw another graph with the values given in your book and compare the two graphs.

The student should be able to do this exercise easily and be able to explain the differences, if any.

Q. 6 What are the features of a senile neutrophil ?

See Q/A 2 above.

Q. 7 Name some conditions that affect the Cooke-Arneth count.

A shift to the left indicates that the bone marrow is actively forming and releasing neutrophils into the circulation. A shift to the right indicates decreased production and release of neutrophils.

Shift to left occurs in:

1. Acute pus-producing infections.
2. Tuberculosis: Though there is lymphocytosis, a shift to the left may be due to removal of older neutrophils from the blood.
3. Hemorrhage.
4. Low-dosage irradiation is said to stimulate bone marrow while heavy doses cause a shift to the right.

Shift to right occurs in

1. Bone marrow depression (hypoplasia and aplasia) due to any factor (see Q/A 17, Expt. 1-11).
2. Drugs, toxins, chemical poisons. (See Q/A 17, Expt. 1-11).
3. Megaloblastic anemia, septicemia, uremia, etc.

1-14

Absolute Eosinophil Count

<table>
<tr><td colspan="2">STUDENT OBJECTIVES</td></tr>
<tr><td colspan="2">After completing this practical you should be able to:
1. Describe the significance of doing absolute eosinophil count.

2. Describe the morphology and functions of eosinophils.

3. Carry out eosinophil count, and name the precautions taken by you.</td></tr>
</table>

4. List the composition of Pilot's solution and the function of each component.

5. Explain the physiological basis of changes in their count.

Relevance

Absolute eosinophil count is required when the differential count shows a high percentage of these cells. This is especially true in cases of bronchial allergy, asthma, urticaria, intestinal parasites pulmonary eosinophilia, etc.

Counting Methods

The absolute count of eosinophils can be done by two methods:

1. **Direct *method*.** The cells are counted directly by employing hemocytometry.
2. **Indirect method.** As mentioned in Expt 1-12 (DLC), the percentage of eosinophils is determined from a blood smear counting of leucocytes. If TLC is done simultaneously, the absolute count can be calculated.

Note
The direct method of hemocytometry will be used in this experiment.

PRINCIPLE

Blood is diluted 10 times in a WBC pipette using Pilot's diluting fluid that lyses RBCs and leucocytes other than eosinophils. The stained cells are then counted in a counting chamber.

APPARATUS AND MATERIALS

1. Microscope •Counting chamber •WBC pipette •Coverslips •Equipment for finger prick.
2. **Pilot's diluting fluid** for eosinophil counting:
   Stock solutions:
   a. Propylene glycol.
   b. Phloxine: 1 % solution in water (0.5% eosin may be used but phloxine is superior).
   c. Sodium carbonate: 10 % solution in water.

Working solution: It is made by mixing and filtering the following:

Propylene glycol	= 50 ml
Phloxine (1 %)	= 10 ml
Sodium carbonate (10 %)	= 1 ml
Heparin	= 100 units
Distilled water	= 40 ml

Note
The diluting fluid is freshly prepared from stock solution when required. Propylene lyses the red cells, phloxine stains the eosinophil granules, and sodium carbonate solution lyses all leucocytes except eosinophils.

PROCEDURES

1. Get a finger prick under asepsis, discard the first 2 drops, and then fill 2 WBC pipettes with blood to the mark 1.0 (EDTA anticoagulated blood can be used).
2. Suck the diluting fluid to the mark 11 in both pipettes. Mix the contents of each for 2 minutes.
3. Place the pipettes on 2-3 layers of moistened filter papers and cover them with a petri dish. Allow to stand for 15 minutes for proper lysis and staining. (The purpose of moist filter papers is to prevent evaporation of water from the pipettes).
4. Take out the pipettes and mix the contents once again for 30 seconds. Discard the fluid in the stems and charge each side of the chamber from each pipette and bring the chamber into focus in the usual manner.
5. Using HP objective, count the eosinophils in the 4 corner groups of 16 squares each, i.e., in a total of 64 squares that were used for TLC. When the counting has been done, calculate the number of cells in 1 c.mm of undiluted blood. Enter your observations in appropriate squares drawn in your notebooks.

OBSERVATIONS AND RESULTS

Calculations
Volume of 64 squares
$$(\text{each} = 1/160 \text{ mm}^3)$$
$$= 1/160 \times 64 = 4/10 \text{ mm}^3$$
Let the eosinophil count in $4/10 \text{ mm}^3$
(i.e., 64 squares) be = x
Then, 1 mm^3 of diluted blood will contain
$$= x \times 10/4 \text{ cells}$$

Since the dilution is 10 times, 1 mm^3 of undiluted blood will contain

$$= x \times 10/4 \times 10$$
$$= x \times 25 \text{ cells.}$$

- Compare the count from the two pipettes. The difference should not be more than 10%.

Normal absolute eosinophil count= 10-400/mm^3 (Eosinophil count of capillary blood is usually 10-15% higher).

Indirect Method of Counting Eosinophil

This method was mentioned in Expt 1-11. For this both TLC and DLC are required. For example, if the TLC is 8000/mm^3 and eosinophils are 2% in DLC, then the absolute count would be= 2/100 x 8000= 160/mm^3 of undiluted blood. This method can act as a check on the result of direct method.

PRECAUTIONS

1. Observe all precautions for obtaining a blood sample, filling the pipette with blood, diluting it, charging the chamber, and counting the cells.
2. Do the cell counting within 20-30 minutes of charging the chamber because the cells begin to disintegrate in the diluting fluid.
3. If possible, use the indirect method to check on your results.

QUESTIONS

Q. 1 What is the clinical significance of absolute eosinophil count?
Formerly, eosinophil count was considered as an index of ACTH activity in the blood. When ACTH is injected into a person with normal adrenocortical function, there is a drastic reduction in the absolute eosinophil count. This test, called "Thorn's test" used to be employed to assess adrenocortical

function. However, with better hormone assay tests, this test is no longer employed.

However, the absolute count helps in diagnosing various allergic and parasitic conditions.

Q. 2 Can any other diluting fluid be used for the count?
Yes. In *Dunger's diluting fluid*, eosin replaces phloxine, and acetone replaces propylene glycol. This fluid contains: 5 ml of 1% aqueous solution of eosin, 5 ml of acetone (analytic), and distilled water to 90 ml.

In *Randolph's diluting fluid*, which is similar to Pilot's solution, methylene blue is added to stain other leucocytes blue compared to red-orange eosinophils.

Q. 3 Where are eosinophils formed, what are their kinetics, and what are their functions?
Eosinophils, along with other leucocytes, develop from PHSC in the red marrow. Their production is regulated by CSF-GM, interleukins 3 and 5 and possibly by the products of dead and dying cells, which also help in their maturation.

They remain in circulation for an hour or so, and then enter the tissues—especially mucosae of lungs, GIT, and urinary tract. Their granules contain a variety of chemicals: major basic protein (MBP), eosinophil peroxidase, eosinophilic cationic proteins, aryl sulphatase B, lysophospholiase, histaminase, cytokines, etc. (See Q/A 19, Expt 1-12).

Q. 4 Name the conditions in which absolute eosinophil count increases and decreases.
Eosinophilia is seen in: allergic conditions, parasitic infestations, skin diseases, pulmonary eosinophilia, malignant neoplasia (eosinophilic leukemia, Hodgkin's disease), and Addison's disease. (Also see Q/A 31 Expt 1-12).
Eosinopenia is seen in: Cushing's syndrome, acute pyogenic infections, aplastic anemia, (Also see Q/A31; Expt 1-12).

1-15

Study of Morphology of Red Blood Cells

Alterations in the morphology of red cells (their size, shape structure, staining characteristics, etc.) are commonly seen in various types of anemia and other diseases. A careful examination of the peripheral blood film can, therefore, provide important information in the diagnosis of these conditions.

PROCEDURES

Prepare and stain a 'thin' blood film. If a suitable film is available from the previous experiments, it may be used. Study the cells in the area between the tail and the thicker head of the smear, away from the edges, where the RBCs are spread out. Note the following features of the red cells:

Size and shape. Note that there is a moderate variation in the size around the diameter of about 7.5 μm. Most cells are round, though a few may be slightly oval.

Staining. Note the size of the central pallor (it normally occupies the central third) and compare the depth of color of different cells. Note if there are any granules. Though reticulocytes are present (0.5 to 2%), their basophilic network does not take up Leishman's stain, and a special process called 'supravital' staining is required (see next Expt). The nucleated red cells are not normally present in the peripheral blood.

Demonstration slides. Stained slides showing reticulocytes and abnormal morphology of red cells (obtained from pathology department) will be set up on the demonstration table. Examine and compare these smears with your own blood film. Note the descriptions listed on the cards beside the microscopes and enter these in your workbook.

Abnormal red cells. The following terms express some abnormal morphological states and the conditions with which they are associated:

1. **Anisocytosis:** Abnormal variation in size; seen in iron deficiency and megaloblastic anemias.
2. **Basophilic stippling (punctate basophilia):** Bluish granules, seen in lead poisoning, thalassemia.
3. **Burr cells:** Irregularly shaped red cells, seen in uremia.
4. **Cabot's rings and Howell-Jolly bodies:** Bluish remnants of nuclei that persist in iron-deficiency and megaloblastic anemias; rarely leukemias.
5. **Leptocytes (target cells, also called Maxican hat cells):** Central staining, a ring of pallor, and an outer rim of staining, seen in liver disease, thalassemias, sickle cell disease.
6. **Hypochromia:** Less dense staining, wider central pallor; seen in iron deficiency anemia.
7. **Hyperchromia:** More dense staining red cells; seen in pernicious anemia.
8. **Microcytes and macrocytes:** Small or large cells; seen in iron deficiency and pernicious anemia.
9. **Normoblasts:** Immature, nucleated red cells; seen in hypoxia, hemolysis.
10. **Pappenheimer bodies:** Visible in lead poisoning, carcinomatosis, after splenectomy.
11. **Poikilocytosis:** Variable shaped cells, seen in iron deficiency anemia.
12. **Polychromasia:** RBCs of different ages stain unevenly, younger cells being bluer. This is a response to bleeding, hemolysis, hematinics (e.g., ferrous sulphate, B_{12}).
13. **Rouleaux formation:** Stacking of red cells on each other; the "visual analogue" of high ESR.

14. **Schistocytes:** Fragmented RBCs, sliced by fibrin bands; seen in intravascular hemolysis.
15. **Spherocytes:** Smaller, spherical cells, appearing more dense, seen in congenital hemolytic anemia or, rarely, in hereditary spherocytosis.
16. **Sickle cells:** The RBCs are shaped like a sickle; it is due to the HbS which alters the shape of red cells.

1-16

The Reticulocyte Count

STUDENT OBJECTIVES

After completing this practical, you should be able to:
1. Indicate the significance of doing this count.
2. Describe the theory of reticulocyte staining and the special stains that are used.
3. Perform the relative and absolute reticulocyte counts.
4. Indicate the origin, kinetics and fate of these cells.
5. Define the terms reticulocyte response, reticulocytosis, and reticulocytopenia.
6. Describe the electronic method of counting these cells.

Introduction. Reticulocytes are the non-nucleated immediate precursors of red cells that develop in the red marrow from the PHSCs. They contain large amounts of the remnants of RNA and ribosomes. They are slightly larger (Diameter= 9.0 μm) than RBCs, and are present in large numbers in bone marrow and in small numbers in blood. Their cell membranes are sticky which plays an important role in their controlled release from the bone marrow. Most of them, because of their larger size and stickiness, are trapped in the trabeculae of the spleen. Here they ripen and mature in a day or two before entering the circulation once again.

Relevance

The reticulocyte count, which is 1-2% of circulating red cells, is an indicator of erythropoietic activity of red bone marrow. It is indicated in all conditions where high counts are expected, such as in hemolytic anemias. It can also help in assessing the effectiveness of a drug being used in the treatment of anemia.

PRINCIPLE

A mixture of blood and a dye (stain) is spread in the form of a thin smear on a glass slide and suitably counterstained to bring out their reticulum. They are then counted per 1000 red cells and their percentage calculated.

APPARATUS AND MATERIALS

1. Microscope. • Glass slides. • Equipment for finger prick. • Petri dish. • Blotting paper.
2. **Reticulocyte stains (supravital stains).** These stains are used for staining unfixed, "living" cells and tissues *in vitro* (outside the body).
   i. *Brilliant cresyl blue.* 1.0 g of this dye dissolved in 100 ml of citrated saline (1.0 volume of 3.8% sodium citrate and 4 volumes of normal saline). The dye stains the RNA of reticulocytes, citrate prevents clotting of blood, and normal saline provides tonicity (1.0% solution of the dye in methyl alcohol can also be used).
   ii. *New methylene blue.* While methylene blue does not stain the reticulum, new methylene blue (which is chemically different) stains this material more deeply and uniformly. 1.0 g of the dye is dissolved in 100 ml of citrate saline.

Theory of Reticulocyte Staining

The basophilic remnants of RNA and ribsomes in the cytoplasm of reticulocytes cannot be stained by the basic dye methylene blue, which is a component of Leishman's stain. The material can only be stained with certain dyes such as brilliant cresyl blue. The dye enters the cells and stains the basophilic material to form bluish precipitates of dots, short strands, and filaments. This reaction can occur only in supravitally (or vitally) stained cells, i.e., in "unfixed" and "living" cells. The more the immature cells, greater is the amount of precipitable ribosomal material present in them.

PROCEDURES

1. Take 2-3 clean, grease-free glass slides and place a drop of reticulocyte stain in the center of each slide about 1 cm from its end.
2. Get a finger prick under aseptic precautions and add an equal-sized drop of blood to each drop of stain. Stir with a pin and put the slides on moist filter paper and cover with a petri dish. Allow the mixture to remain on the slides for 1 minute. (The slides may be incubated at body temperature for 15 minutes to simulate the living conditions so that the stain may better penetrate the reticulocytes).
3. Spread a smear of the blood-dye mixture on each slide, then counterstain with Leishman's stain in the usual manner. (This will stain all cells).

Note
Alternately, take 1 ml of anticoagulated blood in a small test tube; add an equal amount of the dye. Mix gently, and incubate at 37 °C for 15 minutes. Mix the mixture gently to re-suspend the blood cells and prepare smears in the usual manner. Choose the best-stained smear for reticulocyte counting.

OBSERVATIONS AND RESULTS

1. Using oil-immersion objective, bring the blood cells into focus and identify reticulo-cytes. They stain lighter than the red cells and also contain dots, strands, and filaments, etc of bluish-stained material.
   Identification of Reticulocytes. These non-nucleated cells are slightly larger (diameter about 8 µm) than the red cells (average diameter = 7.5 µm). They also stain lighter than the red cells, and contain dots, strands, and filaments of bluish-stained material.
2. Count the reticulocytes in 100 alternate fields, i.e., move one uncounted field before counting them again. (In some fields you may not see any such cells.)
3. Count the red cells in every 5th field, for a total of 10 fields. (When counting red cells in a field, divide the field into 4 imaginary quadrants. This will make the counting easier).

Calculations

If, say, the number of reticulocytes in 100 fields is = 72,
and the number of red
  cells in 10 fields is = 450
The number of red cells
  in 100 fields $= 450 \times 10 = 4500$
Percentage of reticulocytes $= 72/4500 \times 100 = 1.6\%$

Normal values
1. Newborns = 30-40%. Their number decreases to 1-2% during the first week of life.
2. Infants = 2-6 %
3. Children and adults
   a. 0.2-2.0% (average = 1%)
   b. Absolute count = 20,000-90,000/mm^3.

Absolute Reticulocyte Count

A direct reticulocyte counting by hemocytometry is not possible. An indirect absolute count can be obtained from the relative percentage by doing a total red cell count.

= Reticulocyte percent x red cell count/100
    Normal value = 25,000 – 100,000 / mm^3

PRECAUTIONS

1. Observe all precautions as for differential leucocyte count.
2. The blood film should be thin so that the red cells lie separately from each other without any crowding or overlapping.
3. There should be no rouleaux formation on the slide.

QUESTIONS

Q. 1   What are the indications for doing reticulo-cyte count?
See page 94.

Q. 2   What are reticulocytes? Are they normally present in blood? Did you see these cells in the Leishman-stained blood films?
See above.

Q. 3   What is the chemical nature of reticular material?
It is the remnant of RNA and ribosomes.

Q. 4   What is meant by the term "vital" staining? How does it differ from Leishman's staining you employed for blood films?
The term **"vital"** suggests that this method has to do with living cells. Vital staining is a special method of staining employed for unfixed, "living cells" (or as nearly living as possible), including tissue cultures. There are 2 types of vital staining:

1. **Supravital staining.** It is an *in vitro* method where the living cells are stained by immersing them in a dye solution.
2. **Intravitam staining.** It is an *in vivo* method where a dye is injected into a living organism for selective staining.

Q. 5   How does a reticulocyte differ from a red cell?
See page 95.

Q. 6   What are the normal counts in newborns, infants, children and adults?
See page 95.

Q. 7   What is a reticulocyte response? Is its determination of any practical value?
Reticulocyte response is an increase in the number of reticulocytes in the circulating blood. It indicates a high rate of erythropoiesis. Its practical importance is as follows:

1. It is useful in assessing the erythroid activity of the red marrow.
2. It can be employed to check if the diagnosis and treatment of an anemic patient is proceeding on correct lines. For example, if iron deficiency is diagnosed, treatment with iron should produce a prompt reticulocyte response.
3. The potency of a particular drug can also be assessed. The response starts 2-8 days after the therapy is started and reaches a peak in the next 8 to 10 days. After that there is a gradual fall in the response while the RBC count continues to rise steadily (it needs pointing out that reticulocyte response by itself must be interpreted very critically either as evidence of therapeutic efficacy of a drug, or as a prognostic sign, or for assessing the bone marrow efficiency).

Q. 8   What is meant by the term reticulocytosis? Name the physiological and pathological conditions that cause an increase and decrease in the number of reticulocytes.
Reticulocytosis. The term indicates an increase in the number of reticulocytes in the blood.

Physiological variations. Increased count is seen in:

1. **Newborn infants.** The blood contains immature red cells, both nucleated and reticulocytes. After 1 year there are no nucleated RBCs, and not more than 2% reticulocytes.
2. **High altitude.** Erythropoiesis is stimulated by the hypoxic stimuli via erythropoietin.

Pathological variations. Increased count due to disease is seen in:

1. **Reticulocyte response during treatment of deficiency anemias.** There is increase in Hb and RBC count.

2. **After hemorrhage.** The count increases due to hypoxia.

3. **Chronic hemolytic anemias,** disorders of bone marrow (nucleated RBCs present), leukemias, secondary deposits in malignancies and miliary tuberculosis.

4. **Disorders of spleen and after splenectomy.** The response is irregular.

5. **Arsenic and foreign proteins,** etc. produce irregular response without increase in Hb and RBC count.

Reticulocytopenia. Decrease in reticulocyte count may be seen in aplastic anemia, hypopituitarism, myxedema, and after splenectomy. There is no physiological situation in which their number decreases.

Q. 9 Is there any automated (electronic) method for counting reticulocytes?
The automated method for this count employs the following principle: The cells are stained with a fluorochrome dye that specifically stains RNA. The reticulocytes fluoresce when exposed to ultraviolet light and the cells can then be calculated.

1-17

Erythrocyte Sedimentation Rate (ESR)

STUDENT OBJECTIVES

After completing this practical, you should be able to:
1. Describe the clinical importance of doing ESR.
2. Explain why red cells settle down when blood is kept in a tube, and indicate the factors that affect their rate of settling.
3. Name the methods employed for its determination.
4. Describe the sources of error and precautions to be taken.
5. Name the various conditions in which ESR increases or decreases and their physiological basis.

Relevance

The determination of the rate at which the red cells settle or sediment (ESR) is often required by a physician to rule out the presence of organic disease, or to follow the progress of a disease. ESR is generally done as part of complete blood tests.

PRINCIPLE

In the circulating blood the red cells remain uniformly suspended in the plasma. However, when a sample of blood, to which an anticoagulant has been added, is allowed to stand in a narrow vertical tube the red cells (sp.gr. = 1.095) being heavier (denser) than the colloids plasma (sp.gr. = 1.032), settle or sediment gradually towards the bottom of the tube. The rate, in mm, at which the red cells sediment, called ESR, is recorded at the end of one hour.

Sedimentation of red cells

The settling or sedimentation of red cells in a sample of anticoagulated blood occurs in 3 stages:
  i. In the *first stage*, the RBCs pile up (like a stack of coins), and form rouleaux that become heavier during the first 10-15 minutes.
 ii. During the *second stage*, the rouleau (pleural of rouleaux) being heavier (see below) sink to the bottom. This stage lasts for 40-45 minutes.
iii. In the **third stage,** there is packing of massed bunches of red cells at the bottom of the blood column. This stage lasts for about 10-12 minutes.

Thus, most of the settling of the red cells occurs in the first hour or so.

WINTROBE'S METHOD

APPARATUS AND MATERIALS

1. Disposable syringe and needle • Sterile swabs moist with 70% alcohol • Container (discarded penicillin bottle, etc.) with double oxalate mixture, or sequestrene.
2. Pasteur pipette with a long thin nozzle.
3. Wintrobe **tube and stand. Figure 1-13** shows a Wintrobe tube (recall that it is also used for hematocrit or PCV; as was done in Expt.1-9). Check out its dimensions and markings once again. It is graduated 0 to 10 cm from above downwards on one side (for ESR) and 10 to 0 cm on the other side (for Hct). The Wintrobe stand can hold up to 3 (or 6) tubes at a time. It is provided with a spirit level to ensure that the tubes are held vertical throughout the test.

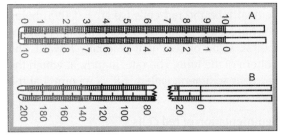

Figure 1-13. (A) Wintrobe's tube. The tube is 12 cm long and closed at its lower end. The markings are in cm and mm, from 0 to 10 from above downward on one side (these are for ESR) and from 10 to 0 on the other side (these are for PCV or Hct). (B) Westergren's tube (Westergren's pipette). This tube is 30 cm long, and open at both ends. The markings are in cm and mm, from 0 to 200. Only ESR can be estimated with this tube

PROCEDURES

1. Draw 0.2 ml of venous blood and transfer it to a container of anticoagulant. Mix the contents gently but well by inverting the vial a few times, or by swirling it. Do not shake, as it will cause frothing.
2. Using the Pasteur pipette, fill the Wintrobe tube from below upwards as was done in Expt. 1-9. Ensure that there are no air bubbles.
3. Transfer the tube to its stand and adjust the screws so that it will remain vertical. Leave the tube undisturbed in this position for one hour, at the end of which read the mm of clear plasma above the red cells.

Express your result as: .....mm 1st hour (Wintrobe).

> **Note**
> The result is not expressed as mm per hour. Do not take the reading after ½ hour and then double it to arrive at 1 hour.

Normal values

Males	:	2-8 mm 1st hour.
Females	:	4-10 mm 1st hour

WESTERGREN'S METHOD

APPARATUS AND MATERIALS

1. 2 ml disposable syringe with needle • Sterile cotton/gauze swabs moist with alcohol • Container (discarded penicillin bottle).
2. Sterile solution of 3.8 percent sodium citrate as the anticoagulant.
3. **Westergren pipette (tube) and stand. Figure 1-13** shows a Westergren pipette. It is 300 mm long and has a bore diameter of 2.5 mm. It is calibrated in cm and mm from 0 to 200, from above downwards in its lower two-thirds. The Westergren stand can accommodate up to 6 tubes at a time. For each pipette, there is a screw cap that slips over its top, and, at its lower end, the pipette presses into a rubber pad or cushion. When the pipette is fixed in position, there is enough pressure of the screw cap to prevent leakage of blood from its lower end. There is a spirit level to ensure vertical position of the pipette.

PROCEDURES

1. Draw 2.0 ml of venous blood and transfer it into a vial containing 0.5 ml of 3.8% sodium citrate solution. This will give a blood: citrate ratio of 4:1. Mix the contents by inverting or swirling the vial. Do not shake, as it will cause frothing.

2. Fill the Westergren's pipette with blood-citrate mixture by sucking, after placing the tip of your finger over the top of the pipette to control the flow of blood into and out of it, or with a rubber bulb. Bring the blood column to exact zero mark. (If there is a difference of 1-2 mm, it should be noted and taken into account before giving the final report at the end of one hour).

3. Keeping you finger (or the rubber bulb) over the pipette, transfer it to the Westergren stand by firmly pressing its lower end into the rubber cushion. Now slip the upper end of the pipette under the screw cap. Confirm that there is no leakage of blood and that the pipette will remain vertical.

4. Leave the pipette undisturbed for one hour at the end of which read the mm of clear plasma above the red cells.

   Express your results as:............ mm 1st hour (Westergren).

Normal values

   Males: 3-9 mm 1st hour
   Females: 5-12 mm 1st hour

Modified experiment. The above procedure is standardized for clinical use. However, you can modify it as an extension of the standard procedure. Instead of taking just one reading at the end of one hour, take ESR readings (to the nearest mm) every 15 minutes from the zero time for 3-4 hours. Using these figures, plot a graph of the distance of fall of red cells against time. Note if the rate of settling of RBCs is constant or not.

For comparison. Using this method, you can compare the ESR of **"normal"** blood with that of "abnormal" blood. Place 0.5 ml citrate in each of 2 dry containers. Draw 5 ml blood from a suitable vein and gently expel 2 ml blood into each container (citrate: blood ratio = 1:4). Add enough glucose to one container to make its blood "abnormal". Set up 2 separate Westergren pipettes containing "normal" and "abnormal" blood samples and take the readings at the end of one hour.

OBSERVATIONS AND RESULTS

Note that if there is no hemolysis, there is a sharp line of demarcation between the red cells and the clear, cell-free, and straw-colored plasma. The bore of the pipette if not less than 2 mm has no effect on ESR, but inclination from the vertical gives false high values. Higher values are also obtained at extremes of temperature, in anemia, and after ingesting food.

Sources of Error. These include: tilting of the tube and high temperature lead to high values while low temperature gives false low values. Hemolysed blood may obscure the sharp line separating red cells and the plasma.

PRECAUTIONS

1. Proper anticoagulant should be used for each method.
2. The blood should be collected in the fasting state.
3. The test should preferably be done within 2-3 hours of collecting the blood sample, and at a room temperature of 20-35°C.
4. The hematocrit should be checked and correction factor applied in cases of anemia (nomograms are available for this purpose).
5. Clotted or hemolysed blood must be discarded.
6. The Wintrobe tube or Westergren pipette should not be disturbed from the vertical position for the duration of the test.

QUESTIONS

Q. 1 Why do the red cells settle down in a sample of anticoagulated blood?

Since the blood is not moving the red cells settle down because they are heavier (sp. gr. = 1.095) than the plasma (sp. gr. = 1.032) in which they are suspended.

Q. 2 Can you use oxalate mixture in Westergren method and citrate in Wintrobe method?

No. The anticoagulants employed for each method cannot be interchanged because both methods have been standardized and employed in clinical practice for the last many years. (Sodium citrate cannot be used in Wintrobe method because the blood will be too much diluted as compared to the height of the tube; and this will give high false values for ESR).

Q. 3 What are the advantages and disadvantages of Wintrobe method?

The **advantage** of this method is that the same sample of oxalated blood can first be used for ESR and then, after one hour, for hematocrit (PCV) by centrifuging it. Thus, in cases of anemias, the appropriate correction factor can be applied.

The **disadvantage** is that this method is less sensitive because the column of blood is not as high as is desirable for good results, and chances of error are high, especially when the ESR is increased, say to over 50 mm.

Q. 4 What are the advantages and disadvantages of Westergren method?

The Westergren method is more sensitive since the tube is sufficiently long and its diameter is also larger. The higher sensitivity and the longer tube is particularly important in cases where ESR is high (> 80 mm).

The **disadvantage** is that the citrate solution dilutes the red cells which by itself tends to raise the ESR. But the fibrinogen and globulins of plasma are also diluted which tends to lower the ESR. These two opposing effects, however, tend to neutralize each other.

Q. 5 Why is ESR reading taken after one hour?

The reason for this is that more than 95-98% red cells settle down by the end of this time. After one hour the rate of sedimentation does not significantly affect the ESR. Further, the method has been standardized for one hour and in clinical practice for long.

Q. 6 What are the factors on which the rate of sedimentation of red cells depends?

Rate of settling of red cells depends on:
1. A downward gravitational force acting on the red cells due to their weight (mass) and,
2. An upward force due to viscosity of plasma, and the area of surface of red cells where viscous retardation occurs, i.e., the plasma-red cell interface.

Thus, the rate of settling of red cells will depend on a balance between these two opposing forces.

Factors Affecting ESR

The factors that affect the ESR include the following:

1. Technical and Mechanical Factors. Factors like the length of the tube. Diameter of the bore (if less than 2 mm), and the anticoagulant used (liquid anticoagulant in Westergren's method gives somewhat higher values.

2. Physiological Factors. The red cell count, their size and their shape, raised body temperature, viscosity of plasma, and tendency to rouleaux formation, all affect the ESR.

Rouleaux Formation

In the circulating blood, the red cells remain separate from each other due to their constant movement and due to their mutual repulsion resulting from their negative electrostatic charge imparted by sialic acid moieties on the cell membranes. This repulsion force is known as *zeta potential*. However, fibrinogen (see below) neutralizes these charges and makes the RBCs sticky so that they tend to adhere to each other and form lager rouleaux.

In health, the rouleaux (in a blood film or in a test tube) are small and settle slowly. But under certain conditions (described below), rouleaux formation increases and thus it is the main factor that increases the ESR. The importance of the size and the rate of rouleaux formation is as follows:

The surface area of a single red cell is about 150 μm², and 10 red cells would have a surface area of 1500 μm²—when they do not form a pile. But when these 10 red cells form a rouleaux (pile), their surface area is only 600 μm² while their mass has increased 10 times. Thus, when the red cells form rouleaux, there is a greater increase in the masses of these red cells as compared to increase in their surface area. This decreases the retardation caused by plasma viscosity, which, in turn, increases the rate of settling of red cells, and thus the ESR.

Factors Affecting Rouleaux Formation

a. **Concentration of large, asymmetric molecules of fibrinogen and globulins.** An increase in the concentration of these plasma proteins promotes rouleaux formation (and hence ESR); this is seen in almost all infections (acute and chronic, tissue destruction due to any cause, and wasting diseases.

b. **Bacterial proteins and toxins, and products of inflammation and tissue destruction** such *as acute- phase* reactants (e.g., C reactive proteins of acute rheumatic fever), released into the blood neutralize the surface charges of red cells. This promotes stickiness of these cells, rouleaux formation, and faster settling.

c. *Number of red cells.* A decrease in RBC count promotes rouleaux formation, while an increase in count (e.g., polycythemia) decreases ESR.

d. *Size and shape of red cells.* Biconcave shape of red cells favors rouleaux formation, while an increase in MCV, hereditary spherocytosis and in sickle cell disease, ESR is decreased.

3. *Viscosity of Blood.* Increased viscosity of blood, whether due to increase in RBC count or plasma protein concentration, decreases ESR while a decrease in viscosity increases ESR. (Viscosity of water: plasma: blood = 1:3:5).

4. *Nature of Anticoagulant Used.* Fluid anticoagulant (e.g., sodium citrate in Westergren method changes red cell/plasma ratio, which increases the ESR.

Q.7 What is rouleaux formation? What are the factors that increase the rate of rouleaux formation and hence the ESR?
See Q/A 6 above.

Q.8 Name the physiological and pathological variations in ESR.

A. *Physiological Variations in ESR.*
1. **Age.** ESR is low in infants (0.5 mm 1st hour Westergren) because of polycythemia. It gradually increases to adult levels in the next few years. However, it starts to increase after the age of 50 years.
2. **Sex.** The ESR is somewhat higher in females, probably due to lower hematocrit (PCV).
3. **High altitude.** People living at high altitudes have relatively higher ESR. (Polycythemia due to hypoxia actually should decrease ESR).
4. **Pregnancy.** The ESR begins to rise after about 3rd month of pregnancy and returns to normal a few weeks after delivery. Hemodilution during pregnancy and increased fibrinogen: albumin ratio are probably the cause of increased rouleaux formation.
5. **Body temperature.** Within limits, ESR varies with body temperature, which tends to affect viscosity.

B. Pathological *Increase in ESR.*
ESR is increased in any condition that is associated with inflammation and tissue damage. It is seen in:
1. *All acute and chronic infections (localized or generalized):* For example, pneumonia, tuberculosis, and acute episodes in chronic infections.

2. All *anemias* except spherocytosis, sickle cell anemia, and pernicious anemia.

3. *Bone diseases:* Tuberculosis, osteomyelitis.

4. *Connective tissue diseases (collagen vascular diseases):* Systemic lupus erythematosis, an rheumatoid arthritis.

5. *All malignant diseases (cancers):* For example, carcinoma of breast, leukemias, especially when they have spread to other parts of the body.

6. *Acute non-infective inflammation:* For example, gout.

7. *Nephrosis:* Marked decrease in albumin level (due to loss in urine), and increase in fibrinogen and globulins raise the ESR.

8. *Trauma, surgery, etc.* Any large-scale tissue injury raises ESR.

C. Pathological Decrease in ESR

1. **Polycythemia.** High red cell counts associated with hypoxia due to heart and lung diseases, such as congestive heart failure (CHF), congenital heart diseases, sever emphysema, etc., show a low ESR.

2. **Anemias:** spherocytosis, pernicious anemia, sickle cell anemia.

3. **Afibrinogenemia.** Decrease or absence of fibrinogen in plasma, which is a genetic disorder, shows a low ESR.

4. **Other diseases.** Reduction of ESR in other diseases is quite rare, though it may be seen in association with sickle cell anemia, spherocytosis, and acholuric jaundice.

5. Severe allergic reactions.

Q. 9 What is the clinical significance of ESR?

1. **As an indicator of bodily reaction to tissue injury and inflammation.** The ESR values are not diagnostic i.e., they will not tell the name of the disease that is causing a raised ESR. It is a sensitive indicator of tissue damage, just as leucocytosis and fever are not diseases but indicate tissue damage, infection, etc. Thus, ESR is raised in all **organic (pathological) conditions** in contrast to **functional disorders** (e.g., anxiety neurosis, hypochondria) where it is normal.

In fact, when ESR is raised, a diagnosis of functional disease should never be made. One must try to exclude organic disease by all possible tests. (In such cases ESR test is repeated). There may be patients where vague symptoms may only require reassurance—if the ESR were not raised. In such cases the cause may turn out to be a cancer, collagen disease, or some other serious condition.

2. **Value of ESR as a prognostic tool.** ESR is a valuable prognostic test in following the course of a disease, such as tuberculosis, rheumatoid arthritis, etc., while a patient is on treatment. If a weekly ESR shows a trend towards a decrease, it would indicate an improvement. But if the ESR shows an increase, it would mean that the disease is deteriorating.

3. **Since ESR increases with age,** the upper limit of normal can be calculated as:

Males   = Age ÷ 2,
Females   = Age + 10 ÷ 2.

Note

If the ESR is near the upper limit, the test is repeated after a month or so. Also, the correction factor to allow for anemia should be applied.

Blood Grouping
(Syn: Blood Typing)

Relevance.

Principle.

Apparatus and materials.

Procedures.

   Preparation of red cell suspension.

   Determination of blood groups.

Observations and results.

Agglutination.

No agglutination.

Precautions.

Questions.

Relevance

Blood transfusion is a life-saving procedure in all cases of severe loss of blood, and in life-threatening anemias. However, blood can only be given after blood grouping which is an essential requirement before blood is given to any individual. Blood grouping is also done to settle paternity disputes and other medicolegal purposes.

PRINCIPLE

The surfaces of red cell membrane contain a variety of genetically determined antigens, called **isoantigens** or **agglutinogens**, while the plasma contains antibodies **(agglutinins)**. To determine the blood group of a person, his/her red cells are made to react with commercially available antisera containing known agglutinins. The slide is then examined under the microscope to detect the presence or absence of clumping and hemolysis (agglutination) of red cells which occurs as a result of antigen-antibody reaction.

APPARATUS AND MATERIALS

1. Microscope. •Glass dropper with a long nozzle. •Sterile blood lancet or needle. •Sterile cotton/gauze swabs. •Alcohol. •5 ml test tube. •Toothpicks.
2. Clean, dry microscope slides. (A special porcelain tile with 12 depressions is available for this purpose and may be used in place of glass slides.)
3. 1% sodium citrate in normal saline (or normal saline alone).
4. **Anti-A serum:** [contains monoclonal anti-A antibodies (against human); these antibodies are also called anti-A or alpha (α) agglutinins]. The anti-A serum can also be obtained from a person with blood group B. (see Q/A 6).
5. **Anti-B serum:** [contains monoclonal anti-B antibodies (against human); these antibodies are also called anti-B or beta (β) agglutinins]. The anti-B serum can also be obtained from a person with blood group A. (see Q/A 6).

6. **Anti-D (anti-Rh) serum:** [Contains mono-clonal anti-Rh (D) antibodies (against human). These antibodies are also called anti-D agglutinins.]

Note

The antibodies against Rh factor do not occur naturally (see below)

Note

These antisera are available commercially. For a quick identification, the anti-A serum is tinted blue, anti-B serum yellow, while the anti-D serum is colorless.

CAUTION
Do not interchange the droppers provided with antisera bottles.

PROCEDURES

1. Using a glass-marking pencil, divide 3 slides, each into two halves by a line drawn down the middle (the left sides will act as "test sides" and right sides as the "control sides"). Mark the left corner of 1st slide anti-A, left corner of 2nd slide "anti-B, and the left corner of 3rd slide "anti-D". Mark the right corners of these 3 slides 'C' (for control).

2. Mark another slide (4th) 'S' (for only red cell suspension in saline, i.e., no antiserum will be added on this slide).

3. Place 8-10 drops of saline in the center of slide 'S'.

4. Preparation of red cell suspension. A suspension of red cells in saline should preferably be prepared and used instead of adding blood drops directly from the fingerpick to the antisera for the following reasons:

a. Dilution of blood permits easy detection of agglutination and hemolysis, if present. (Red cells in undiluted blood tend to form large rouleaux and masses. These may be difficult to disperse and may be mistaken for agglutination).

b. Plasma factors likely to interfere with agglutination are eliminated.

5. Get a finger-prick under aseptic conditions, and add 2 drops of blood to the saline on the slide marked 'S'. Mix the saline and blood with a clean glass dropper to get a suspension of red cells. You may use a toothpick for this purpose.

- A better method is to place 2 ml of saline in a small (5 ml) test tube. Then get a finger pricked and allow a blood drop to form. Now place the pricked fingertip on top of the test tube and invert it. Mix the blood and saline by inverting the tube 2 or 3 times. A suspension of red cells is now ready.

- Washed red cell suspension gives the best results. The red cells are "washed" in saline by centrifuging the diluted blood, removing the supernatant, and adding fresh saline to get a suspension of "washed" red cells.

6. Determination of Blood group.
Put one drop of anti-A serum on the left half ("test side") of 1st slide (marked anti-A), one drop of anti-B serum on the left half of 2nd slide (marked anti-B), and one drop of anti-D serum on the left half of 3rd slide (marked anti-D).

7. Put one drop each of normal saline on the "control" sides (right halves) of the 3 slides (i.e., areas marked 'C').

8. Add a drop each of red cell suspension (from the slide 'S', or from the test tube of red cell suspension) on anti-A, one drop on anti-B and one drop on anti-D sera, and one drop each on the normal saline taken on the "control" sides of the 3 slides.

In this way, the red cells-saline mixture on the "control" sides of each slide will act as a control to confirm *agglutination* or *no agglutination* on the corresponding test side.

9. Mix the anti-sera and red cells, and saline and red cells on each slide by gently tilting it first one way and then the other a few times. Take utmost care that the "test" mixtures and "control" mixtures do not flow into each other and get mixed up.

- The red cells and sera can also be mixed by gently blowing on them. You may use 3 separate toothpicks to transfer red cell suspension to the three anti-sera, and for mixing them, and 3 toothpicks to transfer red cells to saline drops taken on the "control" sides of the 3 slides.

10. Wait for 8-10 minutes, then inspect the 3 antisera-red cell mixtures ("test" mixtures) and "control" mixtures, first with the naked eye to see whether agglutination (clumping and hemolysis of red cells) has taken place or not. Then confirm under low magnification microscope, comparing each "test mixture" with its corresponding "control mixture".

OBSERVATIONS AND RESULTS

It is essential that you should be able to distinguish between "*agglutination*" and "*no agglutination*". The features of each are:

Agglutination.

  i. If agglutination occurs, it is usually visible to the naked eye. The hemolysed red cells appear as isolated (separate), dark-red masses (clumps) of different sizes and shapes.
 ii. There is brick-red coloring of the serum by the hemoglobin released from ruptures red cells.
iii. Tilting or rocking the slide a few times, or blowing on it does not break or disperse the clumps.
 iv. Under LP objective, the clumps are visible as dark masses and the outline of the red cells cannot be seen.

Grading of Agglutination Reaction. The agglutination reaction may be graded according to whether there is a single large agglutinate (4+), or a number of large (3+), medium or small masses with no free red cells (2+), or many small aggregates in the background of free red cells (1+).

No Agglutination

  i. In the "control" mixtures, the red cells may form a bunch, or rouleaux. These sedimented red cells give an orange tinge of a suspension of red cells rather than "isolated dark red masses" of ruptured red cells.
 ii. The red cells will disperse if you gently blow on the slides, or tilt them a few times.

Confirm all these features of "no agglutination" under the microscope.

PRECAUTIONS

1. The slides should be dry, dust-free and grease-free.
2. Identify and mark all slides, containers, and test tubes clearly and legibly. Double-check every step of the procedure.
3. The droppers supplied with the antisera bottles should not be interchanged.
4. Examine the slides with the naked eye and then under the microscope after 8-10 minutes but before the sera-blood mixtures dry up.
5. Do not add undiluted blood from the finger-prick directly on to the antisera for 2 reasons, one, the sera may get intermixed, and two, false positive reaction may develop. Sometimes it is not possible to say with certainty whether agglutination has occurred or not. In such cases the grouping must be repeated with diluted blood.

QUESTIONS

Q. 1 What is a blood group system? What is the physiological and genetic basis of blood grouping?
The surfaces of human red cells contain a variety of genetically determined glycolipids and glycoproteins that act as antigens. The plasma contains antibodies that can react with these

TABLE 1.3

Determination of blood groups					
(+) denotes agglutination				*(–) denotes no agglutination*	
Agglutination		*Your blood group is*	*Your RBCs contain agglutinogens*	*Your Plasma contains agglutinins*	*Your plasma will agglutinate RBCs of group*
Anti-A serum	*Anti-B serum*				
+	–	A	A	Anti-B	B, AB
–	+	B	B	Anti-A	A, AB
+	+	AB	A, B	None	None
–	–	O	O	Both anti-A and anti-B	A, B, AB

Similarly, for Rh(D) blood group:

Agglutination   +   Your RBCs contain
                                            Rh(D) antigen.   You are Rh(D) +ve

No agglutination   –   No Rh(D) antigen
                                            in your red cells.   You are Rh(D) –ve

Note
- Agglutinin against agglutinogen not present in the red cells is present in the plasma of each type.
- There are no naturally occurring antibodies against Rh(D) antigen.
- It is obvious from the above that if a known type of 'A' or 'B' blood is available, it is possible to determine the blood group of any unknown person.

antigens when the two are mixed. Since the red cell antigens cause agglutination of RBCs in the presence of suitable antibodies, they are also called *agglutinogens*; the antibodies in the plasma are called *agglutinins*.

Blood Group Systems

A group of related red cell antigens that show similar chemical, genetic, and reactivity properties constitutes a *"blood group system"*. Within a blood group (e.g., ABO system), there may be more than two or more different *"blood types"* (e.g., A, B, O, AB). However, the terms blood groups and blood types are often used synonymously.

There are at least 30 commonly occurring antigens and hundreds of rare antigens that have been found on the surfaces of human red cell membranes. Of different blood group systems, only two are of great clinical importance. These are the *ABO system* and the *Rh system.* Other blood group systems are: MN, Lutheran, Kell, Colton, Duffy,

Kid, Diego, Lewis, Li, Yt, Xg, P, C, etc. These groups are of little importance because they are not antigenic, though they are of value in anthropological and genetic studies. Some of these function as cell recognition molecules.

Physiological Basis of ABO System

The antigens A and B are complex oligosaccharides differing in their terminal sugars. Those found on red cells are glycolipids, while those found in tissues and body fluids are, soluble glycoproteins. The fucose-containing **H antigen is the basic antigen and is found in all individuals.** In the case of antigen A, a transferase places N-acetylgalactosamine as the terminal sugar on antigen H. In antigen B, the terminal sugar is galactose. In AB persons both transferases are present, while group O individuals have none of the enzymes so that the **antigen H persists in them.** Normally, H antigen has no antigenic activity and, as a result, it is identified by the capital letter O. Since

H antigen is not antigenic, there are no corresponding antibodies. (It seems that group O persons produce a protein that has no transferase activity; this results from single base deletion in the corresponding gene).

Genetic Basis of ABO System

The blood group (type) of a person is determined by two genes, one on each of two paired chromosomes. These genes can be any one of 3 types— A, B, or O, but only one type is present on each of the two chromosomes. The O gene is functionless and does not produce O antigen on red cells, while A and B genes produce strong antigens on red cells. Thus, there are 6 possible combinations of genes – AA, BB, AB, OA, OB, and OO—and each person is one of these 6 genotypes. A person with genotype O has no antigen on red cells and so the blood group is O. A person with genotype AA or OA is blood group A, while genotype BB or OB is blood group B.

Subgroups of A and B blood groups have been described, the most important being A_1 and A_2. The difference between these two, however, is said to be quantitative: each A_1 red cell has about 1 million copies of A antigen, while each A_2 red cell has about 250,000 antigen molecules.

Agglutinins of ABO System

The antibodies in the plasma (they are gamma globulins) are the reciprocal of the A and B antigens. The agglutinin reacting with antigen A is called anti-A (or alpha, α), that reacting with B antigen is called anti-B (or beta, β). The antigen O (H antigen) has no corresponding agglutinins. *These antibodies are present without any specific red cell antigenic stimulus.* For example, they are absent in a newborn; the ABO antibodies start appearing in the plasma by the age of 3-4 months due to cross reactivity of ABO antigens present in naturally occurring bacteria, viruses, pollen, etc. present in the environment (See Q/A 3 for details).

Q. 2 What is meant by the terms "secretors" and "non-secretors"?

The antigens A and B are present not only on red cells, but also in other tissues such as: liver, salivary glands, kidney, pancreas, etc. and body fluids such as: saliva: pancreatic juice, semen, amniotic fluid of some persons. Individuals who have high concentrations of these antigens in their body fluids are called "secretors". Those with low concentrations are called "non-secretors".

It may be noted that A, B, and H antigens are also present in blood platelets, endothelial cells, plant products, the cell walls of bacteria, and in house dust. (As pointed out in Q/A 21 in Expt. 1-12 the HLA antigens, also called MHC, are present on the surfaces of all body cells except red cells. The RBCs have blood group antigens as discussed above).

Q. 3 How can antibodies be present in a person when the corresponding antigens are absent? (i.e., why are anti-A antibodies present in a person whose blood group is B, while the Antigen A is absent in that person).

The specific blood group antibodies are absent at birth. However, they are produced in the next few weeks/months, reaching a maximum by the age of 10 years. These antibodies are produced in response to A and or B antigens (or antigens very similar to these) which are present in intestinal bacteria, or are taken in foods, such as seeds, plants, and in house dust. These antigens are absorbed into blood and stimulate the formation of antibodies against **antigens not present in the infants' red cells,** i.e., those antigens that are recognized as "non-self" by the body's immune system.

(An example will show how specific antibodies appear during infancy and perhaps continue to be formed later on. An adult of blood type A has agglutinogen A on the red cells, and anti-B antibodies in plasma. Now, where did these antibodies come from when there was no antigen B in that person? During infancy, ingestion of antigens A and B in food caused the formation of anti-A and anti-B antibodies. The soluble antigen A in the blood and tissue fluids neutralized anti-A antibodies which disappeared from plasma while anti-B antibodies persisted. Similarly, in blood type O, both anti-A and anti-B antibodies are formed and persist since neither antigen A nor B are present to neutralize either of the antibodies.

Q. 4 What is Landsteiner Law? How does it apply to all blood groups?

The Landsteiner Law (1900), which has 2 major components, states that:

1. If an agglutinogen is present on the red cells of an individual, the corresponding agglutinins must be absent in the plasma.
2. If an agglutinogen is absent in the red cells, the corresponding agglutinins must be present in the plasma.

The first part of the statement is a logical outcome of the situation because if both agglutinogen and agglutinins were present, the red cells would be agglutinated. The second part of the statement is a fact (for ABO system) but not a necessary outcome because if the agglutinogen is absent from the red cells, the agglutinins might well be absent. The exception to this component of the law is that absence of Rh agglutinogen from the red cells in Rh -ve persons is not accompanied by the presence of anti-Rh agglutinins. Obviously, this component of the law was enunciated before the discovery of Rh factor in 1940 by Landsteiner and Weiner.

Q. 5 What are cold and warm antibodies?

The terms 'cold' and 'warm' antibodies are applied to the antibodies of the ABO and Rh systems of blood groups respectively. Their important features are:

ABO system anti-bodies	Rh system anti-bodies
1. The antibodies anti-A and anti-B are of the larger IgM type. They cannot cross the placenta.	1. Rh antibodies are of the IgG type. They can easily cross the placenta.
2. These antibodies react best with the antigens at low temperatures of 5-20°C. They are, therefore, called 'cold' antibodies.	2. The antigen-antibody reactions occur best at body temperature. Hence they are called 'warm' antibodies.

Contd...

Contd...

ABO system anti-bodies	Rh system anti-bodies
3. ABO incompatibility between a mother and her fetus rarely causes any problems.	3. Rh incompatibility between a mother and her fetus may cause serious complications.

Q. 6 How are antisera A and B obtained?

The antisera can be obtained from the humans or from animals:

1. Antisera can be obtained from the clotted blood of individuals of blood group A (anti-B serum), and of blood group B (anti-A serum). However, since an antigen has many epitopes, a variety of antibodies against the antigen are produced. Also, since the titre (concentration) of antibodies is variable, monoclonal antibodies are used.

2. **Monoclonal antibodies.** If a single plasma cell could be isolated, it could be made to proliferate in a tissue culture and produce large quantities of identical antibodies. However, plasma cells and lymphocytes are difficult to grow in culture. The problem is solved as follows: Animals are immunized with a particular antigen, then they are sacrificed. The antibody-producing plasma cells are extracted from the spleen and fused with myeloma cells. (The myeloma cells are B lymphocytes that are easy to grow and they proliferate endlessly). The fused cells are separated by special techniques and each starts a clone of cells descended from a single cell. Thus, large amounts of antibodies can be obtained.

Q. 7 What is the importance of using a control on each of the 3 test slides? What are false positive and false negative results?

The control in each case is only a suspension of red cells in saline. Its purpose is to avoid "false positive" and "false negative" results.

False Positive Reaction. It means that though here is no actual agglutination, the reaction appears to be so. Formation of large rouleaux (this may happen if undiluted blood is used) may give a false impression of agglutination, but the cells will quickly disperse on tilting the slide a few times. Bacterial contamination of an antiserum, or of normal saline, may show agglutination in all tests or in all controls.

False Negative Reaction. It may occur due to loss of potency of the antisera because of faulty storage. All tests will come out negative with such an antiserum.

> **Note**
> In hospitals and blood banks where blood is to be collected for transfusion, the antisera are tested every day before using them for blood grouping/typing.

Q. 8 What is the difference between agglutination and Rouleaux formation? How will you confirm that agglutination has occurred on the microscope slide?

See page 105 for the difference between agglutination and rouleaux formation. The agglutination is always confirmed under the microscope.

Q. 9 What is zone phenomenon?

For agglutination to occur, the concentration of agglutinogens and agglutinins has to be about the same. If the difference is too much, there may be a doubtful reaction.

Q. 10 Why should you wait for 8-10 minutes before checking for agglutination?

This much time is required for antigen-antibody reaction to occur.

Q. 11 Why should the red cell-antiserum mixture be examined before it dries up?

If the mixture dries up, the dried red cells may form masses which may be confused for agglutination.

Q.12 What is agglutination and what is its mechanism?

Agglutination, i.e., clumping and hemolysis of red cells, during antigen-antibody reaction occurs in 2 stages:

i. *Sensitization* The antibodies bind (attach) to the antigens on the red cell surfaces without causing clumping and hemolysis. A single ABO antibody (IgM type) has 10 binding sites and can thus cross-link 10 red cells, while the Rh antibody (IgG type) has 2 binding sites and can link 2 red cells.

ii. *Agglutination.* Immediately after sensitization, the red cells form clumps or lattices, which is followed by hemolysis. The antigen-antibody reaction also activates the compliment system that releases proteolytic enzymes (the lytic complex) which ruptures the red cells and releases hemoglobin. (The hemolysis in circulating blood is more severe due to larger amounts of complement system proteins, as compared to that occurring on the slides).

Q. 13 What is cross matching?

The red cells and the plasma of the donor and recipient blood are separated by centrifugation. The donor red cells are then treated (tested) with the recipient plasma (**major side cross match**), and the donor plasma is tested against the red cells of the recipient (**minor cross match**). The whole process is called **"cross matching'**. If there is no agglutination in either case, the donor blood can safely be given to the recipient.

> **Note**
> Cross matching must always be done before every blood transfusion.

Q. 14 Why is the reaction between donor red cells and recipient plasma called "major cross match" and what is its significance?

The donor red cells are tested against recipient plasma to ensure that the recipient plasma does not contain antibodies that would react with the antigens on the donor red cells. In the case of a mismatch, the donor red cells will start to hemolyse with serious consequences as soon as they enter the recipient's circulation during a transfusion. Since the reaction between donor red cells and recipient plasma is of prime importance, it is called "major side cross match" or "major cross match".

Q. 15 Why is the reaction between donor plasma and recipient red cells called "minor cross match"?

The donor plasma is tested against the recipient red cells to test the potency (strength; ability to cause a reaction) of donor agglutinins. This reaction is not very important and usually does not occur even in a mismatch, because the agglutinins are greatly diluted in the recipient plasma. For example, about 200 ml of plasma in one unit of O group donor blood (which contains both anti-A and anti-B agglutinins) gets diluted in about 3000 ml of recipient plasma, and that also at a slow rate. Furthermore, the donor agglutinins are neutralized by the soluble antigens in the body fluids of the recipient. Thus, the donor agglutinins can usually be ignored, if their potency is not too high. It is for these two reasons that this reaction is called "minor cross match".

Q. 16 What is meant by the terms universal donor and universal recipient?

Since type O persons do not have either A or B antigens on their red cells, they are called "universal donors" because their blood can, theoretically, be given to all 4 blood types. Type AB persons are called 'universal recipients" because they do not have circulating agglutinins in their plasma and can, therefore, receive blood of any type. (Recall that it is the reaction between donor red cells and recipient plasma that is important in transfusion of blood).

In practice, however, the use of these terms was found to be misleading and dangerous. Transfusion reactions were common until the discovery of Rh factor in 1940 by Landsteiner and Weiner (see next Q/A). Then it was realized that the blood contains antigens and antibodies of blood groups other than the ABO system.

Note
Though it is a rule never to give blood without cross matching, an exception could be made in a most extreme emergency, where group O Rh –ve blood may be given immediately.

Q. 17 What is Rh factor and what is its clinical significance?

In addition to antigens of ABO system, the red cells of 80-85% of humans also contain an additional antigen, called Rh antigen (or Rh factor). The Rh factor is so named because this antigen was discovered in the rhesus monkey by Landsteiner and Weiner in 1940. They injected red blood cells of rhesus monkey (the common Indian variety with red ischial callosities) into rabbits. The rabbits immune system reacted by forming antibodies against rhesus red cells, and when the rabbit' plasma was tested against human red cells, agglutination occurred in 80-85% of individuals.

Persons whose red cells contain this additional antigen are called **"Rh positive" (Rh +ve, Rh +)** while those who lack this antigen are called **"Rh negative" (Rh –ve, Rh –).**

There are several varieties of Rh antigen—C, D, E, c, d, and e—but the D antigen is the most common, and antigenically, the most potent. Therefore, Rh +ve persons are also called D +ve and Rh –ve are called D –ve. The antibody of D antigen is called anti-D antibody (anti-Rh antibody). **However, there are no naturally occurring antibodies against Rh (D) antigen. The Rh (D) antigen is not present in body fluids and tissues, but only on red cells.** This antigen is 'warm' antigen and can cross the placenta easily) .

Clinical Significance of Rh factor

Although there are no natural anti-Rh antibodies, and they never develop spontaneously, they can be produced only in Rh –ve persons. This can happen in either of 2 ways: one, when an Rh –ve person is given Rh +ve blood, and two, when an Rh –ve mother carries an Rh +ve fetus.

1. *In transfusions.* When an Rh –ve person receives Rh +ve blood, there is no immediate reaction since there are no antibodies. But during

the next few weeks/months, he/she may produce anti-Rh antibodies that will remain in the blood. (Even 0.5 ml of Rh +ve blood is enough to produce immune response). However, if within a few weeks, or even years later, a second Rh +ve blood is injected, the newly donated red cells will be agglutinated and hemolysed, thus resulting in a serious transfusion reaction.

2. In pregnancy. The most common problem due to Rh incompatibility may arise when an Rh –ve mother (phenotype dd) carries an Rh +ve fetus (phenotype DD or Dd).

Normally, no direct contact occurs between maternal and fetal bloods. However, if a small amount of Rh +ve blood leaks from the fetus through the placenta into the mother's blood, the mother's immune system will start to make anti-Rh antibodies.

This happens at the time of delivery when small amounts of fetal blood leak into the mother as the placenta separates from the uterine wall. As a result, some mothers develop high concentration of anti-Rh antibodies during the period following delivery. Therefore, the first-born baby will not be affected, unless the mother has previously received Rh +ve blood transfusion.

There are cases of fetal-placental bleeding during pregnancy itself when fetal blood may enter the mother's circulation. During the first pregnancy, however, the anti-Rh antibody levels do not reach high enough levels to cause complications. However, during the second and subsequent pregnancies, the mother's anti-Rh antibodies cross the placental membrane into the fetus where they cause agglutination and hemolysis. The clinical condition that develops in the fetus is called " *hemolytic disease of the newborn (HDN)'* or *"erythroblastosis fetalis"*

Chief Clinical Forms of HDN The chief clinical forms (syndromes) of HDN are:

1. *Hydrops fetalis.* If the hemolysis in the fetus is severe, it may die in the uterus, or the fetus may develop anemia, severe jaundice, and gross edema.
2. *Icterus gravis neonatorum* (grave jaundice of the new born). Though the infant is born at term, there is jaundice (hemolytic jaundice), or becomes so within a day or so. Anemia may be absent for a few days though reticulocyte count is high, and many nucleated red cells (erythroblasts) are present (hence the term "erythroblastosis fetalis").
3. *Kernicterus.* In the adults, the bile pigments cannot cross the blood-brain barrier (BBB) but in infants the BBB is not fully developed so that these pigments may pass into the brain and get deposited in the basal ganglia, giving them a bright yellow color. The neurological syndrome of kernicterus is rarely a complication of "physiological jaundice of the new born" because there is no hypoxic stimulus. Also the bilirubin level is not as high as in HDN (The physiological jaundice is due to immaturity of the liver and disappears in a few days).

Q. 18 If an Rh –ve mother carries Rh +ve fetus, what are the complications that are likely to occur?
See Q/A 17 above.

Q. 19 When an Rh +ve mother carries Rh –ve fetus, why are there no complications?
The Rh +ve red cells of the mother cannot cross the placenta into the fetus. But even if small amounts of maternal blood do leak into the fetus as a result of placental hemorrhage at any time during pregnancy, the fetus cannot respond by forming anti-Rh antibodies. The reason for this is that **the ability to respond to foreign antigens develops after birth.** However, when it does develop in later life, transfusion of Rh +ve blood will evoke anti-Rh antibody production.

Q. 20 What is hemolytic disease of the newborn? What are the forms in which this condition may be manifested?
See Q/A 17 above.

Q. 21 What is the probability of the occurrence of hemolytic disease of the newborn when the father is Rh +ve and the mother is Rh –ve?
The blood group antigens are a result of gene action. The gene related to D antigen is called **D.**

When **D** is absent from a chromosome, its alternate form (allelomorph), called **d**, takes its place. The Rh genes of a person are inherited from both parents. If the genes carried by the sperm and ovum are identical, the offspring is homozygous (**DD** or **dd**). Thus, if both carry **D** gene, all the offspring will be DD (homozygous D+; Rh +ve). If one carries **D** and the other carries **d**, the offspring will be heterozygous D+ (Rh +ve). If both ovum and sperm carry **d**, the offspring will be homozygous D –ve (Rh –ve).

Therefore, if the father's genotype is Dd, the offspring may be Rh +ve (Dd) or Rh –ve (dd), but if the genotype is DD, all offspring will be Rh +ve. Thus, the probability of HDN when the father is Rh +ve will depend on whether he is Dd (Rh +ve) or DD (Rh +ve).

Q. 22 How can hemolytic disease of the new-born be prevented? What is the treatment of severe HDN?

The hemolysis of red cells (HDN) is due to the crossing over of anti-Rh antibodies from the Rh –ve mother (through the placenta) into the Rh +ve fetus. The condition can be prevented by desensitizing all Rh –ve mothers by giving them injections of massive doses of anti-Rh antibodies called **anti-Rh gamma globulin (RhoGAM)** after every abortion, miscarriage, or delivery. These antibodies bind to and inactivate the fetal Rh antigens (on fetal red cells) present in maternal circulation. In this way, the Rh antigens from the mother's blood are cleared (removed) before they have had time to stimulate production of anti-Rh antibodies.

(Fetal Rh typing is now possible with samples of amniotic fluid or chorionic villi, and treatment with a small dose of Rh immune serum can prevent sensitization of mother during pregnancy. It is not known how this is achieved but one effect of anti-D antibody is to inhibit antigen-induced B lymphocyte antibody production. It also attaches to D antigen sites on fetal red cells in mother's blood).

Treatment of severe HDN. The best treatment for a severe case of HDN is to successively withdraw small amounts of fetal blood and to replace them with equal amounts of **compatible Rh –ve blood**. Of course, this **exchange transfusion** does not change the inherited blood group of the infant. It only removes the red cells that are destined to be hemolysed.

Q.23 Why does the ABO-incompatibility rarely produce hemolytic disease of the newborn?

The ABO-incompatibility between the mother and fetus rarely causes HDN. The reason is that the anti-A and anti-B (anti-ABO) antibodies belong to IgM type of gamma globulins (cold antibodies) that do not cross the placenta.

Q. 24 What is the incidence of blood types in Indian and a few other populations?

The frequency distribution of blood groups is shown in Table 1.4.

	TABLE 1.4

Frequency distribution of blood groups						
Population	*ABO system (%)*				*Rh system (%)*	
	A	*B*	*AB*	*O*	*Rh +ve*	*Rh -ve*
Indians	21	39	9	31	95	5
White	45	40	11	4	85	15
Black	49	27	20	4	95	5
Chinese	42	27	25	4	100	-
British	42	9	3	46	85	15

Q. 25 What is the importance of blood grouping?

Blood grouping/typing is important in:-
1. Blood transfusion for treatment purposes.
2. Determination of Rh incompatibility between the mother and child.
3. **Paternity disputes.** The ABO, Rh, and MNS blood grouping is used to settle cases of disputed paternity. Antigens A and B are dominant, whereas O is recessive. It is possible to prove that a person

could not have been the father, but nor that he was/is the father. (**"DNA finger printing"** is now a recognised procedure for settling such disputes. It can prove fatherhood with 100% accuracy).
4. Choice of a donor in tissue/organ transplantation.
5. **Genetic studies.**
6. **Medico legal use.** Any red stain on a clothing may be claimed to be blood by a supposed victim. Therefore, it is first confirmed that it really is human blood. Blood grouping of the extracted sample can then prove or disprove the claim of the victim. In doubtful cases, the DNA fingerprinting can decide the claim one way or the other.
7. **Susceptibility to disease.** The people of blood type O are more susceptible to peptic ulcer. Blood type A is more commonly seen in carcinoma of stomach, and to some extent in diabetes mellitus.

Q. 26 How is blood volume supplemented?
The total blood volume, plasma volume, or packed cell volume may be greatly reduced under certain circumstances. Thus, (i) The blood volume may be greatly reduced in cases of severe hemorrhage, (ii) plasma volume may be reduced in severe burns (plasma seeps out), prolonged vomiting or diarrhea, or excessive sweating, and, (iii) red cell volume may be reduced in cases of anemia. The blood volume can be supplemented by various solutions, plasma or whole blood (see Q/A 36).

Q. 27 What are the indications for blood transfusion?
1. **Acute hemorrhage.** Acute loss of blood resulting from accidents, during surgery, ruptured peptic ulcer and aortic aneurysm, ectopic pregnancy, etc. are some of the conditions which may cause hemorrhagic shock, and therefore, need immediate blood transfusion. Cross-matched blood is always given, but if the situation is desperate, group O blood may be given to raise blood pressure. In burns, blood may be given though plasma is preferred.
2. **Chronic anemias that cannot be treated with diet and drugs.** Packed red cells (Hct about 70%) can be transfused when a quick restoration of Hb

is required, as in pregnancy, emergency surgery, etc.
3. **Exchange transfusion.** It is employed in hemolytic disease of the newborn (consult Q/A 22).
4. *Bleeding disorders.* Fresh blood or platelet concentrates are given in purpura. Fresh frozen plasma, or cryoprecipitate is given in hemophilia and other clotting factor deficiencies.
5. **Granulocyte transfusion.** It is needed in cases of neutropenia (TLC < 500/mm^3) with severe bacterial infection.
6. *Bone marrow depression* due to any cause and infiltration by carcinoma cells.
7. **Autologous transfusion** (see below;Q/A 28).

Q. 28 What is autologous transfusion?
In addition to receiving blood from a donor, an individual may also receive one's own stored blood, (i.e., during elective surgery on a pre-selected day in the future), a procedure called **predonation.** (The popularity of this procedure is that it avoids the hazards of AIDS, hepatitis, etc as well as risk of transfusion reaction).

Predonation. It is a form of autologous transfusion and is a common practice in some hospitals. After starting a course of iron tablets, two units of blood are collected, one 16 days before the operation, and the other eight days later. An important technical innovation is the cell-saver machine which sucks up blood from the wound during the operation, recycles it, and returns it to the patient's body.

Q. 29 What is blood doping? When is it employed?
Blood doping is the procedure in which some athletes used to get a unit or two of their own blood (or red cells) removed and stored for a few weeks. It was then reinjected in 2-3 sessions a few days before an event. Since oxygen delivery to active muscles is the limiting factor, increased red cell count was expected to enhance their performance, especially in endurance event. The procedure was (and is) dangerous since it increases the load on the heart due to increased blood volume or

viscosity. The International Olympic Committee has banned blood doping.

Q. 30 What are the hazards (dangers) of blood transfusion?

1. *Transmission of disease.* The donated blood has the potential of transmitting some serious diseases. It is therefore mandatory to test the blood for HIV antibodies (for AIDS), hepatitis B surface antigen, HCV antibodies, syphilis (VDRL test), and malarial parasite.

2. *Incompatibility due to mismatched transfusion* This is the most serious and potentially fatal complication. Whether the transfusion reactions are immediate or delayed, as well as their severity is determined by the speed and extent of hemolysis of donated red cells.

   i. *Body aches and pains.* Within a short time of starting the transfusion, the patient complains of severe pain in the back, limbs, or chest, and a sense of suffocation and tightness in the chest. These symptoms are due to blockage of capillaries by clumps of agglutinated cells. Chills and fever generally accompany pains.

   ii. *Renal failure.* Acute renal failure (kidney shutdown) appears to result from 3 main causes:

      a. Substance of immune reaction and toxic substances released from hemolysing blood cause powerful renal vasocons-triction.

      b. These substances and decrease in circulating red cells frequently cause circulatory shock. The arterial blood pressure falls to very low levels, and renal blood flow and urine output decrease.

      c. If the amount of free Hb in plasma is small, then whatever is filtered is reabsorbed. If this amount is large, it gets precipitated in and blocks many tubules. The result of all these factors is acute renal failure and death may occur in 8-10 days, if the shutdown is not resolved or treated with dialysis.

3. *Faulty technique of transfusion.* Cardiac arrhythmias, cardiac arrest, or circulatory overload may occur, especially in elderly patients of chronic anemia, heart or kidney diseases, if repeated transfusions are given, say, in 24 hours. *Thrombophlebitis* may occur if the intravenous needle remains in the same site for many hours. *Air embolism,* i.e., entry of air into blood via the intra-venous needle is much less likely to occur because of the use of plastic bags (instead of glass bottles) which collapse down as they empty out of blood.

4. *Allergic reactions.* Reactions such as skin rashes and asthma may occur if the donor blood contains substances to which the patient is sensitive.

5. *Pyrogen reactions.* Reactions such as chills and fever are probably due to the presence of antibodies to leucocytes and platelets.

6. *Tetany.* With massive transfusions, the normal conversion of citrate to bicarbonate in the tissues may be delayed. This will result in fall in plasma ionic calcium and hence tetany.

7. *Iron overload.* Repeated transfusions in the absence of blood loss may lead to hemochromato-sis.

Q. 31 What precautions are taken while selecting a blood donor?

The following precautions are observed:

1. The donor should be healthy, and aged between 18 and 60 years. Pregnant and lactating women are excluded.

2. The donor should be screened for com-municable diseases such as AIDS, hepatitis, syphilis, malaria, etc). The malarial parasite can survive at 4° C for 3 weeks.

3. The donor's Hb should be within the normal range (usually above 12.5 g%). Its level is tested with the copper sulphate specific gravity method.

4. Professional donors must be discouraged for reasons that are well known.

Q. 32 What are blood banks? How is donated blood stored? What is the fate of transfused citrate in the body?

With the modern surgical and medical procedures, the demand for blood has greatly increased. It is for this reason that blood banks were started where blood from voluntary donors could be stored, so that it was always available on demand. Most blood banks have lists of would-be donors so that they may be contacted when required.

Storage of blood. After a donor has been screened for donation, one unit of blood (450 ml) is collected, under aseptic conditions, from the antecubital vein directly into a special plastic bag containing 63 ml of CPD-A (citrate-phosphate-dextrose-adenine) mixture. The blood bag is suitably sealed, labeled, and stored at 4° C, where it can be kept for about 20 days. (Faulty storage, i.e., overheating or freezing can lead to gross infection and hemolysis).

The *citrate* prevents clotting of blood, *sodium diphosphate* acts as a buffer to control decrease in pH, *dextrose* supports ATP generation via glycolytic pathway and also provides energy for Na^+- K^+ pump that maintains the size and shape of red cells and increases their survival time, and *adenine* provides substrate for the synthesis of ATP, thus improving post-donation viability of red cells.

Blood is stored at low temperatures for 2 reasons: one, it decreases bacterial growth, and two, it decreases the rate of glycolysis and thus prevents a quick fall in pH.

Changes in red cells during storage. Changes occur due to decreased metabolism, and include increase in their Na^+ and decrease in K^+ concentration due to reduced Na^+-K^+ pump activity, the result being a net increase in total base and water content of the cells that swell and become more spherocytic. The ATP content decreases and inorganic phosphate content increases.

Changes after transfusion. These changes occur within a day or so, the red cells lose sodium and gain potassium, with the volume, shape and fragility returning to normal. Their survival time increases if blood is given within a week of donation.

Fate of transfused citrate. The citrate (in the form of trisodium citrate) that is used to store blood can

safely be injected intravenously (oxalates are toxic). Within a few minutes, the liver removes citrate from blood and polymerizes it into glucose, or metabolizes it directly for energy. But if the liver is damaged, or if large amounts of citrate are injected too quickly, the citrate may lower the calcium level in blood to result in tetany, or even death from convulsions.

Blood substitutes Separate components of blood—packed RBCs, whole plasma (fresh frozen plasma, FFP) to provide clotting factors, platelets, leucocytes, plasma and plasma expanders are now available.

Q. 33 What is the only certain way of avoiding blood incompatibility?
1. The slides and containers must be properly labeled.
2. Cross matching is the only certain way of avoiding the dangers of mismatching.
3. Rh +ve blood should never be given to an Rh –ve female of any age before menopause.

Q. 34 Name the precautions you will observe before and during blood transfusion?
1. Blood should be transfused only when absolutely required.
2. It should be confirmed that cross matching has been done to exclude mismatching of groups other than ABO system.
3. The blood bag should be checked for the blood type indicated on it.
4. It should be confirmed that the blood has been checked for infections especially AIDS.
5. Rh +ve blood should never be given to an Rh –ve person.
6. Blood should never be transfused at a fast rate—usually not more than 20-25 drops per minute, unless otherwise indicated (as in acute and severe loss of blood where blood may have to be pumped into the patient). A rapid transfusion, under normal conditions, may cause chelation of calcium ions and tetany.

7. The condition of the recipient should be checked carefully for the first 10-15 minutes of starting the transfusion, and from time to time later on. The transfusion must be stopped if there is a rapid rise of temperature, (> 40°C), or any other reaction.

Q. 35 What are the earliest effects of a mis-matched transfusion?

Within a short time of starting the transfusion (i.e., when a few ml of blood have entered the recipient's body), there may be severe pain anywhere in the body, a sense of suffocation and tightness in the chest. There may be chills and shivering, fever, etc. (Consult Q/A 30 for details).

Q. 36 Which blood substitutes may be used to restore blood volume if suitable donor blood is not available?

The blood volume may be reduced due to hemorr-hage; plasma volume may be reduced due to burns, vomiting, or diarrhea. Therefore, the ideal treatment would depend on which body fluid needs replacement.

Whole blood. Though it is the ideal medium to replace lost blood because it replaces cells and plasma in physiological ratio, it may not be available. In such a situation, an intravenous drip of a crystalloid or colloid solution is immediately started. (This route is also available for any drug that may be needed, and of course, for later transfusions).

Crystalloid solutions. A commonly-used intra-venous fluid is glucose saline (6% glucose in 0.9% sodium chloride). However, since crystalloids leave the circulation within a short time, this solution restores the blood volume temporarily.

Colloid solutions. Various colloid substitutes are available to increase the plasma volume. They are called plasma expanders, and include human albumin, dextrose and dextrose with NaCl, and a polymer from degraded gelatin. Plasma separated from donated blood can be stored in a liquid form (fresh frozen plasma) for many months, and for a year if it is dried (it is reconstituted with distilled water just before use).

Q. 37 What is Bombay blood group?

This blood type is a rare phenomenon in which the H antigen is absent. Since there is no H antigen, there is no antigen A or antigen B on the red cells. However, the plasma contains anti-A, anti-B and anti-H antibodies. As a result, such a person can receive blood only from a person having Bombay blood type.

Q. 38 What is reverse blood typing?

The blood grouping (typing) procedure (already described) in which the red cells of a person (whose blood type is to be determined) are tested against anti-A and anti-B sera, is called "blood typing" or "forward blood typing".

In another but related procedure called "reverse blood typing" (also called "serum typing" or "backward blood typing") the serum of the would-be recipient is tested against red cells containing known antigens, i.e., red cells from persons with blood types A, B, AB, and O. If agglutination occurs with A and AB red cells, the blood type is B; if agglutination occurs with B and AB red cells, the blood type is A; if agglutination occurs with A, B, and AB red cells, the blood type is O and if there is no agglutination in any RBCs, the blood type is AB. [In AB blood type there are no antibodies in the plasma (serum)].

The serum typing is done along with blood typing as a precaution because in leukemias, the RBC antigens may become considerably weak. Also, in pseudomonas infection, the RBCs become agglutinated by all antisera due, probably, to unmasking of hidden antigens.

Tests for Hemostasis
(Bleeding time; coagulation time; Platelet count; and other tests)

Relevance
Coagulation time
Hemostasis.
Physiological basis of bleeding disorders.

Tests for hemostatic disorders.
Bleeding time.
 Duke bleeding time.
 Ivy bleeding time.
 Simplate method.
 Capillary fragility test

Platelet count
 Capillary blood clotting time.
 Venous blood clotting time.
 Clot retraction time
 Clot lysis time

Prothrombin time
Other tests
Questions.

Relevance

Bleeding after injury is a common experience for most of us. But bleeding stops automatically within a few minutes. However, suspicion of a disease arises when there is frequent and prolonged bleeding with minor injuries, such as during shaving, cutting of nails, or a fall on the knees. In others, there may be spontaneous bleeding (without any apparent trauma) in the skin, gums, or into joints, and muscles, etc. It is in all such cases that various tests are carried out.

Hemostasis

The term hemostasis (Gr. Haema= blood; stasis= halt) refers to the process of stoppage of bleeding after blood vessels are punctured, cut, or otherwise damaged. Hemostasis, which is a homeostatic mechanism to prevent loss of blood, is a result of a complex, natural, physiological response. The term is also used for surgical arrest of bleeding.

Hemostasis involves the following 4 inter-related steps:
1. Vasoconstriction (contraction of injured blood vessels).
2. Platelet plug formation.
3. Formation of a blood clot.
4. Fibrinolysis (dissolution of the clot).

PHYSIOLOGICAL BASIS OF BLEEDING DISORDERS

Excessive and prolonged bleeding with small injuries, or spontaneous bleeding my result from defects of:

i. Platelets.
ii. Blood vessel walls.
iii. Coagulation of blood.

DEFECTS OF PLATELETS AND VESSEL WALLS

Defects of platelets (i) and vessel walls (ii) typically cause spontaneous bleeding from small vessels, or during cuts and bruises (e.g., pinpoint or petechial hemorrhages and purpuric lesions in the skin (blue-red patches), and bleeding in the gums.

DEFECTS OF CLOTTING

Defects of clotting are of 2 types:
a. *Excessive bleeding into tissues* (muscles, joints, viscera, etc) is usually due to injury to relatively large vessels. The delay in the formation of a clot fails to support the normal action of platelets in checking blood loss. Deficiency of clotting factors—inherited or in liver disease (hepatitis, cirrhosis, vitamin K deficiency) are the usual causes.
b. *Thrombosis.* It is clotting of blood that occurs within unbroken blood vessels. A roughened endothelium due to arteriosclerosis, infection, or injury is the common cause.

TESTS FOR HEMOSTASIS

1. Bleeding time (BT).
2. Ivy bleeding time (hemostasis bleeding time).
3. Capillary fragility test of Hess (tourniquet test).
4. Platelet count.
5. Clotting time.
6. Clot retraction time (CRT).
7. Clot lysis time.
8. Prothrombin time.

Other tests. These include: platelet aggregation and adhesiveness tests, prothrombin consumption test, partial thromboplastin test, thrombin time (TT), plasma recalcification time (PRT), activated partial thromboplastin time (APTT), kaolin cephalin clotting time (KCCT), and special tests, including assaying of clotting factors.

BLEEDING TIME (BT) AND CLOTTING TIME (CT)

Bleeding Time (BT) is the time interval between the skin puncture and spontaneous, unassisted (i.e., without pressure) stoppage of bleeding. *The BT test is an in vitro test of platelet function.*

Clotting time (CT) is the time interval between the entry of blood into the glass capillary tube, or a syringe, and formation of fibrin threads.

Note
The BT and CT are two simple tests that are used as a routine before every minor and major surgery (e.g., tooth extraction), biopsy procedures, and before and during anticoagulant therapy, whether or not there is a history of bleeding.

BLEEDING TIME (BT)

[I] "Duke" Bleeding time (finger-tip; ear-lobe)
- Since the skin of the fingertip is quite thick in some persons, a small cut in the skin of the earlobe with the corner edge of a sterile blade gives better results. The earlobe method is the original "Duke" method for BT.
- Ask your partner to fill the capillary tube with blood from the same skin puncture from where you are doing the BT (see below for CT).

Materials • Equipment for sterile finger-prick. • Clean filter papers. • Chemically clean, 10-12 cm long, glass capillary tubes with a uniform bore diameter of 1-2 mm. • Stopwatch.

PROCEDURES

1. Get a deep finger-prick under aseptic conditions to get free-flowing blood. Start the stop watch and note the time.
2. Absorb/remove the blood drops every 30 seconds by touching the puncture site with the filter paper along its edges, without

pressing or squeezing the wound. Number the blood spots 1 onwards.

3. Note the time when bleeding stops, i.e., when there is no trace of blood spot on the filter paper. Encircle this spot and number it as well. This is the end point. (Do not keep the filter paper on the table and then press your wound on it).

4. Count the number of blood spots and express your result in minutes and seconds.

Note
Observe that the size of the blood spots gets smaller and smaller after the 1st or 2nd spot until there are none. This is so because bleeding may increase in the first minute or so after which it decreases and then stops.
• Put the title of the experiment and your name and date on the filter paper, get it signed from your tutor and paste it in your workbook.

Normal bleeding time = 1-5 minutes.
• The test is simple and quite reliable in spite of the fact that the depth of the wound cannot be controlled.
• The BT is prolonged in purpura (platelet deficiency, or vessel wall defects) while it is usually normal in hemophilia.
• Lack of several clotting factors may prolong BT, though it is especially prolonged by lack of platelets.

PRECAUTIONS

1. The skin site chosen for BT should be scrubbed well with alcohol to increase the blood flow.
2. The skin should be dry and the puncture should be 3-4 mm deep to give free-flowing blood. Do not squeeze.
3. Do not press the filter paper on the puncture site.
4. If bleeding continues for more than 10-12 minutes, stop the test and press a sterile gauze on the wound. Inform your teacher about the bleeding.

[II] Another method is to get a finger-prick and dip the finger in a beaker containing normal saline at 37°C. The blood drops will be seen falling to the bottom in a continuous stream. Note the time when bleeding stops.

[III] "Ivy" Bleeding Time (Hemostasis Bleeding Time).
This method is more reliable than the "Duke" method. However, it requires some practice to apply the BP cuff and maintain the pressure.

PROCEDURE

1. Clean the skin over the front of the forearm with 70% alcohol.
2. Apply a blood pressure cuff on the upper arm, raise the pressure to 40 mm Hg and maintain it there till the end of the experiment.
3. Clean the skin area once again. Grasp the underside of the forearm tightly, make a 1-3 mm deep skin puncture, about 5-6 cm below the cubital fossa. Note the time.
4. Remove the blood every 30 seconds by absorbing it along the edges of a clean filter paper by gently touching the wound with it, till the bleeding stops. This is the end-point.

Note
Instead of one prick, two lancet stabs may be given, 5 cm apart, one after the other, and the BT noted in them separately.

Normal bleeding time with this method is upto 9 minutes.

[IV] Simplate method. Though the "Duke" and the "Ivy" bleeding time methods are fairly reliable, it is not possible to control the depth of the wound made by a lancet or a blade. However, by careful standardization, it has become possible to do so. The most widely used technique uses a 'template' or an automated scalpel to control the depth and length of the wound—usually 1 mm deep and 9 mm long—and a blood pressure cuff inflated to 40 mm Hg to distend the capillary bed of the forearm.

Normal bleeding time = < 7 minutes.

Note
Although a BT of over 10 minutes has a slightly increased risk of bleeding, the risk becomes great when the BT exceeds 15 or 20 minutes.

[V] Capillary fragility test of Hess (also called "Tourniquet" test). This is an important test to assess the mechanical fragility of the capillaries (and formation of a platelet plug) by raising the pressure within them. It may reveal latent purpura.

1. Mark a 1 inch diameter circle on the front of the forearm, and using blue ink, mark any pink, purple, or yellow spots within the circle.
2. Apply a blood pressure cuff on the upper arm and note the systolic and diastolic pressures. Then, after a pause of about 2 minutes or so, raise the pressure to midway between systolic and diastolic levels and maintain it there for 15 minutes. Appearance of more than 10 new petechiae (pink or red spots in the skin) is a positive test, which may be seen in various types of purpura and vessel wall abnormalities.

Comments
The BT test is an *in vivo* test of platelet function, and "Ivy" method is probably the most reliable. However, a peripheral blood film is always examined for the number of platelets and their morphology. The students should note that platelets are involved both in BT and CT tests and one is normally affected without the other. If the BT is prolonged due to low platelet count (thrombocytopenic purpura), the platelets that are available are sufficient to give a normal clotting time.

PLATELET COUNT

Despite their small size (2-4 μm) and being non-nucleated fragments of cytoplasm, the platelets contain a wide variety of chemical substances that play an important role in vasoconstriction, hemostatic plug formation, activation of factor X, conversion of prothrombin to thrombin, and in clot retraction that results in permanent sealing of a ruptured vessel.

Platelet counting. There are two methods for this count: *direct method* and the *indirect method*. Automated counters are also available.

A. DIRECT METHODS

You will require: • Microscope • RBC pipette • Counting chamber with cover slip • Equipment for fingerpick • Rees-Ecker diluting fluid—OR— Freshly prepared 1.0% ammonium oxalate solution.

PROCEDURES

I. Ammonium Oxalate Method. This fluid destroys red cells but preserves platelets; it also acts as an anticoagulant.

1. Get a finger- prick and draw blood up to the mark 1.0. Suck the diluting fluid to the mark 101.
2. Mix the contents thoroughly and wait for 20 minutes. The red ells will be hemolysed, leaving only the platelets. Mix the contents once again and charge the chamber on both sides.
   Place the charged chamber on wet filter paper and cover it with a petri dish to avoid evaporation.
3. Focus the RBC square under HP; adjust the diaphragm and position of condenser till you see the platelets – which appear as small, round or oval structures lying separately, highly refractile bodies with a silvery appearance. Rack the microscope continuously and count the platelets in 5 groups of 16 squares each, as was done for red cell count.
   Knowing the dilution (1 in 100) employed and the dimensions of the squares, calculate the number of platelets in 1 mm^3 of undiluted blood.

II. Rees-Ecker Method. The Rees-Ecker fluid contains the following:

Brilliant creseyl = 0.1 g   (The dye stains plate-
blue   lets,formalin prevents
Sodium citrate = 3.8 g   fungal growth and
                            lyses RBCs, citrate
                            prevents clotting and
Formalin   makes the fluid
                            isotonic
(40% formaldehyde) = 0.2ml with blood).
Distilled water = 100 ml

1. Draw freshly filtered diluent to the mark 0.5 in the RBC pipette. Get a finger-prick and draw blood in the pipette so that the diluent reaches the mark 1.0. Wipe the tip and fill the pipette with diluent once again to the mark 101. This gives a dilution of 1 in 200.
2. Roll the pipette gently between your palms for 3-4 minutes. Taking the diluent first in the pipette prevents clumping and disintegration of platelets which occurs if blood is taken directly into the pipette.
3. Discard the first two drops and charge both sides of the chamber in the usual manner. Place it on a wet filter paper and cover with a petri dish, and wait for 10 minutes to allow the platelets to settle.
4. Count the platelets (which appear as bluish, round or oval bodies, highly refractile on racking the microscope) in 5 groups of 16 squares each, as was done for red cells. Calculate their number in 1 mm^3 of undiluted blood.

Note
The chamber and the pipette must be cleaned with absolute alcohol to remove any dust particles, etc. to which platelets could adhere. Use a lint-free piece of cloth for final cleaning.

B. INDIRECT METHOD

1. Place a drop of 14% magnesium sulfate solution on your finger tip, and get a prick through this drop. Blood oozes directly into the solution which prevents clumping, and disintegration of platelets.

2. Spread a blood film with the diluted blood, dry it, and stain it with Leishman's stain.
3. Examine the stained film under oil immersion lens. Count the platelets and red cells in every 5th field until 1000 red cells have been counted. Determine the *"platelet ratio"*, i.e., the ratio of platelets to red cells (usually, there is 1 platelet to 16-18 red cells).
4. Do the RBC count from a fresh finger-prick in a counting chamber, and calculate the count in 1 mm^3 of undiluted blood.

Calculation of platelet count. With the knowledge of platelet count, and the RBC count, the actual number of platelets per mm^3 blood can now be calculated.

(While doing DLC in a stained blood film, the platelets appear in groups of 3-15, and most of them show different degrees of disintegration. In the present case, however, the platelets lie separately from each other and their morphology can also be studied).

Normal platelet count = 250,000 - 500,000/mm^3.

C. AUTOMATED METHOD

It is a very accurate method. It is carried out on an electronic cell counter (See page 1). The red cells and platelets in the diluted blood sample pass through an aperture. The particles between 2 and 10 μm^3 (fl; femtoliters) are counted as platelets., the measuring range being 0-99.9 x 10^3/fl, and the coefficient of variation being within 1.5%. A platelet distribution graph can also be plotted.

CLOTTING TIME (CT)
COAGULATION TIME

[I] Capillary Blood Clotting Time (Wright's Capillary Glass Tube Method)

(While your partner is doing BT on your finger prick, you can proceed with your CT.

1. Absorb the first 2 drops of blood on a separate filter paper and allow a large drop to form.

Now dip one end of the capillary tube in the blood; the blood rises into the tube by capillary action. This can be enhanced by keeping its open end at a lower level.

2. Note the time when blood starts to enter the tube. This is the zero time.
3. Hold the capillary tube between the palms of your hands to keep the blood near body temperature (in winter, you may blow on it).
4. Gently break off 1 cm bits of glass tube from one end at intervals of 30 seconds, and look for the formation of fibrin threads between the broken ends. The end-point is reached when fibrin threads span a gap of 5 mm between the broken ends ("rope formation"). Note the time.

Normal clotting time = 3-6 minutes.

Comments

(i) The clotting of blood with this method involves both the intrinsic and the extrinsic systems of clotting. There is injury to the blood (coming in contact with glass, intrinsic pathway), and the injury to the tissues (extrinsic pathway).
(ii) The CT is prolonged in hemophilia and other clotting disorders, because thrombin cannot normally be generated. Yet, the BT, which reflects platelet plug formation and vasoconstriction, independently of clot formation, is normal.

[II] Drop Method

This method is less accurate than the above method. Place a large drop of blood from a skin puncture on a clean and dry glass slide. Draw a pin through the drop every 30 seconds, and note the time when fibrin threads adhere to the pin and move with it out of the blood drop. The time elapse between placing the blood drop on the slide and the formation of fibrin threads is the clotting time.

Normal clotting time = 2-4 minutes.

- In the original Duke's Drop Method for CT, two drops of 4-5 mm diameter are placed on a glass slide. The slide is tilted at 30 second intervals. The end-point is absence of change in the previous shape when the slide is held vertical.

[III] Venous Blood Clotting Time (Lee and White Test-tube Method)

A. Single test-tube method. This is the most widely used method for the determination of clotting time.

1. Draw 5 ml venous blood by a clean, non-traumatic venepuncture. Note the time when blood starts to enter the syringe. This is the zero time. Transfer the blood to a chemically clean and dry test tube.
2. Holding the test tube in a water bath at 37°C, take it out at 30 second intervals and tilt it. The end-point is when the tube can be tilted without spilling the blood.

Normal clotting time with this method = 5-10 minutes.

B. Multiple test-tube method. The CT can be determined more accurately by using 3 test tubes rather than one only.

1. Rinse 3 test tubes of 8 mm diameter with normal saline, drain them and place them in a metal rack kept in water at 37°C. Transfer 1.5 ml blood into each test tube.
2. Take out the first tube after 1 minute, tilt it to 45° and return it to the rack. Repeat every 30 seconds until clotting occurs, i.e., where the test tube can be tilted without spilling the blood. Note the time.
3. Repeat the tilting on the second test tube and note the time when clotting occurs, (this happens a few seconds later because tilting the tube hastens clotting). The third tube acts as a control and a check on the end-point in the 2nd test tube.

If a siliconized test tube is used at the same time, a delayed clotting time (40-70 minutes) can be shown.

Normal clotting time with this method = 5-10 minutes.

- The CT depends on the condition of the glass itself, and even on the size of the test tube. Therefore, a high degree of standardization is needed.

Comments

This method is more reliable than the capillary blood CT method, because there is no admixture of blood with tissue fluid which contains tissue thromboplastin (extrinsic system). Thus, this method tests only the intrinsic system of blood clotting. However, this method is non-specific because the CT can theoretically increase due to deficiency of any of the factors in the intrinsic system. But, in actual practice, a prolonged CT nearly always means hemophilia in which the CT may exceed 1 hour in severe cases.

Note

Since the CT varies widely and depends on the method, many clinical laboratories measure the clotting factors by using sophisticated chemical procedures.

CLOT RETRACTION TIME (CRT)

Transfer the larger test tube containing clotted blood to an incubator at 30°C., Normally, the clot starts to shrink (retract) in about 30 minutes (leaving behind straw-colored serum), becomes half its size in 2-3 hours, and complete in 24 hours. Note if there is any digestion of the clot or discoloration of serum.

Comments

Clot retraction (tightening or consolidation) depends on the release of many factors from the platelets, and so the CRT depends on the platelet count. The *fibrin-stabilizing factor* causes more and more cross-linking bonds between nearby fibrin fibers. Their spicules also release *contractile proteins*—actin, myosin, and thrombosthenin. The contraction (retraction) of the clot is activated by thrombin, and calcium ions stored in the

endoplasmic reticulum, Golgi apparatus, and mitochondria.

In addition to forming a meshwork and entrapping blood cells and plasma, the fibrin fibers also adhere to the edges of the wound. When the clot contracts, it stitches the edges of the wound and thus prevents further loss of blood.

CLOT LYSIS TIME (CLT)

The dissolution (dissolving; also called fibrinolysis) of a clot is the process by which a clot becomes fluid so that the trapped red cells sink to the bottom of the test tube.

Normally, the clot lysis time is about 72 hours. If it occurs within 24 hours, it is considered abnormal.

PROTHROMBIN TIME (PT)

The patient's blood is quickly oxalated (or citrated) to remove calcium ions so that prothrombin cannot be converted to thrombin. The sample is then centrifuged. Then to the oxalated plasma, a large excess of calcium ions (as calcium chloride solution) and rabbit brain suspension (to provide tissue thromboplastin; tissue factor, TF) is added. The excess calcium neutralizes the effect of oxalate and the TF converts prothrombin to thrombin via the extrinsic clotting pathway (i.e., factor VII).

The time required for clotting to occur is called the prothrombin time (PT).

Normal PT = 15-20 seconds.

Clinical Significance. Since the potency of tissue thromboplastin (TF) may vary, blood from a normal person is used as a control when the test is used for controlling anticoagulant dose, or in a hemorrhagic disease. Bleeding tendency is present when the prothrombin level falls below 20% of normal (normal plasma prothrombin = 30-40 mg/dl). Prolonged PT suggests the possibility of deficiency of factors II (prothrombin), V, VII and X (See Q/A 17). Prothrombin level is low in vitamin K deficiency and various liver and biliary diseases.

TESTS FOR OTHER CLOTTING FACTORS

Tests similar to prothrombin time have been devised to estimate the quantities of other clotting factors. In each test, excess of calcium ions and all the other factors, except the one being tested, are added to the oxalated blood (or plasma) all at once. The time required for clotting to occur is determined in the same way as for prothrombin time. The clotting time will be prolonged if the factor being tested is deficient. The time itself is used to quantitate the concentration of the factor.

QUESTIONS

Q. 1   What is the clinical importance of doing BT and CT?
BT and CT are important in the following situations:
 i. History of frequent and persistent bleeding from minor injuries, or spontaneous bleeding into tissues.
 ii. Before every minor and major surgery (tooth extraction, etc.).
 iii. Before taking biopsy, especially from bone marrow, liver, kidney, etc.
 iv. Before and during anticoagulant therapy.
 v. Family history of bleeding disorders.

Q. 2   How does BT differ from CT? What is the interrelation between them, and which aspects of hemostasis are tested by them?
Both BT and CT are done together in all disorders of hemostasis. They are interrelated in the sense that platelets are involved in both tests. The BT tests the platelet plug formation and the condition of the microvessels (arterioles, capillaries, venules), while CT tests the formation of the clot. Increase in BT (e.g., in purpura), or CT (e.g., in hemophilia) usually occur independently of each other.

Q. 3   What are the factors on which BT and CT depend?
Bleeding time depends on:
 i. Breadth and depth of the wound.
 ii. Degree of hyperemia of the skin puncture site.
 iii. Number of platelets and their functional status.
 iv. Functional status of the blood vessels.
 v. Temperature: In cold weather, low temperature promotes vasoconstriction and thus shorten BT.
Clotting time is depends on:
 i. Nature of contact surface (glass in this case; siliconised surface would prolong the CT.
 ii. Presence or absence of clotting factors.
 iii. Temperature: Low temperature may prolong the CT.

Q. 4   What is meant by the term hemostasis? What are the steps by which it is brought about?
This term refers to the process of stoppage of bleeding from the injured blood vessels. Bleeding from small vessels stops automatically within a few minutes due to low pressure in these vessels besides other factors. But if a large artery is cut, surgical repair may be required. (Tying the bleeding vessels during a surgical operation by the surgeon is also called 'hemostasis').

Hemostasis involves the following interrelated steps.
1.   Contraction of Injured Blood Vessels. The immediate response of the injured vessels is the contraction (spasm) of the circular smooth muscle fibers in their walls. This spasm is due to:
 i. Mechanical stimulation of smooth muscle fibers by the injury.
 ii. Local reflexes produced by stimulation of pain and other sensory receptors.
 iii. Release of potent vasoconstrictors from platelets (serotonin, epinephrine, thromboxane A2, prostaglandins, and from damaged endothelium (endothelins).

Note
The mechanical stimulation of smooth muscle of arteries. {(Even large arteries like the radial),

arterioles, and venules may be so strong that bleeding stops for many minutes. Capillaries do not have smooth muscle in their walls; precapillary sphincters, which, of course, can contract and relax, regulate the blood flow through them}. During this time, the other factors described above go into action and further strengthen the vasoconstriction.

2. Formation of Platelet Hemostatic Plug. The repair of the openings in the vessel walls depends on many important functions of platelets. Their initial reaction is adhesion followed by release reaction. As the injury exposes collagen fibers in the walls of blood vessels, receptors in the platelets interact with these fibers. They swell, become irregular in shape, and throw out many pseudopodia (spicules) and become more and more sticky. They adhere to each other and to collagen fibers in vessel walls. Therefore, at the site of injury, more and more platelets are activated and aggregated by platelet- activating factors—PAF (a cytokine secreted by platelets, monocytes, and neutrophils) and form a growing plug of platelets, which is enough to effectively seal the openings in small vessels.

The adhesiveness (stickiness) of platelets is promoted by ADP (released by them), and by von Willebrand factor (vWF), as described below.

3. Formation of Blood Clot in the Ruptured Vessel. If there is a large hole in the blood vessel, a blood clot is additionally required. The extrinsic and intrinsic pathways of coagulation form a meshwork of very sticky fibrin threads. They reinforce the platelet plug and stitch the wound edges together thus permanently sealing the ruptured vessel.

4. Dissolution of Clot by the Fibrinolytic System. A fibrin clot has a tendency to grow in size due to amplification and positive feedback cycles of the clotting factors. The fibrinolytic system does not allow the fibrin clot to grow and block a vessel, which would cause serious complications. The dissolution of a clot, called fibrinolysis (dissolving of fibrin fibers), is brought about by the formation of the active enzyme **plasmin** from **plasminogen** (a plasma protein) by the action of *tissue plasminogen activator* (tPA) released from injured issues (see Q/A 22 also).

Q. 5 How does bleeding stop from a skin-prick?
Bleeding from small vessels stops due to: (i) low pressure inside the vessels, and the natural elasticity of the tissues, (ii) contraction of smooth muscle in the microvessels, (iii) formation of platelet plugs, and (iv) clotting of blood (if a larger vessel is cut).

Q. 6 Name the conditions in which only the bleeding time is prolonged while the clotting time is normal.
Pronged BT, with normal CT is seen in the following conditions:
A. Low Platelet Count (Thrombocytopenia). It may be due to:
  i. Decreased production of platelets
  ii. Increased destruction of platelets. (See Q/A 12 for details).

B. Functional Platelet Defects. Prolonged BT with normal platelet count suggests the following defects:
  i. Drugs: aspirin, large doses of penicillin, other drugs.
  ii. von Willebrand disease: Inherited as an autosomal dominant trait, this condition is associated with a deficiency of a component of factor VIII called " factor VIII related antigen (VIII R: Ag; vWF) which acts as a carrier of factor VIII (See Q/A 19 also).

    The vWF in the injured vessel wall, along with ADP released from platelets, promotes platelet adhesion and plug formation. So when there is deficiency of vWF, the decreased platelet adhesion to connective tissue leads to traumatic and mucosal bleeding. The BT is prolonged while platelet count is normal. Variants of this disease are also seen.
  iii. Other diseases: uremia, cirrhosis, leukemia, etc.

C. Vessel wall defects. These defects are generally acquired, but may be inherited.

 i. **Prolonged treatment with corticosteroids:** Also other drugs penicillin, sulphas, and aspirin, etc. may damage vessel walls. There may be severe bleeding in a known case of purpura if aspirin is inadvertently administered.

 ii. **Allergic purpura:** There is damage to capillary walls by antibodies.

 iii. **Infections:** Infections such as typhus, bacterial endocarditis, hemolytic streptococci.

 iv. **Deficiency of vitamin C:** Petechia, and bleeding from gums occur due to decreased intercellular substance and less stable capillary basement membrane.

 v. **Senile purpura:** In the elderly, purpuric hemorrhages occur on the back of the hands and forearms due to prolonged pressure or mild trauma. Small vessels rupture due to increased mobility of skin resulting from loss of elastic and connective tissues around blood vessels.

 vi. **Connective tissue diseases:** Some of these diseases may be associated with purpuric bleeding.

Note

In all cases of purpura due to vessel wall defects the platelet counts are normal, but BT is prolonged and the capillary fragility test is positive.

Q. 7 What is the relation between the platelet count and the severity of bleeding?
Broadly speaking, the relation between the platelet count and the severity of bleeding is as follows:

Above 100,000/mm^3	No clinical symptoms, bleeding is rare.
50,000-100,000/mm^3	Bleeding may occur after major surgery.
20,000-50,000/mm^3	Bleeding occurs with minor trauma of everyday life or gentle sports.

Contd...

Contd...

Below 20,000 mm^3	Spontaneous hemorrhages in urinary and GI tract, nose bleeds, etc.
At very low counts.	Fatal hemorrhages may occur in the brain.

Q. 8 What is the normal platelet count? Describe their site of formation, life-span, and kinetics.
Normal platelet count is = 250,000-500,000/mm^3.

Site of formation. Under the influence of the hormone TPO (thrombopoietin), the platelets are formed in the red bone marrow. The myeloid stem cells develop into CFU-GM, which, in turn, develop into megakaryoblast and megakaryocytes. The platelets are formed by the pinching off of the cytoplasm of megakaryocytes (the largest cells of bone marrow—about 100 μm), each cell producing 2000-3000 fragments. Each fragment, enclosed by a piece of cell membrane, is a platelet (thrombocyte), disc-shaped and 2-4 μm in diameter.

About 60-70% of platelets formed in the bone marrow are in the circulating blood while the rest are in the spleen. Their life-span is 7-10 days, about 20% being consumed each day in the repair of micro-vessels (see below). The aged and dead platelets are removed by tissue macrophages (RES) mainly in spleen, but also in the liver. Their number is kept remarkably constant, their production being regulated partly by the circulating platelets but mainly by TPO, and possibly interleukins 1, 3 and 6.

Platelet reactions. Though the circulating platelets are functionally inactive, they contain a variety of chemical, substances. They contain 2 types of granules: **(i) alpha granules**—which contain clotting factors, and platelet-derived growth factor (PDGF) which can repair damaged vessels by proliferation of endothelial cells, smooth muscle, and fibroblasts which lay down collagen fibers;

(ii) dense granules—which contain ADP, ATP, serotonin, Ca^{2+}, etc. There are enzymes for the synthesis of thromboxane A_2, fibrin-stabilizing factor, lysosomes; a few mitochondria, and membrane systems for storing calcium.

The earliest response of platelets is adhesive reaction and their aggregation. This may be followed by either dispersal of the collected platelets, or irreversible agglutination and release reaction.

1. **Adhesive reaction.** The platelets, because of ADP and vWF (von Willebrand factor (the latter also produced by endothelium), stick to each other and to foreign surfaces (to form platelet plugs).

2. **Reversible agglutination.** After they have performed their function, their further aggregation is prevented by adrenalin, serotonin, and possibly other agents (e.g., prostacyclin from endothelial cells) which also promote their dispersion.

3. **Irreversible agglutination.** This is triggered by thrombin, ADP and exposure to foreign surfaces.

4. **Release phenomenon.** Irreversible agglutination is often followed by degranulation and release of many substances—such as platelet factor 3, platelet factor 4 (it can inactivate heparin), etc. In addition to factor V, other factors, especially factors VII, X and XII are also probably adsorbed on other platelets.

Q. 9 How does Aspirin act as an anti-platelet agglutinating agent and what is its clinical value?
Prostacyclin produced by endothelial and smooth muscle cells in the walls of blood vessels, and **thromboxane A_2** formed in the platelets before they enter the circulation, are both prostaglandins and synthesized from arachidonic acid (an essential fatty acid) via the enzyme cyclo-oxygenase.

Prostacyclin prevents platelet aggregation and causes vasodilation. On the other hand, thromboxane A_2 promotes platelet aggregation and causes vasoconstriction. Normally, there is a balance between these two opposite effects and the blood vessels remain patent.

Small doses of aspirin irreversibly inhibit cyclo-oxygenase so that both prostacyclin and thromboxane A_2 are reduced. However, endothelial cells form new enzyme in a few hours, while circulating platelets cannot do this. New platelets capable of forming thromboxane A_2, have to enter circulation, which is a slower process. Thus, the balance shifts in favor of prostacyclin for many hours so that platelets are prevented from aggregating at the sites of endothelial damage—a process which precedes formation of clots.

Aspirin is widely used, on a long-term basis, to prevent formation of clots in the coronary and cerebral vessels.

Q. 10 Enumerate the functions of platelets.
The functions of platelets are:

1. **Hemostatic Plug Formation.**
2. **Role in Blood Coagulation.** Platelets are essential for clotting of blood. They release platelet phospholipid (PPL), which takes part in activating factors XII, XI, and X of the intrinsic system (see below), and factor VII of extrinsic system. Platelets also play an important role in *conversion of prothrombin to thrombin* because most of the prothrombin fist attaches to prothrombin receptors on the platelets that are already bound to damaged tissues.

   The role of fibrin stabilizing factor (Factor XIII) released by platelets was mentioned earlier (Platelet-free plasma takes a long time to form a clot, which is friable and does not retract normally.

3. **Clot Retraction.** As already mentioned, the release of contractile proteins from platelets in a clot helps in clot retraction.

4. **Physiological function.** Even when there are no obvious injuries to blood vessels, minimal stress to capillaries and venules in the legs and feet by hydrostatic pressure of blood when we stand upright, or when these vessels are subjected to knocks and bumps when we run or jump, opens up many gaps and holes in the endothelial cells hundreds of times a

day. These multiple, small ruptures are sealed by platelets, which fuse with the injured endothelial cells and contribute their own cell membranes for repair. They also provide platelet-derived growth factor (PDGF) to help in the growth of new vessels to replace the damaged ones (about 20% of platelets are used up for repair purposes every day. It can thus be visualized how platelet deficiency can lead to hemorrhages typical of purpura).

5. **Phagocytosis.** The platelets can ingest carbon particles, immune complexes, and viral particles.

6. **Transport.** They synthesize, store, and transport a number of substances. They can take up 5-HT against a concentration gradient and transport large amounts from the argentaffin cells of the intestinal glands.

7. **Role in local blood flow regulation.** Products of platelet aggregation (and many other stimuli) also cause the release of nitric oxide (NO), a powerful vasodilator, from the intact endothelial cells. Thus, platelets may have a role in dilating the vessels in the vicinity of vasoconstriction and plug formation in micro vessels as described above.

Q. 11   What are the physiological variations in the platelet count?

Variations in platelet count under physiological conditions are uncommon. However, minor variations occur as mentioned below:

- Increased counts may be seen after severe exercise, and sometimes at high altitudes.
- Decreased counts, near the lower side of the normal, may be seen in the newborns and in females, during menstruation.

Q. 12   What is meant by the terms thrombocytopenia and thrombocytosis? Enumerate the pathological variations in platelet count.

Thrombocytopenia. The term refers to a decreased count of platelets. It may be due to decreased production or increased destruction.

Thrombocytosis. The term refers to an increase in platelet count.

Thrombocytopenia

A. **Decreased production**
1. **Bone marrow injury/depression/failure:** Drugs (sulphas, chloramphenicol, cytotoxic drugs); irradiation, acute septic fevers, toxemias, and aplastic anemia.
2. **Bone marrow invasion:** By leukemias, and secondary deposits of malignant disease.
3. **Periodic thrombocytopenic purpura (purpura hemorrhagica):** Cause not known.

B. **Increased destruction (i.e, decreased survival time).**
1. **Drugs:** Thiazides, quinine, ethanol, estrogens, methyldopa, quinidine.
2. **Immune thrombocytopenic purpura (ITP):** Autoimmune destruction of platelets. May be idiopathic, or associated with some disease, e.g., AIDS.
3. **Sequestration in spleen:** There is increased trapping and/or destruction by enlarged spleen.
4. **Disseminated intravascular coagulation (DIC):** Platelets are depleted and coagulation factors consumed during widespread clotting, e.g., severe infection (especially meningococcal, pneumococcal), severe and extensive burns, trauma (crush injuries), mismatched transfusion, and retained dead fetus. There may be severe bleeding in some cases.
5. **Hemorrhage with extensive transfusion.**

Thrombocytosis

A. **Primary thrombocytosis** (thrombocythemia: count > 800,000/mm^3). It is a myeloproliferative disease involving megakaryocytes. Bleeding and thrombosis may occur.

B. **Secondary (or reactive) thrombocytosis:** count > 500,000/mm^3): This condition occurs after removal of spleen or after severe hemorrhage.

Q. 13   What is purpura and what are its causes?

The term purpura is derived from the purple-colored petechial hemorrhages and bruises in the skin. The blood that leaks out from the capillaries, etc. changes color from red to purple to dark blue to green over a period of time. These colors are due to changes in the pigments derived from hemoglobin.

Causes of purpura: These include thrombo-cytopenia, functional platelet defects, vessel wall defects, allergy, and old age (consult Q/A 6 above on conditions where BT is increased). Perhaps the most common cause of **acquired platelet functional failure** is ingestion of drugs, aspirin being the commonest. Purpura may be primary or secondary.

A. Primary purpura (idiopathic; cause not known). In many cases, antibodies develop against platelets [immune thrombocytopenic purpura (ITP)], causing their excessive destruction. The ITP may be acute or chronic. The acute variety is seen in children, commonly after infection. The onset is sudden, with fever, and purpuric lesions, epistaxis, etc. Steroids help but in some fresh blood has to be given, (one unit raises the count by 10,000/mm^3). Splenectomy cures many.

B. Secondary purpura. It is much more common than the primary form. The causes include: drugs and chemicals, bone marrow depression/destruction, hypersplenism, etc.

Q. 14 What do the platelets look like in a blood film stained with Leishman's stain?
The platelets appear as round or oval bodies, 2-4 µm in diameter. They lie here and there in clumps, (aggregates) of 2-12 in number, which is an *in vitro* appearance. (They do not form clumps in the circulating blood). They stain pink-purple, somewhat darker in the centre. But being fragments of cytoplasm, they do not contain nuclei. On careful study, granules may be seen.

Q. 15 Which other diluting fluid may be used for counting platelets?
In "direct methods", 1% ammonium oxalate solution is used while the other fluid is " Rees-Ecker solution"

In the case of "Indirect method", 14% magnesium sulphated solution is used to prevent aggregation and disintegration of platelets before a blood film can be examined. It is not a diluting fluid.

Q. 16 What is meant by the term clotting of blood? Name the various clotting factors, their sources, and their role in clotting.
Clotting. Within the blood vessels, the blood remains in a fluid state. But when it is drawn out from the vessels, a series of chemical reactions occur. During the next few minutes, the blood thickens, and forms a gel called a clot. The clot consists of a network of insoluble threads called fibrin. The blood cells get entangled in this meshwork and give it a red color. Over a time the clot retracts and serum is expelled out.

Clotting Factors
The blood contains many inactive proteolytic enzymes, also called "factors". **Surface contact or injury to blood (intrinsic system)** and/or **injury to the tissues (extrinsic system)** starts a chain of reactions in which an inactive enzyme precursor is converted into an active enzyme. The activated enzyme, in turn, acts on the next inactive enzyme to form the next active enzyme and so on in a fixed sequence—a process called **enzyme cascade**. Each clotting factor activates many molecules of the next and so on. Thus, the enzyme cascade is an amplifying system so that at the end of the process, i.e., when the cascade comes to an end, a large amount of the final product (fibrin) is formed.

Note
The activated enzyme is designated by the letter "a" after the numeral (e.g., factor XII to XIIa).
• The Roman numerals (also called "factors") given to clotting substances, in order of their discovery, are given below (Table 1.5), though some substances have not been given any such numerals.

TABLE 1.5

	Clotting factors		
Number	Name/s	Source	Pathways of activation
I	Fibrinogen	Liver	Common
II	Prothrombin	Liver	Common
III	Tissue thromboplastin (TPL) (tissue factor, (TF)	Damaged tissues and activated platelets	Extrinsic
IV	Calcium ions (Ca^{2+})	Diet, bones, platelets	All
V	Proaccelerin (accelerator globulin, AcG; labile factor)	Liver and platelets	Extrinsic and intrinsic
VI	There is no such factor.		
VII	Proconvertin; stable factor; serum prothrombin conversion accelerator (SPCA)	Liver	Extrinsic
VIII	Antihemophilic factor (AHF); anti-hemophilic factor A; antihemophilic globulin (AHG)	Platelets and endo-thelial cells	Intrinsic
IX	Christmas factor (CF); antihemophilic factor B (AHF-B) plasma thromboplastin component (PTC)	Liver	Intrinsic
X	Stuart factor, Prower factor Stuart-Prower factor; thrombokinase	Liver	Extrinsic and Intrinsic
XI	Plasma thromboplastin antecedent (PTA); antihemophilic factor C	Liver	Intrinsic
XII	Hageman factor; glass contact factor; glass factor; contact factor; antihemophilic factor C	Liver	Intrinsic
XIII	Fibrin stabilizing factor (FSF); Laki-Lorand factor	Liver and platelets	Common

- 11 of the 12 known clotting factors (including fibrinogen) are globulins
- Prothrombinase (prothrombin activator, PTA) is a combination of factors V and X
- Prekallikrein (Flechner factor)
- High mw kininogen (HMWK; Fitzgerald factor)

Note. Arabic numerals are sometimes used for platelet activities affecting clotting, for example, the terms:

- Platelet factor 3 (PF-3) is used for platelet phospholipid (PPL) procoagulant activity.
- Platelet factor 4 (PF-4) is used for heparin neutralizing activity of platelets.
- Though there are other Arabic numerals mentioned in literature, they are no longer used.

Q. 17 What is the mechanism of clotting of blood?

The clotting of blood involves the following 4 types of chemical substances:

1. Plasma clotting factors.
2. Platelet clotting factors.
3. Tissue factor—present on all the plasma membranes.
4. Calcium ions.

Basic Theory of Coagulation

More than 50 substances that cause or affect clotting of blood have been found in blood and in the tissues. Those that promote clotting are called *procoagulants*, and those that inhibit clotting are called *anticoagulants*. The balance between these two groups of substances decides whether blood will clot or not. Normally, the anticoagulants in the blood prevent blood from clotting as long as it is circulating in the undamaged blood vessels. However, when a blood vessel is ruptured, procoagulants in the damaged area become "activated" and clotting occurs—which is a homeostatic process to prevent further loss of blood.

ESSENTIAL STAGES OF BLOOD CLOTTING

The 3 essential stages of the process of blood clotting are:

Stage (1) Generation of prothrombin activator (PTA; prothrombinase). The PTA is a complex of Xa + Va + phospholipids + calcium ions. Its formation can begin in either or both of the following 2 pathways:

  i. **The extrinsic pathway:** Injury to cells/tissues outside (extrinsic to) the blood vessels (e.g., skin, subcutaneous tissue, etc.).
  ii. **The intrinsic pathway:** Injury to the blood, cells within the blood (e.g., platelets), or injury to cells in direct contact with blood (e.g., endothelial cells and underlying collagen fibers). Outside damage is not needed.

Stage (2) Formation of Thrombin from Prothrombin: The PTA, which is a proteolytic enzyme, splits prothrombin (an alpha-2 globulin present in the plasma) into the active enzyme thrombin.

Stage (3) Formation of Fibrin Threads from fibrinogen: Thrombin acts as a proteolytic enzyme and splits off insoluble fibrin monomers from the soluble fibrinogen. The monomers polymerize to form fibrin thread, which are stabilized (cross-linked) by factor XIII (Loki-Lorand factor) and calcium ions.

Stage (1) Generation of PTA

The Extrinsic Pathway. The extrinsic pathway (system) has fewer steps and is explosive, i.e., it occurs within 10-15 seconds of injury. It is so named because a tissue protein called **tissue factor (TF; tissue thromboplastin TPL; or factor III)** is released from the cells outside (extrinsic to) the blood vessels (e.g., cells of skin, subcutaneous tissue, etc). It is a specific phospholipid-lipoprotein complex present on the surfaces of all cells, including platelets. The TF, which is released when cell membranes are damaged or perturbed (as by a cut, prick, or crush injury) activates factor VII to VIIa **(Figure 1-14)**. The complex of tissue factor + VIIa + calcium ions activate factor X to Xa. Factor Xa combines with factor V and calcium ions to form the active enzyme PTA (prothrombinase). This pathway is inhibited by a tissue factor pathway inhibitor that forms a quaternary structure with TPL, factor VIIa, and factor Xa.

The Intrinsic Pathway. This pathway is more complex and occurs more slowly, usually needing several minutes. It is so named because its activators are present either within (intrinsic to) the blood (e.g., platelets), or the cells in contact with blood (endothelial cells). Injury to blood, such as by a contact with a "foreign" electronegatively charged, water-wettable surface, may occur when blood comes in contact with:

  i. Roughened or damaged endothelial cells and the exposed collagen fibers under them (injury *in vivo*),

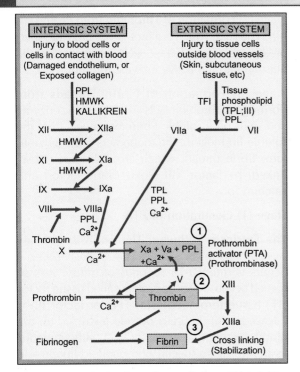

Figure 1-14. Mechanism of coagulation of blood. The intrinsic and extrinsic pathways for blood clotting are shown
Stage 1. Generation of prothrombin activator (PTA).
Stage 2. Formation of thrombin from prothrombin.
Stage 3. Formation of fibrin from fibrinogen.
HMWK: High molecular weight kininogen.
TFI: Tissue factor pathway inhibitor.
PPL: Platelet phospholipid.
(See text for details).

ii. The slippery glass surface of a test tube or any other water-wettable surface (injury *in vitro*).

In both cases, the damaged platelets release phospholipids (PPL), which initiates the initial reaction of conversion of factor XII to XIIa. Factor XIIa converts XI to Ixia and IX to IXa **(Figure 1-14)**. Factor IXa then forms a complex with VIIIa, PPL, and calcium ions. This complex activates factor X to Xa to form PTA.

Interaction Between Extrinsic and Intrinsic factors
It is clear from the above description of the two systems that when a blood vessel is damaged / ruptured, coagulation involves both pathways at the same time. The tissue factor starts the extrinsic system while contact of platelets and factor XII with collagen fibers in vessel walls starts the intrinsic system.

As mentioned above, the extrinsic system is explosive and with severe tissue injury, clotting can occur in 10-15 seconds. The intrinsic system requires 2-6 minutes to cause clotting.

Stages (2) and (3). The Common Pathway
Once PTA (prothrombinase) is formed, the common pathway of blood clotting follows. *In the 2nd stage, PTA+ calcium converts prothrombin to thrombin. In the 3rd stage,* thrombin+ calcium converts fibrinogen to fibrin.

Thrombin also activates factor XIII to XIIIa. It also has 3 positive feedback effects, one on factor V, second on factor VIII, and the third on platelets, which clump together and release PPL.

Q. 18 How does clotting occur in the glass capillary tube in your experiment?
The first reaction that occurs when blood comes in contact with the glass surface is injury to blood. This injury damages the platelets which release phospholipids (PPL). The PPL, along with high m.w. kininogens and kallikrein, converts factor XII to XIIa which starts the intrinsic mechanism of clotting. This pathway is supported by the extrinsic pathway in which tissue factor is released from damaged tissues at the site of skin wound.

Q. 19 Name the conditions where the clotting time is increased and those where it is decreased.
The coagulation time is increased in the following conditions:
A. Hereditary Coagulation Disorders
1. **Hemophilias**—A, B, C, D (see below).
2. **von Willebrand disease.** Though usually a bleeding disease, variant forms show reduced factor VIII activity and an increase in CT. Acquired forms are caused by antibodies which inhibit vWF. The laboratory and clinical features are similar to hemophilia A.

3. **Afibrinogenemia and dysfibrinogenemia.** The concentration of fibrinogen may be greatly reduced (normal = 250 to 300 mg%) or absent or it may be chemically abnormal, though both may be present at the same time.
4. **Deficiency of factor XIII and defective cross-linking** is a rare disorder.

B. Acquired Coagulation Disorders. These may develop in a variety of diseases as mentioned below:

1. **Vitamin K deficiency.** Deficiency of vitamin K (major sources: green vegetables, also gut bacteria) may be due to inadequate intake, intestinal malabsorption (obstructive jaundice), or loss of storage sites in liver. Since it acts a cofactor in the synthesis of prothrombin, and factors VII, IX and X, its deficiency leads to fall in their levels.
2. **Liver diseases.** There is a decrease of all clotting factors except VIII. There is also a reduced uptake of vitamin K, and abnormalities of platelet function.
3. **Intravascular clotting.** Clotting factors are used up and bleeding may occur.
4. **Anticoagulant therapy.** Patients receiving heparin or warfarin show an increased CT.

C. Newborns. Newborns, especially premature babies sometimes have a tendency to bleed because the plasma levels of certain factors are low, especially prothrombin. Usually, these levels reach normal by the 2nd or 3rd week after birth. Vitamin K is given if bleeding persists.

The Clotting Time is decreased in:
Physiological conditions: malnutrition, parturition.
Pathological conditions: There is no pathological condition in which the CT is decreased.

Q.20 What is Hemophilia?
Hemophilia (-philia = loving) is a group of bleeding disorders that result from deficiency of factors VIII, IX, X, or XII. The 4 types have been called hemophilia A, B, C, and D. All are inherited— A and B are sex-linked, being transmitted by females (they act as carriers of the disease) to males who suffer from the disease. (Females are protected by the second X chromosome, which is usually normal.

Hemophilia A, which is also called *classical hemophilia*, is the most common hereditary coagulation disorder. The clinical features of repeated bleedings from nose, into subcutaneous tissues, joints. muscles, etc. either spontaneously or on minor injuries, start early in life, or after surgery or injuries later in life. The severity of clinical features, however, depends on the severity of factor VIII deficiency.

Hemophilia B, called Christmas disease, was discovered in 1952 in a family with the surname Christmas. Hemophilias C and D are rare.

Hemophilia has been called a royal disease because some of the children of queen Victoria of England and Czar Nicholas II of Russia had this disease. (All hemophilias are treated with fresh blood transfusions, or concentrated clotting factors).

Q. 21 Why does calcium deficiency not cause a bleeding disorder though it is essential for many steps of blood coagulation?
The reason why deficiency of calcium does not cause bleeding is that only minute amounts of ionic calcium are required for clotting. A condition of bleeding due to this deficiency is not compatible with life. However, tetany may result due to lack of this mineral.

Q. 22 How is blood maintained in a fluid state within the body?
A balance between clotting and anticlotting mechanisms is required to prevent hemorrhage,

and at the same time, to prevent intravascular clotting.

Hemofluidity within the body is maintained by the following factors:

1. Continuous motion (circulation) of blood does not allow clotting factors to accumulate at one point.

2. Endothelial surface factors:

 a. Smoothness of endothelial surface prevents contact activation of factor XII of the intrinsic pathway (damage to endothelium causes this activation).

 b. The glycocalyx layer on the endothelium repels clotting factors and platelets.

 c. Thrombomodulin secreted by these cells removes thrombin as soon as it is formed. The complex of these two activates protein C which, along with a cofactor, inactivates factors V and VIII.

 d. Prostacyclin secreted by endothelium counteracts platelet aggregation.

3. Antithrombin action of antithrombin III-Heparin complex and fibrin. Antithrombin III, an alpha globulin synthesized in the liver and normally present in plasma in a concentration of 15-30 mg/dl, is called the *antithrombin-heparin cofactor*. A protease inhibitor of intrinsic clotting system, it is one of the most important anticoagulants in the blood.

Heparin, due to its low concentration in the blood, has little or no anticoagulant activity. But when it combines with antithrombin III, it increases the effectiveness of antithrombin III in removing thrombin hundreds of times. This complex also removes activated factors IX, X, XI, and XII.

The fibrin fibers that are formed when a clot is forming adsorb 85-90% of thrombin that is formed. This reduces the local concentration of thrombin, thus preventing its spread into the remaining blood and spreading of the clot.

4. Fibrinolytic system (The Plasmin System). Plasminogen (profibrinolysin), a plasma protein, when activated by tissue plasminogen activator (tPA) that is slowly released from injured tissues and endothelium, is changed into plasmin. Plasmin, a strong proteolytic enzyme resembling trypsin, digests and dissolves fibrin fibers, fibrinogen, prothrombin, and factors V and VIII.

The activated protein C (APC), described above, in addition to inactivating the 2 major clotting factors (V and VIII) not blocked by antithrombin III, also enhances the activity of tPA by inhibiting the activity of a tPA inhibitor.

Thus, once the clot has formed and succeeded in stopping blood loss, the blocked vessel is reopened by the process of fibrinolysis over the next few days, and the blood flow is restored.

Note
Human plasminogen consists of a heavy chain of 500 amino acids and a light chain of 241 amino acids. Receptors of plasminogen are present on many cells, but especially on endothelial cells. When plasminogen binds to its receptors, it gets activated into plasmin that provides a mechanism that prevents clot formation in intact vessels.

Human tPA, produced by recombinant DNA methods, is commercially available and employed for dissolving clots in coronary arteries in early treatment of myocardial infarction. Streptokinase, a bacterial enzyme and a fibrinolytic agent, is also used for the same purpose.

Q. 23 What is the physiological importance of clotting of blood?
Coagulation of the blood is a homeostatic process, i.e., it maintains the integrity of the body, including its internal environment.

1. Clotting prevents further loss of blood by sealing the injured vessels.

2. The wound edges are drawn together by the fibrin threads as the clot shrinks and retracts.

3. It provides a framework for repair of the wound. Scab formation protects against loss of body fluids and drying of tissues. Finally, it forms a scar.

Q.24 What is meant by the terms thrombosis and embolism? What are the dangers associated with these conditions?

Thrombosis. Though the anticoagulating and fibrinolytic systems keep the blood in a fluid state, clotting may occur spontaneously within an unbroken vessel—a process called thrombosis (thromb- = clot; osis = a condition of). The clot thus formed is called a thrombus, (pl = thrombi). Thrombosis must be distinguished from extravascular clotting that occurs in a test tube, in wounds, or in blood vessels after death. Generally, thrombosis can begin in either of the following 2 ways:

i. **Local damage or roughness of endothelial surfaces,** e.g., atheromatous patches in arteries (e.g., coronaries, carotid, cerebral), on damaged cardiac valves, or in veins of the lower limbs. Platelets are activated and start the intrinsic system of clotting.

ii. **Slowing of blood flow (stasis)** in the pelvic and leg veins causes accumulation of clotting factors. This may happen as a complication of pregnancy, prolonged confinement to bed (fractures, surgery, severe burns), or during long flights in aeroplanes.

Embolism. The thrombus may dissolve spontaneously, or it or its fragments may get loosened and be carried away in the downstream blood. A blood clot, an air bubble, fat from broken bones, or a piece of tissue debris, transported by blood is called an embolus (em- = in; bolus = a mass). Emboli in arteries may get lodged in smaller arteries of any vital organ (e.g., brain), while emboli from the veins reach lungs and cause pulmonary embolism. Cases of thrombosis/embolism are treated with fibrinolytics and anticoagulant agents. (See Q/A 22 above).

1-20

Osmotic Fragility of Red Blood Cells (Syn: Osmotic Resistance of Red Blood Corpuscles)

STUDENT OBJECTIVES

After completing this experiment, you should be able to:

1. Define the osmotic fragility of red cells and describe the utility of this test.

2. Define the terms osmosis, exosmosis, and endosmosis.

3. Explain how hemolysis of RBCs occurs when they are exposed to hypotonic saline.

4. Explain the effect of hypertonic saline on red cells.

5. Name the conditions in which fragility of red cells is increased and decreased.

Relevance

In certain hemolytic anemias, the red cells become more fragile, i.e., they are likely to burst and release their hemoglobin into the plasma. The osmotic fragility test assesses their ability to withstand hypotonic saline without bursting. It is employed as a screening test for hemolytic anemias.

PRINCIPLE

The normal red cells can remain suspended in normal saline (0.9% NaCl solution) for hours without rupturing or any change in their size or shape. But when they are placed in decreasing strengths of hypotonic saline, they imbibe water (due to osmosis) and finally burst. The ability of RBCs to resist this type of hemolysis can be determined quantitatively.

APPARATUS AND MATERIALS

1. Wood or metal test tube rack with 12 clean, dry, 7.5 cm × 1.0 cm glass test tubes. •Glass marking pencil. •Glass dropper with a rubber teat.
2. Sterile swabs moist with alcohol. •2 ml syringe with needle.
3. Freshly prepared 1 percent sodium chloride solution. •Distilled water.

PROCEDURES

1. Number the test tubes from 1 to 12 with the glass-marking pencil and put them in the rack.
2. Using the glass dropper, place the varying number of drops of 1% saline in each of the 12 test tubes as shown in Table 1.6. Then, after thorough rinsing of the same dropper with distilled water, add the number of drops of distilled water to each of the 12 tubes, as shown in Table 1.6.

   Mix the contents of each test tube by placing a thumb over it and inverting it a few times. Mark the tonicity of saline on each of the test tubes. Note that tube # I contains

normal saline, which is isotonic with plasma, while tube # 12 contains only distilled water which has no tonicity.

3. Draw 2 ml of blood from a suitable vein and gently eject one drop of blood into each of the 12 tubes. (The blood may be put into a container of anticoagulant, and a drop can be put into each tube with a pipette). Mix the contents gently by placing a thumb over it and inverting the tube only once.
4. Leave the test tubes undisturbed for one hour. Then observe the extent of hemolysis in each tube by holding the rack at eye level, with a white paper sheet behind it.

OBSERVATIONS AND RESULTS

While judging the degree or extent of hemolysis from the depth of the red color of supernatant saline, tube # 1 (normal saline), and tube # 12 (distilled water) will act as controls, i.e., no hemolysis in normal saline (# 1) and complete hemolysis in distilled water (# 12).

a. The test tubes in which no hemolysis has occurred, the RBCs will settle down and form a red dot (mass) at the bottom of the tube, leaving the saline above clear.
b. If there is some hemolysis, the saline will be tinged red with Hb, with the unruptured cells forming a red dot at the bottom. The color of the saline will be seen to be increasingly deeper with decreasing tonicity of saline.

TABLE 1.6

Preparation of saline solutions for testing the osmotic fragility of red cells											
Test tube number	1	2	3	4	5	6	7	8	9	10	11	12
No. of drops of 1% NaCl	22	16	15	14	13	12	11	10	9	8	7	0
No. of drops of distilled water	3	9	10	11	12	13	14	15	16	17	18	25
Tonicity strength of NaCl (in%)	0.88	0.64	0.60	0.56	0.52	0.48	0.44	0.40	0.36	0.32	0.28	0

Note Use the same dropper, after thorough rinsing each time, for measuring saline and distilled water. This will ensure that the volume of all drops is equal for all test tubes.

c. The test tubes in which there is complete hemolysis, the saline will be equally deep red with no red cells at the bottom of these tubes.

Results. Carefully observe each tube for depth of red color of the supernatant and the mass of red cells at the bottom.
- Note the start of hemolysis (also called onset of fragility) and record the test tube number. Express your result in % saline.
- Note the start of complete hemolysis, i.e., the test tube in which there are no red cells at the bottom (hemolysis will be complete below this saline strength). Express your result in % saline.

Hemolysis begins in   ..... % saline.
Hemolysis is complete in   ..... % saline.

If there is doubt about the presence of intact RBCs at the bottom of a test tube, the solution can be centrifuged and the sediment examined under the microscope.

Normal Range of Fragility

Normally, hemolysis begins in about 0.48% saline (tube # 6 in this case). No cells hemolyse in solutions of 0.5% saline and above.

Hemolysis is complete at about 0.36 % saline (tube # 9). It is also complete in tubes 10, 11, and 12.

Note

When the test is done on a patient, it is always checked against a normal sample of blood, which is tested on a separate series of saline solutions.
- When red cells become more fragile, hemolysis may begin at about 0.64% saline and be complete at about 0.44% saline.
- When red cells are less fragile, hemolysis starts and is complete at lower strengths of saline.

Modified Experiment

In this test, the red cell fragility is tested by counting the cells in a hemocytometer, using 0.45% saline for diluting the blood in one pipette, and using

Hayem's fluid for diluting blood in a second pipette. Both pipettes are shaken for about 2 minutes and counts are made from both pipettes. The percent of red cells hemolysed in 0.45% saline is thus determined. Less than 20% of normal RBCs are hemolysed by this method. In hereditary spherocytosis, the abnormal increase in fragility may cause hemolysis of more than 70% of red cells.

PRECAUTIONS

1. Use the same dropper, after thorough rinsing each time, for measuring saline and distilled water.
2. The test tubes should not be shaken vigorously after adding blood, because this is likely to cause mechanical hemolysis.
3. The test tubes should be left undisturbed for one hour before making the observations.

QUESTIONS

Q. 1 What is meant by the terms fragility and hemolysis?
Fragility. This term refers to the susceptibility of red cells to being broken down by osmotic or mechanical stresses.
Hemolysis. This term refers to the breaking down (bursting) of red cells resulting in release of Hb into the surrounding fluid.

Q. 2 Define osmosis and osmotic pressure. How much osmotic pressure is exerted by the blood and what is its importance?
Osmosis. It is the process of net movement of water from a weaker solution (of a solute and solvent) to a stronger solution through a selectively permeable membrane, that is permeable only to water but not to solute (salts, proteins, etc.).
Osmotic pressure. It is the pressure required to be applied to the stronger solution to prevent the movement of solute (water) from the weaker solution to the stronger solution. (It should be noted that the osmotic pressure does not produce the movement of water during osmosis).

Osmotic pressure of blood. The total osmotic pressure of blood (or plasma) due to all crystalloids and colloids is about 5000 mm Hg (6-7 atmospheres). But since the crystalloids (mainly NaCl) are equally distributed across (on the two sides) the capillary walls, it is only the colloidal osmotic pressure exerted by plasma proteins (about 25 mm Hg) that takes part in tissue fluid exchanges. The colloid osmotic pressure opposes hydrostatic pressure (blood pressure) within the capillaries— about 32 mm Hg at their arterial ends and 12 mm Hg at the venous ends. As a result, filtration occurs at the arterial ends and reabsorption at the venous ends. Changes in these forces, called Starling forces, can cause edema (accumulation of fluid in the tissues).

Q. 3 What will be the effect of vigorous shaking of the test tubes after adding blood to each of them?
Vigorous shaking, in an attempt to mix the contents of the test tubes, is likely to cause mechanical rupture of RBCs with release of Hb into the saline.

Q. 4 How do red cells behave in hypotonic and hypertonic saline solutions? How do they resist hemolysis in hypotonic saline?
The red cell membrane is selectively permeable membrane which allows water to pass through easily while the movement of various solutes is restricted to varying degrees.
Red cells in hypertonic saline. In hypertonic solutions, the RBCs , like other body cells, shrink (crenate) due to movement of water out of the cells (exosmosis).
Red cells in hypotonic saline. In hypotonic saline, water moves into the red cells (endosmosis). They swell up and lose their biconcave shape, becoming smaller and thicker. When they swell and become completely spherical, further increase in volume is not possible without an increase in their surface area. However, the surface area cannot increase because the cell membrane is "plastic" but not "elastic", i.e., it can change shape but is not able to stretch. A completely round shape is reached

when the red cell volume increases to about 150 percent of their original volume (say, from 90 μm^3 to 140 μm^3). It is clear that biconcave cells can resist greater hypotonicity as they can accommodate more and more water. Flat cells, on the other hand, can accommodate very small amounts of water before getting stretched and bursting.

Thus, osmotic fragility is an indicator of the shape of the cells. The more fragile the cells, the greater is their degree of spherocytosis. Also, fragility of red cells is greater in venous blood.

Comments
The red cell membrane has protein pumps and ion channels. Its structural proteins, including spectrin, actin, tropomyosin, adducin, etc. are attached to the transmembrane skeletal protein meshwork by the protein ankyrin. (The Hb molecules are not present free within the cells but absorbed on to the protein meshwork). The structural proteins give the red cells the remarkable property of "deformability" so that they can easily change their shape and squeeze through the 4-5 μm tissue capillaries and the still narrower and tighter meshwork and trabeculae of the spleen (in the spleen, which is an important blood filter which detains large and abnormal-shaped and rigid cells, part of the blood flows through the microvessels, while the rest 'percolates' through the phagocytes and lymphocytes of the splenic pulp before entering the sinusoids).

Q. 5 Give the normal range of fragility of red cells.
See page 137.

Q. 6 What will be the effect of waiting for 5-6 hours before observations are made on the test tubes?
If observations are made after, say, 5-6 hours, hemolysis is likely to occur in all hypotonic solutions. The reason is that without energy supply, various membrane pumps (especially Na^+-K^+ pump) will fail to function. Sodium chloride will enter the cells, they will swell up, and finally rupture.

Q. 7 What is the clinical significance of doing fragility test?

Though the fragility test is not done as a routine test, it is employed as a screening test in hereditary spherocytosis.

Q. 8 Name the conditions where red cell fragility increases and those where it decreases?

A. Increased red cell fragility is seen in the following conditions:

1. **Hereditary spherocytosis.** It is one of the commonest causes of hemolytic anemias. A defect in the structural proteins causes them to become spherocytes (in normal plasma), and more fragile. Some red cells are trapped and broken up in the spleen, while others hemolyze in blood.

2. **Autoimmune hemolytic anemia.** Auto-immune antibodies damage the structural proteins.

3. **Toxic chemicals, poisons, infections, and some drugs (aspirin).** These agents make the red cells more fragile in some individuals.

4. **Deficiency of glucose 6-phosphate dehydro-genase (G6PD).** This enzyme is required for glucose oxidation via hexose monophosphate pathway which generates NADPH. Normal red cells fragility is somehow dependent on NADPH. Deficiency of G6PD, which is the commonest human enzyme abnormality, increases the tendency of the red cells to hemolyze by antimalarial drugs and other agents.

5. **The venom of cobra and some insects** contains lecithinase which dissolves lecithin from red cell membranes, thus making them more fragile.

B. Decreased red cell fragility. It is seen in acholuric jaundice and some anemias. The increase in red cell size in pernicious anemia makes them less osmotically fragile as compared to normal red cells (as tested with the above method). However, their mechanical fragility is greater than normal, as a result of which they hemplyze in blood and in spleen.

Q. 9 What are the complications of hemolysis occurring in the circulating blood?

The Hb released from red cells will increase the osmotic pressure of blood thereby affecting tissue fluid exchanges. Further, if the tubular fluid is acidic, acid hematin crystals may be precipitated in the renal tubules and cause renal damage.

Q. 10 Name some hemolytic agents.

Some of the hemolytic agents are:

1. Hypotonic saline
2. Incompatible blood transfusion
3. Snake venom
4. Severe infection
5. Reaction to certain drugs. Aspirin is a common drug that may cause hemolysis at any time.

Q. 11 What is the effect of 5% glucose, 10% glucose, urea solution of any strength, and urine on red cells?

a. **5% glucose.** It is isotonic with blood (and plasma). The RBCs do not show any change in size or shape.

b. **10% glucose.** Since it is hypertonic, the red cells will shrink due to exosmosis (water moving out). However, in the intact body, when 10% or even 20% glucose is given intravenously, the RBCs will shrink in the beginning. But later on, after some time, glucose gets metabolised and there are no harmful effects.

c. **Urea solution.** As urea tends to move into the red cells, this is followed by water. The final result is hemolysis.

d. **Urine.** Since urine is hypotonic, the red cells imbibe some water and swell up. In a highly concentrated urine sample, the red cells shrink to some extent.

Q. 12 How does hemolysis occur in the body?

Hemolysis of red cells within bloodstream may occur in many different ways. It may be due to structural abnormalities (hereditary spherocytosis, sickle cells), mismatched blood transfusion, bacterial toxins, chemicals, adverse drug reactions, venom of snake and insects.

Q.13 Name some isotonic solutions for mammals.

Isotonic solutions of medical interest are:

1. Sodium bromide: 1.5%
2. Magnesium sulphate: 3.3%
3. Sodium chloride: 0.9%
4. Sodium nitrate: 2.5%
5. Dextrose: 5%
6. Sucrose: 10%
7. Sodium bicarbonate: 0.9%

Specific Gravity of Blood and Plasma (Copper Sulphate Falling Drop Method of Philips and van Slyke)

STUDENT OBJECTIVES

After completing this experiment, you should be able to:

1. Define specific gravity and indicate the specific gravities of blood, plasma, and serum.
2. Indicate the utility of this test.
3. Name the various fractions of plasma proteins and their functions.
4. List the different lipoprotein fractions and their clinical significance.

Relevance

The "copper sulphate falling drop method" is a rapid and accurate procedure for estimating plasma proteins and hemoglobin concentrations, and hematocrit values in a large number of cases. The test is useful in screening blood donors, and in handling emergency burn cases requiring plasma transfusions. The test is routinely done in many laboratories, and was used extensively during second world war.

PRINCIPLE

The procedure essentially involves comparing the specific gravity of blood, plasma or serum against the specific gravity of a series of copper sulphate solutions. After the specific gravity has been determined, line charts (or tables) are consulted to read off the concentration values.

APPARATUS AND MATERIALS

1. Well-stoppered bottles of 150 ml capacity—20 in number.
2. **Stock solution of copper sulphate** (sp gr = 1.100) is prepared by dissolving 159.0 g of $CuSO_4. 5 H_2O$ in 1.0 liter of distilled water at 25°C. Its specific gravity can be checked by weighing 100 ml of the solution in a volumetric flask, against distilled water.
3. Syringe and needle • Pasteur pipette. • Sterile swabs moist with alcohol.
4. **Standard copper sulphate solution for protein concentration.** Table 1.7 shows the amounts of stock solution and distilled water to prepare 100 ml portions of the test solutions. The bottles are numbered 1 to 12, and the serial number, specific gravity, and protein concentration (g%) of each solution is indicated on the labels pasted on the bottles. Once prepared, the solutions can be used for 40-50 estimations.
5. **Standard copper sulphate solutions for hemoglobin concentration.** Table 1.8 shows

TABLE 1.7

Preparation of standard copper sulfate solutions for the determination of plasma protein concentration

Bottle number	ml stock per 100 ml d.water	Specific gravity	Protein conc. g%	Bottle number	ml stock per 100 ml d.water	Specific gravity	Protein conc. g%
1	14.90	1.016	3.3	7	23.70	1.025	6.7
2	16.80	1.018	4.0	8	24.70	1.026	6.9
3	18.80	1.020	4.7	9	25.70	1.027	7.3
4	20.70	1.022	5.5	10	26.70	1.028	7.7
5	21.70	1.023	5.8	11	27.70	1.029	8.0
6	22.70	1.024	6.2	12	28.70	1.030	8.3

TABLE 1.8

Preparation of standard copper sulfate solutions for the determination of specific gravity of blood and hemoglobin concentration

Bottle number	1	2	3	4	5	6	7
Stock solution (ml)	49	51	54	57	59	61	64
Distilled water (ml)	51	49	46	43	41	39	36
Specific gravity	1.050	1.052	1.055	1.058	1.060	1.062	1.065
Hb conc (g%)	8.5	10.5	12.5	13.5	14.5	15.5	17

the amounts of stock solution and distilled water to prepare 100 ml portions of test solutions. The bottles are numbered 1 to 7, and the serial number, specific gravity, and Hb concentration of each solution are indicated on each bottle.

PROCEDURES

The procedure for plasma proteins and hemoglobin concentrations is the same. Plasma or serum is obtained from a sample of venous blood.

1. Arrange the bottles of copper sulfate solutions in order of increasing specific gravity from left to right, on a table of convenient height.
2. Starting in the middle of the row, allow a drop of plasma (serum or blood) to fall from a pasteur pipette, into the solution from a height of about 1 cm. (The size of the drop need not be constant.) The drop breaks through the surface, sinks to about 2-3 cm, and loses its momentum in 3-4 seconds. The drop then behaves according to its specific gravity; observe its behavior during the next 15 seconds, i.e., **after it has lost its momentum.** If its specific gravity is lesser than that of the solution, it rises to the surfaces; if it is greater than that of the solution, it sinks to the bottom. If its specific gravity is the same as that of the solution, it becomes stationary and floats in the middle of the solution.

If the drop continues to sink, move to the next higher specific gravity solution; if it begins to rise, move to the lower specific gravity solution, till you come to a solution where the drop remains stationary for about 15 seconds. Note the concentration of proteins indicated on the label.

3. The Hb concentration is measured by using blood, and determining its specific gravity by the "Falling Drop" method. The Hb in g% is then read off from the label on the bottle.

OBSERVATION AND RESULTS

When the plasma or blood drop falls into the solution, it becomes encased in a layer of copper proteinate and there is no change in its specific gravity for the next 15-20 seconds. This is the reason why the behavior of the drop is to be observed during this period. Within a short time, however, the drop becomes heavier and sinks to the bottom as a precipitate. In fact, the drops which initially float on the surface, ultimately become heavier and settle down.

QUESTIONS

Q. 1 Define specific gravity. What is the specific gravity of serum plasma, blood and red blood corpuscles. What does the specific gravity of blood depend on?

Specific gravity is the ratio of the weight of a given volume of a fluid to the weight of the same volume of distilled water, measured at 25°C. The specific gravity of serum, plasma, blood and red cells is as follows:

Serum	1.022-1.024
Plasma	1.028-1.032
Blood	1.058-1.062
Red cells	1.092-1.095

If water and plasma protein concentration are normal, the specific gravity of blood is dependent on the red cell volume (Hct), and therefore, the Hb concentration. The specific gravity of serum and plasma depends on the protein concentration.

Q. 2 What are the other methods of determining the specific gravity of blood?

1. Direct method. Equal volumes of blood and water are taken in special capillary tubes, called pyenometers, and are weighed. The ratio of their weights gives the specific gravity of blood.

2. Indirect methods

a. Hammer Schlag's method (Chloroform-benzene mixture). Chloroform (sp. gr. = 1.480) and benzene (sp. gr. = 0.877) are mixed in a urine glass. A drop of blood is allowed to fall into the mixture and benzene or chloroform are added as required till the blood drop float in the middle of the mixture. The specific gravity of the mixture is then determined with a hydrometer, which will indicate the specific gravity of the blood sample. The mixture, however, is inflammable and hence not preferred.

b. Glycerine and water mixture Glycerine (sp.gr. = 1.225) and water (sp. gr. = 1.000) may be used. The procedure is similar to that of chloroform-benzene mixture. However, since glycerine is hygroscopic (absorbs water), the method is not accurate.

Q. 3 Why is copper sulphate method preferred over the other mixtures?

This method is chosen because the chemical is cheap, and it is not hygroscopic. Also, its temperature coefficient of expansion is about the same as that of blood. No correction factor for temperature is, therefore, required.

Q. 4 What is the clinical significance of determining the specific gravity of serum, plasma, and blood?

The specific gravity test is a quick and accurate method for the estimation of serum and plasma protein concentration as well as hemoglobin concentration and hematocrit. The test is employed in the screening of blood donors, mass surveys for anemia, and in handling emergency cases of burns requiring repeated transfusions of plasma, plasma expanders, or blood. The method was extensively used during World War II for assessing battle casualties requiring blood transfusions.

Use of Specific gravity test in blood banks.
A working solution (sp.gr. = 1.053 is prepared by adding 48 ml of distilled water to 52 ml of stock solution of copper sulphate (described above). A drop of blood is allowed to fall into it from a height of 1 cm. if the drop sinks, the Hb in that sample is over 12.5 g%, and the potential donor is bled for blood donation. If the drop floats for more than 15 seconds, the Hb level is less than 12.5 g% and the donor is considered unsuitable for blood donation.

Q. 5 What are the physiological and pathological conditions in which the specific gravity of blood is increased and decreased?
The specific gravity of blood is affected by:
1. Red cell count.
2. Hemoglobin concentration.
3. Plasma (or serum) protein concentration.
4. Water content of blood.

Physiological conditions. The specific gravity of blood is high in newborns, and at high altitude due to polycythemia. It is decreased during pregnancy (due to hemodilution) and after excess water intake.

Pathological conditions. The specific gravity is **increased** in polycythemia due to any disease (e.g., congenital heart disease, cardiac failure), polycythemia vera, severe dehydration (diarrhea, vomiting and hemoconcentration (loss of plasma due to burns).

The specific gravity **decreases** in anemias, hemodilution (excessive secretion or prolonged treatment with glucocorticoids), and kidney disease (loss of albumin and water retention).

Q. 6 Name the various fractions of plasma proteins? What are their functions?
The normal plasma protein concentration is 6-8 g%. Some of the proteins present in plasma are also found elsewhere in the body. Because of the large size of their molecules, plasma proteins tend to remain within the blood stream. The various fractions of plasma proteins are:

Albumin	=	4.0-5.5 g%
Fibrinogen	=	0.3-0.5 g%
Globulins	=	1.5-3.0 g%
Prothrombin	=	30-40 mg %

Using filter paper electrophoresis, the patterns of serum proteins are:

Albumin	=	57%
Alpha-1 globulin	=	4.7%
Alpha-2 globulin	=	8.45%
beta-1 and beta-2 globulins	=	11.33%
Gamma globulins	=	18.52 %

With the exception of gamma globulins, which are synthesized in the plasma cells in lymphoid tissue, all the other proteins (albumin, fibrinogen, some globulins) are synthesized in the liver.

Functions of plasma proteins. The proteins perform the following functions:
1. **Osmotic pressure.** The osmotic pressure of plasma proteins, called oncotic pressure, is involved in tissue fluid exchanges (see Expt. 1-20).
2. **Protein metabolic pool.** Though these proteins form part of the protein metabolic pool, they are not ordinarily used for providing energy.
3. **Buffering function.** They exert about 15% of the buffering action of the blood (all proteins, including Hb are buffers). They function to convert strong acids or bases into weak acids or bases. Strong acid or bases ionize easily and can contribute many H^+ or OH^- ions, which can affect the pH to a great extent. Weak acids or bases do not ionize as much and thus contribute fewer H^+ or OH^- ions.
4. **Viscosity of blood.** The plasma proteins contribute to the viscosity of blood and so affect the blood pressure (see next experiment).
5. **Coagulation of blood.** Fibrinogen, prothrombin and many clotting factors form part of the clotting mechanism.
6. **Role as carriers.** They act as carriers in the transport of many substances, such as hormones, metals, calcium, ions, amino

acids, bilirubin, vitamin B12, drugs, etc. Binding these substances prevents their rapid clearance from the body by the kidneys. Major lipids do not circulate in the free form but in combination with plasma proteins, (see below).

Q. 7 What are lipoproteins? What are their functions and clinical significance?

The major lipids in plasma (cholesterol, triglycerides, TGs) do not circulate in the blood in free form. Since they are nonpolar and thus hydrophobic molecules, they must first be made water-soluble in order to be transported in watery plasma. This is achieved by binding them to proteins formed in liver. Free fatty acids are bound to albumin, while others are transported in the form of round particles called lipoproteins that are made up of hundreds of molecules.

In a lipoprotein particle, there is an outer coat of proteins, amphipathic phospholipids, and cholesterol that surrounds the inner core of hydrophobic triglycerides and cholesterol ester molecules. The proteins in the outer shell are called **apoproteins** (or simply **APO**). The APOs are designated by letters (A, B, C, D, and E) plus a number. **APO B** has 2 forms: a low m.w. form, APO B-48 that transports ingested lipids, and a high m.w. form, APO B- 100, which transports endogenous lipids. Their levels have clinical significance in atherosclerosis. APO E concentration greatly increases in nerve injuries and is concerned with the repair process.

Functions of lipoproteins. There are several types of lipoproteins each having a different function. However, all are mainly transport vehicles functioning as a sort of pick-up and delivery service. They are classified on the basis of density that varies with the ratio of lipids (they have low density) to proteins (they have a high density). Thus, the lipoproteins are grouped in, from largest and lightest to smallest and heaviest, the following groups: **very low**, **low**, **intermediate**, and **high density lipoproteins.**

Clinical Significance. Their clinical significance lies in relation to coronary artery disease, and atherosclerosis (a form of arteriosclerosis).

The **LDLs** carry about 50% of cholesterol. They transport cholesterol from the liver to body cells for use in repair of cell membranes and production of steroid hormones and bile salts. However, excess of LDLs promote atherosclerosis, so that their cholesterol is called "bad cholesterol".

The **HDLs** contain about 20% cholesterol. They remove and carry excess of cholesterol from body cells to liver for elimination. Since they lower blood cholesterol level, their cholesterol is called "good cholesterol".

The desirable levels of various lipoproteins are:
Triglycerides:

    Males   = up to 165 mg/dl.
    Females   = 40-140 mg/dl.

VLDL cholesterol = < 40 mg/dl.

LDL cholesterol = < 130 mg/dl.

IDL cholesterol = 5-50 mg/dl.

HDL cholesterol = > 40 mg/dl.

Total cholesterol = < 200 mg/dl

1-22

Determination of Viscosity of Blood

Viscosimeter (viscometer). The viscosimeter is a U-shaped glass tube, one limb of which is wider with a bulb near its lower end. The other limb has a bulb near its upper end and a narrow capillary bore below it. There are two markings, 1 and 2, above and below the bulb in this limb.

PROCEDURES

The limb with the wide tube is filled with anticoagulated blood; the blood is then sucked up into the narrow limb to above the mark 1. The time taken by the blood to fall from mark 1 to mark 2 is noted. The procedure is then repeated with water and is compared with that of blood. The apparatus must be kept vertical throughout the experiment.

Normal viscosity of blood = About 3-4 times that of water, i.e., its relative viscosity is 3-4.

Viscosity of Blood

Viscosity, which represents the mutual attraction between the particles of a fluid, is the internal friction or "lack of slipperiness" between the adjacent layers, especially between the outermost layer of the flowing blood and the walls. The shape of the molecules rather than their size determines the viscosity.

The viscosity of blood depends mostly on the ratio of red cells to plasma (fluid) volume and to a lesser extent on the plasma protein concentration. The viscosity of blood *in vivo,* especially in the microvessels, is about 1.2 (water = 0.695; see below) because of axial streaming of red cells (Fahreus-Lindqvist effect).

Effect of temperature on viscosity. Temperature has an important effect on viscosity. Water has a viscosity of 1 cP [centipoise (after Poiseuille)— the unit of viscosity] at 20.3°C and about 1.8 cP at 0°C. The viscosity of plasma and blood is even more sensitive to changes in temperature. Thus, the temperature of skin and subcutaneous tissues exerts an important effect on the viscosity of blood.

Significance of Viscosity of Blood

The **viscosity** of blood is one of the three factors on which the resistance (i.e., the opposition) to flow of blood in the blood vessels depends, the other two being: **average radius of the blood vessels**, and, the **total blood vessel length**. Since resistance, in fact, peripheral resistance to blood flow is directly proportional to the viscosity of blood, any factor that affects viscosity will increase or decrease the blood pressure. In this way, variations in viscosity of blood influence the load to which the heart is subjected during contraction.

Increased viscosity is seen in polycythemia due to any cause, congestive heart failure, diabetes mellitus, multiple myeloma, icterus, profuse sweating when water intake is limited, severe vomiting and diarrhea, and leukemias.

Decreased viscosity is seen in anemias, edematous states, and sometimes in malaria.

Human Experiments

Although ideas about the human body owe a great deal to thinkers like Charak, Sushruta, and Aristotle, they are based on innumerable observations made by a number of investigators on phenomena encountered during the daily course of life. In many short experiments included in this section, the students are invited to perform these tests/experiments on themselves and/on their work partners, both inside as well outside the laboratory.

During the last few decades, there has been a significant change in the thinking and outlook of the physicians on illness—a trend which is essentially physiological in approach. Many of the experiments included here provide an account of various physiological principles underlying tests and investigations employed in clinical medicine.

Unit I
Respiratory System

2-1

Stethography
Recording of Normal and Modified
Movements of Respiration

STUDENT OBJECTIVES

After completing this experiment, you should be able to:
1. Explain how the movements of breathing can be recorded.
2. Define various terms used in connection with respiratory movements.
3. Give an account of the physiological basis of how normal breathing is maintained and controlled.
4. Describe the effect of hyperventilation and breath holding on respiration.
5. Explain why ventilation increases during muscular exercise.
6. List the factors that cause 'breaking point' after voluntary breath holding.

APPARATUS AND MATERIALS

1. **Stethograph.** It consists of corrugated canvas-rubber tubing, about 60 cm long and 3-4 cm in diameter. It has two side clips and an open link chain. One end of the stethograph is

closed while the other end can be connected, via pressure rubber tubing, to an air-recording system, as shown in **Figure 2-1**.

2. **Marey's or Brodie's tambour.** The tambour is a metallic cup or a small flat saucer, with a rubber diaphragm stretched over its top. A light-metal capillary writing lever is mounted on a small metal disc that rests on the diaphragm. A rubber tube attached to an outlet connects the tambour to the stethograph.

3. **Kymograph.** •Stop watch. •Tap water in a cup •Time marker •Polythene bag of 5-6 litres capacity.

PROCEDURES, OBSERVATIONS AND RESULTS

Consult Expt 4-1, Section 4 for a description of the electric kymograph ("drum").

1. Seat the subject on a stool with her/his back to the recording apparatus, and ask her to relax and breathe normally. Tie the stethograph around the subject's chest at a level where respiratory movements are maximum (usually midchest, at 4th-5th intercostal space). Slightly stretch the stethograph so that respiratory movements can cause adequate pressure changes within the stethograph.

Mount the tambour on the stand and connect the stethograph to it. Bring the writing point in contact with the drum surface at a tangent.

2. Recording the respiratory movements. Set the kymograph at a slow speed of 1.2 mm/sec, and record a few respiratory movements. Note that as the chest expands during inspiration, the stethograph gets stretched and its length increases. And, since its mean radius remains unchanged, the increase in its volume leads to a fall in pressure within it. This is transmitted to the tambour where the higher atmospheric pressure pushes the diaphragm, and along with it, the writing lever, downwards. Thus the downstroke of the lever is inspiration while upstroke is expiration. Note the following:

i. Rate of breathing (this you will record after obtaining a time tracing).

ii. Relative duration of inspiration and expiration.

iii. Presence or absence of a gap between one inspiration and the next expiration, and between one expiration and the next inspiration.

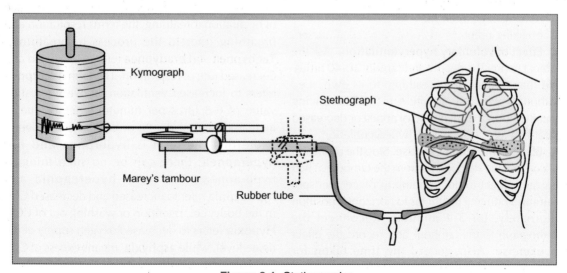

Figure 2-1. Stethography

3. Effect of deglutition (swallowing). Ask the subject to take a mouthful of water, and while movements are being recorded, to swallow it. After a few respiratory movements, ask him/her to drink water from the cup in one go. Note that there is a temporary stoppage of breathing in both cases—a condition called **"deglutition apnea"** (apnea= temporary stoppage of respiration).

4. Effect of modified respiratory movements. Record the effect of coughing, sneezing, talking, singing, laughing, yawning, sobbing, and Valsalva maneuver on respiratory movements, giving a 2-3 minute interval between each act.

5. Effect of breath holding. (also see next experiment on breath holding time). Ask the subject to take a deep breath, close the nose and mouth, and then to hold breath for as long as he/she can. (The drum may be stopped after a few seconds and then restarted near the end of this act). After a variable interval of 30 to 70 seconds or more, the subject 'tries' to make respiratory movements but can still hold breath. However, within a few seconds, breath can no longer be held and a deep breath is taken, a point called **"breaking point"**. Note the following:

- Duration of breath holding
  (after a deep inspiration)   = ... sec.
- Duration for which breathing
  remains high after the
  breaking point   = ... sec.

6. Effect of voluntary hyperventilation. Ask the subject to breathe deeply and rapidly 30-40 times, and then to leave the breathing 'to its own' (i.e., without paying any attention to it). The tracing usually shows a short period of apnea or decreased breathing after stoppage of hyperventilation.

7. Effect of muscular exercise. Stop the drum and disconnect the stethograph from the tambour. Then ask the subject to do "running in place" or "spot running", bringing the thighs to horizontal position alternately, for 3-4 minutes. Reconnect the stethograph to the tambour and record the effect of exercise. Also, record the time taken for respiration to return to resting levels.

8. Ask the subject to breathe into and out of the polythene bag for a few times and note the effect; but discontinue if there is much discomfort.

9. Record a 5-sec time interval below the graph obtained, keeping the kymograph speed unchanged. Indicate various events with arrows and number them. Remove the graph and fix it in the usual manner.

PRECAUTIONS

1. The stethograph applied to the chest should not be too tight nor too loose.
2. Do not let the subject look at the tracings being obtained.
3. Do not allow the subject to hyperventilate for more than 2 minutes or so. Record a few normal movements before each maneuver.

QUESTIONS

Q. 1 What is meant by the terms; ventilation, eupnea, tachypnea, bradypnea, hyperpnea, hypercapnia and hypocapnia, hypoxia, and asphyxia?

The term **ventilation** means movement of air into and out of the lungs. The term **eupnea** means normal breathing. **Apnea** is temporary stoppage of respiration (breathing; the terms respiration and breathing refer to the process of breathing). **Tachypnea** and **bradypnea** refer to increased and decreased rate of respiration. The term **hyperpnea** refers to increased ventilation (above the resting value of 6-8 litres per minute) whether due to increased rate, or depth, or both rate and depth. (Note that the term is **hyperpnea and not hyperapnea**; there can be no such thing as hyperapnea). The terms **hypercapnia** and **hypocapnia** refer to increased and decreased CO_2 in the body, i.e., retention or washing out of CO_2. **Hypoxia** refers to decreased oxygen supply at the tissue level, while **asphyxia** means excess of CO_2 and lack of oxygen in the body.

Q. 2 Is breathing (respiration) an automatic process or a voluntary act? How is normal respiration maintained and controlled?

Respiration is both a spontaneous (automatic) process (i.e., without any conscious effort or being aware of it), as well as a voluntary activity. When we are not/or do not become aware of our breathing (such as during sleep and while we are at our daily tasks), it goes on automatically and spontaneously. However, we can become aware of our breathing whenever we want to or think about it; then we can increase or decrease, or even stop our breathing, at least for a short time.

Spontaneous or automatic breathing. The alternate contraction and relaxation of respiratory muscles (diaphragm, intercostals, etc.) brings about changes in the size of the thorax; as a result of which air enters and leaves the lungs. These muscles, which are striated, skeletal, or voluntary, are rhythmically stimulated by impulses in their motor nerve supply (phrenics and intercostal nerves). These motor nerves have no activity of their own but are activated by a rhythmic discharge of impulses (depolarization and repolarization) from the **"medullary rhythmicity area"**, which is a part of respiratory centre in the brain stem. Thus, the medullary rhythmicity area sets up the basic rhythm of inspiration and expiration.

Voluntary control of respiration. The voluntary control over breathing is exerted via the cortico-spinal (pyramidal) tracts that control voluntary muscle activity throughout the body. The axons of these tracts (upper motor neurons) descend from the cerebral motor cortex, bypass the brain stem respiratory centre and end on phrenic and other neurons that innervate respiratory muscles.

Maintenance and control of respiration. Respiration is maintained by the rhythmic discharge of impulses from the medullary rhythmicity area. The activity of this centre is controlled by a variety of inputs. These inputs include: cerebral cortex, hypothalamus (emotions affect our respiration), central and peripheral chemoreceptors, barorecep-

tors, stretch receptors in the lungs, and muscles, joints, and ligaments.

Q. 3 Why should the subject not look at the tracings being obtained?

Respiratory movements are easily affected by our becoming aware of them—their rate, depth, rhythm, etc. If the subject looks at the record being obtained, he/she will become conscious (aware) of it so that the movements are bound to change and not represent the true effects of various maneuvers.

Q. 4 What is deglutition apnea? Describe its mechanism and physiological significance.

This term refers to a temporary stoppage of breathing when we swallow food or fluids. It is a reflex phenomenon, and occurs automatically whether we swallow a sip of a drink, or drink a cupful of water. During the pharyngeal stage of deglutition, which may last for 0.5 sec or more, the food or fluid stimulates the sensory nerve endings of touch in the mucosa of pharynx. Afferent nerve impulses are set up and relayed along the 5th, 9th, and 10th cranial nerves and cause, via the deglutition center, inhibition of respiratory center. This stops the breathing at any point of inspiration or expiration. Simultaneously, there is closure of glottis, the opening between vocal cords.

Physiological significance of deglutition apnea. The stoppage of breathing and closure of glottis prevents the entry of food or fluid into the upper respiratory passages, which would cause aspiration pneumonia or other complications (it is a common experience that whenever a particle of food or fluid tends to enter our respiratory passages, there is a strong bout of coughing till the offending particle is expelled; all this happens reflexly).

Q. 5 What is "breaking point" and what is its cause?

The **"breaking point"** at the end of breath-holding is due to: (i) accumulation of CO_2 in the body and since it is a potent respiratory stimulus, it leads to resumption of breathing, (ii) increased H^+ ion concentration and (iii) decrease in PO_2. (Consult Q/A 1 in the next Experiment for details).

Q. 6 How can breath-holding time be prolonged?

The breath-holding time can be increased by: (i) hyperventilating before holding the breath. (This will decrease the arterial PCO_2 and raise PO_2 a little) and, (ii) breathing pure oxygen before holding the breath.

Q. 7 What is hyperventilation, how can it be caused, and what are its effects? Are there any harmful effects if it is carried on for long?

Hyperventilation refers to increased volume of air moving into and out of the lungs per unit time—whether due to increase in rate, depth or both. It can result from:

1. **Voluntary effort.** This is the most powerful stimulus for increasing the ventilation.
2. **Muscular exercise.** It is the second most powerful respiratory stimulus.
3. **Chemical stimuli.** High PCO_2, low PO_2 or increased H^+ ion concentration, resulting from lung and heart diseases can increase the ventilation.
   - While the chemical stimuli increase the ventilation to about 80-90 liters/minute, (from the resting level of 6-8 liters/minute), voluntary hyperventilation can achieve rates of over 200 liters/minute, at least for short periods.

Effects of voluntary hyperventilation. When a person hyperventilates for 1-2 minutes and then stops and allows respiration to continue on its own, without exerting any control over it, there is a short period of apnea. This is followed by a few breaths and then a period of apnea once again, followed by a few breaths. The cycle may last for a while before returning to normal rhythm. The apnea is due to washing out of CO_2 (hypocapnia), but as CO_2 accumulates, the breathing starts again. (Though CO_2 is a 'waste' product of metabolism, it is a 'stimulus par excellence' for respiration. Thus, while a high PCO_2 stimulates breathing, a low PCO_2 inhibits it until the blood PCO_2 returns to normal).

Harmful effects of hyperventilation. Though a single bout of hyperventilation may have no ill effects, chronic hyperventilation, as seen in neurotic patients, may produce certain ill effects. The arterial PCO_2 may fall from the normal level of 40 mm Hg to 15-20 mm Hg. This degree of hypocapnia produces vasoconstriction of cerebral blood vessels. (CO_2 is a very strong vasodilator, so its lack will result in vasoconstriction). The cerebral ischemia causes dizziness, light-headedness, etc. Constriction of retinal blood vessels may cause blurring of vision.

A more serious effect of chronic hyperventilation and associated hypocapnia is alkalosis which causes precipitation of ionic calcium. If the serum calcium is already low, an attack of tetany may be precipitated. (Calcium stabilizes cell membranes; low ECF calcium increases membrane permeability to sodium ions, which in turn cause spontaneous depolarizations.) As a result, there are extensive tetanic spasms of the skeletal muscles, especially in limbs and larynx.

Q. 8 What is the cause of increased ventilation during exercise?

A variety of factors are involved in increasing the ventilation during exercise.

1. **Psychic stimuli.** Ventilation often increases in anticipation of the exercise, i.e., before the exercise has started. Soon after the start of exercise, and before blood PCO_2, PO_2 and H^+ ions have time to change, there is a sudden and large increase in ventilation (mainly due to increase in depth) due to the next two factors mentioned below.
2. **Impulses from motor cerebral cortex.** As the motor cortex sends impulses, via corticospinal tracts, to the motor neurons of active muscles, it also sends, via collaterals of the tracts, excitatory impulses to the respiratory centre (as it does to vasomotor centre). The result is a sudden increase in ventilation.

3. **Impulses from proprioceptors.** Body movements, especially those of the limbs, stimulate the proprioceptors (stretch receptors) in the active muscles, tendons, ligaments, joints, etc.; these excitatory impulses are also relayed to the respiratory centre (it is important to note that even passive movements of the limbs increase the ventilation.

4. **Chemical stimuli.** Normally, the increased ventilation is enough to supply the extra O_2 to the active muscles, as well as to remove the excess of CO_2 produced without any significant change in arterial PO_2 and PCO_2, especially in trained athletes. In fact, the PO_2 may be higher and PCO_2 lower than the normal. Thus, low PO_2 and high PCO_2 cannot explain respiratory stimulation during exercise.

Sometimes, the neural signals may be too weak to stimulate the respiratory centre; it is then that the chemical stimuli play a role. Also, in later stages of severe exercise, it is the chemical stimuli that increase the ventilation. (Even though there may be no gas changes, the sensitivity of the respiratory center to the normal levels may be involved).

5. **Other factors.** Increased body temperature, increased blood K^+, lactic acidosis, hypoxia in exercising muscles stimulating the sensory nerve endings, fluctuations in blood gases—all help in increasing the ventilation.

Q. 9 Why does ventilation and oxygen utilization remain high after the end of exercise?

During moderately severe and severe muscular exercise, the muscles obtain their energy from anaerobic (i.e., in the absence of O_2) metabolism of glucose, which results in the formation of lactic acid. The buffering of lactate liberates more CO_2 which further stimulates respiration. After the end of exercise, however, ventilation and O_2 utilization remain high until the "oxygen debt" incurred during anaerobic glycolysis is repaid, i.e., the lactate is converted back to pyruvate when O_2 supply is restored after exercise. The cause of increased ventilation after exercise is, thus, not high PCO_2 (which is normal or low), or low PO_2 (which is normal or high) but the increased arterial H^+ ion concentration due to lactic acidemia.

Q. 10 What is periodic breathing?

Periodic breathing is a disturbance of respiratory control where periods of apnea alternate with periods of increased respiration. This waxing and waning of breathing begins with shallow breaths, which gradually increase in depth, each phase lasting 20-30 seconds.

This is called **Cheyne-Stokes breathing.** Various irregular forms such as, Biot's breathing, Kussmaul's breathing, sleep apnea syndrome, etc. are also seen.

Periodic breathing is generally a sign of brain damage, increased intracranial pressure, congestive heart failure, uremia, etc.

Q. 11 What is Valsalva maneuver? Explain its significance, and effect on breathing.

Valsalva maneuver is forced expiration against a closed glottis. Brief periods of straining and forced expiration, such as during defecation, urination, trying to lift a heavy weight, etc., are a common experience. A deep breath is taken, and the expiratory muscles of chest and abdomen are forcefully contracted while keeping glottis closed so that air cannot leave the lungs. The result is a strong compression of abdomen and thorax. The raised pressures have important effects on venous return and blood pressure (see Expt. 2-6 on Blood Pressure).

The record of respiratory movements shows a deeper inspiration than normal, and then stoppage of breathing during expiration. The tracing may show a downwards shift.

Determination of
Breath Holding Time (BHT)

Relevance

Different individuals can hold their breath for variable periods of time depending on the functional status of the lungs, development of respiratory muscles, practice, age and sex. Determination of breath holding time (BHT) is a simple test which can provide useful information in health, and diseases of the lungs. It is also an instructive laboratory exercise.

PROCEDURES

As the students work in batches of two, one becomes the subject and the other acts as the observer.

1. The subject should sit quietly for a few minutes, breathing normally before the breath holding exercises are started. The procedure should be explained to the subject in clear terms. Use a stop watch and note the time for each determination.

2. Ask the subject to pinch his/her nostrils with the thumb and forefinger, and hold his/her breath after a quiet inspiration. Note the time for which the breath can be held. Make 3 observations at intervals of 5 minutes.

3. Using the same procedure, record the BHT after (a) a quiet expiration, (b) a deep inspiration, (c) a deep expiration, (d) hyperventilation (deep and fast breathing) for 1-2 minutes, (e) re-breathing from a polythene bag for 15-20 seconds with a nose-clip on (discontinue if there is discomfort), and (f) 8-10 deep breaths of pure oxygen from Benedict-Roth apparatus.

4. Tabulate your results as shown below. The highest value for each determination is the BHT for that exercise.

OBSERVATIONS AND RESULTS

Explain your results from the following data

Breath holding after.......	Reading (in sec) 1st	2nd	3rd	Maximum value	Minimum value
a. Quiet inspiration	....	....	....	......	.....
b. Quiet expiration ...	...	...	...	......	.....
c. Deep inspiration ...	...	...	...	....	...
d. Deep expiration ...	...	...	...	...	...
e. Hyperventilation ...	...	...	...	...	...
f. Record single readings					
After re-breathing from polythene bag				.......sec	
After 8-10 deep breaths of oxygen				.... sec	

QUESTIONS

Q. 1 Why cannot a person hold his/her breath for periods longer than a minute or so? What is the cause of breaking point?

The normal level of CO_2, in the body (arterial PCO_2 of 40 mm Hg) is just sufficient to maintain a resting ventilation of 6-8 liters/min. This degree of ventilation is enough to supply adequate amounts of O_2 to the tissues at rest. Any increase in ventilation by high PCO_2 (or low PO_2) or other stimuli shows that the "ventilatory drive" has increased (i.e., the medullary respiratory centre has been stimulated). On the other hand, the cerebral cortex can temporarily allow voluntary breath holding, and thus oppose the ventilatory drive.

Thus, two opposing factors are operating during breath holding: the **ventilatory drive**, and voluntary stoppage of breathing. Since the ability to hold breath remains unchanged in a normal person, the "breaking point", i.e., the point when a breath has to be taken, is reached when the ventilatory drive is so strong that it overcomes the desire to continue to hold breath. (It is interesting to note that the world record for breath holding is 5 min 13 sec.) It is also obvious that a person cannot commit suicide by holding breath, because breathing will begin even if that person losses consciousness.

Note
Usually, the breaking point is reached when the arterial (and alveolar) PCO_2 increases from the normal 40 mm Hg to about 60 mm Hg, and the PO_2 falls from the normal 100 mm Hg to about 50 mm Hg.

Q. 2 What is the effect of prolonged hyper-ventilation on breath holding time?
Hyperventilation washes out CO_2 from the body so that both PCO_2 and H^+ ion concentration decrease. At the same time, there is some increase in PO_2. Therefore, it will take some more time for these chemical stimuli to increase the ventilatory drive so that it reaches the breaking point.

Q. 3 What are the factors that increase and decrease the BHT?
The normal BHT after a deep inspiration may vary from 40 sec to over a minute. It can be increased by practicing breathing exercises as part of Yoga training. Breathing pure O_2 before holding breath delays the breaking point. Hyperventilation increases BHT, as described above. Reflex or mechanical factors also affect BHT. Psychological factors, such as motivation (e.g., telling the subject that his performance is improving, increases the BHT).

BHT decreases in many diseases, e.g, chronic bronchitis, emphysema, congestive heart failure and so on.

Q. 4 What are breath holding attacks?
Breath holding attacks occur in infants and young children and are generally precipitated by emotional distress, such as fright, pain, anxiety, or frustration. The child starts crying, and suddenly holds his/her breath, becomes limp or stiff and may become blue and lose consciousness. The attack lasts briefly and recovery is rapid and complete. In some cases, there may be a rigid phase followed by tonic-clonic convulsions. These attacks are harmless and stop by the age of 3 years; they are not considered epileptic in origin.

2-3

Spirometry (Determination of Vital Capacity, Peak Expiratory Flow Rate, and Lung Volumes and Capacities)

STUDENT OBJECTIVES	
After completing this practical, you should be able to: 1. Define vital capacity and name the muscles involved in carrying it out.	2. Record the vital capacity and explain the effect of posture on it. 3. Describe the physiological and pathological factors that affect vital capacity. 4. Explain the difference between the lung capacities and volumes.

5. Indicate the differences between static and dynamic lung volumes and capacities.
6. Define "timed vital capacity" and indicate its significance.
7. Define peak expiratory flow rate and explain its clinical significance.

Relevance

Although many sophisticated tests are available for assessing respiratory functions, vital capacity is a simple and useful measurement for assessing the ventilatory functions of the lungs in health and disease.

Measurement

Vital capacity may be measured either on a simple spirometer or a recording spirometer (spiro- = breathe; meter = measuring device):

A. **Simple spirometer (student spirometer;** also called a **Vitalograph).** It is a common low-cost instrument, either a metallic or a bellows type, used in colleges, hospitals, sports facilities, and gymnasia;

B. **Recording spirometer.** It is a sophisticated, electrically-driven, recording system used in respiratory physiology labs, hospitals, etc. It provides a graphic record of various lung volumes and capacities.

C. **Wright's peak flow meter.** It is a small portable instrument which can give information about the state of respiratory passages (it can be carried in one's pocket for bed-side use by the physician).

Note
In this experiment, the students will use a simple spirometer and the peak flow meter to measure some of the ventilatory functions of the lungs under normal conditions. The working of a recording spirometer will then be briefly described.

DEFINITIONS AND TERMINOLOGY

The rate. The rate of respiration is somewhat variable even at rest, varying from 12-16/min.

However, when one becomes conscious of one's breathing, it may speed up, slow down, or show a temporary disturbance in its rate, depth, and rhythm.

The respiratory cycle. There is a cycle of inspiration, expiration, and a pause. The duration of the pause varies inversely with the rate. (The pause may not be obvious in some cases).

LUNG VOLUMES AND CAPACITIES

The volume of air in the lungs changes considerably during a respiratory cycle. However, for convenience, 4 lung volumes and 4 lung capacities are distinguished, as shown in **Figure 2-2.**

The term **lung volumes** refers to the non-overlapping subdivisions, or fractions of the total lung air, while the term **capacities** refers to combination of two or more lung volumes.

Lung Volumes

1. **Tidal Volume (TV).** It is the amount of air that moves into the lungs with each inspiration (or the amount that moves out with each expiration) during normal quiet breathing (tidal respiration). It amounts to about 500 ml. (It varies greatly in

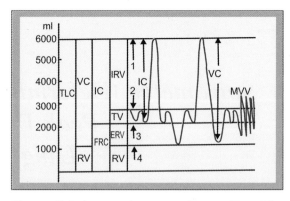

Figure 2-2. Lung volumes and capacities. The volumes do not overlap; the capacities are made up of two or more volumes. Arrows: (1) Maximum inspiratory level; (2) Resting inspiratory level; (3) Resting expiratory level; and (4) Maximum expiratory level. Standard abbreviations used

different persons and in the same person at different times).

2. Inspiratory reserve volume (IRV). It is the extra volume of air that can be inspired over and above the normal (resting, quiet) tidal volume (i.e., from the spontaneous end-inspiratory point), with maximum effort. It amounts to about 2500 ml.

3. Expiratory Reserve Volume (ERV). It is the extra amount of air that can be expelled (expired) by forceful expiration from the spontaneous end-expiratory point, i.e., over and above the normal tidal expiration. It amounts to about 1100 ml.

- (The term 'reserve' in these 2 volumes means this; during quiet breathing (i.e., without effort, spontaneous), we take in 500 ml air and breathe out 500 ml air. In addition to this 500, one can, with maximum effort, take in more air (IRV), or expel more air (ERV).

4. Residual volume (RV). It is the amount of air that remains behind in the lungs after a maximum voluntary expiration. It amounts to 1100 ml. The lungs cannot be emptied out completely of air even with maximum effort because as the pressure outside small air passages increases (i.e., the high intrathoracic pressure due to maximum expiratory effort) they are compressed and thus block the flow of air out of the lungs.

Lung Capacities

1. Vital capacity VC; forced vital capacity, FVC; forced expired (or expiratory) volume, FEV. It is the largest volume of air a person can expel from the lungs with maximum effort after first filling the lungs fully by a deepest possible inspiration. It amounts to 3.5 to 5.5 liters.

2. Inspiratory capacity (IC) It is the maximum amount of air that a person can breathe in with maximum effort, starting from the normal end-expiratory point. It amounts to about 3000 ml. (IRV, 2500 ml + TV, 500 ml = 3000 ml).

3. Functional Residual Capacity (FRC). This is the amount of air remaining in the lungs at the end of a normal (quiet) expiration. It amounts to about 2500 ml. (ERV, 1100 ml + RV, 1100 ml = 2200 ml).

4. Total Lung Capacity (TLC). It is the volume of air that is present in the lungs at the end of a deepest possible inspiration. It is a measure of VC + RV, and amounts to 4500-6000 ml.

Minute ventilation (minute volume, MV). This is the amount of air that is breathed in or breathed out per minute when the person is at rest. It amounts to 6-8 liters/min. (TV × Rate of respiration, i.e., 500 ×12 to 16 = 6-8 liters per minute).

Alveolar Ventilation. Out of a tidal volume of 500 ml, 150 ml air remains in the upper respiratory passages up to respiratory bronchioles (anatomical dead space), while only 350 ml reaches the respiratory zone (respiratory bronchioles, alveolar ducts and alveoli) for exchange of gases. Thus, alveolar ventilation would be = 350 × 12 to 16= 4.2 —5.6 liters per minute.

Maximum voluntary ventilation (Maximum ventilation volume, MVV). It is the mount of air which can be moved into or out of the lungs with maximum effort during one minute. Formerly called **maximum breathing capacity (MBC)**, the MVV amounts to 100-140 liters/min. The subject breathes quickly and deeply for 15 seconds, and MVV is calculated for one minute. (This means that pulmonary ventilation of 6-8 l/min can be increased by 15-20 times with maximum effort, though for short periods).

STATIC AND DYNAMIC LUNG VOLUMES AND CAPACITIES

The lung volumes and capacities may either be **static** or **dynamic,** depending on whether or not time factor has been taken into consideration.

A. Static volumes and capacities. These measurements are those where time factor is not taken into consideration. They are expressed in milliliters or liters, and include:

Static volumes: TV, IRV, ERV, and RV.

Static capacities: IC, VC (FEV, without timing), FRC, and TLC.

B. Dynamic volumes and capacities. These measurements are those where time factor is taken into account, that is, they are time-dependent. They are expressed in milliliters or liters per second or per minute and include:

Dynamic volumes: MV, MVV.

Dynamic capacities: VC (timed vital capacity, FEV_1) maximum mid-expiratory flow rate (MMFR).

A. SPIROMETRY (VITALOMETRY) EFFECT OF POSTURE ON VITAL CAPACITY

Apparatus and Materials. Spirometer; potassium permanganate solution.

Spirometer (Vitalograph; 'student' (or simple) spirometer). It consists of a double-walled metal cylindrical chamber, having an outer container filled with water in which a light-metal gas bell of 6-liter capacity floats. The bell (or float) is attached on its upper surface to a chain which passes over a graduated frictionless pulley. The pulley bears a spring-mounted indicator needle that moves with the pulley and indicates the volume of air present in the bell. The gas bell is counterpoised by a weight (counter-weight) attached to the other end of the chain (**Figure 2-3**). This weight allows a smooth up and down movement of the bell).

The inlet tube, through which air moves into or out of the bell, is corrugated canvas-rubber tubing bearing a mouthpiece. (This tube is attached to a metal pipe fitted at the bottom of the apparatus, the upper end of which lies above the level of water in the outer container). When air is blown into the inlet tube, it raises the bell, the water acting as an airtight seal.

PROCEDURES

Note
One can record not only vital capacity with this apparatus but also a few other lung volumes and capacities, though only approximately. Their accurate recording is done on recording spirometer, as described later.

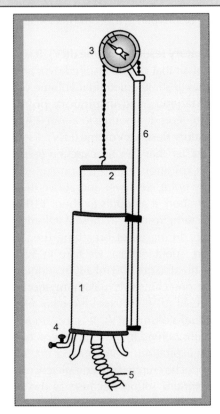

Figure 2-3. Simple spirometer. 1: Outer container; 2: Gas float; 3: Calibrated pulley with spring-mounted indicator needle; 4: Tap for draining water; 5: Wide-bore inlet tube; 6: Counterpoise system

Important
Explain the procedure in detail to the subject and even give her a pilot rehearsal to ensure that the procedure has been fully understood. Also, the subject should be encouraged to exert full expiratory effort during the test. Record the age, height, and body weight before starting the test.

1. Bring the bell to its lowest position by gently pushing it down. Adjust the pointer needle at zero, which indicates that the bell is completely empty.

2. **Measuring VC by collecting expired air in the spirometer (Standard Method).** Ask the subject to stand comfortably, facing the spirometer so that she/he can see the

movement of the bell. Tell her to breathe normally (quietly) for a minute or so. Now direct her to inspire as deeply and as fully as possible to fill the lungs. Then, while keeping the nostrils closed with a thumb and fingers, and the mouthpiece held firmly between the lips, tell him to expel all the air that he can with maximum effort into the spirometer. The bell moves up and the pointer on the pulley indicates the volume of expired air. The forced expiration should be deep and quick but without haste. (Normally, this procedure takes about 3 seconds.) Take 2 more readings at intervals of 5 minutes in the standing position as before.

3. **Effect of posture.** Ask the subject to sit comfortably on a stool and record the VC 3 times as before, at intervals of 2 minutes. Then ask her to lie down on the couch in supine position (face up) and record the VC 3 times. (See Q/A 7 for the effect of posture on VC).

4. **Measuring VC by breathing in from the full spirometer.** This method is a variation of the above method and there is no special name given to it. However, it is an instructive exercise.

   i. Raise and lower the bell a few times, finally raising it to its highest position so that it gets filled with fresh room air. Note the reading.

   ii. Tell the subject to breathe deeply a few times, then to expel air, with maximum effort, from the lungs into the atmosphere. This leaves only the RV in the lungs.

   iii. Now ask the subject to hold the mouthpiece firmly between the lips and then to breathe in maximally from the spirometer (thus breathing in ERV, TV, and IRV in that order, as shown in **Figure 2-2**). Note the reading. The difference between the two readings is the vital capacity. Compare this value with that obtained with the standard method, and explain the difference, if any.

5. **Two-stage Vital Capacity Determination.**
   Stage I Fill the spirometer with fresh room air, and note the reading. Ask the subject to breathe normally a few times. Then, starting from resting end-expiratory position, to take a maximum inspiration from the spirometer bell. Note the reading. The difference will give you inspiratory capacity (IC).
   Stage II Bring the bell to its lowest position (zero level). Tell the subject to breathe normally a few times. And then, starting from resting end-expiratory position, to expel all the air from the lungs with maximum effort into the spirometer. This will give ERV.
   The sum of the above, i.e. IC and ERV will give you vital capacity. Compare it with the value obtained with the standard method and explain the difference, if any.

6. **Measurement of inspiratory capacity.** This can be done in two ways:
   a. **By breathing from the spirometer.** Fill the bell with fresh air as before and note the reading. Carry out the procedure described above for stage I employed for vital capacity. This give IC.
   b. **By breathing out into the spirometer.** Bring the bell down to zero level. Then tell the subject to take a deep breath and to expire forcefully into the spirometer up to the point of resting end-expiratory position. This will give IC, i.e. TV + IRV.

7. **Measurement of expiratory reserve volume.** Carry out the procedure described above for stage II for vital capacity.

8. **Tidal volume.** Only an approximate idea can be obtained by breathing 2-3 times and out of spirometer and taking the readings. This step cannot be repeated for more than 2-3 times because this spirometer is a closed system and there is no provision for absorbing CO_2 from the expired air.

OBSERVATIONS AND RESULTS

Record your observations as indicated below:

Name.... Age.... Sex.... Date of experiment....						
Weight.... kg.... Height........ cm						

1. Rate of respiration ..../min
2. Tidal volume   ..../ml
   Minute ventilation (at rest): ....liters/min

	Readings (ml)			Max value
	1st	2nd	3rd	
3. Vital capacity				
a. Standard method	....	....	....	....
b. Two-stage method	....	....	....	....
4. Inspiratory capacity				
a. Breathing from spirometer	....	....	....	....
b. Breathing out into spirometer				
5. Expiratory reserve volume	....	....	....	....
6. Effect of posture on VC:				
a. Standing	....	....	....	....
b. Sitting	....	....	....	....
c. Supine				

Calculate the vital capacity:
   per kg body weight   ....
   per cm height   ....
   per m^2 BSA (vital index)   ....
(Consult nomogram for body surface area calculation at the end of the book).

B. RECORDING SPIROMETER

The **recording spirometer**, which is electrically driven, is used to provide a graphic record (called **spirogram)** of various lung volumes and capacities. It is used routinely to assess some of the pulmonary functions in health and disease in physiological and clinical studies. It consists of:

1. *Double-walled cylindrical chamber.* It contains water between its two walls (as in vitalograph or simple spirometer) to maintain an airtight seal. A 9-liter lightweight metal "gas bell" dips into the water from above and floats in it. A chain attached to the top of the bell passes over a frictionless pulley and carries a counter-weight and a pen writer. As the volume of air increases and decreases, the writing point moves down and up on the surface of the paper that passes under it. This provides a continuous record of the displacement of air in the bell with each inspiration and expiration.

2. **Soda lime tower.** It is fitted within the spirometer and removes (absorbs) CO_2 from the expired air so that one can continue to breathe into and out of the spirometer.

3. *The kymograph.* There is an on/off switch and a pilot lamp on the front of the apparatus. The paper assembly carries **mm graph paper** calibrated for both *volume of air* and *time.* The paper speed regulator has 3 markings: 60—0—1200.
   i. 60 mm/sec speed is for normal recordings.
   ii. 1200 mm/sec is for recording timed vital capacity.
   iii. The 'zero' mark is for 'neutral' position of the kymograph, at which the paper does not move.

4. *The chart paper.* It is calibrated for time along the X-axis, where 1 mm = 1 sec at the slower speed, and 20 mm = 1 sec at the faster speed. The calibration along Y-axis is for volume, where 1 mm movement of the pen writer (1 mm on the chart paper) represents 30 ml at both speeds. A slot on the side of the unit allows exit of recorded paper.

5. **Breathing assembly.** The breathing assembly has a mouthpiece which is connected to the spirometer, via a Y piece, by 2 rubber-canvas corrugated tubes, one carrying a unidirectional valve for inspiring air from the bell and the other carries a unidirectional valve for expiring air into the atmosphere. The third component of the assembly is a free-breathing valve which has a directional tap. The tap can be turned to permit a person either to breathe room air, or air from the spirometer bell.

6. Also provided are: *Inlet* for filling the gas bell with oxygen or any other gas. A *tap* for draining water out of the apparatus. A *chart reverse knob* can rewind the recorded chart paper by turning the knob clockwise. A *nose-clip* is provided for closing the nostrils during recording.

PROCEDURES

i. Fill 3/4th of the space between the to walls of the chamber with water. Dip the gas bell from above into the water. Connect the valve to the atmosphere and wash and fill the gas bell with fresh room air by slowly raising and lowering it 3-4 times.

ii. Seat the subject facing the spirometer and instruct her/him about the procedures that will be carried out. Insert the mouthpiece between the teeth and lips and apply nose clip on the nostrils. Tell the subject to breathe through the mouth for about a minute to familiarize her with mouth breathing.

iii. Connect the subject to the spirometer and allow her/him to breathe quietly for a short time. Then start the kymograph at the speed of 60 mm/min and record the excursions of the pen writer for about a minute. Note that *the upstrokes are inspirations and down strokes expirations.* The record of tidal breathing will be used for calculating the rate of respiration, tidal volume (TV) and minute ventilation (minute volume; MV).

iv. To record IRV (Consult **Figure 2-2**), ask the subject to breathe in as deeply as possible after a quiet inspiration. IRV + TV will give IC. Record a few tidal breaths.

To record ERV, ask the subject to breathe out as forcefully as possible after a quiet expiration.

v. To record MVV (MBC) ask the subject to breathe quickly and deeply for 15 seconds. Convert the heights of all the excursions of the pen writer in 15 sec into volume per minute to obtain MVV.

vi. To record forced vital capacity (FVC; or forced vital capacity), and timed vital capacity (FEV_1), quickly change the kymograph speed to 1200 mm/min, and ask the subject to first take a deep breath and then expel the air from the lungs as forcefully and as quickly as possible (as for VC). Take 3 readings at intervals of about 2 minutes.

> **Note**
> Residual volume (RV), functional residual capacity (FRC), and total lung capacity (TLC) cannot be determined by spirometry.

C. TIMED VITAL CAPACITY (FEV_1)

The FEV_1 recorded above is a dynamic capacity. In a normal person, a single forced expiration takes about 3 seconds, and the tracing thus obtained is called an **"expiratory spirogram"**. **Figure 2-4** shows such a tracing where the fractions of FVC are: 80% in 1 second (FEV_1), 93% in 2 seconds, and 98% in 3 seconds. The FEV_1 is called the" **first expiratory volume at 1 second (FEV_1)"** or **"forced expiratory volume in 1 second"**.

In addition to FVC and FEV_1, the average expiratory flow rate during the middle 50% of FVC, also called **"maximal mid-expiratory flow rate"** (**MMEFR; or FEF 25-50%**) can also be calculated (**Figure 2-5**).

A horizontal line drawn from 25% (t) and a vertical line from the 75% mark (V) will denote FEF 25-75%. **Figure 2-5** also shows that in the middle 50% of FVC, 2.0 liters of air is expired in 0.5 second (t). Thus, $V/t = 2.0 \, l/0.5 \, sec = 4.0$ liters per second.

Normal range = Males: 1.5—4.5 l/sec.
Females: 1.3—3.0 l/sec.

Clinical Significance of Timed Vital Capacity

FEV_1 and the ratio FEV_1/FVC help in differentiating between two major patterns of abnormal ventilation— **Obstructive** and **Restrictive (constricted)** lung diseases.

I. Obstructive Pattern

The main feature is a decrease in expiratory flow rate throughout expiration (**Figures 2-4** and **2-6**).

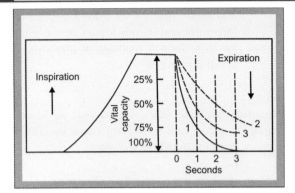

Figure 2-4. The expiratory spirogram: (1) Normal, (2) Airway obstruction, and (3) Restriction

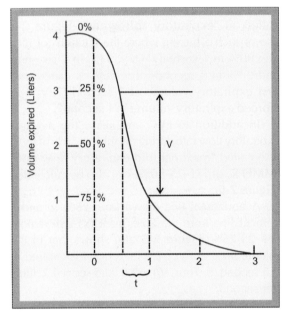

Figure 2-5. Calculation of FEF 25-75% from forced expiratory spirogram. V: volume expired (mild 50%) in time 't'

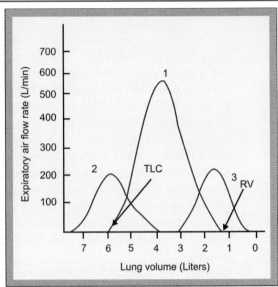

Figure 2-6. Maximum expiratory flow volume curve. 1: normal; 2: chronic obstructive lung disease; 3: restrictive lung disease

PEFR, FEV_1, FEV_1/FVC, and MMEFR are all reduced. Over many years more and more air tends to remain in the lungs, which increases TLC and RV (**Figure 2-6**). This pattern is seen in the following conditions:

1. **Asthma (panting).** It is a partially reversible, chronic obstructive lung disease of the lower respiratory passages. There is inflammation and contraction of smooth muscle (broncho-constriction). This happens in response to inhalation of specific foreign substances in the air (e.g., pollen, house dust, mites, some article of food); or non-specific stimuli (e.g., air pollution in elderly). The IgE antibodies react with basophils and mast cells and release many chemicals (leucotrienes, prostaglandins, chemokines, histamine, etc) that cause contraction of smooth muscle and inflammation.

The symptoms include: coughing, wheezing, difficulty in breathing (especially expiration), tightness in chest, anxiety, etc.

The attacks come at certain times and the patients are generally free from difficulty in breathing in between the attacks. Treatment with inhalation of bronchodilators (e.g., beta$_2$ - adrenergic antagonists, and sometimes with steroids) relieves the breathing problem.

2. **Chronic Obstructive Lung disease (COLD; or Chronic Obstructive Pulmonary Disease, COPD)**

Decrease in expiratory airflow is also seen in *chronic bronchitis* and /or *emphysema*. Air pollution, and cigarette smoking can cause COLD (chemicals in cigarette smoke cause the release of elastases and other proteolytic enzymes which damage elastic fibers; there is also inhibition of alpha-1-antitrypsin which normally inactivates these proteolytic enzymes. The alveolar walls break down and large sacs are formed.

The uneven and inadequate ventilation produces hypoxia and, later, retention of CO_2. The result is dyspnea on exertion or even at rest.

3. **Chronic Bronchitis.** There is an excessive production of tracheobronchial secretions along with cough. Cigarette smoking (and passive inhalation), pollution of air, repeated infections, etc are the usual causes. The condition usually progresses to COLD.

4. **Cystic Fibrosis.** It is an inherited disorder of secretory epithelia in which the lung airways are full of thick mucus, and inflamed. The clogging of these passages causes difficulty in breathing. Other systems like liver, pancreas, and GI tract are also involved. The defect is in a transport protein that transports chloride across plasma membranes.

II. Restrictive Pattern

The main feature is reduced lung volume (mainly TLC and RV), which may be due to *interstitial lung disease (ILD)* or *chest wall deformity* that reduce the air in the lungs. There is no obstruction to the outflow of air. FEV_1 is normal though FVC is low, as shown in **Figures 2-4 and 2-6**.

A. Conditions Involving Lungs.

1. **Interstitial lung disease (ILD).** This term represents a large number of chronic, nonmalignant, noninfectious diseases of the lower respiratory passages. There is interstitial fibrosis, inflammation, and edema. The causes include: idiopathic, immunologic, collagen-vascular disease, rheumatic arthritis, etc.

2. **Pneumonoconioses.** Exposure to and inhalation and deposition of inorganic or organic dust particles, such as coal , silica, asbestos, cotton dust, grain dust, etc. in the lung tissues leads to fibrosis and contracted lungs.

3. **Sarcoidosis.**

B. Conditions Outside the Lungs.

1. **Deformities.** The deformities of vertebrae, ribs, sternum- such as kyphoscoliosis (bending of spine), ankylosing spondylitis, etc cause deficient lung expansion.

2. **Myasthenia Gravis and Muscular Dystrophies.** The weakness of expiratory muscles decreases FEV_1 because the flow rate is reduced due to lowered expiratory pressures that are achieved.

3. **Obesity.** The normal, obstructive, and restrictive patterns of ventilation are shown below:-

Normal	Obstructive		Restrictive
FVC = 4.5 liters	FVC	= 3.0 liters	FVC = 3.0 liters
FEV_1 = 3.5 liters	FEV_1	= 1.2 liters	FEV_1 = 2.8 liters
% = 80	%	= 40	% = 90
FEV_1/FVC	Normal	= > 70%	
	Obstructive	= < 70%	
	Restrictive	= > 70%	

PEAK EXPIRATORY FLOW RATE (PEFR)

Definition The peak expiratory flow rate (PEFR) is the maximum or peak rate (or velocity), in liters per minute, with which air is expelled with maximum force after a deep inspiration.

The Wright's peak flow meter, introduced in 1959, is a simple device for the measurement of ventilatory function of the lungs. A mini version is available which can be carried in one's pocket for bed-side use.

The flow meter is a short cylinder made of plastic material. An indicator (pointer) moves in a slot alongside a scale with numbers on it which indicate liters/min. There is a handle provided near the mouthpiece. The end, opposite the mouthpiece, has holes in it for allowing air to exit from the apparatus.

PROCEDURE

1. Ask the subject to hold the peak flow meter by its handle making sure that the fingers are clear of the scale and the slot, and are not obstructing the holes at the end of the apparatus.
2. Tell the subject to take a deep breath, place the mouthpiece firmly between the teeth and lips, and then to blow out with a short sharp blast. Note the reading on the scale. Bring the indicator back to zero by pressing the button located near the mouthpiece.
3. Take 6 readings at intervals of 1 minute, and select the maximum value for report.

Normal range = 350-600 liters per minute.

Maximum Expiratory Flow-Volume Curve (MEFVC). Figure 2-6 shows a MEFVC in a normal person and in obstructive and restrictive patterns of lung diseases. It should not be confused with a recording of VC or FEV_1. The entire curve represents outflow of air from lungs during a forceful expiration after a deep inspiration. The curve starts at a TLC of about 6.0 liters, quickly reaches a peak of 550 liters/min, and then falls gradually to a residual volume of 1100 ml. The decline in expiratory flow rate is due to compression of airways by the increasing intrathoracic pressure due to compression of chest by the forced expiration.

QUESTIONS

Q. 1 What is meant by the terms lung volumes and capacities? How can they be measured and what are their normal values?
See above.

Q. 2 Name the lung volumes and capacities that cannot be measured on a spirometer.
The lung volumes and capacities that cannot be measured on a spirometer include: Total lung capacity (TLC), functional residual capacity (FRC), and residual volume (RV).

Q. 3 What is the difference between minute ventilation and maximum voluntary ventilation?
See above.

Q. 4 What is the normal vital capacity? Can it be predicted?
The normal vital capacity varies between 3.5 and 6 liters, the value being 20% lower in females. In general, the vital capacity (and other volumes and capacities) are larger in males, taller persons, and in younger adults. Thus, since the VC depends on age, sex, body build, occupation, etc., various formulae have been introduced to predict VC in an individual. Various disorders may then be diagnosed by comparing the actual (determined) values with the predicted normal values for one's age, sex, height, etc.

1. **Relation to height:**
    Males   = Height in cm × 25
    Females = Height in cm × 20
    Athletes = Height in cm × 29

2. **Relation to body surface area (BSA):**
    This is called vital index.
    Males   = 2.5 liters/m^2 BSA
    Females = 2.1 liters/m^2 BSA

3. **Relation to age, sex, and height:**
    Males   = [27.63 – (0.112 × Age)] × Height in cm.
    Females = [27.78 – (0.101 × Age)] × Height in cm.

4. **Relation to body weight:** For an average healthy person, the prediction formula is: Vital capacity (in ml) = $W^{0.72}/0.690$, where W is the body weight in grams.
    The vital capacity is high in athletes, swimmers, divers, etc., but is low in persons who have sedentary habits.

Q. 5 What is the clinical importance of determination of vital capacity?

The VC is frequently determined clinically as an index of lung function and provides useful information about abnormal ventilation due to airway obstruction, fibrosis of the lungs, mechanical interference with chest expansion and compression, strength of respiratory muscles, and so on. However, it cannot help in differentiating between obstructive and restrictive lung diseases, where timed VC is of greater help.

Q. 6 What is two-stage vital capacity?

See above.

Q. 7 Describe the effect of posture on vital capacity?

The VC is maximum in the standing position, less in the sitting position, and least in the supine position. This effect of posture is due to the following factors:

i. In the sitting and supine positions, the muscles of respiration (both primary and accessory) cannot be employed as forcefully and effectively for the expansion and compression of lungs and chest.

ii. In the supine position, the abdominal viscera push the diaphragm up and interfere with its movements. The mobility of the chest is also reduced by the contact of the back with the bed.

iii. There is accumulation of more blood in the blood vessels of the lungs (especially veins) in the supine position. This decreases the total lung capacity, and hence the vital capacity.

Q. 8 Name the factors that affect vital capacity.

The main factors affecting vital capacity are: **the net air capacity of the lungs, condition of the lungs**, and **the compressing force.**

Associated with these aspects, the following factors affect vital capacity:

1. Age. The net air capacity is lower in young children. VC decreases in old age due to loss of elasticity of lungs and weaker compressing forces.

2. Sex. Males have larger chests, greater body surface area, and greater muscle power.

3. Net air capacity of the lungs. This is affected by the volume of blood in the lungs (e.g., pulmonary congestion), condition of the lungs (e.g., loss of elasticity in emphysema), patency of air passages (e.g., asthma), destruction of lung tissue, mechanical interference with expansion (e.g., pregnancy, ascites, deformities of spine, etc.). In the supine posture, the abdominal viscera push up against the diaphragm thus reducing the thoracic space, and interfering with this muscle's action.

4. Magnitude of compressing forces. Swimmers, divers, athletes, and those doing yogic breathing exercises have stronger and better-developed muscles which can compress and expand the chest more efficiently. The common diseases associated with low vital capacity are: emphysema, asthma, chronic obstructive lung diseases, pleural effusion, pulmonary edema, pneumothorax, etc.

Q. 9 What is timed vital capacity (FEV$_1$) and what is its clinical importance?

See above.

Q. 10 What is peak (expiratory) flow rate and what is its significance?

The peak expiratory flow rate (PEFR). The peak expiratory rate is the maximum flow rate, or peak flow rate of air, during a single forced expiration. This estimation is useful in distinguishing reversible (e.g., asthma) from irreversible (e.g., emphysema) diseases. The peak flow meter, which measures PEFR, is of special value in cases of asthma where the effectiveness of treatment with a bronchodilator can be quickly evaluated. For example, a PEFR of, say, 150 liters/min may improve to 300 liters/min within a short time of inhalation of the drug. But the meter is not useful for assessing the degree of disability of patients with lung fibrosis and other restrictive conditions because they may have normal expiratory flow rates.

The measurement of the effect of training in athletes is yet another application of the Wright peak flow meter.

Comments. The major factor that limits expiratory flow rate during most of a maximal forced expiration is the narrowing of small airways. Thus, the flow rate is a function of lung volume rather than the effort exerted. This condition is called "effort-independent flow".

Q. 11 What is the physiological significance of functional residual capacity (FRC)?

Functional residual capacity (FRC), the air that remains in the lungs at the end of a normal (quiet) expiration, is important for the gas exchange function of the lungs. The FRC amounts to about 2200 ml, half of which is residual volume which cannot be expired into the spirometer.

Of the 500 ml of tidal volume (fresh air), 150 ml remains in the dead space while only 350 ml reaches the depths of the lungs. There, it is added to the large amount of 2000-2500 ml of FRC. This causes dilution of the gases and a steady gas exchange throughout the respiratory cycle. The steady exchange prevents sudden changes in arterial PO_2 and PCO_2 which would make the control of breathing extremely difficult.

The FRC is increased when lungs are over-inflated with air as in old age, emphysema (due to loss of elasticity), asthma, etc.

Q. 12 Name the precautions that must be observed during spirometric recording?

1. It should be ensured that the subject/patient has fully understood what he/she is required to do.
2. Make sure that there is no leakage of air anywhere from the mouthpiece to the gas bell.
3. The indicator must be brought to zero reading before each determination.

Q. 13 What is breathing reserve and what is its clinical importance?

Breathing reserve = MVV − MV = 100 − 10
$$= 90 \text{ liters.}$$

This means that breathing (ventilation) can be increased by 90 liters, i.e., from 8-10 liters to 100 liters or more. This is a large reserve for ventilation.

$$\text{Breathing reserve \%} = \frac{MVV - MV}{MVV} \times 100 = \frac{100 - 10}{100} \times 100$$
$$= 90\%$$

The breathing reserve percent is also called **dyspnea index**. Dyspnea is present when this index falls to 60-70 percent which is called the **dyspnea point**.

An example taken from a patient of emphysema will clarify it:

- MVV has decreased from 100 liters/min to 40 liters/min, while MV has increased from 10 liters/min to 20 liters/min (due to respiratory stimulation by increased PCO_2 and low PO_2). Therefore

$$\text{Breathing reserve \%} = \frac{40 - 20}{40} \times 100 = 50\%$$

This means that the dyspnea point has been crossed, so that the patient is experiencing dyspnea (unpleasant awareness of increased breathing).

2-4

Pulmonary Function Tests

STUDENT OBJECTIVES	
After completing this experiment you should be able to: 1. Classify pulmonary function tests and describe the purpose of doing them.	2. Perform some simple tests for assessing lung functions. 3. Demonstrate the effect of posture on vital capacity on a simple spirometer. 4. Record various lung volumes and capacities.

5. Explain the importance of timed vital capacity in differentiating between obstructive and restrictive lung diseases.
6. Describe the diffusing capacity of the lungs.

Though a large number of pulmonary function tests (PFTs) are possible, many of them highly sophisticated and carried out in special cases for research work, a few comparatively simple tests can provide useful information in most cases of lung diseases. These tests help the physician to make a physiological assessment of lung function rather than a pathological diagnosis, which the physician has, in most cases, already arrived at during clinical examination.

Note
Patients of pulmonary edema are not subjected to PFTs, because the condition is serious and easy to diagnose clinically and by X-ray chest if required.

PULMONARY FUNCTION TESTS

The PFTs are employed to assess the 3 basic processes involved in the supply of O_2 to and removal of CO_2 from the body—*ventilation, diffusion,* and *perfusion* of lungs.
  a. **Ventilatory Function.** These tests measure lung size (VC), patency of airways (MVV; FEV_1), and alveolar ventilation.
  b. **Gas Exchange Function.** The efficacy of gas exchange in the lungs is measured by analysis of respiratory and blood gases.
  c. **Perfusion Function.** Special procedures are employed for the study of blood flow through the lungs.

Purpose of Lung Function Tests

Tests for pulmonary functions are employed:
  1. To reach a diagnosis when a patient complains of dyspnea (breathlessness) and to assess the degree of disability.
  2. To follow the progress of disease and the effectiveness of treatment.
  3. To assess respiratory status before anesthesia

and cardio-thoracic surgery, especially if a lung is to be removed.
  4. To assess physical fitness and effects of physical training.
  5. To determine the incidence of respiratory dysfunction in the community and workers in hazardous industries.
  6. To obtain medico legal information and opinion in certain situations, e.g., claim for lung damage in a hazardous occupation.

Classification of Pulmonary Function Tests

I. Simple Tests

These include the following:
1. **Chest expansion.** Measure the chest expansion with a tape placed around the chest just below the level of nipples. The normal chest expands by 5-10 cm following a deep inspiration after a forceful expiration.
2. **Breath holding time.** (Consult Expt 2-2).
3. **Respiratory endurance test (40 mmHg test)** A BP apparatus is required for this test. Disconnect the rubber tube leading from the mercury reservoir to the BP cuff. Ask the subject to take a deep breath pinch his nostrils, and exhale into the tube, raising the mercury to 40 mm level and to hold it there for as long as possible.
Normal = 40-70 seconds or more.
4. **Expiratory blast test.** Using the same procedure as above, ask the subject to take a deep breath and then raise the mercury column to as high a level as possible. A normal person can raise the mercury column to 55-100 mm or more during a single forceful expiration.
5. **Snider's test.** Hold a burning match stick about 12 inches in front of the subject's face and ask him to blow it out with a single forceful expiration.

II. Tests of Ventilatory Function

1. VC and FEV_1 (Consult Expt 2-3).
2. Mid-expiratory flow rate (MEFR, or FEF 25-75%).
3. Peak expiratory flow rate (PEFR; Expt 2-3).

4. Minute ventilation (MV) at rest and maximum voluntary ventilation.

5. Functional residual capacity (FRC). The volume of air remaining in the lungs at the end of a quiet expiration (FRC) cannot be determined directly by spirometry.

Determination of FRC (Nitrogen washout Method)

The FRC cannot be determined by spirometry. However, nitrogen washout method, a simple procedure is used that requires a gas bag (called Douglas bag), a nitrogen meter, and pure oxygen.

Procedure. The subject breathes pure O_2 for 5 minutes and the expired gas is collected in the Douglas bag that has previously been washed out with pure O_2. The concentration of nitrogen in the expired air is determined with the nitrogen meter. Since it is known that the alveolar air contains 80% nitrogen, the FRC can be calculated from *the total volume of expired air and its nitrogen concentration*. For example, if 40,000 ml of expired air contains 5% nitrogen then 2000 ml of nitrogen must have been washed out of the lungs, and as the lungs contains 80% nitrogen, the FRC must be 2000 x 100/80 = 2500 ml. The FRC changes with changes in posture (as does VC).

Note
When spirometry is combined with a determination of FRC, it is possible to calculate TLC and RV.

6. Ventilation Scan. (See below)

III. Tests of Gas Exchange Functions

The single most important function of respiratory system is supply of sufficient amount of O_2 to the tissues and to remove the CO_2 produced by cell metabolism. Obviously, the analysis of blood gases and pH, and respiratory gases are the most fundamental tests of lung functions.

A. *Blood Gases.* Miniature glass electrodes can quickly estimate the blood gases and pH on a very small arterial blood sample.

Normal levels:	Arterial Blood	Venous Blood
O_2:	20 ml/dl at a PO_2 of 100 mm Hg.	15 ml/dl at a PO_2 of 40 mm Hg.
CO_2:	48 ml/dl at a PCO_2 of 40 mm Hg.	52 ml/dl at a PCO_2 of 45 mm Hg.

Note
The venous blood gas levels are given for comparison. The arterial levels mainly depend on the level of alveolar ventilation. Decreased PO_2 of arterial blood may be due to hypoventilation, defective diffusion, abnormal ventilation/perfusion ratio, and right to left shunts.

B. *Respiratory Gases.* Medical gas analyzers that respond rapidly and accurately can provide specific and continuous measurements of respiratory gases. These instruments are used extensively in pulmonary research, diagnosis of lung disorders, and for monitoring patients under anesthesia.

Diffusing Capacity/Transfer Factor for Gases

The diffusion of gases across the alveolo-capillary membrane (respiratory membrane; surface area= 60-80 m^2; thickness= 0.1-0.4 μm) depends not only on pressure gradients of O_2 and CO_2 across the membrane, but also its surface area and thickness, ventilation/perfusion balance, volume of blood in pulmonary capillaries, and the concentration of Hb concentration in the blood. Therefore, the term **transfer factor (TF)** rather than diffusing capacity is used these days.

CO Method for measuring TF for O_2. Since it is technically difficult to measure the diffusing capacity of lungs (TF) for O_2 directly, CO is used instead. A small amount of CO and helium mixture is inhaled and breath held for 10 seconds. A sample of expired air is then analyzed and TF for CO is read from the computer, which is about 17 ml/min/mm Hg. Since the diffusing coefficient for O_2 is 1.23 times that for CO, the diffusing capacity for O_2 is = 17 × 1.23 = 21 ml/min/mm

Hg. {Since time-integrated pressure gradient for O_2 across the respiratory membrane is 11 mm Hg (and not 100-40= 60 mm Hg), a normal resting person picks up about 21 × 11= 230 ml of O_2 per minute}.

Since the TF for CO_2 is about 20 times that for O_2, diffusion problem commonly affects O_2 but not CO_2 (i.e., uptake of O_2 is decreased while there is no CO_2 retention).

IV. Tests for Perfusion Functions

Special methods (e.g., lung scan and catheterization) are employed to determine blood flow through different zones of the lungs. The ventilation/perfusion balance can also be determined.

V. Special Techniques

Some of these tests are the following

1. **Plain X-ray chest, and screening** for evidence of lung disease.

2. **Determination of pulmonary vascular pressures** by catheterization.

3. **Computerized axial tomography (CAT, or CT scan).**

4. **Magnetic resonance imaging (MRI).**

5. **Bronchoscopy.** A fiberoptic (flexible) bronchoscope is introduced through the nose or mouth, through the larynx and trachea into the bronchial tree. A local anesthetic is sprayed at every step. This instrument allows the inside of trachea and lower branchial passages to be directly visualized. A biopsy of a growth can also be taken.

6. **Lung scan.** This test is employed to determine any blockage in the blood flow from the heart into the lungs. A radioactive substance is injected into a vein and detected in the lungs by a scanning camera. In this way, cold spots (areas of decreased blood flow), and hot spots (areas of high flow) can be detected as the scanner converts this information into an image.

7. **Ventilation scan.** This test measures the flow of air into and out of the lungs. A radioactive gas is inhaled; once it is in the lungs, a scanning camera produces an image. Normally the gas is equally distributed in both lungs.

8. **Computerized Multifunctional Spirometers.** Computerized spirometers that can monitor lung volumes and capacities from breath to breath are employed in research labs and hospitals. They can graphically display the results, and show predicted values, and their interpretations, if so desired.

QUESTIONS

Q. 1 What is the purpose of testing lung functions?
See page 165.

Q. 2 Demonstrate any two simple lung function tests.
The student may perform vital capacity estimation and respiratory endurance test (or any other two function tests of his/her choice).

Q. 3 How will you assess gas exchange functions of the lungs?
The gas exchange functions can be tested by analyzing respiratory and blood gases.
Questions/Answers of Expt 2-3 may be gone through as any of these may be asked.

Q. 4 What is the structure of alveolo-capillary membrane? What are the factors that affect the diffusion of gases through it?
This membrane, about 0.1-0.4 μm thick, consists of: a thin layer of fluid, a layer of type I and type II cells and macrophages of alveolar wall, epithelial basement membrane, capillary basement membrane, endothelial cells of capillary, and a thin layer of fluid plasma. (See above for factors affecting gas diffusion).

Q. 5 What is meant by the term ventilation? Name the forces that oppose the movement of air into the lungs during inspiration.
The term ventilation refers to the movement of air into and out of the lungs. The forces that oppose expansion of lungs (and air inflow) include:

i. Elastic recoil of thorax and lungs (elastic resistance).

ii. Non-elastic (viscous) resistance due to movement of tissues.

iii. Airway resistance due to friction between the air passages and the moving column of air.

The contraction of inspiratory muscles must overcome all these forces before lungs can expand and pull air into their depths.

Q. 6 Name some non-respiratory functions of the respiratory tract.

The term "respiratory functions" refers to gas exchange in the lungs. In addition, the respiratory tract performs many other functions that may be called "non-respiratory functions" These include:

air conditioning of the inspired air; role in phonation, smell and venous return; excretion of ketones, alcohol, and methane from the intestines; absorption of general anesthetics and drugs; function as blood reservoir; temperature regulation by panting in some animals, such as dogs.

The protective mechanisms of lungs include: ciliary escalator, pulmonary alveolar macrophages, and alpha-1 antitrypsin released by airway epithelium.

Many biological substances are associated with lungs: activation of angiotensin-I to angiotensin-II (by the angiotensin converting enzyme, ACE), production of surfactant, partial removal of serotonin, prostaglandins E and F, acetylcholine, bradykinin, etc.

2-5

Cardiopulmonary Resuscitation (CPR) (Cardiopulmonary-Cerebral Resuscitation (CPCR)

CPR is a first aid, but life-saving, emergency procedure, and must be started without losing a second. It is not the treatment, however.

Cardiopulmonary Arrest (CP Arrest) is said to have occurred when there is a sudden stoppage of heart or breathing or both. It is an extreme emergency that threatens life. Consciousness is lost within 10-15 seconds of stoppage of oxygen supply to the brain and some brain damage occurs in 5-6 minutes. Circulatory arrest for more than 10-15 minutes causes permanent damage to the brain.

Important

Artificial respiration (AR) alone may be needed if breathing has stopped suddenly though the heart is still beating (as it happens in many cases). However, if breathing is not re-started within 3-4 minutes, the heart will also stop. In this case, both AR and external cardiac compression will be required. (See general plan below).

Note

The survival rates of out-of-hospital CP arrest (say due to a heart attack on a roadside, or in a building) are, sadly, very low. The main reason is ignorance of the value of CPR in saving lives, but even in trained health personnel and bystanders, there is unwillingness to provide CPR for fear of catching AIDS, hepatitis, or tuberculosis through mouth-to-mouth respiration. Also, when professionals do CPR, it is often not done well.

It is for this reason, that medical/dental, and other life-sciences students must be seriously trained in this life-saving procedure.

AIM OF CPR

The aim of CPR is to "artificially" push oxygen-containing blood to the brain and other vital organs (when the heart and lungs fail to do this vital job), till the heart and lungs regain their normal function, or the victim is shifted to the hospital.

THE ABC OF CPR

Airway: Establish an airway, or maintain it if it is open.

Breathing: Provide artificial ventilation if breathing has stopped.

Circulation: Re-establish circulation if there is insufficient heart beat, or if the heart has stopped.

Note
These procedures must be performed in that order.

CAUSES OF CARDIOPULMONARY ARREST

A. *Acute conditions*
1. Drowning.
2. Hanging.
3. Electric shock.
4. Massive, acute myocardial infarction (MI) leading to cardiac standstill (asystole) or fibrillation.
5. Inhalation of poisonous gases (e.g., carbon monoxide).
6. Overdose or sensitivity to an anesthetic agent, poisoning with narcotics and drugs (accidental or suicidal) (e.g., barbiturates, opium, etc), acids, other chemicals.
7. Head injuries.
8. Obstruction of respiratory passages by inhalation of a foreign body (e.g., a fish bone).
9. Anaphylactic shock.

B. *Chronic conditions*
1. Poliomyelitis.
2. Diphtheria.
3. Ascending paralysis.
4. Obstruction of air passages by a tumor of pharynx, larynx, etc.

SIGNS AND SYMPTOMS OF CARDIO-PULMONARY ARREST

1. The victim is unconscious, the lips, face, ear lobes, fingers and toes are blue; and there is death-like appearance.
2. The skin is pale, cold and moist, and the pupils are dilated and fixed, i.e., non-responsive to light. (These features are due to sympathetic stimulation).
3. **Absent or weak arterial pulse.** The carotid artery must be palpated because the radial pulse may be too weak to be felt.
4. **Absence of heart sounds.** Put your ear on the chest of the victim and try to confirm presence or absence of heart sounds.
5. **Breathing is absent.** There is no movement of the chest or the alae nasi (nostrils). There is no air coming out of the nose or mouth.
6. **Blood pressure is not recordable.**

WHAT TO DO IMMEDIATELY

1. Assess
   - **Thump the chest** (if there is no carotid pulse). This may stop fibrillation. Re-check pulse. If absent, start CPR.
   - Make sure you are in a safe place. Trying CPR on the road may risk your life as well.
   i. **First Establish Unresponsiveness.**
   - Determine the responsiveness of the victim by tapping him/her on the shoulder and asking" Are you all right?"

- Check carotid pulse and breathing (see below) *to make sure that the heart and breathing have really stopped.* Because if the heart is still beating, there will be enough muscle tone so that external cardiac massage may cause fracture of the ribs.

Note
CPR is never demonstrated on a normal waking person for the same reason. Demonstration dummies are available for CPR training.

2. **Start CPR routine** after confirming CP arrest, and find out if a bystander can help.
3. **Ask a bystander to phone the hospital emergency** for an ambulance because you do not have time to do so yourself. If no one is available, continue CPR till the victim is revived.

What Not To Do

1. Do not delay resuscitation; immediate intervention is required after establishing unresponsiveness.
2. The victim must not be made to sit or stand. No pillow should be placed under the head or neck, as this will bend the head and close the trachea.
3. The feet and legs should be raised by placing a pillow, etc. under the hips/legs. This will help promote venous return to the heart.
4. Nothing should be given by mouth to a semiconscious or unconscious individual for fear of aspiration of the fluid into the lungs.
5. There should be no crowding around the victim.

GENERAL PLAN FOR CARDIOPULMONARY RESUSCITATION

Management of a case of cardiopulmonary arrest involves 2 phases:
Phase I: Emergency procedures.
Phase II: Definitive treatment.

Phase I: Emergency Measures

If unconscious, but breathing and pulse are present:
   A—Airway: Tilt the head back with a hand under the neck to maintain an open airway.

If not breathing:
   B—Breathe: Give mouth-to-mouth respiration (or mouth-to-nose). Inflate lungs 14-16 times/min to provide adequate oxygen supply. Maintain head tilt to avoid flaccid tongue from falling back into pharynx.
   - Feel carotid pulse. If pulse present, continue lung inflations.

If pulse absent (deathlike appearance, fixed, dilated pupils):
   C—Circulate: Give external cardiac massage. One operator: (2:15). Alternate 2 quick lung inflations with 15 cardiac compressions. Two operators: (1:5). Interpose 1 lung inflation after every 5th sternal compression.

Phase II: Definitive Treatment

This phase of treatment is carried out in the hospital, and includes:
   D—Drugs (adrenaline; intravenous sodium bicarbonate for acidosis, etc.);
   E—ECG monitoring;
   F—Fibrillation treatment with a defibrillator, lidocaine or procaine;
   G—Gauging and restoration of normal breathing and circulation;
   H—Hypothermia; and
   I—Management of the patient in the intensive care unit (ICU) of the hospital.

ARTIFICIAL RESPIRATION (PULMONARY RESUSCITATION)

Artificial respiration (AR; assisted ventilation) may be given by *manual methods*, **mouth-to-mouth method** *(sometimes called "kiss of life" or "rescue breath"),* or by *mechanical methods.*

Note

Though mouth-to-mouth respiration has been found to be the best general first-aid procedure, but which method to use in a given case will depend on the cause of CP arrest. For example, in a case of drowning or near drowning, face injuries, fracture of jaw, chemical burns on lips and in the mouth, it may not be possible to give mouth-to- mouth respiration. In such cases, International Red Cross recommends Holger-Nielson method.

A. Manual Methods

The old prone or supine position methods— *Schafer's* prone-position, back-pressure, *Sylvester's* supine position arm-lift, and *Thomson's* hip-lift chest-pressure methods are no longer employed since they rely on compressing the thorax to cause expiration, and then allowing lungs to expand passively. The Holger-Nielson method described below is used when mouth-to-mouth respiration is not possible.

Holger-Nielson Method (Back-pressure arm-lift, BPAL method)

1. Place the victim, face downwards, on a hard surface, with the arms bent, and the head turned to one side and resting on the hands.
2. Kneel down on one knee at the victim's head, with the opposite foot placed near the elbow.
3. Place your hands, with fingers widespread, on the victim's back just below the scapulae. Now rock forward, with the arms held straight at the elbows, until your arms are vertical and pressing down on the back. This compresses the chest and produces expiration.
4. Slide your hands sideways and outwards on to the victim's arms just above the elbows. Now rock backwards, lifting the victim's elbows until some resistance is felt at her/his shoulders. This movement expands the thorax, decreasing the intrathoracic pressure and causing inspiration.

5. Repeat this cycle of compression and expansion (that lasts for about 3 seconds each) for about 12 times a minute.

B. Mouth-to-Mouth Respiration (Rescue breath; Exhaled-air ventilation)

Mouth-to-Mouth respiration has proved to be superior to all the manual methods in all age groups. Comparative studies have proved it to be the only technique capable of producing satisfactory ventilation.

Advantages and Disadvantages of mouth-to-mouth Respiration. The method is simple, safe, and easy to perform, even by a layman with minimum instruction. Above all, it does not require any apparatus. The only disadvantage is that the victim's flaccid (toneless) tongue tends to fall back into the pharynx and thus obstruct the airway. However, this can be avoided by extending the neck and turning the head slightly to one side.

PROCEDURES

1. Place the victim on his/her back on firm ground, and loosen the clothing around the neck, chest and waist.
2. Remove any mucus, food, saliva, or any foreign material (e.g., grass, dentures, etc) from the mouth and nose with your fingers wrapped in a handkerchief.
3. Open the airway by tilting the head back. Kneel by the right side of the victim. Place your right hand under the neck and lift it, while keeping a pressure on the forehead with the heel of the other hand. (The extension of the neck lifts the flaccid tongue from the back of the throat).Using your right thumb and fingers, lift the chin and angle of the jaw upward and forward. This simple procedure keeps the airway open.
4. Clamp the nostrils with your left thumb and fingers, take a deep breath, apply your mouth firmly on the victim's mouth (or nose if the

pharynx cannot be cleared), and blow a liter of air into the victim's lungs, watching the expansion of the chest at the same time. (Remember, the expired air contains 15% oxygen).

5. Remove your mouth, turn your head to one side and take another deep breath as the elastic recoil of the chest causes expiration. You may feel and hear the expiratory airflow from the victim's mouth and nose.

Note
If the airway is clear, only a moderate resistance will be felt when you exhale air into the victim's lungs.

6. **Repeat the cycle of:** blowing out— turning the head – breathing in—about 14-16 times a minute, till spontaneous breathing returns or the victim is shifted to the hospital.
7. **Important.** Feel the carotid pulse. If, after 6-8 lung inflations, there is no improvement in the color of the victim, suspect cardiac arrest, and start external cardiac massage as well.

C. Mechanical Respirators

Mechanical ventilation is employed when AR has to be given for long periods, e.g., during chronic respiratory failure. Air-tight metallic or plastic devices are placed around the chest and negative pressure is applied at intervals; this draws air into the lungs. The elastic recoil of the lungs and chest causes expiration.

Alternate positive and negative pressures are also employed.

1. **Drinker's Tank Respirator (also called the "iron lung").** It is an iron chamber in which the subject is placed, with the head kept outside, an air-tight collar sealing the body inside. The pressure in the chamber is alternately raised (2-3 cm water) for expiration, and lowered (–10 to –14 cm H_2O) for inspiration, by means of a pump.

2. **Sahlin's jacket model, Brag Paul Pulsator,** and their modifications employ inelastic chest jackets

in which pressure can be increased and decreased at intervals.

3. **Eve's rocking method.** The victim is laid on a stretcher or a plank and the shoulders and ankles are fastened to it. A rhythmic rocking up and down like a see-saw causes the abdominal viscera to push up against the diaphragm (expiration) or pull it down (inspiration).

Note
In operation theaters and critical care units, the acute respiratory failure patients are intubated (an endotracheal tube put in the trachea via the mouth) and pulses of air, or a mixture of gases, are delivered through an Ambu Bag/ machine. It is common to maintain positive end expiratory pressure (PEEP) to help in expansion of the lungs.

EXTERNAL CARDIAC MASSAGE (CARDIAC RESUSCITATION)

Rationale. One may doubt the efficacy of external cardiac massage in causing blood to circulate when the heart has stopped or fibrillating. However, there are two reasons for believing that cardiac output and coronary perfusion can be partially maintained by CPR.

1. When the heart stops suddenly, the pulmonary veins, left heart and the arteries are full of oxygenated blood. Cardiac massage causes this blood to start flowing.
2. Since the heart is situated between two rigid structures—sternum in front, and vertebrae behind—pressure (compression) applied on the chest in front of it squeezes it, thus producing a mechanical systole. The right and left ventricular pressures exceed the pulmonary and aortic pressures, which cause a forward flow of blood. When the pressure is released, it causes diastolic filling of the ventricles due to the pressure gradient between the large peripheral veins and intrathoracic structures—especially the thin-walled right ventricle.

PROCEDURES

1. Lay the victim on a firm surface. Kneel beside him and place the heel of your left hand (fingers extended and not touching the chest) on the junction of upper 2/3rd and lower 1/3rd of the sternum. Place the heel of the other hand over the first, parallel to it.
2. Keeping the elbows straight, bend forward and depress the sternum towards the spine by 4 to 5 cm at a rate of 80-90/min. The movement should be at the shoulders so that the force can be transmitted through the hands to the chest.
   a. CPR by one person (2:15). Alternate 2 quick lung inflations with 15 cardiac compressions.
   b. CPR by 2 persons (1:5). Interpose 1 lung inflation after every 5th cardiac compression.

Note
If the CPR is being given correctly, you will quickly see an improvement in skin color of the victim; pupils will return to normal size, and neck pulsations will be visible, and heart sounds will be heard.

In Infants

Press the sternum with two fingers of a hand, or with a thumb, with the fingers supporting the back of the infant. Compress by 2-3 cm and maintain cardiac compressions at a rate of 100-110/min.

Internal or Open Cardiac Massage

This procedure is employed in hospitals. The chest is opened in the left intercostal space in the midclavicular line; a hand is inserted into the thorax and the heart is compressed against the chest wall. There is a trans-diaphragmatic approach as well.

CPR for Oneself

What to do when one gets an attack of myocardial infarction (MI) when alone. Coughing very vigorously and repeatedly can save life. A breath and a forceful cough, repeated every 3 seconds, without let up till help arrives or the heart is felt to be beating normally.

Reasons for Failure of CPR

In every case you must try your best to get the heart and lungs functioning again. However, in some cases, all efforts at CPR may fail. It may be that:–
   i. The injury to the heart is very severe, or
   ii. Acid-base disturbances (lactic acidemia) and electrolyte imbalance do not allow the heart rate and rhythm to be restored.

Ventricular Fibrillation (VF)

Ventricular fibrillation is the commonest cause of cardiac arrest because a fibrillating ("trembling") heart cannot act as an effective pump. It is most frequently caused by acute myocardial infarction as a result of which an 'ectopic' irritable focus starts to discharge action potentials (APs) in a fast and irregular manner. The heart responds to these APs and goes into fibrillation. If VF is not stopped within 2-3 minutes, it almost always leads to death. The specific treatment includes:

1. **Electroshock defibrillation (cardioversion).** While a weak AC current (as in accidental shock, or in death penalty) causes VF and death, a strong, high voltage current applied to the chest via large, flat electrodes, can stop fibrillation. All action potentials stop and the heart remains quiescent for 4-5 seconds, after which it starts to beat at the normal rate and rhythm. The shock may have to be repeated a couple of times.
2. **Intravenous injection of 100 ml of 8% sodium bicarbonate** is used to neutralize lactic acidemia.
3. **Intravenous injection of 5-10 ml of 1% calcium chloride.**
4. **Intravenous or intracardiac injection of 0.5 ml of 1:1000 adrenalin** often revives the heart.

INHALATION OF FOREIGN BODY HEIMLICH MANEUVER (ABDOMINAL THRUST)

This procedure can be life-saving when a person begins to choke on something he/she is eating (e.g., a fishbone), or in a child who puts something in his mouth and inadvertently 'inhales' it, e.g., a coin, a marble, etc.

Important
Choking must not be confused with an attack of myocardial infarction (MI). A person who chokes on something cannot speak but only make gestures, while a heart attack victim can. (And, of course, choking is likely to occur while eating. Therefore, ask, "can you speak?")

PROCEDURES

1. Stand behind the person, place your clenched fist below his epigastrium (between the costal margin and the umbilicus); and grasp this fist with the other hand.
2. Now give a sudden upward and inward thrust. It is important the thrust be applied to the upper abdomen and not to the thorax.
3. The sudden thrust pushes the diaphragm up so that the forceful blast of air from the lungs carries the foreign body out of the respiratory passages. The maneuver may be repeated until the foreign object is expelled.

Important
In many cases of choking, the respiratory passage is not completely blocked (though there may be laryngeal spasm), so that if the person breathes quietly and without panic, enough air may reach the lungs to keep him alive until he is shifted to the hospital.

If you happen to choke on something, when alone, position yourself over the high back of a chair, or some other suitable furniture, and thrust your abdomen suddenly and forcefully against it. Repeat if necessary.

Emergency Procedure in Children

Bend the head of the victim forward and downward so that it is lower than the chest. Then, with the heel of a hand, give a few blows on the child's back between the scapulae till the offending object is expelled.

Note that the head must be kept lower than the chest, otherwise the foreign object is likely to be pushed further down into the lungs rather than upwards.

QUESTIONS

Q. 1 Name the indications for cardiopulmonary resuscitation.
CPR is a first-aid measure and is indicated when there is a sudden stoppage of breathing or heart, or both.

Q. 2 What are the causes and signs of cardiopulmonary arrest?
See page 169.

Q. 3 Name the advantages and disadvantages of mouth-to-mouth respiration.
See page 171.

Q. 4 How will you handle a case of drowning?
1. As soon as the victim is brought out of the water, check carotid pulse and breathing. If both present but unconscious, press on lower abdomen to expel water from stomach, if any. Then place the victim in "recovery position", i.e., partial supine position, head turned to one side, left arm under left thigh, right arm above the head, and right leg bent.
2. If the pulse is present, but the victim is not breathing—start mouth-to-mouth breathing or Holger-Neilson method of AR.
3. If both pulse and breaching are absent— start CPR, till the victim recovers or is shifted to the hospital.

Q. 5 How does defibrillation help in ventricular fibrillation?
A strong, high-voltage AC current applied to the chest can stop a fibrillating heart. However, within a few seconds, normal heart beat usually returns.

Q. 6 What is Heimlich maneuver?
It is an emergency procedure to clear the upper respiratory passages after a foreign body has been accidentally inhaled.

Unit II
Cardiovascular System

2-6

Recording of Systemic Arterial Blood Pressure

STUDENT OBJECTIVES

After completing this practical, you should be able to:
1. Define blood pressure, and explain why blood exerts a pressure on the walls of blood vessels.
2. Define systolic, diastolic, pulse, and mean arterial pressures. Indicate their significance.
3. Determine blood pressure by palpatory, oscillometric, and auscultatory methods. Name the advantages and disadvantages of each method
4. Indicate the precautions that must be taken before and during recording of blood pressure.
5. Describe the Korotkoff sounds, and their cause. Name the criteria for systolic and diastolic pressures.
6. Detect the appearance and muffling/disappearance of Korotkoff sounds while recording blood pressure.
7. Name the factors that maintain and control blood pressure.
8. List the physiological variations in blood pressure.
9. Explain how blood pressure is regulated on short-term and long-term basis.
10. Define auscultatory gap and explain its significance.
11. Describe the clinical conditions of hypertension and hypotension and their pathophysiology.
12. Explain the importance of sino- aortic mechanism (baroreceptor reflex).

INTRODUCTION

The cardiovascular system (CVS) is slightly overfilled with blood, i.e., its contents are more than its capacity. As a result, the blood exerts an outward force against the vessel walls as it flows through them.

The term **blood pressure** refers to the force exerted by the blood as it presses against and attempts to stretch the walls of blood vessels.

Although blood exerts this outward force throughout the CVS, the term blood pressure, used unqualified, refers to systemic arterial blood pressure (others are: venous, capillary pressure, etc).

Measurement of blood pressure is an important clinical procedure as it provides valuable information about the cardiovascular system (CVS) under normal and disease conditions.

Measurement of Blood Pressure

Direct Method

The direct method of recording blood pressure (BP), in which an artery is punctured with a cannula connected to a manometer, was first used by Rev Stephen Hales, a British priest, in horses and dogs, in 1733. When he inserted a cannula into the femoral artery of a mare and connected it to a long glass tube, the blood rose to a height of 8 feet 3 inches. When he put the cannula in the femoral vein, the blood rose to a height of only 12 inches. Stephen Hales first expressed blood pressure in terms of weight of blood. His estimate in man was 7½ feet of blood which corresponds to 176 mm Hg.

The direct method was first employed in man in 1856 by Favre, a French physician. He employed Poisseulle manometer and recorded pressures in 3 patients prior to amputation—in the upper part of brachial artery in 2 patients and in femoral artery in 1 patient. In each case, pressure of about 120 mm Hg was recorded, which he thought was the mean aortic pressure.

Note

These days, direct method is used in research work in animals, and during cardiac and arterial catheterization in man.

Indirect Methods

Obviously, the direct method is not suitable as a routine clinical procedure. Indirect methods were, therefore, introduced; methods that are variations of a procedure called sphygmomanometry.

PRINCIPLE

A sufficient length of a single artery is selected in the arm (brachial artery), or in the thigh (femoral artery). The artery is first compressed by inflating a rubber bag (connected to a manometer) placed around the arm (or thigh) to stop the blood flow through the occluded section of the artery. The pressure is then slowly released and the flow of blood through the obstructed segment of the artery is studied by:

i. Feeling the pulse—the palpatory method.
ii. Observing the oscillations of the mercury column—the oscillometric method, and
iii. Listening to the sounds produced in the part of the artery just below the obstructed segment—the auscultatory method.

APPARATUSES

Stethoscope
(Steth = chest, scope = to inspect)

Though introduced in its present form by Laennec in 1819, it was not until 1905 that Korotkoff used it for recording the blood pressure. The sounds produced in the chest and elsewhere in the body are heard with a stethoscope. The instrument has the following 3 parts:

a. **The chest-piece.** The chest-piece has two end pieces—a bell and a flat diaphragm, though some have only the diaphragm.

b. **The rubber tubing.** In the commonly used stethoscope, a single soft-rubber pressure tube (inner diameter 3 mm) leads from the chest-piece to a metal Y-shaped connector. The plastic diaphragm causes magnification of low-pitched sounds though it distorts them a little. The bell-shaped chest-piece conducts sounds without distortion but with little magnification. Murmurs which precede, accompany, or follow the heart sounds are better heard with the bell.

c. **The ear-frame.** It consists of two curved metallic tubes joined together with a flat U-shaped spring which keeps them pulled together. The upper ends of the tubes are curved so that they correspond to the curve of the external auditory meatus, i.e., they are directed forwards and downwards. Two plastic knobs threaded over the ends of the tubes fit snugly in the ear. Two rubber tubes connect the Y-shaped connector to the metal tubes.

Sphygmomanometer
(Commonly called the "BP apparatus")

The sphygmomanometer is the instrument routinely used for recording arterial blood pressure in humans. The term "sphygmomanometer" is derived from three Greek roots with Latin equivalents "sphygmo" means pulse, "manos" means thin, and "metron" refers to measure. In early procedures when physicians used to feel the pulse during measurement of BP, they described its first appearance as "thin", hence the term. Different types of BP instruments are in use, but the one in common use is the mercury sphygmomanometer. It consists of the following parts:

a. **Mercury manometer.** The manometer is fitted in the lid of the instrument. One arm of the manometer is the reservoir for mercury—a broad and short well that contains enough mercury to be driven up in the other limb— the graduated glass tube.

b. **Graduated tube.** The manometer glass tube is graduated in mm from 0 to 300, each division representing 2 mm, though actually slightly less than 2 mm. The reason for this is the greater diameter of the mercury reservoir than that of the glass tube. For example, when mercury is driven up the tube for, say, 20 mm Hg, the meniscus in the reservoir falls less so that the actual pressure on its mercury is slightly greater than 20 mm Hg. And, to compensate for this, the tube is calibrated with divisions that are slightly less than 2 mm apart.

A stopcock between the two limbs, when closed, prevents the mercury from entering the glass tube. The one-way valve fitted at the top of the mercury well prevents spilling of mercury when the lid is closed, while allowing pressure to be transmitted from the rubber bag to the mercury reservoir. A spring-loaded clip at the top of the tube keeps it firmly pressed into a rubber washer at its lower end to prevent leakage of mercury.

c. **The armlet (rubber bag; Riva Rocci cuff).** The "cuff" as it is usually called, consist of an inflatable rubber bag, 24 cm × 12 cm, which is fitted with 2 rubber tubes—one connecting it to the mercury reservoir and the other to a rubber bulb (air pump). The bag is enclosed in a long strip of inelastic cloth with a long tapering free end. The cloth covering keeps the rubber bag in position around the arm when pressure is being measured. In some cuffs, 2 velcron strips are provided in appropriate locations for the same purpose.

The rubber bag is 12 cm wide which is enough to form a pressure cone that reaches the underlying artery even in a thick arm. As a general rule, the width of the bag should be 20% more than the diameter of the arm, though it should be wider in an obese person. The recommended width of the bag in different age groups is as under:

Infants (below 1 year)	: 2.5 cm
Below 4 years	: 5 cm
Below 8 years	: 8 cm
Adults	: 12 cm

d. **Air pump (rubber bulb).** It is an oval-shaped rubber bulb of a size that conveniently fits into one's fist. It has a one-way valve at its free end, and a leak-valve with a knurled screw, at the other where the rubber tube leading to the cuff is attached. The cuff can be inflated by turning the leak valve screw clockwise, and alternately compressing and releasing the bulb. Deflation of the bag is achieved by turning this screw anticlockwise.

Aneroid manometer. In this manometer, in which metal bellows, mechanical links, and a calibrated dial replace the mercury manometer, is also in common use. However, it should be calibrated against a mercury manometer from time to time.

PROCEDURES

The subject may be lying down (supine) or sitting, but should be mentally and physically relaxed and free from excitation and anticipation.

Lay the arm bare up to the shoulder and record the blood pressure first with the palpatory method, followed by auscultatory method. The upper arm on which the BP cuff is to be tied must be at the level of the heart. (In the supine position, the arm resting on the bed will be nearly at the heart level. In the sitting position the arm resting on the table of a suitable height will be at the correct level).

In obese subjects, the cuff may be applied on the forearm with the stethoscope placed over the radial artery for auscultatory method. (If no sounds are heard a reasonably reliable determination can be obtained by palpation at the wrist).

A. Palpatory Method (Riva Rocci 1896)

1. Make the subject sit or lie supine and allow 5 minutes for mental and physical relaxation.

2. Open the lid of the apparatus until you hear the "click". Release the lock on the mercury reservoir and check that the mercury is at the zero level. If it is above zero, subtract the difference from the final reading. If it is below zero, add the required amount of mercury to bring it to zero level.

3. Place the cuff around the upper arm, with the centre of the bag lying over the brachial artery, keeping its lower edge about 3 cm above the elbow. Wrap the cloth covering around the arm so as to cover the rubber bag completely, and to prevent its bulging out from under the wrapping on inflation. The cuff should neither be too tight nor very loose.

4. Palpate the radial artery at the wrist and feel its pulsations with the tips of your fingers. Keeping your fingers on the pulse, hold the air bulb in the palm of your other hand and tighten the leak valve screw with your thumb and fingers.

5. Inflate the cuff slowly until the pulsations disappear; note the reading then raise the pressure another 30-40 mm Hg.

6. Open the leak valve and control it so that the pressure gradually falls in steps of 2-3 mm. Note the reading when the pulse just reappears. **The pressure at which the pulse is first felt is the systolic pressure**. (It corresponds to the time when, at the peak of each systole, small amounts of blood start to flow through the compressed segment of the brachial artery). Deflate the bag quickly to bring the mercury to the zero level.

Note

It is easier to detect the reappearance of radial pulse than its disappearance. The first 2-3 beats being thin, may be missed so that the actual systolic pressure is 4 to 6 mm Hg higher than the recorded value.

7. Record the pressure in the other arm. Take 3 readings in each arm, deflating the cuff for a few minutes between each determination.

Advantages of palpatory method. This method avoids the pitfall of the auscultatory method in missing the auscultatory gap.

Disadvantages of palpatory method:

i. This method measures only the systolic pressure, the diastolic pressure cannot be measured.

ii. This method lacks accuracy because the systolic pressure measured by it is lower than the actual by 4-6 mm Hg. It assumes that the first escape of blood under the cuff will cause pulsations in the peripheral artery (radial in this case). However, there is no evidence that the amount of blood that escapes when the artery first opens is enough to produce a pulse wave detectable by the fingers. Thus, definite pulsation may not occur until the cuff pressure has been reduced by 6-8 mm Hg.

B. Oscillometric Method

Riva Rocci, in 1896 (i.e., before Korotkoff sounds were described) measured systolic pressure (SP) by the palpatory method while the diastolic pressure (DP) was recorded from the oscillations of the mercury column. As the cuff pressure was raised and then lowered, oscillations appeared which became maximum and then disappeared. Some workers took the midpoint of maximum oscillations as the DP while others considered the lower level of these oscillations as the DP (oscillations are best seen with an aneroid manometer). The students must have seen these oscillations in the mercury column.

In a modification of the above method, a cuff is placed on the upper arm and a lightly-inflated one on the lower arm. As the pressure in the upper cuff is raised and lowered, pulsations can be recorded from the lower cuff.

1. **Digital Blood pressure Monitor.** It is a small, compact, battery-operated, palm-top unit

with an LCD display screen and memory function. The recorder works on the 2-cuff *"oscillometric measuring"* principle described above, and automatically translates pulse wave oscillations into SP and DP. The advantage of this method is that it can be easily used by a layperson. The pressure measuring range is 0-280 mm Hg, while the HR range is 40-180/min. There are 2 input sockets, one on either side of the unit.

Connect the rubber bulb to one socket and the cuff (wrapped on the upper arm) to the other. The procedure is the same as that for auscultatory method except that you do not auscultate for Korotkoff sounds.

As the pressure is raised and then lowered, the pressure and pulse readings appear on the screen and the final readings remain there until you switch off the unit.

Note
The terms oscillatory and oscillometric are synonymous; except that when you get a record you call it oscillometric (as you do in "dog experiments" where the BP recorded by mercury manometer on a kymograph paper shows oscillations around the mean arterial blood pressure.

2. Wrist Digital Blood Pressure Monitor
This innovative, compact, battery- operated BP monitor also works on the oscillometric principle. It fits over the wrist with a Velcro cuff. The controls include: Mode/set : for date and time; Start/stop, and Recall buttons.

PROCEDURE

1. Wrap the cuff on the wrist, with the palm of that arm facing up. Ensure that the wrist is at the level of the heart.
2. Press the start button. The cuff starts inflating immediately and automatically, and the readings show a gradual increase. Soon after the artery gets occluded, the readings begin

to decrease in steps of 4-6 mm Hg till the final readings for SP, DP and Pulse rate appear on the screen.

Important
Both the palm-top and the wrist BP monitors should be checked against standard sphygmomanometer from time to time.

C. Auscultatory Method (Korotkoff, 1905)

Note
Before recording the BP by the auscultatory method, it should always be first recorded by the palpatory method so as to avoid missing the auscultatory gap.

Note
Ordinarily no sound are heard when the chest-piece of a stethoscope is applied over the brachial (or any other) artery. However, if the cuff pressure is raised above the expected systolic pressure and then gradually lowered, a series of sounds, called Korotkoff sounds, are heard over the artery just below the cuff.

1. Place the cuff over the upper arm as described above, and record the BP by the palpatory method.
2. Locate the bifurcation of brachial artery (it divides into radial and ulnar branches) in the cubital space just medial to the tendon of the biceps which can be easily palpated in a semiflexed elbow as a thick, hard, elongated structure. Mark the point of arterial pulsation with a sketch pen.
3. Place the chest-piece of the stethoscope on this point and keep it in position with your fingers "and thumb of the left hand (if you are right-handed).

Note
The chest-piece should not rub against the cuff, rubber tubes, or the skin in this area because these disturbing noises will interfere with auscultation of sounds.

4. Inflate the cuff rapidly, by compressing and releasing the air pump alternately (sounds may be heard as the mercury column goes up). Raise the pressure to 40 to 50 mm Hg above the systolic level as determined by the palpatory method.
5. Lower the pressure gradually until a clear, sharp, tapping sound is heard. Continue to lower the pressure and try to note a change in the character of the sounds.

These sounds are called Korotkoff sounds and show the following phases:

Phase I This phase starts with a clear, sharp tap when a jet of blood is able to cross the previously obstructed artery. (Sometimes this phase may start with a faint tap, especially when the systolic pressure is very high). As the pressure is lowered, the sounds continue as sharp and clear taps. This phase lasts for 10-12 mm Hg fall in pressure (**Figure 2-7**).

Note
Criterion of systolic pressure The level at which the first sound (clear, sharp, or faint), is heard is taken as the systolic pressure.

Phase II The sounds become murmurish and remain so during the next 10-15 mm Hg fall in pressure when they again become clear and banging.
Phase III It starts with clear, knocking, or banging sounds that continue for the next 12 to 14 mm Hg pressure, when they suddenly become muffled.
Phase IV The transition from phase III to phase IV is usually very sudden. The sounds remain muffled, dull, faint and indistinct (as if coming from a distance) until they disappear. The muffling of sounds and their disappearance occurs nearly at the same time, there being a difference of 4-5 mm Hg (i.e., phase IV lasts for 4-5 mm Hg).

Important
Note the reading at muffling and another at disappearance of sounds, after which deflate the cuff quickly.

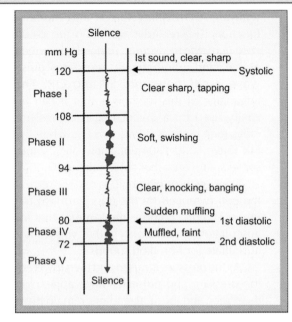

Figure 2-7. Phases of Korotkoff sounds, showing the changes in their character during each phase as the mercury column is gradually lowered. Systolic pressure: 1st appearance of sounds. Diastolic pressure: sudden muffling of sounds

Phase V This phase begins when the Korotkoff sounds disappear completely. If you reduce the pressure slowly, you will note that total silence continues right up to the zero level.
6. Take 3 readings with the auscultatory method and repeat 3 readings on the other arm.
7. Effects of posture, gravity, and muscular exercise on blood pressure are discussed in the next experiment.

COMMENTS, OBSERVATIONS AND RESULTS

1. It may be noted that the Korotkoff sounds are not heard equally well in all individuals. Indeed it may be difficult to identify any phases at all except the first appearance of sounds—the criterion of systolic pressure.
2. Sometimes muffling of the sounds (1st diastolic pressure) may not be distinguished

though their disappearance is clear. In such cases 5 mm are added to the level at which they disappeared (2nd diastolic pressure). In cases like aortic regurgitation, the Korotkoff sounds may continue right down to the zero level. In others, the sounds may disappear only after 15-20 mm Hg after muffling. In these cases, placing the stethoscope over an artery and pressing its rim on the vessel may produce sharp tapping sounds, called "pistol shot" sounds.

3. **Criterion of diastolic pressure.** The criterion for diastolic pressure is the muffling of the sounds or their disappearance?

Simultaneous recordings of BP with auscultatory method and intra-arterial recordings with pressure transducers have shown that the diastolic pressure correlates better with the disappearance of sounds. However, in adults after exercise, and in children, the diastolic pressure has better correlation with muffling. Therefore, the blood pressure may also be expressed as: 120/80/76, the last figure indicating the disappearance of sounds (1st and 2nd diastolic, **Figure 2-5**).

Note
The BP readings are seldom identical in the two arms. It has been suggested that both arms be used, preferably the right arm and then the left arm.

Tabulate your results as shown below (Table 2.1):
For report, express your result as:
Right arm: Systolic/lst diastolic/2nd diastolic ;
(e.g., 120/80/76).
Left arm: Systolic/lst diastolic/2nd diastolic;
(e.g., 118/76/72).

TABLE 2.1
Record of systemic arterial blood pressure

A. PALPATORY METHOD (mm Hg)

	Right arm	**Left arm**
1st reading		
2nd reading		
3rd reading		

Maximum value =	.... mm Hg
Heart rate =	.... mm Hg

B. OSCILLATORY METHOD

C. AUSCULTATORY METHOD (mm Hg)

	Systolic pressure	Diastolic pressure	Mean arterial pressure	Pulse pressure
Right arm				
1st reading	....	.....	......	....
2nd reading	....	.....	.....	.....
3rd reading	....	.....	.....	.....
Left arm				
1st reading	.....	......	......	.....
2nd reading	......	......	......	.....
3rd reading	......	......	......	......
Maximum values:				
Right arm =				
Left arm =				

PRECAUTIONS

1. The subject should be physically and mentally relaxed and free from tension and anxiety. He/she should be assured and rested for 5 minutes or so to avoid the condition of "**white coat hypertension**" (i.e., some people have higher BP readings in the clinician's office than during their normal daytime activity). It is good practice to compare the pressures in the two arms when recording BP for the first time. If the readings are above the upper normal limits, the measurement must be repeated under basal conditions, i.e., early in the morning before the subject gets up from the bed. A diagnosis of hypertension must never be made lightly and in haste.

2. The arm, with the cuff wrapped around it, should be kept at the level of the heart to avoid the influence of gravity. The cuff tubing should lie anterolateral to the cubital fossa so that they do not rub against the chest-piece of the stethoscope.

3. The cuff should not be too tight nor too loose.

4. The cuff should not be left inflated with high pressures for any length of time, because the discomfort and reflex spasm of the artery and its branches will give false high readings.

5. Do not apply pressure on the artery with the chest-piece as this may produce partial obstruction of the artery and a fake low reading.
6. Check the pulse rate at the time of recording BP as the heart rate affects the BP.
7. The palpatory method must always be employed before the auscultatory method.
8. In suspected and known cases of hypertension, the pressure should always be raised well above 200 mm Hg; or above the level estimated by palpatory method.
9. In obese subjects, a cuff that is wider than the standard should be used. Similarly, when measuring the pressures in the thigh, the cuff should be wider, because the thick layer of fat in the obese, or the large amounts of tissues in the thigh dissipate some of the cuff pressure, thus giving false high results. (The BP may be recorded with the cuff on the forearm while palpating and auscultating the radial artery).

QUESTIONS

Q. 1 Define blood pressure. Why does blood exert a pressure on the walls of the blood vessels? Is this pressure constant throughout the cardiac cycle? What are the units employed for blood pressure?

The vascular system is "overfilled" with blood so that it is slightly stretched by the blood. As a result, the blood exerts an outward lateral force on the inside of the vessels; this force is known as blood pressure. Although blood exerts a force (pressure) throughout the vascular system, the term blood pressure, used unqualified, refers to systemic arterial pressure. (Thus, other pressures would be capillary pressure, venous pressure, pulmonary pressure, etc).

Relation between contents and capacity—the cause of blood pressure. The relation between the contents and capacity of a distensible container determines whether or not the fluid will exert a pressure. So long as the contents are equal to or less than the capacity, no pressure is exerted i.e., the pressure is zero, or atmospheric. (All pressures in the body are described with reference to the atmospheric pressure which is taken as zero. Thus, a pressure of 120 mm Hg means a pressure of 760 + 120 mm Hg; a pressure of -5 mm Hg is equal to 760 - 5 = 755 mm Hg). A pressure is exerted only when the volume of contents exceeds the capacity, i.e., when extra fluid is injected into the container. (An example will clarify the point: we have a rubber ball of 200 ml capacity. When we inject 200 ml water into it, say, with a syringe, the pressure exerted will be zero or atmospheric. Now, if we inject another 20 ml water, the water will exert a pressure. Introduction of another 20 ml water will further increase the pressure. Thus, **pressures are created when the contents become more than the capacity.** The arterial tree of an adult has a capacity of about 500 ml, while this space contains 750 ml blood; the blood therefore, exerts a mean pressure of 100 mm Hg. If the volume of blood decreases to 500 ml (say, due to hemorrhage), the blood pressure will fall to zero). If we suddenly stop the heart in an experimental animal, the blood redistributes itself throughout the vascular tree, and now it exerts a pressure of 8-10 mm Hg, which is called the **mean circulatory filling pressure.**

How much pressure would be exerted by blood on the vessel walls is determined by:
1. The degree of stiffness of the aorta and its large branches.
2. The inflow of blood into the arterial tree (controlled by cardiac output).
3. The outflow of blood from the arterial tree controlled by arteriolar tone (i.e., peripheral resistance), and
4. The volume of blood (see **Figure 2-8**).

Arterial blood pressure is pulsatile. The BP does not remain constant at one level but rises and falls rhythmically with systole and diastole of the heart, i.e., it is pulsatile. It reaches a maximum during systole and falls to a minimum during diastole (See next Q/A also).

Units employed for blood pressure. Pressure is a force acting on a unit area (e.g., dynes/cm^2). The pressure exerted by blood is usually expressed in terms of the height of a column of fluid that the pressure will support. The SI unit of pressure is the pascal (Pa). This is the pressure exerted by 1 Newton force on an area of a square meter (1 Pa = 1 N/m^2); 1 mm Hg = 133.3 Pa = 0.1333 kPa).

Q. 2 What is systolic blood pressure? How is it produced and what is its significance?
With each systole of the left ventricle, 70-80 ml of blood is ejected into the aorta and its branches and the pressure sharply rises. These vessels, which are highly elastic, get stretched (expanded) and accommodate some of this stroke volume, while the rest runs off down the arterial tree. During diastole of the heart, (when the ventricles are relaxing and getting filled with blood from the atria), the large elastic vessels recoil and the blood that was accommodated earlier, now moves down the arterial tree. Thus, these vessels act as **"secondary pumps"** which produce a pressure and blood flow during diastole of the heart.

The periodic entry of blood into the arterial tree causes the pressure within to alternately rise to a maximum and fall to a minimum. **The maximum pressure is reached during the maximum ejection phase of systole and is called the systolic pressure.** The minimum pressure is reached during diastole and is called the **diastolic pressure.**

Note
It may be pointed out that during systole, the pressure rises to a maximum and then begins to fall as blood runs off down the arteries. The pressure would fall to zero but for the next systole when another stroke volume is ejected into the aorta and the pressure rises again. This rise and fall of blood pressure is repeated over and over again.

Significance of systolic pressure. The systolic pressure indicates the force of contraction of the heart and thus it represents the work done by the heart in overcoming the resistance of the vessels.

Q. 3 What is diastolic pressure and what is its criterion and significance?
Diastolic pressure is the **minimum pressure** reached in the arteries during diastole of the heart, i.e., just before the next systole. The relaxation of the heart cannot be a cause of a pressure in the aorta because the left ventricle itself is getting filled with blood. Two factors, both outside the heart, combine to produce a pressure in the arteries during diastole.
   i. Elasticity of aorta and large branches (i.e., recoil of aorta), and
   ii. Peripheral resistance.
   If the aorta and large arteries were rigid, there would be no diastolic pressure; also the systolic pressure would rise to a much higher level (thus, the elasticity buffers the systolic pressure and does not allow it to rise very high). Similarly, there would be no diastolic pressure if there were no peripheral resistance, as most of the blood would run off into the periphery.
Criterion of diastolic pressure. See page 181.
Significance of diastolic pressure. Clinically, greater importance is attached to the DP because this pressure is being exerted all the time during systole and diastole, while systolic pressure is reached only momentarily during systole. Since a sustained high pressure causes damage to the vessel walls, diastolic hypertension is much more dangerous than systolic hypertension.

Q. 4 What is mean arterial pressure and what is its significance?
The mean arterial pressure (MAP, or mean arterial blood pressure, MABP) is the average of all the pressures measured during the cardiac cycle. Since the duration of systole is shorter than that of diastole, the MAP is slightly less than the average of systolic and diastolic pressures. (The true MAP can be determined only by integrating the areas of the pressure curves). However, a reasonable approximation is: one-third of pulse pressure plus diastolic pressure (e.g., SP = 120; DP = 80; so

MABP is equal to 13 + 80 = 93 mm Hg). Another approximation is 40% SP + 60 % DP (e.g., 40% of 120 = 48, and 60% of 80 = 48; thus 48 + 48 = 96 mm Hg).

Significance of mean arterial pressure. The MAP of about 95 mm Hg provides the pressure head, or the driving force (vis a tergo) for the flow of blood through the arteries, capillaries, and veins, etc. The MAP in medium-sized arteries (e.g., radial) is about 90 mm Hg. Thus, most viscera, muscles, and other tissues are perfused at a relatively high pressure. The mean pressure of about 85-80 mm Hg at the start of arterioles falls to about 32 at their capillary ends. (Thus, maximum fall in pressure occurs in the arterioles). The pressure then continues to fall progressively till it reaches zero in the right atrium. The pressure gradient of about 95 mm Hg is responsible for the circulation of blood.

Q. 5 What is pulse pressure and what is its significance?

Pulse pressure (PP) is the difference between systolic and diastolic pressures, the average PP being about 40 mm Hg. Other factors remaining unchanged, the magnitude of PP indicates the stroke volume. Thus, it provides information about the condition of cardiovascular system. For example, conditions such as atherosclerosis (hardening of blood vessels) and patent ductus arteriosus generally increase the PP. The normal ratio of SP to DP and to PP is about 3:2:1.

Q. 6 Name the precautions you will observe while recording blood pressure?

See page 181.

Q. 7 What are the advantages and disadvantages of palpatory method of recording blood pressure?

See page 178.

Q. 8 What will be the effect of using a wrong-sized blood pressure cuff in different age groups, or a standard cuff in a very obese person?

If an over- or under-sized cuff is used, the reading will be higher than actual because more pressure would be required in the cuff to overcome tissue resistance and to form a cone of pressure.

When a standard cuff is used in an obese individual, the reading will be higher than actual because of loss of pressure in overcoming tissue resistance.

Q. 9 What are Korotkoff sounds and how are they produced?

Normally, the blood flow through the arteries is laminar or streamline, and no sounds are heard when a stethoscope is placed on them. When the cuff pressure is raised above the expected systolic pressure, and then gradually lowered, a time comes, when at the peak of each systole, the intra-arterial pressure just exceeds the cuff (extra-arterial) pressure. But, in between these peaks, the artery is still constricted. Now, it is known that constriction of an artery increases the velocity of blood flow through the constricted part. Thus, when the small amounts of blood are jetted through the partially constricted artery, their velocity increases and then exceeds the critical velocity. This produces **intermittent turbulence** that in turn produces Korotkoff sounds (beyond the constriction) which have a staccato quality (tapping intermittent sounds).

Also, the blood column in the distal part of the artery, i.e., below the cuff, is set into vibration by the jets of blood striking against it, which contributes to the sounds. (The velocity of blood has to increase beyond a certain critical level before turbulence and hence sounds are produced. This velocity is sometimes normally exceeded in the ascending aorta at the peak of systolic ejection. Turbulence also occurs commonly in anemia because the viscosity of blood is low. This probably explains the systolic murmurs in these cases).

When the cuff pressure is near the diastolic level, the artery is still partially constricted, but **the turbulent flow is now continuous rather than intermittent,** and sounds from continuous turbulent flow have a muffled quality rather than a tapping or staccato quality. As the cuff pressure further falls, the blood flow becomes laminar once again and the sounds disappear. The change in the character of sounds during early phases is related to the degree of turbulence.

In aortic regurgitation (leaking of blood back from the aorta into the ventricle through an incompetent valve), the sounds may continue right down to near zero and only muffling of sounds can indicate diastolic pressure. In fact, a slight pressure with a stethoscope   alone (without the cuff on the upper arm) may produce sharp, clear, snapping sounds, called "pistol shot" sounds, in this condition.

Q. 10 What is auscultatory gap, and what is its significance?

In some patients of hypertension, there may be a gap in the Korotkoff sounds. As the mercury is lowered, a few faint sounds are heard which soon disappear only to reappear once again at a lower pressure. This brief interruption, which may range from 40 to 60 mm Hg, is called the **"auscultatory" or "silent" gap**. If the mercury column is raised to this gap, and then the pressure lowered, one may miss the first appearance of sounds, which indicate systolic pressure, and thus record a false low systolic pressure.

To avoid this mistake, the BP should always be recorded by the palpatory method first. Then during auscultatory method, the mercury column must be raised 30-40 mm Hg above the level found by palpatory method.

Q. 11 When recording blood pressure, why should the upper arm with the cuff wrapped around it, be kept at the level of the heart?

The force of gravity exerts an important effect on the blood pressure readings. The degree of its effect varies with the vertical distance above and below the level of the heart. Consult next Expt on the effect of gravity on blood pressure.

Q. 12 What is the effect of muscular exercise on blood pressure?

Consult next Expt for the effect of exercise on blood pressure.

Q. 13 What is oscillometric method of recording blood pressure?

See page 178.

Q. 14 How does the blood pressure recorded in the femoral artery differ from that recorded in brachial artery?

A cannula inserted in an artery, with the artery tied off beyond this, records an end pressure. (Flow in the artery is interrupted and all the kinetic energy is converted into pressure energy). If a T tube is inserted in an artery and pressure is measured in the side arm of the tube, it records the side pressure, which is lower than the end pressure.

The subclavian and the brachial arteries represent the side arms from the wall of the aorta. The pressure recorded in the brachial artery, thus, represents the side pressure or the lateral pressure in the aorta. On the other hand, the femoral arteries are the direct extensions of the aorta. When pressure is recorded from a femoral artery, the end pressure is represented in the recording. For this reason, even in the supine position, pressures recorded in the lower limbs are somewhat higher than those in the upper limbs. A low pressure in the femoral artery with hypertension in the arms is the basic clue to the diagnosis of coarctation of aorta. With the normal person standing, the femoral pressure is higher than brachial pressure.

Q. 15 What are the physiological variations in blood pressure?

Normally, variations in BP occur as mentioned below:

1. **Age.** The average SP at birth is about 40 mm Hg, reaches 70 at 2 weeks and 80 at one month. The SP/DP averages 90-100/60-70 mm Hg between 4 and 10 years and adult levels are reached by 18-20 years. Both SP and DP rise with age; at 60 years the BP may be 160/90 mm Hg.

2. **Sex.** The BP is generally lower in females by about 8-10 mm Hg. It remains so till the age of menopause, after which it remains slightly higher than the male average.

3. **Body build and obesity.** Overweight individuals tend to have higher blood pressure. Since

resistance to blood flow through a blood vessel depends on its length, increased length of blood vessels is bound to increase the resistance and hence blood pressure. (Each extra kg of adipose tissue is associated with the development of an additional 400 km of blood vessels).

4. Diurnal variations. The BP is lowest under basal conditions, the peak being seen in the late afternoon, mainly in the systolic level. The SP shows a significant fall during sleep.

5. Digestion. The systolic pressure shows a rise of 8-10 mm Hg after meals and lasts for about 1 hour. Diastolic is little affected, though it may decrease a little due to vasodilation in the viscera.

6. Emotional stress. Hypertension is a natural response to pain, and stress in nonhypertensive individuals. The systolic pressure rises during anger, apprehension, excitement, etc. Some hypertensives, because of nervousness, have higher BP in the clinician's office than during their normal daytime activity—a condition which has been called **white coat hypertension.**

7. Posture. See next Experiment.

8. Muscular exercise. See next Experiment.

9. Sleep. The blood pressure, both systolic and diastolic, tend to be low during the early restful stage of sleep, especially systolic pressure which may fall by 15-20 mm Hg due to general relaxation, decrease in sympathetic tone, etc. Meditation has the same effect.

Q. 16 How is arterial blood pressure maintained and controlled?

Establishing and maintaining blood pressure. There are 5 basic factors involved in establishing and maintaining systemic arterial blood pressure. They include: pumping action of the heart, peripheral resistance, elasticity of large blood vessels, the volume of circulating blood, and the viscosity of blood. Normally, the last 3 factors do not take part in the control of blood pressure on a short-term basis. This leaves the first 2 factors, i.e., cardiac output and peripheral resistance (**Figure 2-8**) for the regulation of blood pressure.

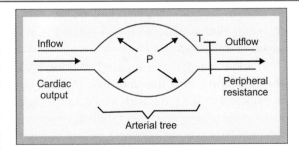

Figure 2-8. Relation between inflow, outflow, and pressure (P) in the arterial tree. With each systolic input, the pressure raises to a maximum (during systole) and then falls to a minimum (during diastole). The arterioles act as taps (T) and control the outflow of blood from the arterial tree. (The capacity of arterial tree is about 500 ml but it contains about 750 ml blood; therefore, it exerts a pressure)

It is commonly stated that **blood pressure is the product of cardiac output and peripheral resistance.** This does not mean that the two values are to be multiplied. It only means that any BP reading is the result of the interaction of these two factors. Cardiac output controls the inflow of blood into the arterial tree, while peripheral resistance controls the outflow.

1. Pumping action of the heart. The rate and force of cardiac contraction determines the cardiac output, i.e., the volume of blood ejected into the arteries by each ventricle separately. The heart rate and force of contraction are controlled by the cardiovascular centres in the medulla, ventricular end diastolic volume, and myocardial contractility. (See chart 5-10, Section 5).

2. Peripheral resistance. This refers to the resistance (opposition) that the blood encounters while passing through small vessels, especially arterioles (two-thirds of the peripheral resistance lies here). All the arterioles, except a few, are innervated by the sympathetic nervous system, which maintains them in a state of slight constriction (a phenomenon called vasomotor tone). Thus, these vessels can further constrict by increase in sympathetic activity, or relax by decrease in sympathetic activity. Increase in peripheral resistance raises blood pressure while decrease in resistance has the opposite effect.

3. Elasticity of large arteries. The elasticity of aorta and its major branches determines both systolic and diastolic blood pressure. With increasing age, these vessels become less elastic (arteriosclerosis). This results in an increase in systolic pressure with a normal diastolic blood pressure (systolic hypertension). (But since peripheral vessels also harden, the diastolic pressure may also rise).

4. Volume of circulating blood. Increase in blood volume, as during salt and fluid retention, raises the BP, while loss of body fluids, such as due to severe diarrhea and vomiting, and hemorrhage result in a fall in blood pressure. (Of course, changes in blood volume are not involved in short-term regulation of BP).

5. Viscosity of blood. The viscosity of blood partly determines resistance to blood flow through the small vessels. Polycythemia increases viscosity while anemia decreases it.

Q. 17 How is blood pressure regulated on short-term, intermediate-term, and long-term basis?

An adequate pressure of blood is required to perfuse vital organs and other tissues. On the other hand, a high BP can damage the blood vessels in vital organs and can cause serious complications. Under normal conditions, therefore, many different but interdependent negative feed-back subsystems control BP by adjusting heart rate, stroke volume, peripheral resistance, and to some extent, blood volume.

The BP regulatory mechanisms may be divided into: **short-term**, **intermediate-term** and **long-term** processes.

I. Short-term Regulation of BP. This mechanism is **life- saving**, and functions from moment-to-moment and minute- to- minute. (e.g., sudden standing from supine position may decrease the BP significantly and cause fainting; see next Expt). It involves baroreceptors, chemoreceptors, and CNS ischemic response.

a. ***Sino- aortic mechanism.*** Baroreceptors (stretch receptors) in the walls of heart, large arteries and veins of the thorax monitor (sense) *the pressure within these structures. They are stimulated by distension* (stretching) of their walls by the pressure inside. They oppose sudden increase or decrease in BP.

The most well known baroreceptors are present in carotid sinus and aortic arch. The APs from these receptors affect cardiovascular center in medulla. A sudden rise in BP sends APs from these receptors via IX and X nerves to the nucleus of tractus solitarius (NTS). They are relayed to the medulla where they inhibit tonic discharge of vasoconstrictor nerves and excite vagal nerves to the heart. The result is vasodilatation, venodilatation, decrease in cardiac output, and bradycardia—and thus a fall in BP.

A fall in BP has the opposite effect because it decreases the inhibitory APs from the baroreceptors so that the vasoconstrictor nerves are released from inhibition while cardiac vagal nerves are inhibited. The result is tachycardia, increase in CO, and vaso-and venoconstriction. (Consult Expt2-9 for more details).

b. ***Baroreceptors in Atria and Pulmonary Veins.*** These are low pressure receptors so that they cannot detect changes in blood pressure. However, they detect and respond to changes in blood volume (degree of fullness), and control the release of ADH, atrial natriuretic peptide (ANP), and rennin-angiotensin-aldosterone system.

c. ***Chemoreceptors.*** When the BP falls below a critical level, the blood flow to carotid and aortic bodies chemoreceptors decreases. The increased CO_2 and H^+ and decrease in O_2 stimulate these receptors and the BP is restored to some extent. (These chemoreceptors play a much more important role in the regulation of respiration).

d. *CNS Ischemic response.* This response, in which the vasomotor center is stimulated (by increased CO_2 and decreased O_2), is the last ditch effort to raise the BP when it falls below 60 mm Hg.

II. Intermediate-term Regulation of BP. This mechanism is **life-sustaining** and functions from day-to-day and from week-to week. It involves movement of tissue fluid into circulation by *capillary fluid shift* and *stress relaxation* of vessels.

III. Long-term regulation of BP. This mechanism is **life-stabilizing** and functions over months and years. It involves *renal-body fluids volume system* because the kidney is the major organ that regulates extracellular, and thus intracellular, fluid volume. The hormones involved include: rennin-angiotensin-aldosterone, catecholamines, vasopressin (ADH), ANP, and nitric oxide (NO).

Note

The sino-aortic baroreceptors are not effective for intermediate and long term regulation of BP because they become "reset" at a higher level in 1-2 days.

Q. 18 What is hypertension, and what are its causes and complications?

Chronic elevation in blood pressure beyond 140/85 is generally labeled hypertension (HT). The higher the BP, the greater the risk of complications. A diagnosis of HT requiring treatment with potentially toxic drugs is usually made on the basis of more than 3 high pressure readings on different days.

Students are often unclear as to which pressures—systolic or diastolic—should be considered as abnormal; and how to label different degrees of HT. A recognised classification is given below:

With DP below 90 mm Hg:

SP below 140 mm Hg = Normal
140-159 mm Hg   = Borderline isolated systolic hypertension.

160 or higher   = Isolated systolic hypertension.

Diastolic pressures

Below 85 mm Hg   = Normal
85-90 mm Hg   = High normal.
90-104 mm Hg   = Mild hypertension.
105-114   = Moderate hypertension.
115 and above   = Severe hypertension.

Classification of hypertension. The disease is grouped into the following two main categories:

1. Essential hypertension. About 90-95% of hypertensives belong to this category in which the cause of the high pressure is not known—although obesity, high salt intake, alcohol ingestion, heredity, and mental make-up (tense, irritable and over-ambitious individuals; the Type I personality) are believed to play a role.

2. Secondary hypertension. The remaining 5-10% of hypertensives belong to this group, in which the cause of high BP is known. Secondary hypertension, which is curable, should always be considered in patients under age 30 years or those who develop hypertension after age 55 years.

a. **Renal diseases.** Parenchymal disease; polycystic kidney; narrowing of renal artery.

b. **Coarctation of aorta**

c. **Endocrine diseases.** Pheochromocytoma (catecholamine-secreting tumor of adrenal medulla); hyperaldosteronism; Cushing syndrome; hyperthyroidism; oral contraceptives; acromegaly.

d. **Toxemias of pregnancy.**

Malignant hypertension. In some patients, the blood pressure, especially the diastolic pressure, is accelerated and rises to very high levels within a short time (diastolic pressure above 120 mm Hg is a medical emergency). If untreated, the patient may di.e., within 1-2 years.

Complications of Hypertension. Hypertension has been called a "silent killer". It may go unnoticed and undiagnosed for years when permanent damage has already occurred in vital organs. (This shows the importance of regular medical checkups). The common causes of death are myocardial infarction ("Heart attack"), hemorrhage or occlusion of a blood vessel in the brain ("brain attack"), and renal failure. Hemorrhages in the retina may cause blindness.

Q. 19 What is hypotension and what are its effects?

Hypotension, or low blood pressure, is hardly, if ever, considered a disease or a cause of alarm in otherwise healthy individuals. However, the BP may show low readings under certain conditions.

 a. *Sudden fall in BP.* This may be due to myocardial infarction, acute loss of large amounts of blood, severe diarrhea and vomiting, and excessive intake of diuretics. The person may go into a state of shock.

 b. *Postural hypotension.* When the SBP falls by 20 mm Hg or more on sudden standing from supine position, it is called postural hypotension. It is usually due to autonomic insufficiency as a result of diabetic polyneuropathy, and during treatment with sympatholytic drugs in hypertension. Rising from bed after prolonged illness may also cause fall in BP.

 c. *Chronic primary hypotension.* It is seen in some elderly persons, but its cause is not known.

2-7

Effect of Posture, Gravity and Muscular Exercise on Blood Pressure and Heart Rate

Note

The effect of posture, gravity and muscular exercise can best be studied by using palm-top or wrist digital BP described in the previous practical.

Changes in posture, gravity, and exercise all affect BP and HR in different ways and to different extents. In order to study these effects, the following precautions must be taken:

PROCEDURAL PRECAUTIONS

 1. Record the BP with the arm, with the cuff wrapped around it, at the level of the heart except when studying the effect of gravity.
 2. Do not remove the cuff in between the estimations but leave it in position by disconnecting the metal connection between the cuff and the mercury reservoir.
 3. Record the pulse rate and blood pressure as soon as possible after a change in posture (or after the exercise is over), preferably within 10-12 seconds because the changes in BP are rapid and short-lasting.
 4. If during exercise, the subject feels discomfort and fatigue in the legs, breathlessness, giddiness, suffocation, etc., tell the subject to discontinue the exercise.

EFFECT OF CHANGE IN POSTURE

The effect of changes in posture depends on whether these are recorded immediately after standing from supine position, or after prolonged standing. They also depend on whether a person stands against a support (e.g., a wall), or is standing 'free' and still.

Immediate Effect. As the person assumes erect position, blood tends to pool in the lower parts of the body (especially in the veins) due to gravity. This decreases the venous return, and hence CO and BP. A pooling of 250-300 ml of blood can decrease the systolic pressure by 10-15 mm Hg. However, within some 8-10 seconds the sino-aortic baroreceptor mechanism restores BP to normal level.

Effect of Prolonged Standing. If a person stands still, especially against a support, more than 500 ml of blood may pool in the lower body. Also, increased capillary hydrostatic pressure causes fluid to be filtered out into the tissues, which further reduced venous return. The CO and BP fall, resulting in cerebral ischemia that causes the person to fall down unconscious. The fainting is actually a homeostatic mechanism, as it restores venous return, CO and BP, thus relieving cerebral ischemia.

Note
The problem of prolonged standing is commonly encountered in sentries, soldiers, and traffic policemen. They are, therefore, advised to tense their leg muscles, and walk around from time to time (to promote venous return by the "muscle pump"). They also wear 'wrappings' (tight strips of thick cloth) around their legs.

PROCEDURES

1. Allow the subject to rest and relax for a few minutes in the supine position. Record the heart rate (pulse rate) and BP by the palpatory method and auscultatory method (later on by auscultatory method alone). Disconnect the cuff from the BP apparatus.
2. Ask the subject to sit up and immediately record the BP and heart rate (HR). Repeat the determinations after 1 min, 2 min, and 5 minutes.

3. Make the subject lie down again and rest for a few minutes. Then record the BP and HR. Now ask him to suddenly stand up, and record the BP and HR.
4. Record your observations in your work-book.

EFFECT OF GRAVITY

The proper procedure for studying the effect of gravity on BP would be to put the subject on a turn table and to record intra-arterial and intra-venous pressures (with catheters) in the feet, near the heart level, and carotid vessels. The pressures can then be recorded in the supine position and then immediately after standing). However, for student experiments, the effect of gravity may be studied in the upper arm by recording the BP with the arm kept at heart level, then above the head and then hanging it below the heart level.

PROCEDURES

1. Make the subject sit comfortably and record the HR and BP with the arm at heart level.
2. Record the BP with the subject's arm raised above the head, while your work-partner holds the BP apparatus at heart level.
3. Record the BP with the subject's arm hanging down below the heart level.
4. Record the BP in the brachial artery with the subject in the standing position. Then wrap the cuff over the lower part of the thigh and record the BP by auscultating the popliteal artery behind the knee.
5. Tabulate your results.

Note
It is easier to raise or lower the arm with the "Wrist BP monitor".

EFFECTS OF MUSCULAR EXERCISE

The effect of muscular exercise on BP depends on the following:

1. The type of muscular exercise—whether aerobic or anaerobic, and isotonic or iso-metric.

2. The severity and degree of exercise. Depending on the increase in heart rate, and relative load index (RLI) , i.e., percentage of maximum oxygen utilization, the WHO grading of muscular exercise into light (mild), moderate, heavy, and severe is shown in the next experiment (Expt. 2-8), However, work done may be taken into consideration (Eg; light= 150-250 watts; moderate= 350-500 watts; and heavy= > 550 watts).

3. The duration of exercise.

4. It also depends on whether the subject is a trained athlete or an untrained individual.

Important
If during exercise the subject feels discomfort, fatigue and pain in the legs, breathlessness, giddiness, suffocation, etc., tell him/her to discontinue the exercise.

PROCEDURES

Various types of exercises, of varying degrees, and duration may be devised and their effects may be compared.

1. Make the subject comfortable and explain the procedures to be followed in this experiment. You may employ any of these exercises: "running in place" (spot running) with the thighs brought up to the horizontal alternately, for 3-5 minutes (if a metronome is available the speed of running can be varied); hopping on each foot for 3 minutes, raising the feet 12-15 inches off the ground; climbing up and down the stairs; jogging, or

2. Harvard step test as described in the next experiment.

3. Graded exercises can be given on a treadmill, if available.

OBSERVATIONS AND RESULTS

Enter your findings in a tabulated form as shown below (Table 2.2):

TABLE 2.2

Effect of posture	Pulse rate	Systolic pressure	Diastolic pressure	Mean arterial pressure	Pulse pressure
Effect of posture, gravity and exercise on blood pressure					
Effect of Posture					
Supine position					
Sitting from supine					
Standing from sitting					
Standing from supine					
Femoral Artery					
Prone position					
Standing					
Effect of Gravity					
Arm at heart level					
Arm above head					
Arm below heart					
Effect of Exercise					
Resting					
After exercise					
At 2 minutes					
At 4 minutes					
At 6 minutes					

- The HR returned to resting level after: .... minutes
- The BP returned to resting level after: .... minutes

QUESTIONS

- Read the Questions/Answers in the previous Experiment (Expt 2-6) on "Recording of Systemic Arterial Blood Pressure".

Q. 1 Describe the effect of posture on blood pressure in your experiment.

The effects of changes in posture on blood pressure are due to the effects of gravity. With the arm raised above the head the pressure decreases as compared to the pressure recorded at heart level. The pressure increases when the arm is below the level of the heart.

The pressure recorded in the femoral artery is greater than the pressure recorded in the brachial artery for 2 reasons:

  i. The BP recorded in the femoral artery is the sum of the side pressure (lateral pressure) plus the end on pressure.

  ii. The effect of gravity further adds to this pressure. (See Q/A 14 in Expt 2-6).

Q. 2 What is postural hypotension?

See Q/A 19 Expt 2-6.

Q. 3 What is the effect of gravity on blood pressure?

The pressure in any artery or vein below the level of the heart is increased and that in any vessel above the heart *is* decreased by the effect of gravity. The degree of this effect (the product of the vertical distance above or below the heart, the acceleration due to gravity (980 cm/s/s) and the density of blood), is 0.77 mm Hg/cm. The mean pressure in a large artery at heart level is 100 mm Hg (a few mm Hg in a vein). In a standing person, however, the MAP in a large artery in the foot (about 100 cm below heart) is about 180-200 mm Hg (100 + [0.77 × 100]). (The pressure in a large vein increases to the same extent). The pressure in the head (50 cm above the heart) is about 60 mm Hg, i.e., a drop of about 30-40 mm Hg (100 – [0.77 × 50]). (The pressure in a large vein in the head is negative). (Since the pressures in both arteries and veins are equally affected, the tissue fluid dynamics are not affected).

Q. 4 Why is it important to record the heart rate (pulse rate) when studying the effect of muscular exercise on blood pressure?

The heart rate is noted because the effect of exercise on blood pressure varies with the intensity of exercise. So heart rate gives us information about the intensity of exercise. (See Expt 2-8 on "cardiac efficiency tests").

Q. 5 What are the different types of exercises?

Aerobic and anaerobic exercise. "Aerobics" are those exercises where one "huffs and puffs" to supply oxygen to the exercising muscles (these exercises are beneficial to the cardiovascular and respiratory systems). **Aerobic exercises** include jogging, cycling, spot running, rebounding (running in place on a minitampoline), swimming skipping rope etc. These exercises do not require excessive speed or muscular strength.

Anaerobic exercises are those where oxygen is not used for that duration, e.g., sprinting where

one runs so fast that one does not take a breath. These exercises do not last long.

Isotonic exercises are those where body movements are performed—The two types of isotonic contractions are concentric isotonic where a muscle shortens and produces movement (e.g., flexion of elbow) and eccentric isotonic where a muscle gradually lengthens while continuing to contract (e.g., gradually lowering a weight held in the hand such as in weight lifting).

In **isometric exercises,** much tension is generated without shortening of the muscle.

Q. 6 What are the effects of muscular exercise on blood pressure?

The cardiovascular responses depend on whether the muscle contractions are primarily isometric or isotonic, with the performance of work in the latter.

In **isometric exercise,** the heart rate rises due, largely to decreased vagal tone, and also due to psychic stimuli and sympathetic excitation. Both SP and DP rise within a few seconds (the SP increases with the severity of exercise). The blood flow through the contracting muscles is reduced due to compression of blood vessels.

In **isotonic exercise,** there is a quick rise in heart rate as well as stroke volume due to generalised excitation of sympathetics. The increased rate and force cause an increase in cardiac output and so a prompt rise in systolic pressure (the pressure may rise to 180-200 mm Hg, or even more). There is a net fall in total peripheral resistance due to accumulation of local metabolites in the contracting muscles (CO_2, K^+, H^+, adenosine, increased osmolality, and decreased O_2). This increases the runoff of blood from the arterial system. At the same time there is vasoconstriction in splanchnic region. As a result of these changes, the systolic pressure rises moderately, while the diastolic pressure may remain the same, increase a little, or even decrease somewhat, i.e., it is affected to a much less degree.

After the exercise is over, the heart rate and BP gradually return to the pre-exercise levels over a variable period of time (see next Expt).

2-8

Cardiac Efficiency Tests
(Exercise Tolerance Tests)

The response of the cardiovascular system to standardized exercise (**"exercise tolerance test"**, also called **"stress testing"**) is the single and the best test for assessing the efficiency of the heart.

During exercise, there is a progressive increase in the heart rate (HR) and blood pressure (BP). However, after the exercise is over, these values return to the pre-exercise levels during the next few minutes.

The fact that, compared to a trained person, there is a greater increase in the heart rate and BP in an untrained individual during exercise, and that these values take a longer time to return to basal levels, forms the basis of exercise tolerance tests.

The response to physical exercise depends on the cardiac reserve, (i.e., efficiency of the heart), muscle power, training, motivation, and the state of nutrition. Therefore, the cardiac efficiency tests can also be used to test physical fitness in an individual.

I.   Record the basal pulse rate, then ask the subject to hop 20 times on each foot, raising the shoulders 6 inches at each step.

If the heart is healthy, there should be little disturbance of breathing and the pulse rate should not increase by more than 10-20 beats per minute, and should return to pre-exercise level in about a minute.

Record these timings in your workbook.

II.   Harvard step test.
Caution. This is a test for physical fitness and should not be used in patients.

Protocol. Record the basal pulse rate. Then ask the subject to alternately step up and down, lifting each foot about 20 inches (16 inches in females) off the ground, at a rate of 30 double steps per minute, for a period of 5 minutes. (Alternately, the subject may step up and down a 50 cm bench (40 cm in females), at a frequency of 30 times/min for 5 minutes). Stop the test if the subject feels breathless and exhausted and is unable to continue the test.

Count the pulse rate 1 minute after the end of the exercise. The pulse rate is inversely proportional to the degree of cardiac efficiency. To obtain an approximate idea of the cardiac efficiency index, count the pulse rate at the following intervals:

i.   Between 1 and 1½ minutes = /min (a)
ii. Between 2 and 2½ minutes = /min (b)
iii. Between 3 and 3½ minutes = /min (c)
iv. Time after which the pulse
     rate returns to basal levels   =.........minutes

$$\text{Cardiac efficiency index} = \frac{\text{Duration of exercise in seconds (300)}}{a+b+c} \times 100$$

In normal individuals, the cardiac efficiency index is nearly 100 percent, but is more in sports persons.

Efficiency Index

Over 90%   Efficiency is excellent.
81-90%   Efficiency is good.
55-80%   Efficiency is average.
Below 55%   Efficiency is poor.

III. Master's Step Test. The Master's step test, employed in the past, was a two-step wooden bench, each step being 9 inches high. The subject steps on and off the steps 12 times a minute and the pulse rate is noted. The time of recovery is about 5 minutes. (The test also used to be repeated with stepping rates of 18 and 24 times a minute).

QUESTIONS

Q. 1 How is physical exercise graded?

Grading of exercise. The WHO grading of muscular exercise, according to heart rate and relative load index (RLI; i.e., percentage of maximum O_2 utilization) is as follows:

Grade	Heart rate (per minute)	Relative load index (RLI) (% of max O_2 consumption)
Light (mild)	< 100	< 25
Moderate	100-125	25-50
Heavy	125-150	51-75
Severe	> 150	> 75

Q. 2 What is the purpose of the exercise tolerance tests?

Purpose of exercise tolerance tests. The exercise tolerance tests are the best tests for determining the efficiency of the heart as a pumping organ. These tests take the place of cardiac output measurements which cannot be made with ease in most clinical settings.

Q. 3 What is meant by the term "cardiac reserve"?

Cardiac reserve. The cardiac reserve is the difference between the basal cardiac output of an individual and the maximum cardiac output that can be achieved in that person. It can also be expressed as cardiac reserve percent. For exam-

ple, basal cardiac output = 5 liters/min maximum achievable output = 25 liters/min.

$$\text{Thus, cardiac reserve percent} = \frac{25 - 5 \times 100}{25} = 80\%.$$

Q. 4 Name some other cardiac efficiency tests?

Treadmill test (TMT). A very sophisticated "stress test" employed these days is the one using a treadmill or a bicycle ergometer. The individual is subjected to standardized incremental increase in external workload, according to a definite protocol (Bruce protocol), while the person's 12-lead ECG, arm blood pressure, and symptoms are continuously monitored by a physician present throughout the test. The performance is usually symptom-limited, and the test is discontinued as soon as there is evidence of chest discomfort, severe dyspnea, dizziness, fatigue, ST-segment depression of more than 2 mm, a fall in systolic pressure exceeding 15 mm Hg, or development of ventricular tachyarrhythmias.

The test is also done in cases of coronary artery disease to assess the degree of cardiac disability. The test can be enhanced by i/v radioisotope (thallium 201) to assess regional myocardial perfusion by means of gamma camera. Radio-isotope angiography using technitium-[99] m can also be employed to measure various parameters of ventricular performance.

Note

It may be noted that exercise testing can neither at present definitely exclude the presence of coronary artery disease, nor it is absolutely specific in predicting its presence.

2-9

Demonstration of Carotid Sinus Reflex

Pressure sensitive sensory receptors are present in the walls of carotid sinuses. Since these are located close to the surface of the anterior neck, it is possible to stimulate these baroreceptors thereby exerting pressure on them or massaging them.

PROCEDURES

1. Ask the subject to lie down supine on the examination couch. Loosen his collar and lay the neck bare. Locate the anterior edge of sternomastoid muscle and feel the pulsations of the common carotid artery which lies deeper and medial to it. Locate the upper border of the thyroid cartilage, and feel the pulsations in the carotid sinus which is a small dilation of the internal carotid artery just above the bifurcation of the main trunk (the sinus lies just below the angle of the jaw).
2. Palpate the radial artery with your left hand and, with the thumb of your right hand press the carotid sinus against the vertebral bodies for *2 seconds only*. The pulse can be felt at this site as well as in the radial artery.

> CAUTION
> Do not compress both carotids at the same time.

QUESTIONS

Q. 1 What is the effect of compressing the carotid sinus?

Compressing the carotid sinus stimulates the stretch receptors (presso or baroreceptors) in its tunica adventitia. Impulses from these receptors pass along the sinus nerve, a branch of 9th cranial nerve, to the medulla where the cardioinhibitory center (nucleus ambiguous, the motor nucleus of the vagus) is stimulated and the vasomotor center is inhibited (impulses also pass to the hypothalamus and cerebral cortex). The result is a reflex slowing of the heart, and decrease in peripheral resistance due to inhibition of the tonic discharge in the vasoconstrictor nerves supplying the arterioles.

Q. 2 What is the function of sino-aortic baroreceptor reflexes?

As mentioned in Expt 2-6, this system is a powerful short-term mechanism for the regulation of BP. The inhibitory impulses along the sinus and aortic nerves (buffer nerves) can affect both CO and PR and can thus increase or decrease the BP as required.

Q. 3 If the sino-aortic mechanism is so effective in regulating BP, why do people suffer from hypertension?

This mechanism is very effective on a short-term basis. However, if there are repeated episodes of increased BP (due to stress, anger, etc.), this mechanism is "reset" to maintain blood pressure at a higher level and one gets into a state of hypertension.

Q. 4 What is the practical significance of carotid sinus reflex?

Stretching or putting pressure on the carotid sinus, such as by hyperextension of the head, carrying heavy shoulder loads, and wearing tight collars may decrease the heart rate and blood pressure to cause **carotid sinus syncope**—when a person faints due to inappropriate stimulation of carotid baroreceptors.

Massage of carotid sinus is sometimes taken advantage of to slow the heart rate in cases of paroxysmal atrial tachycardia (PAT).

Demonstration of Venous Blood Flow

The flow of blood through the veins of the forearm and the presence of valves in these veins can be demonstrated by a simple experiment. William Harvery originally described it as one of the proofs for his theory of circulation, in his 68-page book "Exercitatio. Anatomica de motu cordis et sanguinis in Animalibus", published in Latin in 1828.

PROCEDURES

1. Seat the subject on a stool with his arm resting on a table. Apply the BP cuff on his upper arm and inflate it to 30-40 mm Hg. The superficial veins of the forearm will become prominent.

2. Place the tip of your right index finger (call it "R") over one of the veins, and mark the position of the valve (call it "V") above it, with a felt pen.

3. Keeping the finger "R" in the same position, and using your left index finger, squeeze out the blood from this vein towards the elbow. Note that the segment of the vein between points "R" and "V" remains collapsed and that there is no back flow of blood. However, the vein above the valve "V" is distended and the valve becomes prominent.

4. Keeping the finger "R" in position, place the left index finger above the valve "V" and try to squeeze the blood downwards towards the finger "R". It will be noticed that the blood cannot be forced backwards across the valve "V" unless a pressure that would be enough to rupture the valve "V" is applied.

QUESTIONS

Q. 1   What are the functions of the valves in the veins?

The valves in the veins of the limbs (there are no valves in abdomino-thoracic veins) help in venous return, especially during muscular exercise (the "muscle pump" for venous return). They also prevent the exudation of fluid out of the veins of the legs and feet (the pressure in these veins is very high due to the effect of gravity) by breaking the veins into short segments instead of there being a long continuous column of blood below the level of the heart.

Q. 2   What is the function of the veins?

Being thin-walled, the veins constitute the "capacitance" or storage vessels of the circulatory tree and contain about 70% of the blood. Although the amount of smooth muscle in the veins is small, considerable venoconstriction occurs by factors (e.g., sympathetic excitation) which cause vasoconstriction in arterioles. Local factors such as O_2 lack and CO_2 excess can also affect small veins. During hemorrhage, substantial amounts of blood can be translocated from the veins to the general circulation, thus helping in increasing the effective blood volume.

2-11

Recording of Venous Pressure

There is a pressure gradient from the arterial to the venous side in both systemic and pulmonary circuits. The gradient in the systemic circuit is about 95 mm Hg (MAP in aorta = 95 mm Hg; Right atrium = 0-4 mm Hg) and that in the pulmonary circuit is about 12-15 mm Hg (MAP in pulmonary artery = 15 mm Hg; Left atrium = 2-6 mm Hg).

There are three simple experiments to assess venous blood pressure.

PROCEDURES

Experiment I

1. Seat the subject on a stool, with his right arm hanging downwards; the veins of the arm will become distended. While watching the veins on the back of the hand and the wrist, slowly and gently raise the subject's arm till these veins begin to empty out. Determine the vertical height between the wrist and the junction of 3rd costal cartilage with the sternum (this point is the level of entry of superior vena cava into the right atrium). The distance measured in cm is the approximate measure of the right atrial pressure. (In normal subjects the hand will be a few cm above the heart when the veins empty out completely).

2. Repeat the above procedure after asking the subject to close his nose and mouth and then perform a forced expiratory effort (Valsalva maneuver). The venous pressure is now increased i.e., the veins will remain engorged even when the hand is raised to the level of the head. (The Valsalva maneuver increases the intrapleural pressure to + 20-30 mm Hg, which interferes with the venous return. The

normal intrapleural pressure remains negative, i.e., below the atmospheric, during quiet inspiration and expiration).

3. Repeat the same procedure after asking the subject to close his nose and mouth and then to make a deep inspiratory effort (Muller's maneuver). In this case, the intrapleural pressure becomes much more negative, which facilitates venous return.

Experiment II

A flat glass cup with an outlet at the top (a small funnel will also serve the purpose); water manometer; air bulb of a BP apparatus; a glass T-tube; collodion; and rubber tubing will be required for this experiment.

1. Connect the glass cup, the air pump, and the water manometer to the T-tube.

2. Seat the subject on a stool, with his forearm resting on the table, at the level of the heart. Apply the cup over a prominent vein on the forearm, and seal the cup with collodion. After the seal dries, gently increase the pressure in the cup till the vein just empties out. Read the manometer pressure at this point. Express the venous pressure in cm of water or mm Hg (1 mm Hg pressure = 13.6 mm H_2O). Repeat the Valsalva and Muller maneuvers to study their effects on venous pressure.

Experiment III

The venous pressure can also be directly recorded by inserting a wide-bore needle into a vein in the antecubital region, and connecting it to a manometer filled with normal saline containing an anticoagulant.

QUESTIONS

Q. 1 What are the normal venous pressures?

The pressure in the venules is 12-16 mm Hg. The peripheral venous pressure, say in the forearm (at the heart level) is 6-8 mm Hg. The pressure in the great veins near the heart is 3-4 mm Hg, but varies with respiration. The pressure in the dural sinuses (with the head upright) is subatmospheric (i.e., negative) because these venous channels are rigid and cannot collapse.

Q. 2 When does the peripheral venous pressure increase?

The peripheral venous pressure in the abdomen and limbs increases in cases of right heart failure (congestive heart failure). The failure of the right ventricle to effectively pump out all the blood that is returning to it causes back pressure in the systemic veins. Increased pressure in the portal veins causes exudation of fluid, a condition called "ascites". In the limb veins, the back pressure increase the capillary hydrostatic pressure which leads to edema.

2-12

Demonstration of Triple Response

The response of the skin to mechanical injury, described first by Lewis in 1927, is called the **triple response** or the **Lewis' response.** With light injury, only the "white line" is seen, while with a stronger stimulus, all the three stages of the "triple response" can be seen.

White Line (White Reaction)

Seat the subject on a stool with his forearm resting on the table. Draw a blunt-pointed object—a closed forceps, fingernail, a blunt pencil—lightly on the skin of the ventral forearm. The response, which appears in 8-10 seconds, is a pale or white line in the track of the stimulus. The mechanical stimulus causes contraction of the precapillary sphincters, squeezes out blood from the capillaries and small venules, leaving behind a white line.

Triple Response

After the white line disappears in about a minute, use a stronger stimulus with the forceps. The response will vary from person to person. A full-fledged triple response, especially in sensitive skins, consists of the following 3 stages:

1. **The red line (red reaction).** It appears in about 10 seconds, and is due to relaxation of the precapillary sphincters resulting from histamine, kinins, polypeptides etc. that are released locally from injured cells. Passive capillary dilatation and increased blood flow cause the red line.

2. **The flare.** The flare which follows in a few minutes, is an irregular, reddish, mottled area surrounding the red line. It is due to dilatation of arterioles resulting from a local reflex called the **axon reflex.** In this case, impulses originating in the sensory nerve endings by the injury are relayed antidromically (i.e., opposite to the normal direction) down other branches of the sensory nerve fibres which supply the arterioles. This appears to be the only example of a physiological effect due to antidromic conduction in nerve fibres. The axon reflex is not a true reflex as it does not involve some part of the central nervous system.

3. **The wheal.** The flare is soon followed by local edema, (swelling) due to increased permea-

bility of the capillaries and small venules, as a result of which fluid leaks out from these vessels. Histamine (released from local mast cells), kinins, substance P and other polypeptides all contribute to increased permea- bility and edema. Injection of histamine in the skin produces flare and wheal via the H_1 receptors. A common example of the triple response is the finger-marks left on the skin of the face following a hard slap.

Electrocardiography (ECG)

The electrocardiogram (ECG, or EKG) is a graphic representation of the electrical events associated with the heart beat. (It does not represent the mechanical events of the heart, i.e., systole or diastole). The various waves of the ECG reflect the rhythmic electrical depolarizations or repolarizations of the cardiac muscle which precede or follow the contractions.

INSTRUMENTATION

I. The ECG, Machine

The electrocardiograph works on the household current AC-230 volts, or on battery, and has a very sensitive galvanometer. The potentials picked up from the surface of the body are suitably amplified before flowing through the galvanometer. It has the following controls:

a. **Mains switch.** The ON/OFF switch controls the power supply. A filter cuts off unwanted 50 Hz interference.
b. **Calibration.** A commonly used sensitivity is 1 mV/10 mm, so that a calibration signal of 1 mV causes a pen deflection of 10 mm.
c. **Centering.** The baseline control knob is used for bringing the pen to the centre of the paper.
d. **Lead selector switch.** It permits selection of various unipolar or bipolar electrodes.

II. Electrodes

The electrodes for the limbs are flat metal plates which are kept in position by rubber straps. The chest electrode is a metal cup which is kept in position by "suction" produced by a rubber bulb. Electrode jelly is rubbed on the skin at the electrode positions to reduce skin resistance. Cable lead wires connect the subject to the machine.

An esophageal electrode, which can be swallowed and made to lie behind the heart, is employed for special purposes. An electrode at the tip of a cardiac catheter can record events from within the heart, a record called His Bundle Electrogram (HBE).

III. ECG Paper

The standard graph paper is divided into 1 mm squares by thin lines (see **Figure 5-3**) every 5th line being thick, both horizontally and vertically. Each horizontal division of 1 mm represents 0.04 second, so that the time duration between two thick lines is 0.2 second. Each small vertical division represents 0.1 mV, so that 10 mm represent 1 mV. This facilitates quick calculations of the duration and amplitudes of various waves, and intervals of the ECG record. The paper transport system pulls the paper from a roll (or folded stack) and moves it under the pen at the standard speed of 25 mm/second.

IV. Pen Recording System

This system is either an ink writing pen, or an electrically-heated stylus that inscribes on a chemically treated paper. The ECG record may also be displayed on a CRO.

V. Electrocardiographic Leads

The term *lead* is used for the specific points of electrical contact, i.e., electrode position, on the limbs and the chest, as well as for the actual record obtained from any two points.

The two shoulders and the left thigh where it joins the torso, form the Einthoven triangle (consult Chart 5-3). Since the potentials at these points are the same as at the wrists and the left ankle, the limb electrodes can be attached at these locations since they are more convenient to use. The right leg is used as a ground conductor.

The electrodes employed in ECG may be **unipolar**, where one electrode is kept at zero potential while the other is the exploring electrode, or **bipolar**, where potential difference is recorded between two points.

1. Bipolar leads. The bipolar leads may be **bipolar limb leads**, or **bipolar chest leads**.

A. **Bipolar limb leads (Standard leads or "classical" limb leads).** These were the earliest leads to be used. Three leads are formed by measuring the potential difference between any two limb electrodes.

   a. *Lead I* is the potential at the left arm (LA) minus the potential at right arm, or LA–RA.

   b. *Lead II* is the potential at the left leg (LL) minus the potential at the RA, or LL–RA.

   c. *Lead III* is the potential at LL minus the potential at LA, or LL–LA.

B. **Bipolar chest leads.** One electrode is placed on the different locations of the chest, while the other electrode is placed on the right arm (CR 1-7); left arm (CL 1-7); and left leg (foot) (CF 1-7) [These leads are not used routinely].

2. Unipolar leads. These leads record the potentials from a single region of the body. One of the electrode, the *indifferent electrode*, is kept at zero potential by connecting the three limb leads to a common (or central) terminal in the machine where the currents from the limbs neutralize each other. The other electrode, the *exploring electrode*, can be on the limbs (unipolar limb leads), or on the chest (unipolar chest leads). (There can be no "true" unipolar electrode).

a. **Augmented unipolar leads.** Any of the limb electrodes can be used to record cardiac potentials in comparison to the common terminal (kept at zero potential). For example, the voltage recorded at right arm (RA) can be determined by the equation: RA – (RA + LA + LL). The recorded voltage is small, because the potential difference is reduced by the RA potential in the common terminal. Disconnecting the RA lead from the common terminal increase the potential difference by 50% and results in augmented unipolar limb lead, aVR. Thus, the augmented leads are:

   i. *aVR* is the potential difference between RA and (LA + LL).

   ii. *aVL* is the potential difference between LA and (RA + LL).

   iii. *aVF* is the potential difference between LL and (RA + LA).

b. **Unipolar chest leads (also called unipolar precordial leads).** These leads record the potentials from the anterior surface of the heart, from the right side to the left side of the chest, in relation to the indifferent electrode (RA + LA + LL). The standardized sites for the unipolar chest leads are as follows:

V_1 is in the 4th intercostal space (ICS), just to the right of the sternum.

V_2 is in the 4th ICS, just to the left of the sternum.

V_3 is halfway between V_2 and V_4.

V_4 is at the midclavicular line in the 5th intercostal space.

V_5 is in the anterior axillary line at the same level as V_4.

V_6 is in the mid-axillary line in the 5th intercostal space.

V_7 is in the posterior axillary line in the 5th intercostal space.

V_8 is on the infrascapular line, just below the angle of the scapula.

PROTOCOL

1. Ask the subject to lie down on the couch and be comfortably relaxed. Rub small amounts of the electrolyte jelly on the front of the wrists and just above the ankles. Apply the electrodes on these points and fix them in place with straps. Fix the lead wires, identified with the letters RA, LA, LL, and RL, to the electrodes. Connect the connector cable to the machine.

2. Switch on the machine and "center" the stylus (pen). Run the paper and, using the CAL (calibration) push the button 2-3 times, and adjust the pen deflection to 10 mm (see **Figure 5-3**).

3. Using the lead selector switch, record 4-6 ECG complexes in the standard order—Leads I, II, III, lead II on deep inspiration, aVR, aVL, aVF—in this order.

4. Stop the machine, and apply the electrode jelly on the chest positions for V_1 to V_6. Using the chest electrode, record the ECG from these positions one after the other (**Figure 5-3**).

5. Tear off the paper from the machine and label the various leads. Note down the name of the subject and the date (Consult Chart 5-3 for question-answer discussion of ECG).

2-14

Experiments on Student Physiograph

The high cost and relative complexity of multi-channel 'polygraphs' have prevented their adoption for use by the medical students in this country. However, single channel electronic recorders and electronic stimulators are now available in the market and are being used in many medical colleges in group experiments under the guidance of staff members. Many of the experiments which were previously carried out an electro-mechanical apparatuses can now be done on these modern devices. One such apparatus, the 'Student Physiograph' is shown in **Figure 2-9**. It has the following advantages over the electro-mechanical devices:

1. Many more parameters can be recorded on a single apparatus through the use of couplers, matching transducers and pick-ups.

2. The group experiment concept permits more than one physiograph to be used indepen-

dently or interconnected to each other in tandem for the same experimental set-up.

3. Though the controls are kept to a few only the sensitivity and accuracy of these devices are high.

The 'Student Physiograph' consists of:

A. The Main Console

The main console has the following:

1. **Chart drive.** The multispeed chart drive can provide paper speeds ranging from 0.25 mm/sec to 100 mm/sec through the use of a range selector knob and push buttons. The paper, 70 mm in width, is fed through a slot under the writing pens.

2. **Pen recording system.** Two recording pens are provided, the upper for the main recording channel 1 and the lower for synchronised

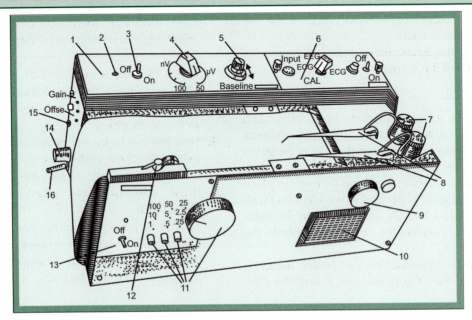

Figure 2-9. Student physiograph. 1: Mains amplifier; 2: Pilot lamp; 3: 50 Hz filter; 4: Sensitivity selector; 5: Pen position control; 6: EKG coupler in position; 7: Ink wells; 8: Pens; 9: Pen lift knob; 10: Paper feed window; 11: Speed selectors; 12: Paper drive bearing and thumb screw for starting and stopping paper; 13: Mains switch; 14: To mains; 15: Fuse; 16: Ground

Time/Event recording. The pen is 120 mm in length to minimise arc distortion. The contact tension of the pens on the paper can be adjusted, if needed, with the help of cradle springs. A pen lift knob lefts the pens from the paper.

3. **The main amplifier.** The main amplifier, which is common to all couplers, is fitted in the console. A 50 Hz toggle switch cuts off unwanted 50 cycles/sec interference. There is a 'baseline' control knob for adjusting the position of the pen and another control for selecting the sensitivity of the amplifier ranging from 50 μV to 500 μV in 4 steps and from 1 mV to 100 mV in 7 steps.

Three screw-driver adjustments are provided on the side of the console. Once adjusted they do not normally require adjustments. The side of the console also has IN and OUT jacks. The OUT jack of one physiograph connected to the IN jack of another unit connects them in tandem and both units will record simultaneously from the same experimental set-up. Another input jack takes the synchronised Event/Time marker of the electronic stimulator.

4. **Coupler housing.** Different interchangeable couplers can be plugged into the coupler housing. An appropriate transducer is to be connected to the coupler in use.

B. Couplers

The following couplers are available for use with the physiograph:

1. **Bio-potential coupler.** The bio-potential coupler is designed to record any AC phenomenon like electrocardiogram (ECG), electroencephalogram (EEG), electromyogram

(EMG), sensory and motor nerve conduction velocities in humans, movements of the eyes (electronystagmogram) and so on. A control knob selects the phenomenon to be recorded. It has a CAL position for the checking of calibration for which a push button is provided.

2. **Electrocardiogram (EKG).** The coupler is used for recording clinical EKG (ECG). There is a knob for selecting various leads-I, II, III, aVR, aVL, aVF, V, CR, CL and CF as described in experiment 2-13. There is another knob for calibration.

3. **Strain Gage Coupler.** This coupler records activity from various strain gage transducers (pressure-volume, volume, muscle-force transducers). The experimental applications of this coupler include: arterial and venous pulse, blood pressure in cannulated dog or rabbit, plethysmography, experiments on frog's gastrocnemius muscle sciatic nerve preparation (simple muscle twitch, strength of stimulaton, effect of two successive stimuli, effect of temperature and load, tetanus, fatigue, isometric contraction etc.) experiments on frog's heart, experiments on isolated tissues (intestine, uterus, rat diaphragm etc.), experiments on isolated perfused rabbit's heart, effect of load on finger movements and so on. Springs of different tensile strength are available with the force transducer.

4. **Pulse-Respiration Coupler.** This coupler is employed for recording arterial pulse with a photoelectric pulse transducer and respiratory movements with a respiration belt transducer. A toggle switch selects pulse or respiration mode.

5. **Temperature Coupler.** This coupler is used for recording rectal or surface temperature. For such recordings the transducer has to be calibrated within the desired temperature range using a water bath.

C. The Stimulator

The electronic stimulator can be used in two modes:
  i. to energise either a time base or act as an event marker, and
 ii. to provide electrical stimuli of up to 30 volts as a single pulse, or as 2 successive stimuli with predetermined intervals ranging from 5 to 250 msec, or as repeated stimuli with frequencies ranging from 0.5 to 100/sec. The electrical stimuli provided by the stimulator are rectilinear with a fixed pulse width of 0.5 msec.

Steps for the Use of the Physiograph

1. Put the stack of paper in the paper receptacle, chart side facing down and the paper end facing the paper-feed window located on the front of the console. Lift the pens by turning the lift knob clockwise. Fold the paper end into a V and with the fingers of one hand pass it through the slot in the console top and then pull it out from the slot with the other hand. Slide the paper under the two perspex guides and then under the ball bearing after lifting the latter by using the thumb screw. Check ink flow by lifting each ink-well top, putting a thumb over the hole, and depressing it down—the ink should flow freely from the pens. (During the experiment, when not recording, lift pens from paper).

2. With the mains switch on the console on the OFF position plug in the desired coupler (let us say you are going to record the ECG in a subject). It is important to remember that a coupler should not be plugged in or removed while the mains switch is ON. Select the standard speed on 25 mm per second.

3. Apply the electrodes on the subject's arms and legs as described in Experiment 2-13. Connect the electrodes through lead wires to the 5-pin junction box and the latter to the EKG coupler.

4. Switch ON the mains console and then the coupler. Adjust the sensitivity on the main amplifier to 1 mV. Adjust pen position to centre. Put the lead selector control on the coupler to CAL position for calibration. Run the paper and press and release the CAL push button on the coupler 3 or 4 times while adjusting the CAL control so that 1 mV may produce a deflection of the pen by 1 cm. Stop paper.

5. Move the lead selector control to lead I position and record 6-8 ECG complexes. Stop paper; move the control to lead II and take recording. Continue this process till all the leads have been obtained.

For experiments on the frog's nerve-muscle preparation and for recording the mechanical activity of the frog's heart the muscle force transducer is employed. This transducer has a hook projecting from its free end. It is fitted to the vertical stand above the chamber or board carrying the preparation and is connected to the strain gage coupler. The electronic stimulator is used for providing the stimuli. Your tutor will demonstrate how the recording are to be obtained.

For recording EEG and EMG from the skin surface over a muscle in a human subject small cup electrodes are used. A thick electrode paste keeps the electrodes in position. Needle electrodes are employed for recording muscle action potentials. Your tutor will demonstrate their application.

Unit III
Special and General Sensations

2-15

Perimetry (Charting the Field of Vision)

STUDENT OBJECTIVES

After completing the following experiments on vision you should be able to:

1. Define field of vision and physiological blind spot.
2. Determine the field of vision in a subject and describe its extent in various meridians.
3. Describe the printed perimeter chart.
4. Name the factors that affect the field of vision.
5. Trace the visual pathway and name the effects of lesions at different places.
6. Explain the physiological basis of stereoscopic vision.
7. Show that it is the anterior surface of the lens that becomes more convex during accommodation for near vision.

The part of the extenal world visible to one eye when a person fixes his gaze on one point is called the **field of vision** for that eye. The process of charting the monocular field of vision is called perimetry. It is employed for the diagnosis of various lesions of the visual pathways.

The Visual Pathway

The optic nerve fibers (axons of ganglion cells of the retina) from the nasal (medial) half of each retina cross to the opposite side in the optic chiasma, while fibers from the temporal (lateral) half of each retina remain on the same side. For example, fibers in the right optic tract come from the temporal half of right retina and nasal half of left retina **(Figure 2-10)**, thus serving the nasal (medial) half of field of vision in the right eye and temporal (lateral) field in the left eye. (Blindness resulting from lesions of the visual pathway are labeled in terms of defects in the visual fields). The optic tract fibers end in 2 ways: (i) Pretectum of midbrain to synapse on the Edinger-Westphal nucleus for light reflexes, and, (ii) Lateral geniculate body (LGB). Fresh relays from LGB pass back in the geniculocalcarine tract (optic radiations), which passes through the internal capsule, where they lie behind the somatic sensory fibres, to reach the *primary visual area (area 17 of Brodmann)* on the medial surface of the occipital lobe. Areas 18 and 19 on the lateral surface are the *visual association areas.*

PERIMETER

Priestley-Smith and Lister perimeters are self-recording. A simple "hand" perimeter is also available. The former consists of the following parts:

1. **Stand.** A heavy stand, on which a metal arc is fitted on a pivot, provides stability to the apparatus. A large black disc with a frame for holding the perimeter chart is provided on the back **(Figure 2-11)**.

2. **Metal arc.** A broad metal arc shaped like a half circle is mounted on the stand and can be rotated in any meridian around its central pivot. One half of the arc, the concavity of which is directed toward the subject, has a scale of 0 to 90 degrees marked on its convex surface, while a source of light is fitted at the

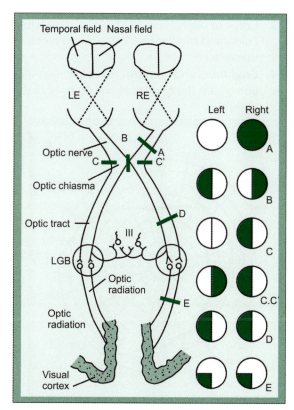

Figure 2-10. The visual pathway. Lesions of the pathway at different locations produce defects in the fields of vision as shown on the right. RE: right eye; LE: left eye; LGB: lateral geniculate body; III: oculomotor nuclei

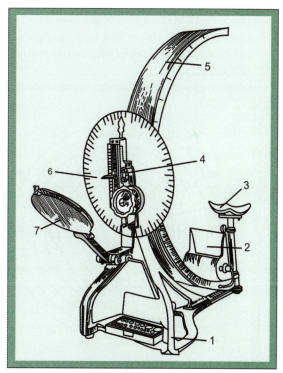

Figure 2-11. Perimeter (Lister model). 1: Stand with object holder; 2: Source of light; 3: Adjustable chin rest; 4: Spring lock; 5: Metal arc; 6: Chart marker; 7: Disc (chart plate) for holding perimeter chart

end of the other limb of the arc. A small plane mirror is fixed in the center of the arc. Test objects of various sizes and colors can be fitted in a carrier which moves in a groove in the graduated limb of the arc. When the test object is moved with a knob, a pin on the back of the apparatus moves correspondingly.

3. **Chin rest.** An adjustable chin rest is provided to keep the head steady. The chin of the subject rests on the right cup when the left eye is to be tested and the left cup is used when the right eye is tested.

4. **Chart** The perimeter chart (**Figure 2-12**) on which the field of vision is to be plotted is divided by circles from 0 to 90°, and by meridians at 15° intervals. Both the angles and the meridians are printed on the chart. The limits for the normal peripheral fields of vision for the two eyes, and the blind spots, are printed on the chart for comparison with the plotted fields of vision. The term "peripheral field" refers to the peripheral or outer limits of the field.

Student Perimeter

In this model the inclination of the arc is read from a plastic dial fitted behind the mirror. When an object, which is moved along the inside of the arc, becomes visible, the angle it subtends at the fixation point (i.e., the mirror) in a given meridian can be read from the scale engraved on the outside of the arc. The readings—the meridian and the angle—are then transferred to the corresponding points on the chart.

Factors Affecting Visual Field

1. **Visual Acuity.** Obviously, the visual acuity should be sufficient to enable the subject to see the test object clearly.
2. **Size of object.** Though the visual field is better with a large object, a standard test object is used.
3. **Color of object.** The field is widest for white color, and smaller for blue, red and green in that order.
4. **Brightness and contrast.** Adequate illumination affects the brightness and contrast of the object.

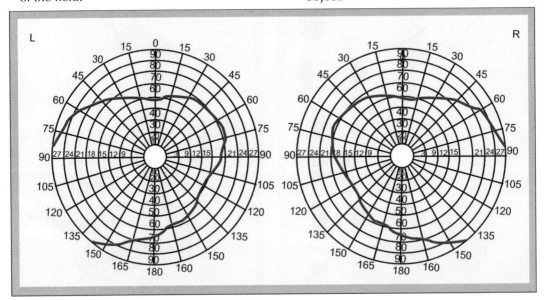

Figure 2-12. The field of vision. Note that the 'binocular segments' of the two eyes overlap and are seen by both the eyes. The mononuclear segments lie outside the binocular segments. The black spot 15° lateral to the center of the field is the blind spot

PROCEDURES

1. Place the perimeter on a table of suitable height and seat the subject in front of it. Fix a chart in the frame. Ask him to place his chin on the chin rest and adjust its height so that his eye (e.g., right eye) is at the level of the mirror. Instruct the subject not to move his eye but to keep looking at the mirror. Tell him to cover his left eye with a cupped hand.

2. Position the arc on zero meridian, on the temporal side. Fix a 5 mm white object in the carrier and take it to the end of the arc; switch on the light. Ask the subject to say "yes" as soon as the object comes into view. Slowly move the object towards the mirror and as soon as the subject says "yes", strike the chart holder against the pin so that it punches a hole in the chart. (The object will be visible beyond $90°$ on this side).

3. Rotate the arc downwards (or upwards) by $30°$, take the object to the end of the arc, and move it towards the mirror. When it becomes visible, mark the angle on the chart paper as before. Repeat the procedure after moving the arc by $30°$ each time until the arc returns back to the starting position, i.e., through 360 degrees.

4. To mark the blind spot, position the arc at $100°$ meridian (i.e., $10°$ below the horizontal) on the temporal side. Move the object from the periphery towards the center. The subject will continue to see the object up to about $20°$, then it will disappear, but reappear once again after about $5°$. Mark both the points on the chart; a small circle around these points will mark the blind spot which is 5-$6°$ in diameter and situated about $15°$ lateral to the fixation point.

5. Plot the field of vision for the other eye in similar manner.

6. Record the peripheral field of vision of one eye for green, blue, and red objects.

7. Remove the chart from its holder and join all the pinholes with a pen to obtain the peri- pheral fields of visions for both the eyes. Note the area that is common to both eyes.

8. Examine the entire field of vision, in addition to mapping only the peripheral field of vision, by bringing the test object right up to the fixation point at the mirror, in all meridians, and noting if the object disappears after appearing at the periphery of the field. This will reveal if there is any scotoma in any part of the field.

PRECAUTIONS

1. The procedure should be explained to the subject, and instructed not to move the eye from the fixation point.

2. Adequate illumination should be provided.

3. If the subject wears glasses, these should be removed as they may restrict the field.

4. Healthy eye should be tested first.

QUESTIONS

Q. 1 What is meant by field of vision? What is the extent of a normal field?

The field of vision, visual field, or field of view, is the cone of space with its apex at the eye, which is seen by the subject, when that eye is kept fixed at one point. Of course, one can see much larger part of the outside world if the eye is moved. The whole of the view of a subject is subdivided into: (1) The right and left visual fields, "seen" by the right and left eyes respectively; (2) The binocular segment which is "seen" by both eyes; and (3) The right and left monocular segments outside of the binocular segment to the right and the left.

The peripheral field of each eye extends upto about $100°$ on the temporal side; about $65°$ downwards (it is limited by the cheek); 55-$60°$ on the nasal side (limited by the nose); and about $50°$ upwards where it is limited by the brow.

The peripheral field is widest for the white color, and smaller for blue, red and green colors in that order.

Q. 2 Which parts of the retina are tested by perimetry?

Perimetry tests most parts of the retina except the macular region which contains the fovea centralis. The fovea contains only the cones and is the region of most acute vision. The acuity of vision is tested with Snellen chart for distant vision (Chart 5-11) and Jaeger chart for near vision.

Q. 3 Are all objects within the field of vision seen equally clearly?

Objects whose images fall on the macula are seen in very minute details, and the colors are bright and distinct. Objects away from the point of fixation becomes less and less clear and colors are difficult to identify. Thus, only a small part of the field is seen in sharp focus. For example, when reading printed material, only about 10 mm of each line is in sharp focus. At a distance of 6 meters, only a person's head and neck are in clear focus. We are normally unaware of this because the eyes are continuously moving over a scene and when they come to rest, much of what was seen in detail remains part of our perception. However, the peripheral part of retina is very sensitive to movement—moving objects, flashes of light, etc. We can see a moving object much more easily through the "corner of the eye" than by directly gazing at it.

Q. 4 What is physiological blind spot and what is its significance?

The *physiological blind spot* corresponds with the optic disc which is the region where the optic nerve leaves and the blood vessels enter the eye. The optic disc is 1.5 mm in diameter and is located 3 mm medial to and slightly above the posterior pole of the eye (the location of macula lutea). As there are no rods or cones in the optic disc, any image falling on it is not visible. Normally, we are not aware of the blind spot even if only one eye is used (see Expt. 2-17).

Q. 5 Describe the visual pathway?

See page 204.

Q. 6 What is bitemporal hemianopia and what is its cause?

Blindness in the temporal fields of vision of both eyes is called bitemporal hemianopia (or hemianopsia). A lesion of crossed fibers in the central part of optic chiasma, commonly due to a pituitary tumor, causes this type of visual defect (**Figure 2-10:B**).

Q. 7 What is binasal hemianopia and what is its cause?

Blindness in the nasal halves of fields of vision of both eyes is called binasal hemianopia. It occurs when the uncrossed optic nerve fibers in the lateral parts of optic chiasma are damaged. Usually, there is right or left nasal hemianopia as a result of a calcified internal carotid artery pressing on one or the other side of the chiasma (**Figure 2-10C:C'**).

Q. 8 What is homonymous hemianopia?

Blindness in the temporal half of field of vision of one eye and the nasal field of the other eye is called *homonymous hemianopia*. A lesion of optic tract or optic radiation by tumors of parietal or temporal lobes produces this type of defect. A lesion on the right side will produce left homonymous hemianopia, and a lesion on the left side will produce right homonymous hemianopia. (Homonymous, because right half of field of one eye and right half of field of the other eye is affected. If right half of field of one eye, and left half of field of the other eye is affected, it is called *heteronymous hemianopia*, e.g., binasal or bitemporal hemianopias). Partial damage to optic radiation will produce superior (lower part of radiation involved) or inferior (upper part affected) homonymous quadrantanopia (**Figure 2-10:D**).

Q. 9 What is stereoscopic vision?

The visual fields of the two eyes overlap, the portion common to both eyes having a diameter of 120 degrees. The images of an object falling on the two maculae are slightly different from each other because of the separation of the two eyes. This is the basis of stereoscopic or binocular vision which is responsible for depth perception.

Q. 10 What is a scotoma?

Generally, the term scotoma (plural, scotomata) is applied to a small area of blindness (except the physiological blind spot) lying within a visual field. It is important clinically to detect the presence of scotomata and to map their location. Due to disease, a patch or patches of retina may get separated (retinal detachment) from the underlying choroid from where it gets its oxygen and other nutrients. The receptors in the affected part/s degenerate and produce scotomata. Just as we are unaware of our own blind spots, similarly the patients are unaware of even quite large scotomata. Therefore, if detected early, the detached retina can be "welded" back into position with laser beams.

Q. 11 Name any other method of determining the field of vision?

The confrontation test can provide a rough estimate of the peripheral field of vision (consult clinical examination of the optic nerve).

2-16

Mechanical Stimulation of the Eye

Close your eyes and press on the outer corner of an eye with your index finger. The pressure produces an impression of a dark circular spot surrounded by a bright circle in the field of vision directly opposite to the point of pressure. These visual sensations are called *"pressure phosphenes"* and are caused by "inadequate" retinal stimulation.

This experiment supports the "Muller's Law of Specific Nerve Energy", which states that different types of stimuli applied to a sensory organ always produce the sensation peculiar to that receptor. In the case of retina, the natural stimulus of light requires minimum of energy to stimulate the rods and cones, while a mechanical stimulus requires many times the energy needed by the normal stimulus.

2-17

Physiological Blind Spot

I. Mariotte's Experiment

Draw a small cross on a blank sheet of your work book, then draw a small spot about 10 cm to the right of the cross (**Figure 2-13**). Cover your left eye with your left hand and hold the figure in front of your right eye. Fix your gaze on the cross (the more nasally located of the two marks), then move the figures towards and away from you until, at a certain distance, the spot disappears. At this moment, the image of the spot is falling on the blind spot. Record the distance of the work-book from the eye. The presence of the blind spot in the left eye can be confirmed by fixing the left eye on the spot and moving the figures towards or away from the eye till the cross disappears.

Figure 2-13. Mariotte's experiment to demonstrate the physiological blind spot

II. Plotting the Blind Spot

1. Seat the subject in front of a blackboard so that his eyes are 1 meter from it. If possible, fix the head to steady it.
2. Draw a small cross on the board, then ask the subject to cover his left eye with a cupped hand, and to gaze fixedly on the cross with his right eye.
3. Move a stick with a small white tip slowly on the board to the right of the cross until he can no longer see the white tip. Mark this spot with a chalk; this is the rough position of the blind spot.

4. Slowly bring the tip of the stick in vertical and oblique directions, from the periphery towards the roughly positioned blind spot, marking all the points when the white tip becomes visible. Join all these marks to obtain the outline of the projected image of the optic disc.
5. By using the method of similar triangles, the distances on the retina, i.e., the diameter of the optic disc, and its distance from the fovea, can be calculated from the distances on the blackboard (i.e., the diameter of the projected image of the optic disc, and its distance from the cross). The point at which the rays intersect in the eye is the nodal point, which can be assumed to lie 17 mm in front of retina. The distance of the nodal point from the board is 1 meter (the small distance from the nodal point to the cornea may be ignored).

$$\frac{\text{Size of object}}{\text{Size of image}} = \frac{\text{Distance of object from nodal point}}{\text{Distance of image from nodal point}}$$

2-18

Near Point and Near Response

I. Near Point

The nearest point at which an object can be seen clearly is called the near point.

PROCEDURE

1. Seat the subject near a window, in good light, and ask him to cover one eye with a cupped hand. Hold a pencil in front of the other eye and slowly move it, preferably along a meter stick, towards the eye until it can no longer be seen in *sharp* focus. Record the distance between the pencil and the eye to determine the near point.

2. Measure the near point for the other eye as well. If glasses are worn, measure the near point with and without glasses. Finally, measure the near point with both eyes open.

II. Near Response

Seat the subject near a window and ask him to fix his eyes on a distant object. Then bring your finger in front of his eyes and ask him to focus his eyes on it. There is convergence of eyes, constriction of pupil, and increase in the curvature of the lens. This three-part response is called the near response or the accommodation reflex.

III. Range of Accommodation

The far point is the farthest point from the eye at which an object is seen clearly.

1. Measure the far point in a manner similar to that used for the near point, remembring that if the subject is emmetropic (having normal vision), it will be infinitely far away. (A distance of 6 meters from the eye is considered the practical far point because light rays coming from this distance are parallel).

2. If the subject wears glasses, record the near and the far points with and without glasses. Calculate the range of accomodation, i.e., the distance between the far and near points for each eye, separately.

QUESTIONS

Q. 1 How does the eye accommodate for near vision?
Consult Chart 5-12 for answer.

Q. 2 What is meant by amplitude of accommodation?
Consult Chart 5-12 for answer.

Q. 3 What is presbyopia?
Consult Chart 5-12 for answer.

2-19

Sanson Images

If a phakoscope is available, it should be employed to show that it is the anterior surface of the lens that becomes more convex during accommodation reflex. However, a simple experiment can be conducted to show this response of the lens.

PROCEDURES

Conduct the experiment in a dark room.

1. Seat the subject comfortably. Hold a burning candle to one side of his eye and observe the images of the candle flame from the other side. The following images are seen:
   i. On the anterior surface of the cornea: the image is bright and upright.
   ii. On the anterior surface of the lens (near the center of the pupil): the image is upright, somewhat larger, and not so bright.
   iii. On the posterior surface of the lens: the image is smaller but inverted, and not so easily seen.

2. Ask the subject to look at the far wall of the room. While observing the images carefully, hold a finger in front of his eye and ask him to look at it.

Result. The image # 2 (i.e., on the anterior surface of the lens) moves closer to the image # 1; it also gets smaller and brighter. This shows that during accommodation for near vision, the *anterior surface* of the lens moves forwards, i.e., this surface becomes more convex.

See chart 5-12 for mechanism of accommodation.

Demonstration of Stereoscopic Vision

PROCEDURES

1. Thread a needle first with both eyes open, and then repeat the experiment with one and then with the other eye. Note the time it takes in each case. Your hands should not touch each other otherwise the touch clues (such as relative position of the hands) will reduce the effect of closing one eye.

2. Hold a matchbox about 20-25 cm in front of your eyes. Draw its appearance as seen with only the right eye, and then with the left eye. Compare the two sketches. The normal mechanism of vision fuses the two slightly different images into one to give an impression of solidity.

Dominance of the Eye

Just as we habitually use one hand more than the other, we unconsciously have some other left-right preferences. Most people have a preferred eye, ear and foot. The dominant eye is the one that a person normally employs to thread a needle or look into a camera.

PROCEDURES

Make a circle with your thumb and index finger and, holding it at arm's length, look through it, with both eyes open, at a small object across the room, say, a door handle. Close one eye and then the other; the eye that sees the object within the circle is your dominant eye.

Subjective Visual Sensations

Procedures

Do this experiment on a clear day. Close one eye and look at the sky with the other and try to concentrate on what you see. You will observe small, circular, semitransparent, grey specks, or zigzag wispy filaments, or hair-like objects, or rows of cell-like structures that drift across the field of vision. These are called *muscae volitantes* or *floaters.* If you try to focus on them, they drift away or sink down; and if you jerk your eye up they rise up, but sink down or float away once again.

Muscae volitantes are a normal phenomenon, especially as age advances. They are the shadows cast on the retina by cellular and other debris in the aqueous and vitreous humors. Images of the retinal blood vessels reflected from the posterior surface of the lens also contribute to the floaters. A sudden appearance of new floaters, if accompanied by bright flashes in the peripheral field of vision, could indicate a retinal tear or detachment.

2-23

Tuning-Fork Tests of Hearing

STUDENT OBJECTIVES
After completing this practical, you should be able to: 1. Explain the importance of doing hearing tests in clinical physiology. 2. Define sound, and name its characteristics that are perceived by the ear. 3. Describe the principle underlying tuning-fork tests. 4. Differentiate between air (ossicular) conduction and bone-conduction. 5. Trace the auditory pathway. 6. Describe the principle of audiometry. 7. Comment on cochlear implants.

INTRODUCTORY

I. Nature and Characteristics of Sound Waves

Sound waves are alternating regions of high- and low-pressure traveling through some medium (e.g., air) in the same direction. They are produced by some vibrating object and are perceived by us as the sound sensation.

The auditory analyzer perceives the following 4 properties of sound:

i. *Pitch.* It is the psychological perception of the sound frequency; the higher the frequency, the higher the pitch. The entire audible range extends from 16 Hz to 20, 000 Hz (1 Hertz = 1 cycle/sec). The term **infrasound** refers to frequencies below 16 Hz, while **ultrasound** refers to frequencies above 20, 000 Hz.

The human ear is most sensitive to frequencies between 500 and 5000 Hz. The average conversation voice frequency is 120 Hz in the males and 250 Hz in the females. The sounds from a distant plane range from 20 to 100 Hz.

Pitch discrimination is possible because different frequencies cause vibrations in different regions of the basilar membrane. Each segment of this membrane is thus "tuned" for a particular pitch—high-pitched sounds near the base of cochlea, and low-pitched sounds near the apex.

Note

While the human ear cannot perceive ("hear") ultrasounds, bats, dogs, and other animals can. Ultrasound is used extensively to study the internal organs of the body. The inaudible sounds are reflected from the organs and analyzed by a computer to provide a picture on the display screen.

ii. *Intensity (loudness).* The intensity or loudness of a sound is the psychological term referring to the amplitude of the sound vibrations. The sound intensity is measured in units called decibels (Db; db). (See below Q/A 1).

iii. *Timbre (quality or pattern).* This property refers to the sensation perceived when we hear a mixture of related frequencies, i.e., harmonics or overtones. (The same note played on different musical instruments is "perceived" or "sounds" differently).

iv. **Direction of Sound.** The ability to detect the position of the source of sound is called binaural effect (Consult Expt. 2-24).

II. Mechanism of Hearing

The sound waves striking the tympanic membrane are magnified by the ossicles and set the basilar membrane to vibrate, which, in turn, causes movement of the hair cells of the organ of Corti. The bending of the cilia of hair cells transducts mechanical vibrations into APs by releasing a neurotransmitter (probably glutamate) at the bases of hair cells where nerve endings of 1st- order sensory neurons synapse. The APs are carried up the auditory pathway to the primary auditory areas of the cerebral cortex (Brodmann's areas 41, 42). Since many fibers cross over from one auditory pathway to the opposite pathway in medulla, the primary auditory areas receive signals from both sides.

III. Auditory Pathway

The **pathway of hearing (Figure 2-14)** from the cochlea to the auditory cortex consists of 4 to 6 neurons. The cell bodies of 1st order neurons (bipolar) lie, in the spiral ganglion. The peripheral processes end on the hair cells of the organ of Corti, while the central processes, which form the auditory nerve, enter the upper medulla to synapse on the dorsal and ventral cochlear nuclei. The 2nd order neurons from these nuclei take different routes through the nearby olivary nuclei and the trapezoid bodies of both sides (some fibres end here), cross to the opposite side and turn upwards to form the lateral lemniscus. The lemniscal fibres synapse on the neurons in the inferior colliculi and medial geniculate bodies from where fresh relays 3rd order neurons spread upward as auditory

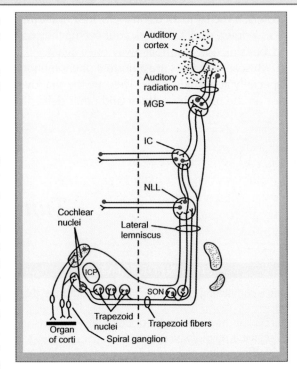

Figure 2-14. The auditory pathway. ICP: Inferior cerebellar peduncle; SON: superior olivary nucleus; MGB: medial geniculate body; IC:inferior colliculus; NLL: nucleus of lateral lemniscus

radiation to terminate in the primary auditory cortex (Brodman's areas 41 and 42).

IV. Tests of Hearing

1. *Whisper test.* (See clinical testing of 8th nerve.
2. *Watch test* for these tests)
3. *Tuning-fork tests.* These are the most commonly used tests in clinical practice.
4. Recording of brain stem auditory evoked potentials (BAEP; see Expt 2-33).

TUNING-FORK TESTS

Before one can understand the principles on which the tuning-fork tests are based, one must understand what is meant by **air conduction** and **bone conduction** of sound.

Air (Ossicular) Conduction (AC)

Normally, most of the energy of incident sound waves is transmitted via the outer ear, tympanic membrane, and middle ear ossicles to the cochlea where it stimulates the sensory hair cells of the organ of Corti. This mode of conduction of sound is called **ossicular conduction**, though it is commonly and **misleadingly called air conduction. True air conduction,** i.e., vibrations of tympanic membrane→vibrations of air in the middle ear→round window of cochlea (that is, where vibrations of the ossicles are not involved) does not play any role in normal hearing.

Bone Conduction (BC)

Since cochlea is enclosed in a bony cavity (bony cochlea), vibrations of the skull bones themselves can be transmitted to the organ of Corti—a type of sound conduction called bone conduction. In this case, sound from a vibrating tuning fork, directly placed anywhere on the skull, can be heard in both ears by bone conduction. However, even loud sounds in the environment do not possess enough energy to cause vibrations of the skull bones and thus stimulate the organ of Corti; they usually take the air and ossicular route.

Principles of Tuning-Fork Tests

Tuning forks, which emit pure tones, allow comparison of AC (air-conducted) hearing and BC (bone-conducted) hearing in an individual.

In *AC hearing*, sound from a vibrating tuning fork held in front of the external ear passes via the external auditory meatus, tympanic membrane, and middle ear ossicles to the organ of Corti.

In *BC hearing*, vibrations from a tuning fork, directly placed on the skull are conducted to the organ of Corti and perceived as sound.

Normally, AC hearing is better than BC hearing (written as AC > BC, or Rinne positive).

Conduction (or, Conductive) Deafness

Pathology in the outer ear (e.g., wax), or damage to the tympanic membrane (e.g., perforation), or pathology in the middle ear (e.g., loss of mobility or destruction of ossicles), reduces AC hearing without affecting bone conduction (BC hearing), a condition called **conductive deafness.**

Nerve Deafness

Damage to the hair cells in the organ of Corti or auditory pathways, will reduce both AC and BC hearing, a condition called **nerve deafness** or **perceptive deafness.** In other words, if BC is normal, the inner ear (cochlea) and auditory pathways must be normal, but if BC is reduced the cochlea or the pathways are at fault.

PROCEDURES

Equipment • Tuning fork (256 or 512 Hz) • Audiometer • Ticking watch.

Important
1. In all tests, the procedure must be clearly explained to the subject/patient. Ask the subject to raise his/her hand or finger when the *sound disappears.*
2. The sense of hearing should first be tested with the whisper test, and then with a tuning-fork.
3. The student is advised to perform all these tests on herself and on her partner.

I.   Rinne's Test

This test compares the subject's AC hearing with his BC hearing, in each ear separately.
  1. Hold the stem of the tuning fork with the thumb and finger and set it into vibration by striking one of its prongs on the heel of your hand. (The other prong will also start to vibrate).

2. Place its base on the mastoid process (the bony prominence behind the ear). The subject will hear a sound. Ask him to raise his hand when the sound stops. Note the time for which the sound is heard.

3. When the sound stops, bring the prongs in front of the ear—the sound will become audible once again. Note the time for which it lasts (E.g., for another 10 seconds; total= 45 seconds).

Results

In normals: For example, sound heard on mastoid process = 35 seconds.
Sound heard in front of ear = 35+ 10= 45 seconds
Thus, AC> DC (Rinne positive).

In Conduction Deafness. BC sound remains normal at 35 seconds, but AC sound not heard after BC sound stops.
Thus, AC < BC (Rinne negative).

In Nerve Deafness. Hearing will be impaired in both BC and AC sounds.
For example, BC becomes 15 seconds, AC becomes 20 sec.
Thus, AC > BC, if nerve deafness is partial.

4. Test the other ear and record the timings for BC and AC sounds.

II. Weber's Test

This test compares the bone conduction of the subject in his two ears.

1. Set the tuning fork into vibration and place its base in the midline on the top of the subject's head or on his forehead. Ask the subject if he hears the sound equally well in both the ears, or louder on one side.

   In a normal subject: Bone conducted sounds are heard equally well on the two sides.

   In conduction deafness: Sound is louder/ better heard in deaf or deafer ear because of masking effect of environmental noise is absent on diseased side.

   In nerve deafness: The sound is louder /better heard on the healthy side i.e., the patient lateralizes the sound to healthy side.

2. Conduction deafness can be artificially created if you close one ear (say, left) of the subject with your finger.

   Set the tuning fork into vibration once again and place it on his head or forehead.

   In a normal person: Sound is better heard in the closed ear due to bone conduction. Closing his ear produces a situation of conduction deafness, and demonstrates the masking effect of environmental noise.

III. Schwabach's Test

This test compares the subject's bone conduction with the examiner's bone conduction. It is assumed that the examiner's hearing is normal.

1. Set the tuning fork into vibration as before and place its base on the subject's mastoid process. Ask him to indicate, by raising his hand, when the sound stops.

2. After the subject stops hearing the sound, place the fork on your own mastoid process.

In a normal person: BC sound in the subject is nearly equal to your own.

In conduction deafness: The subject's bone conduction is better than your bone conduction.

In nerve deafness: BC sound in the subject is reduced as compared to your own. (This means that you will be able to hear BC sound after the subject stops hearing this sound).

Note
The Weber's and Schwabach's tests demonstrate the important masking effect of environmental noise on the auditory threshold.

QUESTIONS

Q. 1 What are the features of sound that are perceived by the hearing mechanism? What is the unit of intensity of sound?
The auditory analyzer perceives the pitch, intensity or loudness, timbre or quality of sound, and the direction of the source of sound.

The **intensity or loudness of sound** is expressed in decibels (db). The standard sound reference (faintest audible sound) corresponds to zero (0) db at a pressure level of 0.0002 dyne/cm^2. This is the minimum sound intensity that can be perceived by a normal person. Thus, a zero db sound is not inaudible, but just audible. Ordinary conversation at 6-8 feet is held at 50-60 db. The sound pressure that can damage cochlear receptors is >10^{14} times, i.e., more than a trillion times the auditory threshold (the db scale is logarithmic). This pressure approximately equals about 140 db. Loud stereo music with headphones on, or prolonged exposure to other loud noises causes selective loss of hearing.

Q. 2 What is meant by the terms ultrasonic, infrasonic and supersonic ?

The audible range for humans extends from 16—20, 000 Hz. *Infrasound* refers to frequencies below 16 Hz and ultrasound refers to frequencies above 20,000 Hz (See above).

The speed of sound at sea level is about 770 miles per hour (about 1250 km/hr). The term **supersonic** refers to an object (e.g., an aeroplane) that travels at a speed faster than that of sound. (The term "mach 1" is used for planes flying at the speed of sound; twice this speed is "mach 2" and so on. Now-a-days, planes can fly at over "mach 5-6").

Q. 3 What are the limitations of the tuning-fork tests? What is audiometry?

The tuning-fork tests often provide valuable information, but cannot give quantitative estimates about the acuity of hearing. Furthermore, bone-conducted vibrations reach all parts of the skull irrespective of where the fork is placed on the head. Thus, when testing bone conduction in one ear, the subject/patient will also be hearing sound in the other ear, which is likely to confuse him.

Audiometry. An audiometer is an apparatus in which selected pure tones of 125—800 Hz can be fed into each ear separately through headphones. The threshold is determined at each frequency and is then plotted as a percentage of normal hearing. Audiometry is thus the only reliable method to determine the nature and degree of deafness in a patient.

Brainstem auditory evoked potentials (BAEPs): The BAEPs' recorded from the scalp after applying a suitable auditory stimulus are employed to localize the site of lesion in the central auditory pathways (Consult Expt 2-33).

Q. 4 Describe the auditory pathway?

See page 214.

Q. 5 What are cochlear implants?

A cochlear implant is a device, which converts sounds into electrical signals that can be interpreted by the brain. It is useful in deafness due to damage to the hair cells of the cochlea.

The *external part* of this device has a *microphone*, a *sound processor* (which can be kept in the patient's shirt pocket), and a *transmitter* (worn behind the ear). The *internal receiver* relays signals to electrodes implanted in the cochlea where they generate impulses in the sensory fibers of the cochlear nerve. These signals are then propagated along the normal pathways to the brain where they are perceived as sounds.

2-24

Localization of Sound

Procedures

Seat the subject in a quiet room, and ask him to close his eyes. Use a forceps to produce clicking noises behind, in front, and to each side of his head, one after the other, and ask him to locate the direction of sound in each case. Enter the results in your workbook, indicating the ability to localize the sound as excellent, good, fair and poor.

Comments

The ability to judge the position of the source of sound with both ears is called the *binaural effect*. Two factors are involved in this process:

1. The difference in the loudness of the sounds at the two ears, and
2. The difference in the interval of sound at the two ears, i.e., the phase difference or the interval between equal phases of sound waves entering the two ears.

The human ear can gauge the direction of a sound's origin on a 0.00003-sec difference in its interval at the two ears. When we want to localize a sound coming from a distance, we turn our head until the sound is equally loud in the two ears. The direction in which we are facing is the direction of the sound's origin.

2-25

Masking of Sounds

That we raise our voice when travelling in a noisy bus or train is a common experience. When the noise suddenly stops, we become aware of the loudness of our voice. This masking effect of noise is employed to detect malingering.

Procedures

Ask the subject to read from a book. After a few seconds, make a rattling noise near his ear by using a tin box containing some metal objects. The subject automatically increases the intensity of his voice. Obviously, this would not occur in a deaf individual. A person malingering deafness, on the other hand, will raise his voice.

2-26

Sensation of Taste

The following material will be required: Strong solutions of sucrose (10%) and sodium chloride (15%), and weak solutions of acetic acid (1%), and quinine sulfate (0.1%) kept in dropper bottles •A hand lens •Small cotton swabs, or toothpicks •Four cards with sweet, salt, sour and bitter printed on them.

PROCEDURES

Instruct the subject that he is to point to a card to indicate the taste felt by him.

1. Seat the subject near your work table. Ask him to protrude his tongue. Using the hand lens, examine and identify the areas which have large concentrations of papillae and taste

buds. Locate the fungiform and circumvallate papillae.

2. Ask the subject to rinse his mouth; then dry it with gauze. Moisten a swab with a few drops of sugar solution, apply it to the tip of the tongue, and ask him to indicate, without withdrawing the tongue, the taste experienced by him.

3. Have him rinse his mouth; dry the tongue with gauze, and repeat the procedure with the salt solution.

4. Repeat this procedure with all the four substances, one by one, on the sides, near the tip, the anterior 2/3rd, and the posterior 1/3rd of the dorsum of the tongue; and taking care that the test solution does not spread across the midline. The tip of the tongue may be held with gauze while testing.

Record the results, and grade the intensity of taste sensation as: intense (+ + + +), moderate (+ + +), mild (+ +), slight (+), or absent (0).

Comments

Though the 7th cranial nerve is almost entirely a motor nerve, it carries taste fibers from the anterior 2/3rd of the tongue. These fibers pass from the lingual nerve into the chorda tympani and then through the geniculate ganglion and the nervus intermedius of Wrisburg to enter the medulla to form the tractus solitarius. Taste fibers from the posterior 1/3rd of the tongue are carried by the 9th nerve. General sensations from the tongue are carried by the 5th cranial nerve.

The sweet taste is better experinced near the tip of the tongue, salt on the sides and top, bitter in the posterior part, and sour sensation in between these areas.

2-27

Sensation of Smell

Vials containing oil of cloves, turpentine oil, and alcohol will be used for testing the sense of smell. Ammonia or acetic acid should not be used because these irritants stimulate the 5th nerve supplying the nasal mucosa. It should be confirmed that the subject's nose is not blocked by common cold.

Procedures

1. Ask the subject to close his eyes, and occlude one of his nostrils. Then have him smell and distinguish the odors of each of the test substances, one by one, in each nostril, separately.

2. Ask him to occlude one nostril, and have him smell the oil of cloves until the odor can no

longer be detected. Immediately after this, ask the subject to try to distinguish, with the adapted nostril, between turpentine and alcohol. Describe the result in your practical workbook.

Pathway for Smell

The pathway of smell is: Olfactory receptor cells → Olfactory nerves → Olfactory bulb → Olfactory tract → Olfactory cortex (uncus and pyriform cortex, for perception of sense of smell). Lesions in this area may be associated with perversion of smell. The olfactory cortex forms part of the limbic system which is concerned with emotions, and instinctual and social behavior.

Laboratory Exercise on Sensations of Touch, Pain, Temperature

The short experiments included here are meant to illustrate some of the features, as well as limitations of our cutaneous sensations, namely, touch, pressure, vibration, proprioception, temperature, and pain. Some of these experiments are employed as clinical tests during the neurological examination of a patient.

Instructions

1. Work in batches of two, one student acting as the subject and the other as the observer. The observer should ensure that the subject's answers are honest and based on the actual sensation arising from the end organ under study. No guess work should be used.
2. When testing a sensation, whether in a student or in a patient, it is important not to suggest the response, either verbally or by allowing him to see the stimulus.
3. The tests may be repeated a few times because of the variability in responses to identical stimuli. However, during any lengthy testing, the attention of the subject should be checked from time to time.

TOUCH, PRESSURE, VIBRATION

Although clinically, touch, pressure and vibration are treated as separate sensations they are all detected by similar types of receptors. The 3 submodalities of touch are: **touch, *pressure*** and **flutter- *vibration.*** *Receptors for touch lie in the cutaneous and subcutaneous tissues and include: Meissner's corpuscles, Merkel discs (also in Iggo domes),* and *basket hair endings. Pacinian corpuscles* located in subcutaneous and deeper tissues detect pressure and vibration frequencies

of 100-500 Hz. *Krause end bulbs* and *Ruffini end organs* seem to detect low frequencies of 20-100 Hz and pressure.

Free nerve endings subserving touch are present in epidermis and dermis, and belong to Aδ and C fibers. The terminal C fibers serving touch are also called C mechanoreceptors.

PROCEDURES

Equipment • Compass. • von Frey's hair esthesiometer • Algometer • Pins • Cotton

A. Touch Perception

1. Seat the subject near a table. Draw 3 cm squares on the palm of the hand near the base of the thumb, back of the hand, and ventral forearm—one hairy and the other hairless. Divide each square into 4 squares each. If Von Frey's hair esthesiometer **(Figure 2-14)** is available, it should be used for testing touch perception. Horse-hairs or nylon bristles mounted in hypodermic needles also give good results.
2. Draw similar grid charts in your workbook, preferably on a larger scale for recording touch-sensitive and touch-insensitive spots within the squares drawn on the skin. The purpose of the grid is spatial location of touch spots and not an indication of their size.
3. Ask the subject to close his eyes, and tell him to respond with a "yes" or "no". Gently touch the skin regions with the test object and note the results in your workbook, showing touch-sensitive spots.
4. Stroke a wisp of cotton lightly over the palm and the back of the hand and ask the subject to compare this sensation with that aroused

by the hair esthesiometer. (A wisp of cotton is used for testing the sensation of touch during clinical examination).

B. *Adaptation time for light touch.* Ask the subject to close his eyes. Using the point of a pencil, or a pin, very carefully displace one hair on his forearm and carefully maintain the displacement. Ask the subject to report the moment he is aware of the displacement (i.e., touch perception) and the instant the touch sensation is no longer present (though the hair is kept displaced). Carefully time the duration of the sensation in at least 5 different hairs. Record the result in your workbook and calculate the average duration.

C. *Localization of light touch.* Ask the subject to close his eyes, and again displace a hair; mark its position with a colored sketch pen. Ask the subject to try to touch with a different color, the base of the displaced hair. Record the distance between the point he touches and the base of the displaced hair. Repeat the test 5 times on the same or nearby hairs and determine the average error for localization of touch. Tabulate your results.

D. *Two-point discrimination (tactile discrimination).* The ability to distinguish two simultaneously applied touch stimuli as separate can be tested with a Weber's compass (it has two blunt and two sharp points, and a scale to read the distance between the two points), or an ordinary pair of dividers, or the heads of two pins.

Ask the subject to close his eyes. Test areas on the fingers, back of hands, forearms, legs and back of the subject for the minimum distance between two points which arouse two distinct touch sensations. Start with a separation of 1 millimeter between the two points, and varying this distance irregularly, find out the minimum distance, until a very slight reduction in the separation of the two points results in the sensation of being touched at only one site. The subject should report "one", "two", or "don't know". Record the minimum separation discriminated with certainty for each site in your workbook.

Discrimination varies greatly in different regions of the body—2 mm at the fingertips, a few cm on the forearms and legs, and many cm on the back. It is related to the density of the touch spots.

E. Localization of touch. Have the subject close his eyes. Lightly touch the skin, with a colored sketch pen, on different areas on the fingers, arms, legs, and back (choose areas which the subject can reach easily), one at a time, and ask the subject to mark the respective spots with a different color. Test at least 5 different sites in each of the skin areas. Measure in mm the error in localization for each of the 5 trials in each of the areas. Tabulate your results to show the average error for these areas.

F. Perception and adaptation of pressure sensation. Half fill a small beaker with mercury and another with water to the same level. Ask the subject to close his eyes. Insert his right index finger in the mercury and the left index finger in water. His arms may rest on the table but his hands and fingers should not touch the sides or the bottoms of the beakers. Ask him to describe the sensations of touch, pressure, temperature, and buoyancy in each case. Determine the time required in each case for these sensations to disappear.

> **Note**
> Consult Section 3 for clinical testing of touch pressure and vibration.

PAIN

I. Superficial Pain

This experiment is concerned with the fast component (or first pain) of the pain sensation. The stimulus for pain is potential or actual damage to the tissues. Note, however, that in the following experiment very little pressure is needed to elicit this type of pain.

Draw a 3 cm square on the back of one of the subject's hands, and divide it into a 4 squares. Blindfold the subject, or have him close his eyes. Using a blood lancet, or a sharp pin, apply brief and light stimuli within the squares. Map out the pain-sensitive spots within the grids (the areas in between the pain spots will be pain-insensitive). Note that the subject should report with a "yes" when the stimulus elicits pain and not when the stimulus can be detected as causing only touch/pressure sensation. Record your results in the grids drawn in your workbook.

II. Pressure-pain (deep somatic pain)

If An algometer is employed to quantitatively test for deep pain. It is a cylindrical, hand-held instrument having a metal rod that can slide into the cylinder when it is pressed against a surface (it resembles the shock-absorber of a car). The rod, which is calibrated in kg and has a slide-clip around it, has an ebony knob at its free end. To test for deep pain, the knob is pressed against a bone or muscle, and the pressure applied, in kg, that elicits pain, can be read from the scale.

III. Clinical testing of pain sensation

Consult section 3 or clinical testing of pain.

TEMPERATURE

I. Prepare three jars of water in the order—hot, warm, and cold. The hot water should be as hot as can be easily tolerated by a finger without evoking pain. Ask the subject to dip his right index finger in the cold water, and the left in the hot water. After about 30 seconds, ask him to dip both index fingers in the warm water. Ask him to describe the sensations resulting from the experiment.

II. **"Cold" and "Warm" spots:** Satisfactory thermal probes can be made by taping the two inches of the blunt ends of pithing needles with electrician's insulation tape (the plastic serves as an insulated handle). Pack 3-4 such probes each in a 500 ml beaker filled with hot water and another beaker filled with crushed ice and water.

Make a 3 cm square with a sketch pen on the dorsum of the subject's hand, and divide this into 4 squares. Ask him to close his eyes. Very gently touch the skin within the squares with a probe. The subject is to report "cold" or "hot" as the case may be. Select hot and cold probes at random and test for hot and cold spots until the entire square has been mapped. Mark the locations where the subject reports hot sensations with red dots and those of cold sensations with blue dots. (Dry each probe before use, and return it to the beaker after use). Several other areas may be tested in a similar manner. Use the same colored dots to show hot and cold spots within the grid drawn in your workbook.

III. Clinical testing of temperature sensation: Consult section 3.

Unit IV
Nervous System,
Nerve and Muscle

2-29

Electroencephalography (EEG)

It was Caton who, in 1875, discovered that when an electrode was placed on the exposed brain of a conscious experimental animal, it was possible to record spontaneous rhythmic changes in electrical potentials. However, it was Hans Berger, a German psychiatrist, who in 1929, made a systematic study of these potentials, or the so-called '*brain waves*'. He introduced the term *electroencephalogram (EEG)* to denote the record obtained from the surface of the scalp of the human subject. The term *electrocorticogram (ECoG)* is employed for the electrical activity recorded from the surface of the exposed brain.

Two types of electrical activity of the brain may be recorded:

i. *Spontaneous Activity (EEG).* This activity appears to arise without any obvious stimulation.

ii. *Evoked Potentials.* These are the electrical potentials that are caused (and recorded) by the stimulation of sensory receptors or sensory nerve fibers.

Relevance

EEG has not only contributed a great deal to our understanding of the functioning of the brain but is also an important tool in the study of patients of epilepsy, brain tumors, head injuries, brain attacks, etc.

Principle

Gold-plated discs or shallow cups are placed on multiple analogous areas on the two sides of the scalp and simultaneous recordings are made from these areas for analysis and interpretation.

FEATURES OF EEG WAVES

Normally, all the recurring oscillations in potentials (EEG waves, or brain waves) recorded from different areas of the scalp are more or less identical in waveform (shape), though their amplitude may wax and wane slightly. The dominant rhythm of the waves is 8-13/sec and an amplitude of about 50 μv which is called the alpha rhythm. Depending on their frequency and amplitude, which are inversely related, the following rhythms are described:

Rhythm	Frequency/sec	Voltage (μV)
delta	1-3.5	100-200
theta	4-7	50-100
alpha	8-13	30-70
beta	14-25	10-20
gamma	20-30	2-8

Alpha Rhythm (Berger Rhythm, 8-13/sec)

The alpha rhythm is the dominant rhythm of a normal EEG, especially from the parieto-occipital region. It is found in almost all normal, waking, and relaxed adults, with the eyes closed. It represents a resting state of cerebral activity, i.e., it is the rhythm of inattention.

The alpha rhythm is called *synchronized EEG;* the synchronization is due to:

  i. The synchronizing effect of neighboring, densely packed, parallel- arranged fibers (dendrites) in the cerebral cortex.
  ii. Rhythmic discharges from thalamus, and possibly other subcortical structures.

Changes in Alpha Rhythm

Alpha rhythm is decreased in: hypoglycemia, low body temperature, high arterial PCO_2, low levels of glucocorticoids, anesthesia, and sleep.

Alpha Rhythm is increased in: hyperglycemia, rise in body temperature, low arterial PCO_2, and hyperventilation.

Note
Alpha rhythm, the rhythm of "inattention", is usually associated with a relaxed state of mind and a feeling of well-being. It can be promoted by "biofeedback" that is employed in the management of stress.

Desynchronization. Desynchronization, or *arousal response,* refers to the replacement of a rhythmic EEG pattern by irregular, low-voltage activity. The ascending reticular activating system (ARAS) is responsible for this desynchronization that follows any type of sensory stimulation, e.g., cutaneous, visual effort at mental arithmetic, etc.

Delta Rhythm (1-3.5/sec)

A rhythm slower than alpha rhythm, i.e., theta or delta rhythm, does not usually occur in a normal waking individual (except in infants). However, the alpha rhythm is replaced by delta rhythm *in normal subjects during sleep.* The presence of delta rhythm during the waking state in adults may indicate the presence of organic brain disease.

Beta Rhythm (14-25/sec)

It is seen in infants instead of alpha rhythm.

Theta Rhythm (4-7/sec)

It may be seen in children where it is blocked by visual stimulation. The frequency of alpha rhythm is decreased by low blood glucose and low temperature.

Cause of EEG Waves

The neural basis of the EEG waves is not fully known (they are not action potentials). However, their rhythmicity indicates that fluctuations in potentials are occurring in a number of neurons. The activity recorded is mainly that of similarly-oriented and densely packed dendrites in the superficial layers of the cortex. These dendrites and the deeper-lying cell bodies function as fluctuating dipoles in response to the ascending inhibitory and excitatory signals from subcortical structures, especially from the thalamus. These oscillating potentials spread to the scalp from where they are recorded as the EEG waves.

INSTRUMENTATION

EEG records may be *unipolar* or *bipolar.* A unipolar tracing records the potential difference between a *sensitive scalp electrode* and a theoretically *indifferent* or *reference electrode* placed at a distance away from the sensitive (or exploring) electrode. A bipolar recording shows the fluctuations in potential between two sensitive electrodes placed on the scalp or on the exposed brain.

1. EEG Machine

A variety of electroencephalographs having different numbers of recording channels (up to 32) are available. The number of channels is important because simultaneous recordings can be made from wide areas of the scalp. (The number of electrodes is fixed). In the present experiment, a 20-channel ink-writing oscillograph (Medicaid NG 8917) was used. The potentials picked up by the electrodes are suitably modified and amplified before being fed to the recording unit. The machine has the following controls:

a. **Mains supply:** The ON/OFF power switch controls 220 volts AC, 50 Hz current supply. A 50 Hz filter excludes interference from the strong sources of AC current near the recording site. A wooden couch is used for the subject/patient (earlier, a grounded wire-cage was employed for the patient).

b. **Filters:** Special filters are provided to select desired frequencies and to modify the output of the amplifiers.

c. **Sensitivity control:** A commonly used sensitivity is 7 µv/mm so that a calibration signal of 50 µv causes a pen deflection of about 7 mm.

d. **Input selector switch:** Various combinations of electrode placements (montages)—unipolar, bipolar, and unipolar plus bipolar—can be selected by this control. Three montages—A, B, and C, are provided in this machine.

e. **Photic stimulation:** A stroboscopic lamp can give light flashes of desired frequency (usually 25/sec) and duration of stimulation (usually 5 sec).

f. **Hyperventilation time clock:** A time clock displays the duration of voluntary over-breathing (usually 3 to 4 minutes) during the EEG recording.

2. Electrodes

The surface electrodes are shallow silver cups, about 10 mm in diameter, and have a central hole. Lead wires connect them to the electrode board. They are applied to the scalp with an electrode jelly which holds them in place and provides good mechnical and electrical contact with the skin. Cotton balls are placed over the electrodes to delay the drying of the conductive paste.

Electrode paste. It is bentonite paste, prepared by thoroughly mixing 100 g of bentonite powder with 100 ml of normal saline and adding glycerin slowly.

3. Electrode or Input Board

It connects the electrodes on the subject's head to the input selector switches of the machine. A diagram of the scalp showing various electrode positions is printed on the board. There is a provision for checking any loose connections. There is a provision in the machine for minimizing skin to electrode impedence (resistance).

4. Electrode Placement

The standard set of electrodes for adults consists of 22 electrodes including one ground electrode. The international *"10-20" ("ten-twenty") system* of electrode placement (**Figure 2-15**) uses the distances between 3 bony landmarks of the skull—nasion (bridge of nose), inion (occipital protuberance on the back of the head), and pre-auricular point—to generate a system of lines which run along and across the head and intersect at intervals of 10% or 20% of their total length. The electrodes are named with a letter and a subscript. The letter denotes the underlying region—frontopolar (Fp), frontal (F), central (C), parietal (P), occipital (O), and auricular (A). The subscript is either the letter z indicating zero or midline placement, or a number indicating lateral placement, odd numbers on the left and even numbers on the right side of the head. Thus, *Cz* is placed at 50% of the nasion-inion distance in the midsaggital plane, while *C3* and *C4* are 20% of this distance to the left and right of *Cz*.

5. EEG Paper

The paper transport system pulls the paper from a folded stack in a storage bin and moves it under the writing pens at the standard speed of 3 cm/sec (it can be increased or decreased). The paper has printed vertical lines at 3 cm intervals, as shown in **Figure 2-15**.

6. Pen Recording System

There are 21 recording pens, the lower-most being for the time tracing. The pens are 120 mm in length to minimize arc distortion. The contact tension of the pens on the paper can be adjusted, if required, with cradle springs. A pen lift knob can lift the pens from the paper.

PROTOCOL

Records are taken simultaneously from multiple analogous areas of the scalp for at least 20-minute period.

1. No special preparation of the patient is required except that the scalp should not be oily. Ask the subject to lie down on the couch comfortably and relax.
2. Apply the reference electrodes on the ear lobes and ground electrode above the bridge of the nose. Place the sensitive electrodes on the scalp as per the "20—20" system. Connect them to the electrode board and check for any loose connections.
3. Sensitivity calibration. Calibrate the machine so that an input of 50 μV gives a pen deflection of 7 mm.
4. Ask the subject to close his eyes and make a test recording. Normally, alpha rhythm is recorded, as shown in **Figure 2-15**.

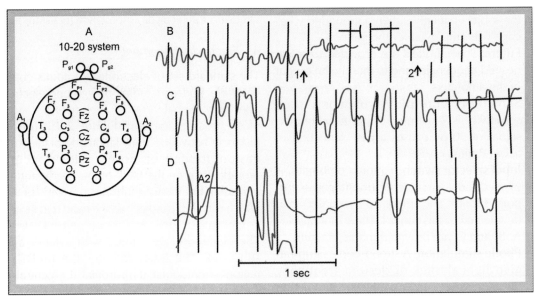

Figure 2-15. Electroencephalogram. (A) The international "10-20" ("ten-twenty") system of electrode placement. (B) Normal record showing alpha rhythm; and the effect of opening the eyes (arrow 1, alpha block) and closing the eyes once again (arrow 2) when the alpha rhythm is restored. (C) Delta rhythm; low-frequency high amplitude waves in a patient of focal epilepsy (channel O_2-A_2 right side). (D) Grand mal epilepsy, spike-wave pattern

5. *Effect of opening the eyes.* Ask the subject to open his eyes. Note that the alpha rhythm is immediately replaced by desynchronization, i.e., by fast, irregular activity. Ask the subject to close his eyes, the alpha rhythm reappears.

6. **Photic stimulation**. As the record is running, deliver light flashes at a rate of 25/sec for 5 seconds, first with eyes closed, then with eyes open.

   Normally, there may be no change, but in abnormal cases (e.g., epilepsy), delta rhythm may appear. In some cases, even an attack of epilepsy may be precipitated. (A flickering television is known to result in an attack of epilepsy).

7. **Effect of hyperventilation.** Ask the subject to breathe deeply and quickly for 3 minutes. Normally, the frequency of alpha waves decreases by low PCO_2 and the record may show theta or even delta rhythm. In epilepsy, an attack may be precipitated, along with abnormal patterns.

Interpretation of EEG

The interpretation of EEG depends on the frequency, amplitude, and distribution of the wave activity in various leads. Each record is then graded according to different systems.

Clinical Applications of EEG

The EEG has its limitations in that a normal record may be obtained in spite of strong clinical evidence of organic disease. Also, an abnormal record may not always indicate an organic disease. Still, EEG is useful in the following disorders:

1. **Epilepsy.** In epilepsy, an excessive discharge from some part of the cerebrum is commonly associated with abnormalities of consciousness. In **grand mal epilepsy,** there are generalized tonic clonic convulsions of the muscles followed by unconsciousness. The EEG shows high-voltage high-frequency synchronous waves during tonic stage and slower and larger waves during clonic stage. In **petit mal epilepsy,** there are brief (lasting a few seconds) episodes of loss of contact with surroundings and the patient has a vacant look. The EEG shows a "spike and dome" pattern. In **psychomotor** or **temporal lobe epilepsy,** there are behavioral changes (they indicate involvement of the limbic system). The EEG may show low-frequency rectangular waves.

2. **Brain tumors and abscess.** Abnormal EEG recorded from a region overlying a tumor or abscess can help in the localization of these lesions.

3. **Head injuries and vascular lesions.** Serial EEG recordings can help in following the course of head injuries, e.g., an expanding hematoma.

4. Encephalitis, meningitis, and congenital defects of brain.

5. **EEG and organic and functional disorders.** EEG may prove useful in differentiating between organic and functional disorders, i.e., non-organic psychiatric disorders. However, its role in functional disorders is doubtful.

Electro-neuro Diagnostic Tests
Nerve Conduction Studies
Motor Nerve Conduction in Median Nerve

The introduction of CRO, amplifiers, various types of stimulating and recording electrodes, single fiber preparations, and the use of computers in medical investigations have tremendously increased our knowledge of the functioning of the nervous system. It has also significantly improved diagnostic methods in clinical neurology.

These techniques involve stimulating, recording, displaying, measuring, and interpreting action potentials and other electrical changes occurring in:

i. *Peripheral nerves (Nerve Conduction Studies; NCS).*
ii. Muscles (Electromyography; EMG)
iii. *Central Nervous System (Evoked potentials).*

Terminology

1. **Voltage.** This term represents the difference of potential between two points. It is measured in millivolts (mV) or microvolts (µV).
2. **Current.** It is measured in milliamperes.
3. **Time.** It is measured in milliseconds (ms, or msec), and microseconds (µsec)

Equipment

1. Cathode Ray Oscilloscope. A beam of electrons emitted by a cathode is focused on a fluorescent screen as a bright luminous spot, and is made to sweep from left to right in a horizontal plane. The amplified potentials from the tissue under study are applied to plates above and below the beam to move it in a vertical plane above and/or below the base line. The movement of the spot traces out the activity as a function of time. The display can be photographed or recorded directly on an ink-writing oscillograph.

2. Amplifiers. A variable degree of amplification is required in most applications because biological signals are very small because of intrinsic impedence (resistance) of the recording electrodes. Also the impedence of the electrode- skin contact point tends to reduce the amplitude of potential changes. Amplification also minimizes distortion of waveforms and improves noise rejection. The sensitivity of the amplifier can be adjusted as required.

3. Filter. It is a device that removes unwanted frequencies (high or low) from a signal and allows only desired frequencies to pass through.

4. Averager. This extracts small signals that are buried or hidden in large noise. For example, evoked potentials buried in EEG noise, sensory nerve action potentials hidden in EMG noise.

5. Stimulators. Stimulators are required in most applications in neurophysiology. They are of two general types:

i. *Electronic/electrical stimulators.* They can provide variable constant current or constant voltage, single pulse or repeated stimuli.
ii. *Magnetic stimulators.* These are employed for non-invasive stimulation of motor cerebral cortex, spinal cord, and peripheral nerves.
   • Low-intensity stimulation causes current flow mainly in superficial soft tissues. With stronger stimuli, more current enters tissues at the cathode which may be painful in some persons.

6. Stimulus artifact. When a stimulus is applied, there is a brief, irregular deflection of the base line; this is called a stimulus artifact and is due to leakage of current from the stimulating to the recording electrodes. (See Chart 5-8 for details). It is employed for measuring the latent period (latency).

7. Electrodes.

a. *Recording electrodes (RE).* Three electrodes are employed for recording potential changes: *active*, *reference*, and *ground*. The AP is measured between active and reference electrodes. The ground electrode serves as a 'zero' voltage reference point.

Electrodes are made of metal—platinum, silver, gold, stainless steel, chromium, nickel, etc. Silver and gold electrodes have the advantage of stable electrode polarizing potentials that give noise-free recordings. (When a metal electrode reacts with an electrolyte such as sweat, or electrode paste, or ECF, an electro- chemical reaction occurs that results in electrode polarizing potentials of 100-500 mV).

The recording electrodes are of 2 general types:

i. *Surface electrodes*. They are in the shape of discs, cups or rings, and are used for recording activity from body surface. They are 'attached' (applied) in place with electrode paste or jelly that is gently rubbed on the skin to reduce the resistance to electrode-skin contact point.

ii. *Concentric needle electrode*. The concentric (or coaxial) needle electrode (usually 24 gauge) is a *bipolar electrode*, one pole of which is formed by the shaft, and the other by a teflon-coated wire threaded through the shaft. The electrode records activity at its tip, the recording area being 150-500 μm^2, thus sampling a restricted area in a muscle.

The monopolar needle electrode is solid steel, 22-24 gauge needle, coated with varnish or Teflon except at its tip. The referenced electrode is placed on the skin.

Note

Microelectrodes with tip diameter of < 1μm can record potentials from single fiber preparations.

b. *Stimulating electrodes (SE).* Stimuli can be applied through cup, disc, or ring electrodes.

PRECAUTIONS

1. The mains supply must be checked to confirm adequate voltage.
2. Proper earthing of the equipment must be ensured. The subject should also be properly grounded.
3. The procedure should be explained to the subject.
4. Loose wire and cable connections as well as the electrode placement may cause distorted APs.

Note

Although both median and ulnar nerves are mixed nerves, **motor nerve conduction** is discussed in median nerve in this experiment, while sensory nerve conduction will be taken up in the ulnar nerve in the next experiment.

NERVE CONDUCTION STUDIES

Nerve conduction studies are carried out in both motor and sensory nerves. The nerves commonly tested are:

a. In the upper limbs: median, ulnar, radial and brachial plexus.
b. In lower limbs: sciatic, femoral, common peroneal, tibial and sural nerves.

Clinical Significance

Testing of conduction velocities in both motor and sensory nerves provides early and accurate diagnosis; there may be an increase in the latency or even complete block of nerve impulses.

Nerve conduction tests are useful in: nerve injuries during accidents, fractures of bones, fracture dislocations of joints, local pressure on nerves by tumors or by ligaments, arthritis, neuropathies in diabetes mellitus demyelination (multiple sclerosis), vitamin B deficiency, leprosy, and so on.

Nerves and Nerve Fibers

The nerves (nerve trunks) dissected by the students during anatomical studies contain thousands of individual nerve fibers packed in bundles. The individual nerve fibers are the protoplasmic extensions of the neurons, their lengths varying from a few mm to over a meter. In the core of a fiber is the axis cylinder- the continuation of cell cytoplasm. The nerve cell membrane extends over the axis cylinder as the axolemma that is the site of all ionic fluxes and electrical processes.

Medullated (myelinated) and non-medullated (non-myelinated) nerve fibers. Fibers larger than 1 μm in diameter have a covering of lipoproteins called myelin (medullary) sheath. This insulating sheath is interrupted at regular constrictions, about 1 mm apart, called the nodes of Ranvier. In peripheral nerves, the myelin sheath is covered with glia-like cells called the cells of Schwann, there being one such cell to each internode. (In the CNS, the cells of Schwann are absent and the myelin sheath is laid down by oligodendroglia.

Nerve fibers, usually less than 1 μm lack myelin sheath, the axolemma being directly exposed to ECF throughout its length.

Nerve Fiber Type and Function. The nerve fibers are classified, according to their diameter, conduction velocity and various features of APs into 3 types: A, B, and C. Type A fibers (12-20 μm) are further divided into Aα (12-20 μm; somatic motor, proprioceptive); Aβ and Aγ (8-12 μm; touch, pressure, efferent to muscle spindles), and Aδ (2-4 μm; touch, pain temperature). Group B fibers

(1-3 μm) are autonomic preganglionic. The C fibers (0.5- 2 μm), are non-medullated pain fibers in the dorsal roots, and postganglionic sympathetic).

A numerical grouping of fibers into I (IA and IB), II, III, and IV takes their functional features also into consideration.

Resting Membrane Potential (RMP).
Consult Chart 5-8.

Action Potential (AP).
Consult Chart 5-8.

Conduction of Nerve Impulses.
Consult Chart 5-8.

Non-medullated fibers.
Consult Chart 5-8.

Medullated Nerve Fibers.
Consult Chart 5-8.

Factors Affecting Nerve Conduction Velocity.
Consult Chart 5-8.

MOTOR NERVE CONDUCTION

Principle

When a current is passed through 2 electrodes placed on the skin, some of it penetrates deep into the tissues. If it is strong enough and in the neighborhood of a nerve, then it will stimulate enough fibers to produce a recordable muscle response.

Nerve conduction velocity determination requires stimulation of a nerve at two places along its length. The velocity in m/sec can be calculated from the difference in the latent periods of the two responses and the length of the nerve segment between the two points stimulated (Refer to Expt 4-6 on Velocity of nerve impulses in frog's nerve muscle preparation).

Median Nerve (C-6, 7, 8; T-1**).** It is a mixed nerve and arises from the brachial plexus. Its motor branches supply most of the flexor-pronator muscles of the forearm. It enters the hand through the carpal tunnel to supply the thenar muscles. It is sensory to the lateral palm and lateral two and one half fingers, and their distal ends. It has no innervation in the upper arm.

Apparatus. • CRO • Preamplifier • Electronic stimulator • Stimulating and recording electrodes • Electrode jelly • Spirit swabs.

PROCEDURE

1. Ask the subject to sit on a chair near a table and explain the procedure to him.
2. Clean the skin over the thenar muscle pad and the areas over the median nerve at the elbow and the wrist. Rub electrode jelly over these areas (**Figure 2-16**).
3. Apply the cup recording (active) electrode (A) over the motor point of abductor pollicis brevis, and the reference electrode (R) about 3 cm away from it. Place the ground electrode (G) between recording and stimulating electrodes (S-1). Connect the recording electrodes to the CRO through the pre-amplifier.
5. Apply the stimulating electrodes on the wrist 3 cm above the distal wrist skin crease (S-1) and apply a supramaximal stimulus. Note the response of the thenar muscles. Now shift the electrodes to the elbow and apply a stimulus (S-2). Note that at both the sites of stimulation (S-1 and S-2), the *cathode* is the stimulating electrode and it is placed distal to the anode.
6. Observations and results

In both cases, there is a stimulus artifact at the beginning of the sweep, followed by a latent period, and a biphasic AP with initial negativity, this is called *a biphasic muscle potential* or *compound muscle action potential (CMAP)*.

Compound Muscle Action Potential (CMAP) It includes the onset latency, duration, and the amplitude of the biphasic AP, as shown in **Figure 2-17**.

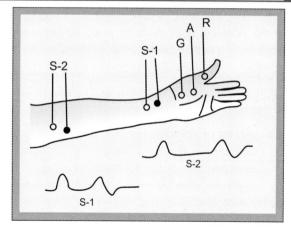

Figure 2-16. Measurement of motor nerve conduction velocity in median nerve. S-1: stimulation at wrist; S-2: stimulation at elbow. A: recording (active) electrode; R: reference electrode; G: ground electrode

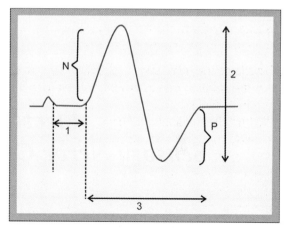

Figure 2-17. Compound muscle action potential (CMAP). N: negative phase; P: positive phase; 1: onset latency; 2: amplitude (peak to peak); 3: duration of CMAP

Onset latency. It is the time from the stimulus artifact to the start of the first negative deflection. It is a measure of speed of conduction in fastest nerve fibers and includes neuromuscular transmission time, spread of AP over the muscle fibers, and the process of excitation-contraction coupling.

Amplitude of CMAP. It is measured from baseline to the negative peak (base to peak) or between negative to positive peaks (peak to peak).

Duration of CMAP. It is measured from onset to the negative or positive peaks, or the final return of the waveform to the baseline.

Calculation of Velocity. For example:

Latent period at S-1 = 5 msec.

Latent period at S-2 = 9.5 msec.

Length of nerve between the two stimulated points = 26 cm.

Distance traveled in 4.5 msec = 26 cm.

Distance traveled in 1 second = 58 meters.

Normal values: The normal velocity in the motor fibers of the median nerve in humans is 55-65 m/sec.

Clinical Significance. The median nerve in entering the hand passes through a tunnel formed between the carpal bones and the flexor retinaculum—a band of connective tissue. The tunnel gets constricted or thickened due to fracture of the wrist or thickening of the retinaculum. The resulting compression can cause pain, paresthesias (sensations of pins and needles), wasting and paralysis of thenar muscles and trophic changes of fingertips. This relatively common condition, called *"carpal tunnel syndrome"* is treated by cutting through the retinaculum to relieve the pressure. Testing the conduction velocity in median nerve provides early diagnosis. (The latent period at the wrist may increase from the normal values of 3-5 msec to 8-10 msec or even more).

Note

Working for long periods at the keyboard of a computer may also cause this type of syndrome.

2-31

Electro-neuro Diagnostic Tests
Sensory Nerve Conduction in Ulnar Nerve

Ulnar Nerve

The ulnar nerve, like the median nerve, is also a mixed nerve. It arises from C-7 to T-1 segments of the spinal cord, passes behind the medial epicondyle of humerus and then down the ulnar side of the forearm. It gives *motor* branches to muscles in the forearm, and in the hand to the hypothenar and other muscles. Its *sensory* branches supply the skin of the medial half of the hand and of the little and ring fingers.

Principle of Sensory Nerve Stimulation. In the body, sensory nerve fibers conduct nerve impulses (APs) only in one direction, i.e., from the sensory receptors towards the CNS (orthodromic conduction). But when they are stimulated artificially, say, through the skin, they can conduct APs in the opposite direction as well, i.e., towards the sensory receptors (antidromic conduction). • **Equipment.** CRO with storage facility. • Electronic stimulator • Stimulating silver ring electrodes. • *Recording* silver cup electrodes • Electrolyte paste • Spirit swabs.

PROCEDURES

1. Clean the areas of the little finger and where electrodes are to be applied and rub electrode jelly over these points.

2. *Stimulating electrodes (SE).* Place silver ring electrodes, one on the middle phalanx (active electrode) and the other on the terminal phalanx.

3. *Recording electrodes (RE).* Apply 2 silver cup recording electrodes about 2-3 cm apart, proximal to wrist skin crease. Apply the ground electrode between the SE and the RE on the palm. Connect all these to the CRO through the preamplifier.

4. Adjust the settings: filter= low cut: 5-10 Hz; high cut: 2-3 KHz; gain= 1-5 μV/div; sweep speed= 1-2 msec/ div, or as desired.

5. Apply a supramaximal stimulus and note the response. Record a time tracing and note the distance between the SE and the RE.

6. For antidromic conduction, simply reverse the connections of SE and RE.

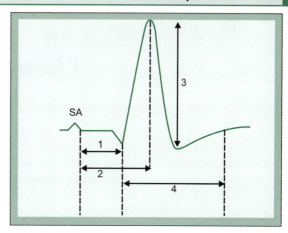

Figure 2-18. Sensory nerve action potential (SNAP). SA: stimulus artifact; 1: onset latency; 2: Peak latency; 3: peak to peak amplitude; 4: Duration of SNAP

OBSERVATIONS AND RESULTS

Figure 2-18 shows a sensory nerve action potential (SNAP). It has a stimulus artifact, onset latency, amplitude, and duration.

Calculate the velocity of sensory nerve conduction velocity as follows:

Velocity = Length of nerve in mm/Latency in msec.
    Normal value: 50-65 m/sec.

Comments
The orthodromic and antidromic conduction velocities provide similar information in clinical practice. The duration of SNAP gives information about the number of slow-conducting fibers, while amplitude reveals the density of nerve fibers. Both are affected in nerve injuries, neuropathies, vitamin efficiencies, leprosy, etc.

Note
Sensory nerve conduction velocity can also be determined in median nerve by placing stimulating ring electrodes on the index finger and recording electrodes at the base of the thumb. This will record orthodromic conduction velocity. Antidromic velocity can be recorded by reversing the locations of the electrodes.

QUESTIONS

1. Name the equipment employed in electro-neuro diagnostic techniques.

2. What is the basis of working of a cathode ray oscilloscope?

3. What are electrodes employed for in these studies?

4. What is a waveform and what are its components.

5. Name some properties of nerve fibers.

    Nerve fibers are excitable; they show resting membrane potential; they can conduct the excitatory state (AP); they show all-or-none response, i.e., either there is a full-fledged AP, or no AP at all. They also exert a trophic influence on the structures innervated by them.

2-32

Electro-neuro Diagnostic Tests
Electromyography (EMG)

Electromyography is a recording of the electrical activity occurring in a muscle during voluntary contraction. It is the sum of action potentials of many muscle fibers. This change of potential sets up a current field that can be recorded either with needle electrodes or by surface electrodes.

Relevance

Although the EMG does not provide a specific clinical diagnosis, it can help in arriving at a diagnosis when its results are interpreted along with the results of other tests and clinical features of the patient. EMG is useful in the detection of lower motor neuron diseases, and disorders of neuro-muscular transmission.

INTRODUCTION

A skeletal muscle consists of a number of anatomically separate, paralelly-arranged, cylindrical, multinucleated fibers (cells), 10-100 μm in diameter, and of varying lengths from a few mm to many cm. They have no activity of their own, but contract only in response to nerve impulses arriving along their motor nerve supply from the CNS.

In normal muscles, the muscle fibers do not contract individually but as part of a motor unit consisting of a variable number of innervated muscle fibers. Thus, the motor unit is the functional unit of muscle activity.

Motor Unit. A motor unit consists of one anterior grey column motor neuron of the spinal cord (or the equivalent motor cranial neuron in the brain stem), its axon and all its branches as it enters a muscle, and all the muscle fibers innervated by

these branches. The number of muscle fibers in a motor unit varies from a few (external ocular muscles) to many hundreds (muscles of the back, thighs, etc). (Consult Expt 4-4 for details).

> **Note**
> While a normal muscle fiber shows a RMP, and an AP when activated for contraction, a denervated muscle fiber shows unstable potential and spontaneous twitching.

MOTOR UNIT POTENTIAL (MUP)

The motor unit potential (MUP) is the potential change produced by the excitation of muscle fibers of a motor unit. Since these fibers discharge synchronously (at the same time) near the needle electrode, the MUP has higher amplitude and a longer duration than the AP produced by a single muscle fiber.

A. Characteristics of MUP. A MUP is characterized by its firing frequency, duration, amplitude, phases, and rate of rise.

   i. *Frequency.* With mild contraction, the MUP shows a frequency of 5-15 Hz. With stronger contractions, there is recruitment of additional motor units (and so of MUPs) that depends on the size principle—the smaller motor units being recruited first, then larger and larger units are brought into action.

  ii. *Duration.* The duration of a MUP is measured from the initial take-off of the potential to the point of return to the base line (**Figure 2-19**). It varies from 5-10 msec, being shorter in children and longer in adults. The duration of MUP is a measure of conduction velocity,

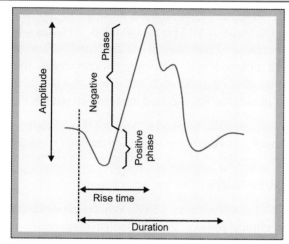

Figure 2-19. Diagram to show normal motor unit potential (MUP) recorded by needle EMG

length of muscle fibers, membrane excitability, and synchronization of response of muscle fibers.

- Short –duration MUP are found in myopathies, myasthenia gravis, and early stage of reinnervation after nerve injuries.
- Long-duration MUP are seen in lower motor neuron lesions and myopathies.

c. *Amplitude.* It is measured from peak to peak and the normal value is 0.5-2.0 mV. It depends on the size, density, and type of muscle fibers, synchrony of firing, nearness of needle to muscle fibers, age of the subject and temperature of the muscle.

d. *Phases.* The MUP recorded by needle electrodes shows a triphasic potentiall, i.e., positive—negative—positive sequence, as shown in **Figure 2-19**. A phase is the part of a MUP between the departure and return of the potential to the base line. A MUP with more than 4 phases is called polyphasic. Some potentials show directional changes without reaching base line—these are called *turns*. Polyphasic potentials and turns are more commonly seen in myopathies when regeneration is occurring.

e. *Rise time.* The rise time of a MUP is the duration from the initial positive to the next negative peak. The usual rise time is up to 500 msec and indicates the distance of the needle from the muscle fibers. A greater rise time indicates increased resistance of the intervening tissues.

B. **Factors Affecting MUP.**

Technical factors. These include: type of needle electrode and its location, (superficial, deep, or near end plate of muscle fiber; the amplitude is smaller when it is superficial); preamplifier and amplifier, and method of recording, etc.

Physiological factors. These are: age—the amplitude and duration increases while firing rate decreases as age advances. Sex and the temperature of muscle also affect MUPs.

METHODOLOGY

Principle

A resting muscle is electrically silent, i.e., it does not show any electrical potentials. When it contracts, however, such changes can be recorded.

Instrumentation

1. CRO • Polygraph (paper recorder) • Preamplifier • Audio amplifier with speaker
2. Electrode paste . 70% alcohol, and cotton and gauze swabs.
3. Recording electrodes • Surface electrodes • Needle electrode.
4. *Equipment settings: Sweep speed* = 5-10 msec/ division; *Filter setting* = 20-10,000 Hz
   Amplitude f= 50 µV/div for spontaneous activity, and 200 µV for MUPs.

Procedure for Surface EMG

1. With the subject lying supine on a couch and the arm extended, clean the skin over the biceps with alcohol. Tell him/her to relax and that the procedure will be painless.

2. Using electrode paste, fix a set of 3 electrodes over a small area of the skin, one for grounding and the other 2 for recording (one active, one reference). Connect the electrodes through the preamplifier to the CRO, the recorder, and the audio amplifier. Observe if there is any electrical activity,

3. Ask the subject to flex the arm, and then pronate and supinate the forearm, first gently, then with greater force. Note the potentials.

Procedure for Needle EMG

1. Clean the skin with alcohol and let dry, and fix the ground electrode on the skin. Tell the subject that an injection needle will be inserted into the muscle.

2. Insert the concentric needle gently into the muscle, and advance it by steps to several depths.

3. Make the following observations *at each depth:*

Activity evoked by insertion; activity produced by moving the needle; activity of relaxed (resting) muscle with the needle undisturbed; and activity during weak and then during stronger and stronger voluntary contractions.

OBSERVATIONS AND RESULTS

Note the following activities and draw diagrams in your notebooks.

1. *Insertion Activity.* There is a brief burst of electrical activity of 0.5-1.0 msec due to mechanical damage by the needle, appearing as positive or negative bursts of high-frequency spikes.

2. *Spontaneous* Activity. There is no spontaneous electrical activity except that when the needle electrode is near the end plate region when miniature end-plate potentials (MEPP) may be recorded. They are monophasic negative waves of up to 100 µV and of 1-2 msec duration.

- Abnormal spontaneous activities include: fibrillation, fasciculation, and cramp potentials, and complex repetitive discharges (CRD).

3. *Voluntary Contractions.* With weak contractions, MUPs of 5-15 Hz are recorded. With stronger contractions, potentials of 0.3-2 mV and 5-15 msec are recorded. With still stronger contractions, the potentials run into each other and the resulting confused tracing is called interference pattern.

Audio signals. As audio signals, the MUPs produce knocking or thumping sounds on the loud speaker.

QUESTIONS

Q. 1 Define the term EMG. What is its relevance in clinical physiology and medical diagnosis?
See page 234.

Q. 2 Why are resting muscles electrically silent?
The resting muscle fibers only show a steady resting membrane potential (RMP) across their cell membranes, negativity on the inside and positivity on the outside. So when the recording electrode lies near them, no potential difference is recorded and they are electrically silent. They show action potentials only when they reactivated by signals arriving along their motor nerves. This electrical activity is then followed by the mechanical activity of contraction.

Q. 3 How is force of contraction graded?
The varying force of reflex or voluntary contraction of skeletal muscles depends on:

1. Number of motor units activated.
2. Frequency of nerve impulses.
3. Synchronization of nerve impulses.
4. Initial length of muscle fibers. (See Expt 4-4 for details).

Q. 4 How can recruitment of motor units be demonstrated experimentally without needle electrodes?
This can be done by placing recording electrodes on the skin over thenar region and then asking the subject to move the thumb slowly at first and then with greater force. MUPs of different amplitude and shape will be recorded.

2-33

Electro-neuro Diagnostic Tests Evoked Potentials Brainstem Auditory, Visual, Somatosensory, and Motor Evoked Potentials

As mentioned earlier, electrical potentials can be produced (evoked) in the cerebral cortex by the stimulation of sensory receptors or sensory nerves. But since these cortical potential changes are small and buried in the background of spontaneous electrical activity (EEG), their details can only be studied and evaluated by repeated stimulation and averaging the responses obtained after each stimulation by a computer.

The commonly tested evoked potentials are:
1. Brainstem auditory evoked potentials (BAEPs).
2. Visual evoked potentials (VEPs).
3. Somatosensory evoked potentials (SEPs).
4. Motor evoked potentials (MEPs).

Note
The brainstem auditory evoked potentials will be taken up to illustrate the technique of evoked potentials, while others will only be briefly mentioned.

BRAINSTEM AUDITORY EVOKED POTENTIALS (BAEPS)

The BAEPs represent an objective test for hearing. They are a series of potentials generated by sequential activation of different parts of the auditory pathway. These APs can not only be recorded from along this pathway but also from the body surface, especially from the scalp.

Auditory Pathway. Consult Expt 2-23 for its description.

Equipment

• CRO • Preamplifier • EEG electrodes • Electrode paste • Alcohol or ether swabs • Headphones.

PROCEDURES

1. The test is carried out preferably in a sound proof room. Ask the subject to sit in a chair, with his back to the apparatus, and relax.
2. Clean the skin where electrodes are to be applied. Place the recording (active) electrodes on both ear lobes, or on the mastoid processes. Place the reference electrode at the vertex (Cz position), and the ground electrode on top of the forehead.
3. Connect the REs to the amplifier. Use amplification of 200,000 to 500, 000; set low filter at 100 Hz and high filter at 3000 Hz.
4. Apply brief click stimuli of 70 db intensity above the subjects threshold, at a rate of 10/sec, and of 0.1 msec duration. (The stimuli are usually square wave pulses; the pulse wave can move the diaphragm of the earphone either towards or away from the ear, i.e., condensation or rarefaction stimuli).
5. The sound clicks stimulate not only the ipsilateral ear but also travel to the opposite ear by bone and air conduction to stimulate that ear at an intensity of 40-50 db lower than the ipsilateral ear.
6. Observe the effect of intensity of stimulation on the BAEPs.

Observations and Results

The auditory nerve and BAEPs are "volume conducted" to the surface recording electrodes. At the vertex and ear lobes, they form vertex positive and vertex negative potentials. A sequence of 5 or more distinct wave forms (vetex positive peaks) labeled I to V (**Figure 2-20**) are recorded within 10 msec of the application of stimulation. If the recording is continued, a few more positive and negative waves are recorded. The origin of the waveforms is: *Wave I*: from the peripheral part of auditory nerve; *Wave II:* from cochlear nuclei; *Wave III:* from superior olivary nucleus; *Wave IV:* from lateral lemniscus; *Wave V:* from inferior colliculi; *Wave VI:* from medial geniculate body; and *Wave VII:* from auditory *radiation.*

Measurement of BAEP Waveforms. The features noted are: absolute latency, amplitude, interpeak latencies, inter-ear-interpeak differences, and amplitude ratio of V/I.

Factors Affecting BAEPs. These include: age, sex, height, temperature, drugs (alcohol and barbiturates prolong the latency of wave V), and hearing loss.

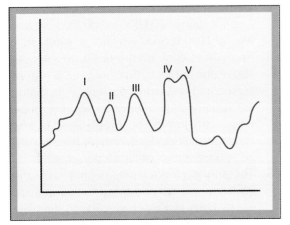

Figure 2-20. Brainstem auditory evoked potentials in normal individual. Interpeak latencies are measured from the top of one peak to the other. Refer to text for the origin of different waveforms

Clinical Significance

1. The auditory responses provide an objective assessment in infants and young children suspected of being deaf.
2. The BAEPs aid in assessing the degree of hearing loss.
3. The latencies of waveforms provide information in patients of vestibular nerve and brainstem tumors, demyelination, and in distinction of various kinds of coma and drug-induced and traumatic disease processes.

VISUAL EVOKED POTENTIALS (VEPS)

The VEPs are the potential changes recorded from the scalp in response to visual stimuli. They represent the resultant responses of cortical and subcortical structures to photostimulation. Normal VEPs indicate the intactness of the entire visual pathway (See Expt 2-14). They can detect abnormality, if any, but cannot exactly locate the site of lesion.

The VEPs primarily represent the activity originating in the central 3° to 6° of visual field that is relayed to the visual cortex (area 17). (Impulses from peripheral retina project to the visual cortex buried in the calcarine fissure).

Photic stimulation by black and white checkered board, or vertical grating at rates of 1,3,6,10,20 flashes per second is employed. One eye is tested at a time, and standard disc EEG recording electrodes at Oz, Fpz, and Cz (See Expt 2-29 for location of these electrodes) are employed. A series of waveforms of opposite polarity, i.e., N (negative) and P (positive) are recorded and their latency, duration, and amplitude determined and evaluated.

SOMATOSENSORY EVOKED POTENTIALS (SEPS)

In humans, event- related, "far field somatosensory evoked potentials" are simultaneously recorded from several electrodes placed over the popliteal fossa, lumbar and thoracic vertebrae (spinal evoked potentials), and over the parietal region of the opposite side.

The SEPs are generated mainly by the large diameter (12-20 μm) fibers in response to repeated stimuli applied to them anywhere along their course in peripheral nerves, or in ascending tracts in CNS. (Large fibers carry mainly proprioceptive impulses, while small diameter fibers (0.5 μm) carry pain and temperature).

Though SEPs can be obtained by stimulation of any large peripheral nerve; in clinical practice they are generally recorded from median nerve (median SEPs) and the posterior tibial nerve (tibial SEPs). The method can prove useful in the evaluation of spinal defects such as multiple sclerosis, spinal injuries, etc.

MOTOR EVOKED POTENTIALS (MEPS)

Sensory evoked potentials (auditory, visual, and somatosensory) are recorded from the scalp or from sensory pathways after sensory stimulation. The motor evoked potentials, on the other hand, are recorded from target muscles as EMG following stimulation of motor cortex or spinal cord.

The stimuli used may be electrical or magnetic. Since electrical transcranial stimuli can be painful, magnetic stimuli are applied over the vertex, and cervical and lumbar regions. The target muscles include deltoid, biceps, thenar muscles, tibialis anterior, and abductor hallucis brevis.

A very important precaution is to ensure that the subject is not using a cardiac pacemaker, a cochlear implant, or has a history of epilepsy.

2-34

Electro-neuro Diagnostic Tests
The Hoffmann's Reflex (H-Reflex)

INTRODUCTION

Tendon jerks or deep reflexes (tested clinically) are reflex contractions of skeletal muscles in response to stimulation of their stretch receptors located in their muscle spindles. The stimulus is the sudden stretch of their muscle spindles that sends impulses via IA (Aα) afferents to the spinal cord where they stimulate the AHC that supply the muscle.

The H-reflex is the electrical equivalent of a tendon jerk. It confirms the integrity of the reflex pathway.

Equipment

• CRO • Electronic stimulator • Stimulating and recording electrodes • Swabs moist with alcohol or ether.

PROCEDURE

1. Apply the stimulating electrodes on the skin over the tibial nerve behind the knee, and recording electrodes on the skin overlying soleus muscle in the calf region.
2. Apply a minimum strength of stimulus. Since the threshold of stimulation of Ia sensory fibers is much lower compared to motor fiber, the H-wave (H-reflex) will be recorded, as shown in **Figure 2-21**. It has a long latency because the Ia signals are conducted orthodromically (arrow 1) to monosynaptically stimulate AHC that innervate soleus.
3. Increase the strength of stimulus to stimulate both sensory and motor fibers. Note that two responses are recorded from the muscle. The first waveform is the *'M wave'* resulting from

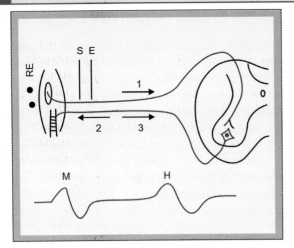

Figure 2-21. Recording of H-reflex. SE: stimulating electrodes on skin over tibial nerve; RE: recording electrodes on skin over the muscle. M: M-wave due to direct (orthodromic) stimulation of muscle. H-wave: due to H-reflex

direct stimulation of motor fibers (arrow 2), while the second response is the *'H-wave'* due to H-reflex resulting from excitation of Ia sensory fibers.

4. Increase the strength of stimulus still further, and note that the H-wave gradually decreases and then disappears, leaving only the M-wave. The APs in motor nerves, in addition to normal orthodromic conduction towards the muscle, are also conducted antidromically (arrow 3) to cause depolarization of AHC so that when Ia signals arrive they find the motor neurons refractory—thus cancelling their reflex response.

Note

Two clinical signs are associated with Hoffmann's name:

Hoffmann's sign. Flicking the distal phalanx of the index finger causes clawing movement of fingers and thumb. This response in the upper limb is equivalent to the Babinski response in the sole of the foot in UMN lesions.

Hoffmann's sign of tetany. Electrical or mechanical stimulation of a sensory nerve produces muscle spasm. (The ulnar nerve is usually selected for this test in parathyroid tetany).

2-35

Study of Human Fatigue Mosso's Ergography

The **erg** is the unit of work and **ergoraph** is the apparatus used for recording voluntary contractions of skeletal muscle in humans. The Mosso's ergograph is employed not only to assess the performance of hand and forearm muscles but also to study the phenomenon of fatigue and the factors that affect fatigue.

EQUIPMENT

1. Mosso's Ergograph. It consists of a flat wooden board with 2 pairs of clamps and curved plates to fix, hold, and steady the forearm of the subject **(Figure 2-22)**. There is a pair of metal tubes into which index and ring fingers are inserted. The middle finger remains free to be connected to a thick cord and hook.

A sliding plate that can move to and fro carries a lever system to record muscle exertions on a kymograph cylinder. A sling fits over the middle finger, and a strong cord bearing a hook on which different weights can be hung. (In some cases the sliding plate can carry a chart paper on which a

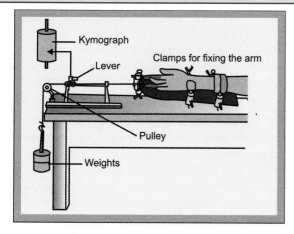

Figure 2-22. Mosso's ergograph

pencil or ballpoint pen can record the contractions).

2. Metronome. It is a clockwork device that functions as a 'variable interrupter' to deliver "tick tock" sounds at a pre-selected frequency of up to 200/minute. There is a thin metal rod bearing a scale on which a sliding clip can set the desired frequency. (The metronome is commonly used to provide "beats" during training in piano playing).

PROCEDURES

1. Place the ergograph on a table such that the weight will hang down over its edge. Explain the procedure to the subject and seat her/him beside the table.

2. Fix the forearm on the ergogrph, and insert the index and ring fingers in the finger holders. With the middle finger extended and the string with the cord attached to it, adjust the position of the forearm and fingers so that the subject is comfortable. Apply a weight of 1-2 Kg on the hook.

3. Ask the subject to flex the middle finger and check that the system works freely.

4. Adjust the beat of the metronome at 30/minute, i.e., one beat every 2 seconds, and set it oscillating. Ask the subject to contract the flexor muscles maximally and

rhythmically, following each beat of the metronome, and to continue (without moving the shoulders) until fatigue is so great that the weight can no longer be lifted.

5. *Motivation*: Give a rest for 15 minutes and then repeat the whole procedure, telling the subject that she/he will do much better this time.

6. *Effect of venous occlusion.* After another rest period, apply the BP cuff on the upper arm and raise the pressure to 40 mm Hg to stop venous return. Repeat the whole procedure. Fatigue sets in earlier because of accumulation of waste products in the exercising muscles.

7. *Effect of arterial occlusion.* After another period of rest, raise the blood pressure to about 160-170 mm Hg to stop arterial blood flow. Tell the subject to repeat the muscle contractions. Fatigue sets in much earlier now because there is not only an accumulation of waste products but also a deficiency of oxygen and other nutrients.

Calculation of work done: Calculate the work done in each case as shown below:

Work done (in Kg meters) = Weight lifted × Distance

The distance through which the weight is lifted is the sum of all the heights of contractions, converted to meters.

Comments

Fatigue is defined as a temporary and reversible loss of the physiological property of contraction of skeletal muscles. There is also a subjective feeling of tiredness so that the onset of fatigue can be somewhat delayed by motivation. With rest however, fatigue is completely reversible.

Factors that Affect Onset of Fatigue

The degree, duration and type of work done is the important factors that in general affect the onset of fatigue.

1. The weight to be lifted.
2. Frequency of contractions.
3. Motivation.
4. Blood supply to contracting muscles.
5. Training.
6. Obesity.
7. Environmental factors such as temperature, humidity and pollution affect the onset of fatigue.

QUESTIONS

Q.1 Define the term fatigue. What are the factors that affect the onset of fatigue?
See above.

Q.2 How does motivation improve muscular performance?
Encouragement improves performance for a short time. This shows that cerebral cortex is involved in fatigue in humans. In sports physiology, motivation plays an important role in enhancing performance.

Q. 3 How will you demonstrate the site of fatigue in an intact muscle?
After the flexors of the fingers are fatigued, they will still contract on peripheral nerve stimulation. This will show that fatigue is a "central" phenomenon involving synapses.

Q. 4 How does fatigue in this experiment compare with fatigue in frog's nerve-muscle preparation?
In frog's preparation (Expt 4-9), there is no blood supply. Hence fatigue sets in early. Also, the seat of fatigue is neuromuscular junction. In the present experiment, the seat of fatigue appears to be a central phenomenon.

Q. 5 Name a condition where venous or arterial occlusion can impair muscular performance.
In thrombosis of leg veins due to thrombophlebitis, the venous return is decreased so that fatigue sets in early. Arterial occlusion occurs in Buerger's disease (said to be due to chronic smoking); there is pain while walking. The narrowed vessels cannot keep pace with increased demands of muscles for oxygen. In coronary artery disease, the ischemic muscle pain has a similar mechanism.

2-36

Autonomic Nervous System (ANS) Tests (Autonomic Function Tests; AFTs)

INTRODUCTION

1. The term *autonomic nervous system* (ANS) was suggested by Langley over 100 years ago for that part of the nervous system that controls visceral activities, i.e., cardiac muscle, smooth muscle, and glands. Most visceral activities are not under our control (hence called autonomic) and cannot be easily altered or suppressed.
2. The main input to ANS is via autonomic sensory nerves from interoreceptors (stretch receptors, chemoreceptors, etc) in blood vessels, and viscera that monitor the internal environment. Mostly, these signals are not consciously perceived.
3. The ANS excites or inhibits visceral structures in response to its continuous sensory input.
4. *Organization of ANS.* Like the somatic nervous system, the ANS is also organized on the basis of reflex, arc.
   a. *Afferent neuron*: Its cell body is in the DRG, the peripheral process being

connected to sensory receptors while the central process enters the spinal cord to synapse with the connector neuron.

b. *Center:* It consists of a connector neuron, the cell body being located in the lateral gray column of the spinal cord (or the visceral components of III, VII, IX, and X cranial nerves). Its axon terminates in a ganglion situated outside the CNS (paravertebral ganglia in sympathetic system (SS) and near or in the viscera in parasympathetic system (PSS).

c. *Efferent pathway.* While somatic efferent pathway consists of a single motor neuron (AHC), the visceral efferent pathway has 2 neurons—preganglionic and post-ganglionic neurons.

5. *Divisions of ANS.* Depending on the anatomical location of connector or preganglionic neurons, the ANS is divided into **cranio-sacral (parasympathetic)** and **thoraco-lumbar (sympathetic)** components (**Figure 2-23**).

6. The preganglionic fibers in both systems are myelinated and cholinergic, while the postganglionic fibers are non-myelinated cholinergic in parasympathetic division and nor-adrenergic in sympathetic division, except those supplying sweat glands and blood vessels in skeletal muscles, which are cholinergic.

7. The parasympathetic system conserves and stores energy and is anabolic while the sympathetic system is catabolic and prepares the body for emergency situations.

8. The effects of PSS are localized and short-lived, the effects of SS are prolonged and widespread.

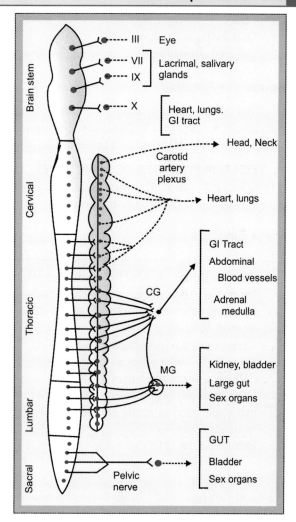

Figure 2-23. Diagram to show the efferent pathways of the autonomic nervous system. The preganglionic neurons are shown as solid lines, postganglionic neurons as dashed lines. CG: celiac ganglion; MG: mesenteric ganglion

AUTONOMIC FUNCTION TESTS

A. TESTS FOR SYMPATHETIC FUNCTIONS

1. QT: QS2 ratio.
2. Sympathetic skin response (SSR).
3. Cold pressor response (CPR).
4. Handgrip test (BP response to isometric exercise).

B. TESTS FOR PARASYMPATHETIC FUNCTIONS

1. Standing test (30:15 RR ratio).
2. Standing to lying ratio (SL ratio).
3. Valsalva ratio test.
4. Tachycardia ratio.
5. Deep breathing test.

Other tests
1. Tests for papillary function.
2. Test for lacrimation.

Equipment Required

ECG machine • BP apparatus • Multichannel polygraph • CRO • Electrodes • Electronic stimulator • EMG machine and preamplifier.

A. TESTS FOR SYMPATHETIC FUNCTIONS

1. **QT-QS 2 ratio.** This test is an index of sympathetic excitation of the heart.

Procedure

1. Ask the subject to lie down supine on the couch and relax. Attach ECG leads, and place the contact microphone on the carotid artery to record heart sounds (phonocardiogram).
2. Record lead II of ECG, and PCG simultaneously at a paper speed of 50 mm/sec.
3. Measure QT interval from the beginning of QRS complex to the end of T wave. Measure QS-2 from the beginning of QRS to the first major vibration of aortic component of 2nd heart sound in PCG.
   Determine the QT/QS-2 ratio.

Comments
QS-2 is the total electromechanical systolic interval. A high value indicates greater sympathetic tone while a low value represents low sympathetic tone.

2. **Sympathetic Skin Response (SSR)**

Rationale

The sweat glands distributed over the entire body are innervated by sympathetic postganglionic cholinergic fibers (except in palms and soles which are innervated by noradrenergic sympathetic fibers). The stratum corneum of the skin, which is punctured by the ducts of sweat glands, offers maximum resistance to the passage of current through the skin. However, when the sweat glands are activated, the ducts get filled with sweat (which is an electrolyte), so that an electric current can easily pass through the skin due to a fall in skin resistance.

Change in skin potential in response to stimuli causing sympathetic activation is called sympathetic skin response (SSR). It is also called galvanic skin response.

Procedure

An EMG machine and a CRO are generally adequate to record the response to application of current. However, a polygraph may be used.

1. Set the preamplifier to GSR and EMG machine: Frequency response = 0.1 to 1000 Hz; gain= 0.5 mV/div, and set the sweep to record 5 seconds after the stimulus.
2. After cleaning the skin and applying small amounts of paste, place the active electrode (disc type) on the palm (or sole of foot), reference electrode on the dorsum of the hand (or foot), with the ground electrode between the two.
3. Apply a constant current of 5 microamperes, and note the response and calculate its latency and amplitude. Estimate the skin resistance in millivolts from the recording pen deflection (The deflection resulting from 1 mV to the amplifier is equal to a resistance change to 10 k-ohm).
4. Give a stimulus in the form of startling sound (say, a sudden hand clap near the head of the subject) and record the response i.e., the SSR potentials, their latency and amplitude. (The stimulus will activate the sympathetic system).

Note
The SSR may be mono-, di-, or triphasic and the potentials may be 1.1-1.5 mV in amplitude and about 1.5 sec in latency in the hands and 0.7 – 0.9 mV and 2.0-2.5 sec in the feet. Abnormal SSR is usually seen in progressive autonomic dysfunction.

3. Cold Presser response

Rationale

Physical or mental stress causes stimulation of sympathetic system. Plunging a hand in cold water acts as a pain stimulus and causes rise in blood pressure. (Since this test is somewhat unpleasant, it is done at the end of ANS testing).

1. Explain the test to the subject and seat him/her in a chair; record the baseline blood pressure.
2. Ask the subject to immerse one hand in cold water at 4-5°C for 2 minutes. Record the BP from the other arm at 30 sec intervals.
3. Note the maximum increase in systolic and diastolic pressures and compare with the pre-test readings. The SP may increase by 20 mm Hg, while the DP rises by 10 mm Hg.

Results

Reduced sympathetic activity is indicated by a smaller rise of BP. In some normal persons, there may be no significant rise in BP.

4. Handgrip Test (Isometric exercise)

Sustained handgrip causes a rise in HR and BP. An ECG machine, a sphygmomanometer, and a hand-grip spring dynamometer will be required for this test.

1. Apply the BP cuff on the non-exercising arm, and lead II of ECG for recording heart rate. Record the resting BP and HR at 30 sec intervals for 4 minutes. Then ask the subject to hold the dynamometer in the dominant hand and take a full grip on it.
2. Ask the subject to exert maximum force and note the maximum tension developed. Repeat 3 times at intervals of 2 minutes. Take the highest reading and note it as *maximum isometric tension (T max).*
3. Now ask the subject to maintain a tension of 30% of T max for 5 minutes. During this procedure record the BP and ECG at 30 sec intervals.

4. Note the diastolic BP (DBP) at the point just before the release of handgrip.
5. Note the mean resting value of DBP readings during the last 3 minutes before starting the exercise.

Results

The rise in DBP in normal subjects is more than 15 mm Hg but less than 10 mm Hg in sympathetic insufficiency.

B. TESTS FOR PARASYMPATHETIC FUNCTION
1. Standing test (30:15 RR ratio)

Rationale

Upon sudden standing from supine, there is pooling of blood in the lower parts of the body. This is followed by a sequence of events: fall of venous return → decrease in cardiac output and BP → decreased baroreceptor activity → increase in sympathetic tone and decrease in para-sympathetic activity. This causes reflex increase in heat rate and peripheral vasoconstriction, after which the heart rate falls.

Thus, heart rate rises immediately on standing and continues to rise for the next 15-20 seconds, after which it slows down to a maximum degree as a result of variations in vagal tone.

Procedure

1. Ask the subject to lie supine on the couch and relax for 15 minutes. Apply ECG leads and the BP cuff (or the wrist BP monitor).
2. Record ECG (lead II) for noting heart rate, and blood pressure. Then ask the subject to stand (without support i.e., leaning against the wall), and remain motionless for 3 minutes, recording the ECG continuously. Record BP at the end of 1st and 3rd minutes after standing. Mark the point of standing on the ECG paper.
3. Calculate the HR from R-R interval at 15th beat (fastest HR; shortest R-R interval) and at

30th beat (slowest HR; longest R-R interval) after standing.

4. Determine the 30:15 ratio, which is considered a cardiac vagal effect. Normal value is > 1.04. An R-R ratio of less than 1.0 indicates autonomic insufficiency.

5. In normal persons, the fall in SBP on standing should not be more than 10 mm hg.
   • In orthostatic hypotension, the SBP and DBP fall more than 20 mm Hg and 10 mm Hg.
   • In vasovagal syncope, hypotension is accompanied by paradoxical bradycardia because cardiac vagal supply is over-active.

Note
Similar responses can be better studied by passively tilting the subject on a tilt-table from supine position to an inclination of 80° (head up) for a period of 3-4 minutes.

2. Standing to Lying Ratio (S/L ratio)

Rationale

When a normal person lies down from a standing position, there is at first a rise in HR which is followed by a slowing of the heart. This rise and fall of HR is due to changes in vagal tone.

Procedure

1. Explain the procedure to the subject. Connect ECG leads for recording lead II. Ask the subject to stand quietly for 2 minutes and then to lie down supine without any support.

2. Record ECG for 20 beats before and for 60 beats after lying down. Note the point of change of position on the ECG paper.

3. Repeat 3 times at intervals of 5 minutes.

4. **Calculation of S/L ratio.** Take the average R-R interval during 5 beats before lying down and shortest R-R interval during 10 beats after lying down. The maximum ratio of the 3 trials

is reported. Any abnormally low ratio indicates parasympathetic insufficiency.

3. Valsalva Ratio

Valsalva maneuver (effort) is forced expiration against a closed glottis. This straining, associated with changes in HR and BP, is a simple test for baroreceptor activity.

Procedure

1. Seat the subject on a stool and explain the procedure. Connect ECG leads and BP cuff to him/her, and close the nostrils with a nose-clip.

2. Disconnect the cuff from another BP apparatus and ask the subject to take a deep breath, blow into the manometer and maintain the pressure a 40 mm Hg for 15 seconds.(recall the 40 mm Hg test for lung functions).

3. Record ECG (lead II) for 1 minute before the straining, for 15 seconds during straining, and for 45 seconds after the release of strain. It may also be calculated as the ratio of longest RR interval after the strain to the shortest RR during the strain.

Observations

During straining there is decrease in venous return, fall in cardiac output, and BP, inhibition of baroreceptors, followed by tachycardia and vasoconstriction. The HR increases throughout straining due to vagal inhibition initially and sympathetic activation later.

At the release of strain, there is a transient fall of BP without significant change in heart rate. After this, the BP slowly rises with decrease of HR. These, in turn, stimulate barorecceptors causing bradycardia and drop in BP to normal levels. The maximum valsalva ratio of 3 trials is taken as the index of autonomic activity. A ratio of greater than 1.45 is normal, 1.20 to 1.45 is borderline, and less than 1.20 indicates autonomic disturbance.

Clinical Significance

Failure of HR to increase during straining suggests sympathetic insufficiency, while failure of HR to slow down after the effort suggests a parasympathetic insufficiency.

4. Tachycardia Ratio

This ratio is related to Valsalva ratio and is defined as the ratio of shortest RR interval during valsalva effort to the longest RR interval before the effort. It is believed to be a better index of vagal activity.

5. Deep Breathing Test

The HR increases during inspiration (due to decreased cardiac vagal activity) , and decreases during expiration (due to increased vagal activity). This is a normal phenomenon and is called *sinus arrhythmia.*

Procedure

There are two methods to show the effect of breathing on heart rate. In one method, a single deep breath is taken and its effect noted. In the other method, the subject breathes deeply for 1 minute.

1. Explain the procedure to the subject, and ask him to lie down supine and relax, with the head raised to 30^0.
2. Attach the ECG leads for recording lead II. Then ask the subject to breathe deeply and slowly at a rate of 6 breaths per minute, with 5 seconds for inspiration and 5 seconds for expiration. Record ECG before and during deep breathing.
3. Determine the maximum and minimum heart rate with each respiratory cycle and note the average HR in inspiration and in expiration.
4. Calculate the expiration to inspiration ratio (E: I ratio). This is the mean of maximum RR intervals during expiration (slow heart rate) to the mean of minimum RR intervals during deep inspiration (Fast HR).
6. In normal persons, the fall in HR should be > 15 beats/min. In vagal insufficiency the HR slows < 10 beats/minute.

C. OTHER TESTS

The smooth muscle of the iris and ciliary body are supplied by both SS and PSS nerve fibers. Sympathetic activity causes papillary dilation while parasympathetic activity causes papillary constriction, accommodation, lacrimation, and salivation.

1. TEST FOR PUPILLARY FUNCTION

Denervation Hypersensitivity

This is the phenomenon in which an effector tissue (muscle, in this case) becomes hypersensitive to a neurotransmitter 2-3 weeks after denervation of that tissue.

i. Put a drop or two of 0.125% pilocarpine drops in the eye of the subject. Normally, this causes minimal papillary constriction. In parasympathetic denervation, there is a strong constriction of the pupil.
ii. In a similar way, 2-3 drops of 0.1% solution of epinephrine put 3 times in the eye at 1-minute intervals causes minimal dilatation of the pupil. But in sympathetic denervation, there is strong papillary dilatation. (Checked at 15, 30, and 45 minutes).

2. TEST FOR LACRIMATION (Schirmer's test)

Take a strip of filter paper, 25 mm long and 5 mm wide, and place its one end between the lower eyelid and sclera, allowing its other end to hang down over the cheek.

Measure the length of its wetting after 5 minutes. In normal persons, the filter paper wets by about 15 mm while less than 10 mm suggests parasympathetic insufficiency.

Unit V
Reproductive System

Semen Analysis

Relevance

Semen (spermatic fluid) is studied for sterility, i.e., the inability of a male to impregnate a normal female. It is a routine test to determine if the sterility is due to a defect in the semen. Study of semen is also done to confirm the completeness of vasectomy, a procedure commonly adopted for controlling birth.

Characteristics of Normal Semen and Comments

A sample of semen collected after 2-3 days of sexual abstinence has the following features:

Volume

Normal volume is 2.5 - 5 ml. It decreases in functional disorders, or inflammation of the male genital tract.

Physical Characteristics

White, opalescent, mucoid, sticky.

pH

7.2- 7.7. The alkaline pH brings the vaginal pH of 3.5-4.5 to about 6-6.5, the pH at which sperms show maximum motility.

Morphology

Normal sperms are actively motile. They are one of the smallest cells (5-6 μm), in contrast to an ovum, which is the largest cell of the body (about 120 μm). They have a head, neck, body, and tail.

Abnormalities in shape include: bifid or absent heads, bifurcated tails, etc. If present in more than 70% of sperms, it indicates some pathology.

Motility

More than 80% sperms show a good forward motility due to "flail-like" movements of their tails. More than 70% of sperms in a specimen should show active motility within 3 hours of collection of specimen. Less than 40% motile sperms indicate sterility.

Count

Normal count is 60-120 million/ml; with an average of 100 million/ml. Counts between 20-40 million/ml indicate borderline infertility. Counts below 20 million/ml indicate sterility.

Clotting and Liquefaction

Normal semen clots within 5 minutes of ejaculation (due to fibrinogen and other clotting proteins) but undergoes secondary liquefaction due to the presence and activation of plasmin and other proteolytic enzymes, such as prostate specific antigen (PSA), pepsinogen, hyaluronidase, and amylase

Fructose

Normal semen contains fructose. It is used by sperms for production of ATP via Kreb's cycle.

- Also present are: calcium, citric acid, clotting proteins different from those of blood clotting, hyaluronidae, acid phosphatase, and prostaglandins.

Principle of sperm counting. Semen is collected from the subject, diluted 20 times in a WBC pipette and the sperms are counted in a Neubauer chamber.

Apparatus and Materials

1. Microscope • Improved Neubauer chamber • WBC pipette • Cover slips • Slides • Plasticine.
2. Diluting fluid: 5%sodium bicarbonate. In 1.0% phenol.

PROCEDURES

1. Collect a fresh sample of semen (after two days of abstinence) in a petri dish or a small beaker.
2. Wait for 25-30 minutes for secondary liquefaction. Observe if the liquefaction is uniform. Measure its volume.
3. *Assessing sperm motility.* Place a drop of semen on a cover slip and invert it on the rim of a small circle of plasticine previously made on a slide. Examine under low- and, high-

power and watch the motility of sperms. Try to assess the percentage of motile to non-motile sperms. Also note their morphology.

4. **Counting the sperms.** Gently shake the sample to assure uniformity.
   i. Draw semen to 0.5 mark in the WBC pipette, then draw the diluting fluid to the mark 11. Mix the contents of the bulb for 2-3 minutes.
   ii. Discard the first few drops, then charge the counting chamber and count the sperms under high power in the 4 WBC squares, as was done for TLC.
5. Calculation
   Number of sperms in 64 squares (volume= $4/10$ mm^3) = N
   Then number of sperms in 1 mm^3 of undiluted semen = N x 10/4 x 20
   To get sperm count in 1 ml = N x 50 x 1000
   Normal count = 60–120 million/ml
   Report: Morphology.............
   Count: .... million/ml.

QUESTIONS

Q.1 What is semen? Where are sperms formed?
Semen (or seed) is a mixture of spermatozoa and a liquid consisting of the secretions of seminiferous tubules, seminal vesicles, prostate and bulbourethral glands. The liquid part provides nourishment and a transport system.

About 60 million sperms are manufactured daily in about 1000 seminiferous tubules in each testis, each tubule being 50-60 cm long. Leydig cells of testis secrete testosterone, the male sex hormone that promotes spermatogenesis, in addition to primary and secondary 'male' sex characteristics.

Q. 2 What are the indications for sperm analysis?
Semen is examined for 3 main purposes:
i. To determine whether a male is fertile or not.
ii. In the investigation of genetic disorders like cryptorchidism and Klinefelter's syndrome.

iii. To diagnose inflammatory or neoplastic diseases of the genital tract.

Q. 3 What is the composition of semen? Name some features of the sperms.
See page 248.

Q. 4 Why is abstinence advised for 2 days before collecting a sample of semen?
Since the volume and sperm count of semen decrease rapidly with frequent ejaculations, it might give a misleading low-count result if this precaution is not taken.

Q. 5 What is he significance of clotting and liquefaction of semen?
These two features of semen—clotting and secondary liquefaction— appear to play a biological role: the initial coagulation helps to retain semen in the vagina, while the subsequent liquefaction aids the sperms to swim up the female genital tract.

Q. 6 When is a male considered infertile?
The male infertility (or sterility) is the inability of a person to fertilize a secondary oocyte. It may be due to a low sperm count (<20 million/ml), or a high percentage of non-motile or abnormal sperms.

Infertility should not be confused with impotence (erectile dysfunction), i.e., inability to perform the sexual act.

Q. 7 For how long can sperms remain capable of fertilization in the female genital tract?
The maximum duration of fertilization capacity of normal sperms varies between 24 hours and 48 hours.

Q. 8 Define the terms oligospermia, azoospermia and necrospermia.
Oligospermia refers to a count less than 20 million/ml, azoospermia means total absence of sperms, and necrospermia refers to dead (non-living) sperms in the semen.

Q.9 When only one sperm is required for the fertilization of ovum, why has nature provided such a huge number of sperms?
The large and extravagant excess of sperms appears to be a reminder of (and a 'fall-back' on) life's origin in the sea. Some fish simply spray their sperms into water on the off chance that a drifting egg will be fertilized.

Q. 10 What is vasectomy and why is it done? For how long sperms may appear in the semen after bilateral vasectomy?
Vasectomy is the chief method for *the sterilization of males* by a simple surgical operation. Incisions are given on each side of scrotum, vas deferens are located, and a piece is removed from each. Sexual desire and performance are not affected since testosterone secretion continues normally. Sperm production also continues but they cannot reach outside. In time, they degenerate and are removed by macrophages.

For the first 2 months after vasectomy, viable sperms may be released from their storage in ampullae of seminal vesicles.

Note
Though 'recanulization' of the ducts is possible, the chances of regaining fertility are very slim.

2-38

Pregnancy Diagnostic Tests

Most of the laboratory tests for pregnancy are based on the detection of the presence of human chorionic gonadotropins (HCG) in the woman's urine. Some tests are so sensitive that the earliest diagnosis of pregnancy can be made within a few days of the conception, i.e., even before the next missed period. These tests can be grouped into *biological, immunological*, and *radiological*.

I. BIOLOGICAL DIAGNOSTIC TESTS

These tests, which involve injection of urine into various animals, are time consuming and costly. They are, however, 99% accurate.

1. *Aschheim-Zondek mouse test:* Urine is injected subcutaneously into immature mice. Appearance of blood-filled ovulated follicles on 5th day confirms pregnancy.
2. *Friedman rabbit test:* Intravenous injection of urine into virgin female rabits causes ovulation in 18 hours.
3. *Galli Mainini frog test:* Injection of urine into the dorsal lymph sac of male frogs or toads causes shedding of sperms in about 3 hours.
4. *Hogben test.* Adult female toads are used in this test. Injection of urine into the lymph space causes ovulation within 18 hours.

II. IMMUNOLOGICAL TESTS

Principle

The HCG (human chorionic gonadotropins) secreted by syncytiotrophoblast cells of placenta is antigenic and antibodies against this hormone can be produced by injecting it into rabbits. These antibodies are available commercially and are employed to detect the presence of HCG in the subject's urine or serum by precipitation, hemaggluination, or complement fixation, etc.

Procedures

Collection of urine. The sensitivity level of HCG in urine is 1.5-3.5 IU/ml in slide test and 0.2-1.2 IU/ml in test tube test. This concentration is reached by 10th day of fertilization (i.e., even before the missed period). The subject is advised to restrict water intake for 12-14 hours, and urine is collected in a clean container in the morning. The specific gravity of urine should be at least 1.015 and it should be free from protein and blood.

A. Latex Agglutination Inhibition (LAI) Test. (Gravindex test)

Basis of test. Small globules of latex (rubber) particles coated with pure HCG, and antiserum to HCG, are available commercially in 'kit' form. A sample of urine is treated with antiserum on a glass slide placed against a black background.

- If the urine contains HCG (i.e., if the woman is pregnant), then the antibodies in the antiserum are all "used up". Then if the coated latex particles are added, they do not get agglutinated.
  Urine (HCG present) + Antiserum + Latex particles = No agglutination.
  Therefore, **"No agglutination"** means a positive result, i.e., the woman is pregnant.
- If the urine sample does not contain HCG, then the antibodies in the antiserum "remain free". Then if latex particles are added, antigen-antibody reaction occurs and the particles get agglutinated.
  Urine (HCG absent) + Antiserum + latex particles = Agglutination.

Therefore, **"agglutination"** means a negative result, i.e., the woman is not pregnant.

B. Hemagglutination Inhibition (HAI) Test (Prognostican test)

In this test, sheep's RBCs coated with HCG are employed in place of latex particles. The test is done in a test tube and observations are made after 2 hours. The principle is the same as LAI.

C. One-step immunoassay test. This test is based on the combination of monoclonal antibody-dye conjugate with polyclonal solid phase antibodies for the qualitative detection of HCG in the urine. A sample of urine is applied to the TEST zone of the card or strip, and if it contains HCG, a pink-purple colored band develops. A control is provided to check the potency of the test reagents. A number of test kits under different proprietary names are available.

D. Radioimmunoassay (RIA)

HCG radio-labeled with iodine (iodine ^{135}) is treated with fixed amounts of antibodies and the urine/serum sample. The method is much more sensitive and can detect as little as 0.003 IU/ml of beta subunit and 0.001 IU/ml of alpha subunit of HCG in the specimen.

E. ELISA (Enzyme Linked Immuno Sorbent Assay)

Elisa has been widely used to detect a variety of antigens and antibodies. The principle of the test is the same as that of RAI except that an enzyme is used in place of a radioactive substance. The enzyme acts on the substrate to produce blue color which is a positive test for pregnancy.

III. ULTRASONOGRAPHY

Pulses of ultrasonic waves at high frequency are generated from a piezo-electric crystal transducer that also acts as a receiver to detect waves reflected back from various parts of the uterus. The echoes (reflected waves) are displayed on the ultrasound screen.

It is the most reliable method for detecting pregnancy. The gestational ring is evident as early as 5th week of pregnancy, cardiac pulsations by 10th week, and fetal movements by 11th week.

The method is particularly useful in detecting fetal viability and position, site of placenta, multiple pregnancy, and fetal-maternal abnormalities etc. The method, however, is being used for the determination of sex of the fetus. If the fetus is a female, many parents get the fetus aborted by unscrupulous doctors.

QUESTIONS

Q. 1 What is the principle underlying biological tests for pregnancy?
See above.

Q. 2 What is the physiological basis of immunological tests for pregnancy?
See above.

Q. 3 Why are immunological tests preferred over biological tests?
Immunological tests are used routinely in all hospitals and clinics. Compared to biological tests, they are less costly , simpler and easy to carry out, take very little time for reporting, and can confirm pregnancy within 10 days of conception.

Q. 4 What are the conditions in which false positive and false negative results may be obtained?
False positive results. These may be obtained due to excessive protein or blood in the urine sample, or at menopause, or at the time of ovulation due to increased secretion of LH. Such a result can also be seen in benign or malignant tumors of the placenta. Drugs such as thiazide, diuretics and steroids my affect early pregnancy tests.

False negative results. Such results may be seen when the concentration of HCG in urine/serum is very low (though the woman is pregnant), or testing too soon, or due to an ectopic pregnancy.

Q. 5 What is the chief advantage of ultrasound method?
See above.

Q. 6 What is the utility of pregnancy tests?

1. Use in diagnosing pregnancy.
2. The tests are also employed in detecting hydatidiform mole (a benign tumor of placenta), and chorioepitheliom (carcinoma of placenta). Repeated tests in these conditions show a high and rising concentration of HCG (the urine diluted 1 in 500 may give a positive test) while in normal pregnancy, the HCG titer falls by 12th week.
3. They are employed in assessing and planning the course of action in cases of repeated abortions.

Q. 7 Name the hormones released from the placenta during pregnancy. What are their chief functions?

1. **HCG.** The most important function of HCG is to prevent degeneration of corpus luteum (which occurs about 2 weeks after ovulation) and maintain its viability. This allows it to continue to secrete estrogens and progesterone—an activity required to prevent menstruation and for continued attachment of embryo and fetus to the uterine endometrium.

HCG is now used for maintenance of pregnancy in women with history of repeated abortions. It is also used for stimulating the release of ova that can be collected and later employed for *in vitro* fertilization (for the so-called "test tube babies").

2. **HCS (Human Chorionic Somatomammotropin;** also called **"human placental lactogen, HPL).**

The rate of secretion of HCS reaches maximum levels after 32 weeks and remains high after that. It prepares mammary glands for lactation, increases protein synthesis in the fetus and its growth, causes retention of nitrogen, calcium and potassium.

3. **Estrogens.** These are secreted by corpus luteum in early stages of pregnancy but placenta becomes the major site of estrogen secretion. Important effects are enlargement of uterus and breasts, protein anabolic effects including building of strong bones, and relaxation of pelvic ligaments for facilitating birth at term.

4. **Progesterone.** It is secreted by corpus luteum during early pregnancy and maintains pregnancy. From 4-9 months, placental progesterone increases. It relaxes uterine muscle by decreasing spontaneous movements and helps in continuation of pregnancy, and promotes growth of alveoli in breasts.

5. **Relaxin.** Secreted from placenta, it relaxes uterus and helps in continuation of pregnancy. In later pregnancy, it relaxes pubic symphysis and dilates uterine cervix to facilitate delivery.

6. **CRH (corticotropin-releasing hormone).** This hormone (normally secreted by anterior pituitary), has recently been shown to be part of the "clock" that establishes the timing of delivery. Its secretion begins at about 12 weeks and greatly increases towards the end of pregnancy. It also increases the secretion of cortisol that is required for the maturation of lungs and secretion of lung surfactant in the fetus.

Q. 8 What is amenorrhea and what are its causes?

Amenorrhea (a- = without; men- = month; -rrhea = flow). The term refers to absence of menstruation, the most common causes being pregnancy and menopause (the latter occurs at age 45-50 years).

In vigorous and competitive women athletes, amenorrhea results from reduced gonadotropin-releasing hormones (GnRH) from the hypothalamus, and thus, LH and FSH from the anterior pituitary. The result is a failure of development of ova and stoppage of ovulation. Low body weight, and low body fat (and low levels of leptin secretion by adipose cells) may be a contributing factor.

Short periods of amenorrhea my be harmless, but long-lasting disruption of reproductive function may cause loss of bone density that is a part of the "female athlete triad" of osteoporosis, disordered eating, and amenorrhea.

2-39

Birth Control Methods

Birth control is the procedure employed to restrict the number of children by various methods that control fertility and prevent pregnancy. **Contraceptives** are temporary or permanent measures employed to prevent pregnancy in spite of sexual intercourse.

With the explosion of population in our country, various methods of planning a small family have been in vogue for the last many decades. However, there is no single, ideal method of preventing pregnancy. The only method of preventing pregnancy with 100% surety is total abstinence, i.e., avoidance of sexual intercourse.

Birth control methods are employed not only for limiting the number of children but also for the spacing of pregnancies because repeated pregnancies pose danger not only to the health of the mother, but also to that of the offspring.

The requirements of different couples vary, so that one or more of the following methods may be recommended.

I. Methods Based on Physiological Principles

1. *Rhythm Method ("Safe Period"; Periodic Abstinence).* Normally, only one viable ovum is released per menstrual cycle and it remains viable for about 24 hours, while the sperms, after entering the uterus survive for about 48 hours. Thus, there is a minimum period of 3 days during which intercourse must be avoided to prevent pregnancy.

For this method to be effective, the time of ovulation must be known. In most women who have regular periods, ovulation usually occurs *14 days before the onset of the next menstruation* (not the 14th day from the 1st day of a cycle). For example, if the cycle starts on the first day of a month and lasts 30 days, the time of ovulation

would be the 16th of that month. Pregnancy is unlikely to occur if coitus is avoided 4 days before and 4 days after the expected day of ovulation.

The determination of the time of ovulation is discussed in Q/A 1 below. Calculation of "safe period", when the periods are irregular is discussed in Q/A 23 of Section 6.

Note

The rhythm method, though physiological, is the most unreliable method because pregnancy has been reported to occur from coitus on every day of the cycle.

2. **Withdrawal method.** Withdrawal of penis just before ejaculation (orgasm or climax) though practiced is not reliable, the failure rate of this method (coitus interruptus) being about 20 percent.

II. Barrier Methods (Condom and diaphragm)

Since it is very cheap and effective, the condom (a rubber sheath worn over the penis during coitus), is the most widely used method by the males. An added advantage is the protection it gives to the male against sexually transmitted diseases (STDs) like AIDS, hepatitis, syphilis, and gonorrhea.

A similar barrier, the rubber diaphragm, is fitted over the cervix by the female.

In addition to these mechanical barriers, a spermicidal jelly is used by many couples at the same time.

III. Use of Spermicidal Agents

Use of creams, jellies, foams, suppositories, etc in the female before coitus, and vaginal douches after intercourse may be combined with barriers.

IV. Interruption of the Normal Paths of Sperms or Ovum (Surgical Sterilization)

Interrupting the normal paths of sperm or ovum by vasectomy in males and tubectomy in females, appear to be the ideal methods suitable for our poor and illiterate population. However, restoration of the patency of these tubes, if required later on, has few chances of success.

V. Intrauterine Devices (IUDs)

IUDs or intrauterine contraceptive devices (IUCDs) are foreign bodies (plastic or metal) that are placed in the uterus and left there. "Copper T" and "Loop D" (stainless steel) are the common devices used. They possibly make the endometrium unsuitable for implantation of fertilized egg by causing" aseptic inflammation" and/or by increasing uterine motility. IUDs have long term use (6-10 years), can be removed when desired, and are as effective as tubectomy. (The copper in "copper T" may also be spermicidal).

VI. Oral Contraceptives (Hormonal Methods)

It has been known for long that various doses of synthetic estrogens and progesterone given during the first half of menstrual cycle inhibit release of FSH and LH by negative feedback. This, in turn, reduces the levels of the normal ovarian estrogens and progesterone, the mid-cycle LH surge does not occur, and ovulation is not triggered. Even if ovulation does occur, changes in cervical mucus and in the endometrium prove hostile for sperms and implantation.

The pills are started early in the cycle, continued beyond the expected day of ovulation, and then stopped to allow menstruation to occur. The contraceptive "pills" are 100% effective and are used by millions world-wide. The hormonal methods include:

a. **The classical pill.** It contains orally active progesterone-like substance—gestagen, and a small dose of estrogen. In addition to inhibiting ovulation, these pills also render the cervical mucus hostile to sperm penetra-tion. They may also induce endometrial changes which prevent implantation of the fertilized egg.

b. **The sequential pill.** It has a high dose of estrogen for 15 days followed by estrogen plus gestagen for 5 days. This pill inhibits ovulation by suppressing both LH and FSH.

c. **Luteal supplementation pill.** These pills contain low doses of gestagen throughout the entire cycle. It controls fertility without inhibiting ovulation. The hormone may be acting on the cervical mucus, or on the endometrium, or perhaps by reducing the motility of the Fallopian tubes.

d. *The "Morning -after Pill" (Emergency Contraception, EC).* These pills have high doses of estrogens and progestin. They inhibit FSH and LH, and stop the secretion of ovarian estrogens and progesterone. The sudden fall of these hormones causes shedding of uterine endometrium, thus blocking implantation.

When two pills are taken within 72 hours of unprotected coitus, and another two tablets after another 12 hours, chances of pregnancy are greatly reduced.

Other Hormonal Methods Include

- Subcutaneous implantation of hormone-containing capsules (they slowly release the drug into the circulation and are effective for about 5 years.
- Intramuscular injection of progestin (e.g., Depo-Provera) every 3 months.
- Once-a-month intramuscular injection of estrogen and progesterone, skin patches containing these hormones, once a week for 3 weeks of the cycle.

QUESTIONS

Q. 1 How can the time of ovulation be determined?

The anterior pituitary hormone FSH is responsible for the early maturation of the ovarian follicle, while LH is responsible for its final maturation. A burst of LH secretion at the midcycle causes the release of the ovum and the initial formation of corpus luteum. It is important to know the time of ovulation for the rhythm method to be effective in preventing pregnancy. The following methods are employed to determine the time of ovulation:

1. **Change in the basal body temperature.** A fairly reliable and convenient indicator of the time of ovulation is a rise in the basal body temperature at the time of ovulation. Using a thermometer with wide graduations, and before getting out of bed in the morning, the oral temperature is recorded every day and charted on a temperature chart. The temperature continues to fall during the first half of the cycle, then it starts to rise from the time of ovulation till the onset of the next cycle, the difference being 0.5 to 1.0°C. The cause of temperature rise is probably the increase in progesterone secretion, since this hormone is thermogenic.

2. **Examination of cervical secretions.** It shows thick, cellular mucus that does not form a fern pattern.

Q. 2 What is meant by MTP? How is it carried out?

The procedure of deliberately evacuating the uterus before 28 weeks of pregnancy is called "induction of abortion". Under certain conditions such as cases of rape, theatened abortion, fetal abnormalities, etc, pregnancy may be legally terminated (aborted)—a procedure called "medical termination of pregnancy (MTP)". Some of the methods employed are:

1. **Dilatation and curettage (D & C; up to 12 weeks).** The cervix is dilated with graduated metal dilators, and a curette is used to evacuate the uterine contents.

2. **Vacuum aspiration.** The cervix is dilated and the uterus is evacuated with an electrical suction pump. The method is suitable up to 12 weeks of pregnancy.

    Menstrual syringe. A plastic syringe and cannula, called menstrual regulator (MR) syringe, is used to aspirate the uterine contents, up to 6 weeks of pregnancy.

3. **Intra-amniotic hypertonic saline solution (13-20 weeks).** About 200 ml of 20% saline, or 80 g of urea in 200 ml of water, are injected into the amniotic cavity to cause abortion.

4. **Extra-amniotic ethacrydine lactate (13-20 weeks).** About 10 ml/week of pregnancy of this dye solution is introduced via a catheter placed in the cervix.

5. **Prostaglandins (13-20 weeks).** Prostaglandin PGE, PGF_2, or their analogues are instilled intra-amniotically to cause strong uterine contractions which cause expulsion of fetus.

6. **Pitocin (oxytocin).** Pitocin drip, 10-20 units in 500 ml of 5% dextrose solution is used for inducing or augmenting abortion.

Clinical Examination

*"Illnesses are experiments of
nature witnessed at the bedside"*

3-1

Outline for History Taking and General Physical Examination

The chief objectives of introducing preclinical students to the art and science of clinical examination of a patient are to impress upon the students the following points:

1. Clinical medicine is essentially a matter of communication between the doctor and the worried and anxious patient. However, a fresh student starting clinical work is likely to be somewhat apprehensive and uncertain when first approaching a patient. And this uncertainly is least likely to generate a bond of confidence in the patient.
2. The students get a chance to "clinically examine" their work partners, an opportunity they will not probably avail of once they get down to examining "real" patients. They should, therefore, make the most of this chance.
3. One of the happy results of increased physiological knowledge lies in that many of the signs, symptoms, and tests which were previously empirical can now be rationally explained. This has increased the reliance that can be placed on clinical evidence while interpreting laboratory tests.
4. The methods of clinical examination may appear to vary somewhat from clinician to clinician, but whatever method you follow you must adhere to it.
5. The value of accurate history taking (interrogation of the patient) and general physical examination cannot be overemphasized. They train the beginner in the habit of thoroughness and exactness at the bedside. They assure that no important point will be missed. You will be taught how to keep a systematic record of the patients you will see in your clinical training.

CLINICAL EXAMINATION

There are two basic steps in clinical examination of a patient/subject:

I. **History Taking (interrogation).** It includes general and special interrogation.

II. **Physical Examination.** It is an orderly examination for evaluation of the patient's body and its functions. It includes the non-invasive methods (see below), along with measurement of vital signs. It has two components"

A. General Physical Examination.
B. Systemic Physical Examination

I. HISTORY TAKING

A. General Interrogation

1. *Personal History.* It includes name, age, marital status, occupation (including type of work), education, financial condition, dependents, and address.
2. *Family and Social History.* State of health of parents and siblings, or cause of death. History of intake of alcohol / drugs.
3. *Chief Complaints.* These are the primary reason for seeking medical help. Allow the patient to tell his chief presenting complaints in his/her own words. Note them in chronological order. All symptoms are not of equal diagnostic importance. Usually there is/are one (or two) symptom/s that trouble the patient more than others.
4. *History of Previous Illnesses, Accidents, Operations.* These should be recorded.
5. *History of Present Illness.* Its mode of origin and when it began. Did it start slowly or suddenly? The order in which the symptoms appeared and how they have progressed. Ask for any treatment received. Enquire about any loss of weight, appetite, and strength. (Note reliability of information).

Ask! "When were you free of any illness?"

B. Special Interrogation

This should follow general interrogation described above. It is only with experience that the student will learn which body system appears to be involved, and what is essential to ask and what to leave out.

Special interrogation includes: asking questions about the particular system (e.g., respiratory, circulatory, etc) that appears to be involved in the disease process. Leading questions may have to be asked.

II. PHYSICAL EXAMINATION

Conditions for a Satisfactory Physical Examination.

1. As mentioned earlier, clinical examination is basically a matter of communication between a patient and the clinician. Therefore, one must try to establish a rapport (sympathy) with the patient as soon as possible. He/she will not only be relaxed and reassured but will also be communicative (and thankful to you).
2. The room should be comfortable, with adequate natural daylight because artificial light can affect skin color. If the patient is a female, the husband, female relative, or a female nurse must be present.
3. The patient should be asked to undress and then covered with a gown or bed sheet (for heart and lung examination).
4. The doctor, if right handed, must always stand on the right side of the patient.

A. General Physical Examination

1. *General appearance.* Does the patient look healthy, unwell, or ill? Apparent age, weight and height, Body build, Nutrition. Note if breathing is comfortable.
2. *Posture in bed and gait.* In congestive heart failure there is orthopnea (ie, the patient is more comfortable sitting rather than lying down). Some diseases are obvious by the gait, e.g., drunken *(zig- zag)* gait of cerebellar ataxia, and the rigid gait of Parkinsonism.
3. *Face and speech.* Note the expression, symmetry, and color of the face. Does he/she speak or is silent? Is the speech hysterical? Eyeballs, facial palsy, exophthalmos, nose, lips.
4. *Skin.* Look for the color, texture, eruptions, petechiae, scars. There is pallor in anemia (color of oral mucosa and creases of palm give a better idea of paleness); yellowish in

jaundice and hypercaroteinemia; and bluish in cyanosis (due to presence of at least 5.0 g of reduced Hb in the skin capillaries).

5. **Neck.** Look for enlarged lymph glands; thyroid; pulsations of vessels, venous distension; position of trachea.

6. **Chest.** Shape; deformities, curvature of spine at the back. Note rate of breathing. (Normal= 12-16/min). Odor of breath; breath may be sweet and sickly in diabetes and ketosis; ammoniacal in uremia; halitosis ('bad breath') in poor dental and oral hygiene.

7. **Abdomen.** Contour, skin, scars, pulsations.

8. **Hands.** Look for attitude, tremors, skin, nails, clubbing of fingers, trophic changes.

9. **Extremities.** Arms, legs, hands, feet, scars, wounds, deformities, edema, prominent leg veins.

10. **Pulse rate.** Count for 1 minute. Note if there is tachycardia or bradycardia.

11. **Temperature.** Keep the thermometer under the tongue for 2 minutes. (Normal range = 97.2°-98.8°F)
(In children, the axillary or groin temperature is less by about 1.0°F)

12. **Bloods pressure.** Record the blood pressure after a short period of rest.

B. SYSTEMIC PHYSICAL EXAMINATION (Common Non-invasive Procedures)

Inspection

Observation, a very essential faculty in medical practice that has to be cultivated rigorously, is the hallmark of inspection. Inspection should be carried out in good light, the part of the body should be fully exposed, and looked at from different angles. Note if there are any changes in the body that deviate from the normal.

Palpation (-palp = gentle touching)
It means touching and feeling a part of the body with the flat surfaces of your palm and fingers. The principle is to mould your hand to the body surface. Place your right hand flat on the body part, with the forearm and wrist in the same horizontal plane. Apply a gentle pressure with the fingers, moving them at the metacarpophalangeal joints. Never "poke" the patient's body with your fingers. The ulnar border of your hand may also be used for palpation.

Percussion (percur- = beat through)
Percussion means giving a sharp tap or impact on the surface of the body, usually with the fingers. Its purpose is to set up vibrations in the underlying tissues, and listening to the echo.

The tip of the bent middle finger of the right hand strikes, two or three times, the middle phalanx of the middle finger (pleximeter finger) of the left hand placed firmly in contact with the skin. Two things are noted:

i. Character of the sound produced.
ii. The characteristic feeling imparted to the pleximeter finger.

Auscultation (auscult- = listening)
It refers to listening to body sounds to assess the functioning of certain organs. A stethoscope is used to amplify the sounds. For example, listening to heart sounds and breath sounds.

COMMONLY USED TERMS

1. **Symptoms.** These are subjective disturbances in the body function resulting from disease, which a patient experiences and which cause him to feel he is not well. These subjective changes that are not visible to an observer are called symptoms.

2. **Physical Signs.** These are objective marks of diseases that a trained person can see and measure using his senses, generally unaided, though the aid of a stethoscope is usually allowed under this definition (e.g., fever, high BP, paralysis).

3. **Disorder.** The term refers to any abnormality of structure or function.

4. **Disease.** It is a more specific term for an illness characterized by specific recognizable set of

symptoms and signs. Thus, it is any specific change from the state of health. A disease may be a local one, affecting a part or limited region of the body. Or it may be a systemic disease affecting either the entire body or several parts of it.

5. **Diagnosis** (Dia- = through; -gnosis = knowing). It is the science and skill of distinguishing one disorder or disease from another. The patient's history of illness and physical examination (and sometimes various tests), and their correct interpretation builds up a picture of the patient's illness. Sometimes the diagnosis is only "provisional", which is usually confirmed after laboratory and/or special investigations.

6. **Prognosis.** After considering all aspects of a patient's illness, the doctor may be able to give an opinion about the possible future course of the disease, ie, the degree of cure possible (or otherwise). This comment on the future course of the disease is called prognosis.

7. **Vital Signs.** This term refers to the 4 signs which can be seen, measured, and recorded in a living person. They include: pulse, blood pressure, respiration, and body temperature. The former 3 are controlled by the 'vital centers' located in the medulla, while the body temperature is controlled by the hypothalamus.

The vital signs must always be checked during general physical examination.

Clinical Examination of the Respiratory System

Important Landmarks. Vertical lines dawn on the front and back of the thorax constitute some of the important landmarks. These are: midsternal line; midclavicular lines; anterior axillary, midaxillary, and posterior axillary lines; midspinal and midscapular lines.

Important Signs and Symptoms of Respiratory Disease

The important signs and symptoms of respiratory disease include **fever, cough** (dry or with sputum, short or paroxysmal, times at which it occurs, and the character of its sound), **expectoration** (amount, color, pus, blood, watery or frothy), **hemoptysis, dyspnea** (breathlessness, unpleasant awareness of the need for greater respiratory effort, present at

rest or on exertion, and effect of posture), **pain, cyanosis, and clubbing of fingers.** Some of these are also encountered in non-respiratory diseases.

INSPECTION

Q. 1 Inspect the chest for its form and respiratory movements in the subject provided.
The subject is examined in good light, stripped to the waist, and preferably in sitting position. The chest should be inspected from all sides, especially from behind and over the shoulders.
A. Form of the chest. The normal chest is bilaterally symmetrical and there are no large bulges or hollows. It is elliptical in shape, the normal ratio of transverse to anteroposterior diameter **(Hutchinson's index)** being 7:5, (the chest becomes

barrel-shaped in emphysema). A depression runs down the sternum, and is most marked at its lower end.

Observe carefully the positions of trachea and apex beat, and note whether engorged veins are present over the chest.

- *Abnormal forms of chest* include: alar and flat chests due to poor posture, rachitic chest in rickets, pigeon breast chest; and barrel-shaped chest in emphysema.

B. Respiratory movements. The rate, depth, rhythm, and type (manner) of breathing should be noted. The rate should be counted surreptitiously, while keeping the fingers on the radial pulse, because a nervous patient may breathe rapidly and irregularly. The normal rate of respiration is 14-20 per minute, one inspiration and one expiration making up one cycle. It is faster in children and in old age. The rate bears a definite ratio to pulse rate of about 1:4, which is usually constant in the same person. The rate and depth usually increase or decrease together. They are regulated by the respiratory center via reflexes arising in the thorax and the great vessels.

Note

Inspiration is an active process and involves elevation of thorax and forward movement of abdomen. Expiration is passive and is associated with depression of ribs and abdominal wall. (The main muscle of inspiration is diaphragm, supplied by phrenics).

Type of breathing. This depends on age and sex. In males, the diaphragm is more freely used than intercostal muscles and its downward movement causes a free outward movement of the abdomen—the *abdominal respiration*. In women, the movements of the chest are greater than those of abdomen—the *thoracic respiration*. Various combinations of these two types—the *thoraco-abdominal* and *abdomino-thoracic*—are also seen. Children have abdominal respiration. It should also be noted if the respiration is similar on the two sides.

A particular note should be taken of the **equality of expansion on the two sides**. Both sides move equally, symmetrically, and simultaneously. Asymmetric expansion of the lungs may be seen when the underlying lung is diseased. Fibrosis, consolidation, collapse, or pleural effusion can all decrease chest expansion on the affected side though other physical signs will also be present.

C. Position of Trachea and Apex beat. Inspection may not show the position of trachea, though cardiac pulsation may be visible; the lowermost and outermost point on which would be the apex beat. (It will be confirmed by palpation).

PALPATION

Q. 2 Palpate the chest for position of trachea and respiratory movements in the subject provided.

Before palpating the chest, it is essential to confirm the:

- a. *Position of trachea.* Feel the rings of trachea in the suprasternal notch with the tip of your index finger, and try to judge the space between it and the insertion of sternomastoid muscle on either side of it.

   Normally, trachea is in the midline or slightly to one side. However, in diseases, it may be pulled to the affected side (fibrosis, lung collapse), or pushed away from the affected side (pneumothorax, pleural effusion).

- b. *Position of Apex beat.* (See next experiment for locating its position). Displacement of trachea and apex beat indicates shifting of the mediastinum.

- c. *Presence of lymph glands.* Note the presence or absence of lymph glands in the axilla and supraclavicular regions, because these may be the only evidence of carcinoma of the lungs.

For successful palpation the hands must be warm and used as gently as possible. The chest is palpated in the upper, middle, and lower regions, on the front and the back.

The movements of the upper zones of the lungs are compared by placing the hands over the two apices from behind, and the thumbs are approximated in the midline on the back. The movement of the thumbs away from the midline, as the subject breathes deeply, indicates equal or unequal expansion.

The middle and lower regions are palpated by placing the hands on either side of the chest, with fingers stretched out and the thumbs just touching in the midline. The excursion of each thumb away from the midline indicates the degree of expansion of the lungs.

Palpation also detects subcutaneous emphysema (air in the tissues) which results from fracture of ribs and gives a characteristic spongy feeling.

Q. 3 Palpate the chest for vocal fremitus.
Vocal Fremitus. The detection of vibrations transmitted to the hands from the larynx through bronchi, lungs and chest wall during the act of phonation is called **vocal fremitus**. The palm, or the ulnar border of the hand which is more sensitive, is placed on the intercostal spaces while the patient is asked to say "ninety-nine", "one-two-three", or "ek-do-teen", once or twice. The vibrations felt by the hand are compared on identical points, from above downward, on the front, axillary region, and on the back of the chest.

Vocal fremitus may be *diminished* if the voice is feeble, or when a bronchus is blocked by a new growth which interferes with the passage of vibrations, or when the vibrations are dampened by fluid or air in the pleural cavity. It is *increased* when the vibrations are better conducted, as through solid lung (consolidation due to pneumonia).

The expansion of the chest should be measured with a tape measure placed around the chest just below the level of the nipples. The chest expands by 4 to 8 cm after a deep breath.

PERCUSSION

Q. 4 Percuss the lungs of the subject provided.
Percussion is the procedure employed for setting up artificial vibrations in a tissue by means of a sharp tap, usually delivered with the fingers.

Percussion is done for determining:
a. The condition of the underlying tissues—lungs, pleura.
b. The borders of the lungs.

Protocol

The rules for percussion are:
i. The middle finger (pleximeter finger) of the left hand is placed firmly in contact with the skin. The back of its middle phalanx is struck with the tip of the middle finger of the right hand, two or three times.
ii. The striking finger should lie, almost over and parallel to the pleximeter finger as it falls, should be relaxed and should not be lifted more than 2 or 3 inches. It must also be lifted clear immediately after the blow to avoid damping of the resulting vibrations.
iii. The movement of the hand should be at the wrist and not at the elbow or shoulder.
iv. If the percussed ogran or tissue lies superficially, the percussion should be light, but heavier if the tissue lies deeper.

The following two things are to be noted while percussing:
a. **The character of the sound produced.** It differs in quality and quantity over different tissues. Air-containing organs, such as lungs, produce a note (sound) called **resonance**. The opposite of resonance, ie, lack of note, called **dullness**, is found over solid viscera like heart and liver, or when the lung becomes solidified as in pneumonia, growth, or fibrosis. An extreme form of dullness is called *stony dullness*, in which a feeling of resistance is felt by the tapping finger along with a dull note; such dullness is found by percussing over the thigh, and is encountered in pleural effusion.

The percussion note changes to *tympani* when air fills the pleural cavity, or when air is contained unloculated in a large lung cyst or in stomach.
b. **The characteristic feeling imparted to the pleximeter finger.** (The student should

practice percussing over different parts of his/her body, and over various objects like wooden and steel furniture, and so on).

The percussion is carried out according to the following rules:

a. When the boundaries of organs are to be defined, percussion is done from resonance to dullness and from more resonant to less resonant areas.

b. The direction of percussion should be at right angles to the edge of the organ.

Apical percussion. It is carried out in the supra-clavicular fossae to determine the upper borders of the lungs which lie 3-4 cm above the clavicles.

Basal percussion. The lower limits of lung resonance are determined by percussion the chest from above downward, with the pleximeter finger parallel to the diaphragm. With light percussion and in quiet respiration, the lower border of the right lung lies in the midclavicular line at the 6th rib, in the midaxillary line at the 8th rib, and in the scapular line at the 10th rib. Posteriorly, on both sides, and anteriorly on the right side, the percussion note changes from resonance to dullness, while anteriorly on the left side, the percussion note changes from resonance to tympani.

AUSCULTATION

Q. 5 Auscultate the lungs and trachea of the subject provided.

Before using the stethoscope for auscultation of the lungs, **one should listen carefully to the patient's breathing**. The breathing of a normal resting subject cannot be heard at a distance of more than a few inches from the face. Audible breathing at rest can be an important sign of airway disease (narrowing, secretions) and in some other conditions. For example, the breathing sounds may be: *stertorous* (snoring like; in coma due to any cause); *gasping, grunting and sighing* (exercise, pain, fear, grief); *wheezing* (usually louder during expiration, as in asthma); *hissing* (Kussmaul's

breathing, as in acidosis of diabetes and uremia); and *stridor.*

> **Important**
> Quietness and a properly-fitting stethoscope are essential. Crackling noises due to hairs on the chest, rubbing of chest-piece on the skin or against clothes, and shivering and heart sounds are to be ignored. Sitting position is ideal; when auscultating at the back, the patient is asked to lean forward, flex the head, and cross the arms in front.
> (For description of a stethoscope, consult Expt 2-6).

Auscultation

Auscultation is done all over the lungs—front, axillary regions and back—and sounds at corresponding points on the two sides are compared. Since breath sounds during quiet breathing are insufficient for study, the patient is asked *to breathe deeply through open mouth* (it is best to show this to the patient). The following points are noted:

a. **The type or character of breath sounds—** whether vesicular or bronchial.

b. **Intensity of breath sounds—**whether diminished or absent.

c. **Added or adventitious sounds—**crepitations, rhonchi, pleural rub, etc.

d. Character of vocal resonance.

Vesicular breath sounds

i. The vesicular breath sounds are produced by passage of air in the medium and large bronchi; they get **filtered** and **attenuated** while passing through millions of air-filled alveoli before reaching the chest wall. These sounds are heard both during inspiration and expiration.

ii. The inspiratory sound is low-pitched and rustling in character, and is always longer than the expiratory sound.

iii. The expiratory sound, which is softer and shorter, follows without a pause and is heard

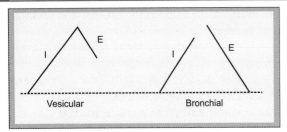

Figure 3-1. The two main types of breath sounds
I: Inspiration, E: Expiration

during early part of expiration (it may commonly be inaudible) as shown in **Figure 3-1**.

iv. Normally, breathing over most areas of the chest is vesicular, and most typically so in the axillary and infrascapular regions.

Bronchial breath sounds

i. Bronchial breath sounds originate probably in the same medium and large bronchi, and replace vesicular sounds when the lung tissue between them and the chest wall becomes airless as a result of consolidation (as in pneumonia), tuberculosis, carcinoma and fibrosis. There is **no filtration and attenuation** of sounds because they pass directly from bronchi through diseased lung tissue instead of passing through air-filled alveoli.

ii. The bronchial breath sounds are loud, clear, hollow or blowing in character and of high frequencies.

iii. The inspiratory sound becomes inaudible just before the end of inspiration while the expiratory sound is heard throughout expiration. Thus, the bronchial breath sounds are loud and clear, the inspiratory and expiratory sounds being of about same duration, and separated by a distinct pause.

Tracheal breath sounds. The bronchial type of breathing resembles that heard over the trachea although tracheal sound is much harsher and louder. In fact, auscultation over the trachea can give the student an idea about bronchial breathing.

In children, the breath sounds normally are harsher than in adults, and are described as **peurile breathing**, and a similar type of breathing is produced by exercise.

Q. 6 Auscultate the areas where bronchial breath sounds can normally be heard.
Bronchial breath sounds can normally be heard over the following areas:

a. **Trachea and larynx:** The sounds are harsher and louder than those heard over diseased lungs.

b. **Interscapular region and the apex of right lung:** There is more of bronchial element than vesicular in these regions because the trachea and bronchi come near to the surface.

c. **Bronchial breathing** may also be heard in the *interscapular*, right *infraclavicular*, and over the *lower cervical vertebrae*.

Q. 7 Auscultate the lungs for vocal resonance in the subject provided.
Vocal resonance refers to the sounds heard over the chest during the act of phonation. The vibrations set up by the vocal cords are transmitted along the airways and through the lung tissues to the chest wall.

The subject is asked to repeat "ninety-nine", or "ek-do-teen" in a normal, clear and uniform voice; and the sounds heard are compared on the identical regions on the two sides.

Intensity of Vocal Resonance. The normal intensity of vocal resonance gives the impression of being produced near the chest piece of the stethoscope.

When the intensity is increased, and the sounds appear to come from near the earpiece of the stethoscope, they are called **bronchophony**. It is heard over consolidation of lung tissue in pneumonia, over tuberculosis, or other resonating cavity or over lung apex when the upper lobe is collapsed and trachea is pulled to that side.

When the words are clear and appear to be spoken (whispered) right into the ears, and the words can be clearly identified, the condition is called **whispering pectoriloquy**.

Vocal resonance may be decreased or even abolished when there is fluid in the pleural cavity, pneumothorax, or emphysema.

Q. 8 What are adventitious or "added" sounds?
The sounds which do not form an essential part of the usual breath sounds are called adventitious (extra) or " "added" sounds. They are generally of 3 types:

a. *Rhonchi (or wheezes)*. These are *"dry sounds"* and are produced by the passage of air though narrowed or partially blocked respiratory passages.

b. *Crepitations (or "moist sounds")*. They are discontinuous "bubbling" or "crackling"

sounds produced by the passage of air through fluid in the small airways and/or alveoli. Crepitations may be "fine" or "coarse". (If you rub your hair between your thumb and a finger near your ear, the sound produced resembles fine crepitations.

c. *Pleural rub (or "friction sound")*. It is a "creaking" or "rubbing" sound produced by friction between the two layers of inflamed and roughened pleura. It is mainly produced during that part of respiration when the rough surfaces rub against each other, i.e., during deep inspiration. The pleural rub disappears when there is accumulation of fluid in the pleural cavity.

3-3

Clinical Examination of the Cardiovascular System

The circulatory system consists of *blood* and *cardiovascular system (CVS)*. The CVS is made up of *heart* and *blood vessels* (arteries, veins etc). The clinical examination of CVS, therefore, involves examination of both of these components.

1. Examination of the vascular system, and

2. Examination of precordium, i.e., the part of the anterior chest wall lying in front of the heart, for heart function.

IMPORTANT SIGNS AND SYMPTOMS OF CARDIOVASCULAR DISEASE

The important signs and symptoms of CVS disease include:

i. **Dyspnea** on effort, paroxysmal dyspnea at rest, orthopnea (i.e., the patient is more comfortable sitting than lying down).

ii. **Palpitation.** This is an unpleasant awareness of heart beat.

iii. **Cardiac pain.** Pain may be present as angina at rest or on effort, or as myocardial infarction.

iv. **Tachycardia** and/or other arrhythmias, headache, dizziness, fatigue, cyanosis.

Occasionally, some symptoms may not appear to be connected with CVS disease. There may be *GI tract symptoms*, such as loss of appetite or even vomiting, *urinary symptoms* such as oliguria in renal failure resulting from heart disease, or *cerebral symptoms*, such as attacks of syncope.

Cardiovascular disease may also be detected during a routine medical examination though the patient may be otherwise symptom-free. Essential hypertension is such a disease and has, therefore, been called a 'silent killer'.

QUESTIONS

Q. 1 How would you proceed to examine the cardiovascular system?

It is the usual practice amongst physicians to proceed with the examination of the CVS according to the following plan before starting examination of the heart.

1. The cardiac impulse—its position, character, rhythm, and duration.
2. Examination of the arterial pulse.
3. Recording of blood pressure.
4. Examination of the jugular veins in the neck.
5. Presence or absence of veins on the chest wall.
6. Any other pulsation—in the suprasternal notch, at the root of the neck, and over the thorax and epigastrium.
7. Examination of the heart: inspection, palpation, percussion, and auscultation.

Q. 2 Examine the arterial pulse in the subject provided and comment on your findings.

Definition. The alternate expansion and recoil of the elastic aorta after each systole of left ventricle sets up a pressure wave. This pressure wave travels along the arteries and causes expansion and recoil of their walls which is palpable as the arterial pulse. In simple words, arterial pulse is the action of the left ventricle felt in a peripheral artery.

The examination of arterial pulse includes: inspection, palpation and auscultation of some important vessels—especially radial, brachial, carotid, temporal, retinal, femoral and popliteal arteries and their branches, especially the dorsalis pedis artery.

Why radial artery is chosen. The routine examination of arterial pulse is done on this artery, (called the 'pulse') because:

i. It is conveniently accessible as it is located in an exposed part of the body.
ii. The artery lies oven the hard surface of the lower end of the radius.

PALPATION OF THE RADIAL ARTERY

The radial artery is palpated with the tips of three fingers compressing the vessel against the head of radius bone. The subject's forearm should be slightly pronated and the wrist slightly flexed. The index finger (toward the heart) varies the pressure on the artery, the middle finger feels the pulse, while the distal finger prevents reflections of pulsations from the palmer arch of arteries. The following observations are made:

1. **Rate of pulse.** The normal pulse rate at rest averages about 72/min. The rate is normally higher in children (90-110/min) and slower in old age (55-65/min). The pulse rate normally increases during deep inspiration and decreases during deep expiration. When this happens during quiet breathing, it is called **sinus arrhythmia**, which is due to irradiation of impulses from the inspiratory center to the cardiac center. Quite trivial factors increase the pulse rate—climbing stairs, a brisk short walk, nervousness, etc. For this reason, the pulse rate should be counted 2 or 3 times at intervals of 10-15 minutes.

   The pulse rate should always be compared with the heart rate, as in some cases the pulse rate may be less than heart rate (pulse deficit; see below).

2. **Rhythm.** The normal pulse waves follow at regular intervals, i.e., the rhythm is regular. The common irregularities in the pulse, which may be occasional, regularly irregular, or irregularly irregular, are extrasystoles (premature beats), atrial flutter and fibrillation, and various degrees of heart block.

3. **Character or form.** By character or form is meant whether the individual pulse wave has a normal *rise, maintenance, and fall*, as the pulse is being palpated. The dicrotic wave (see **Figure 5-1**) which is seen on a record of pulse wave, is not felt on palpation.

Types of arterial pulse. Some special types of arterial pulse are the following:

a. **Collapsing pulse:** In this, both the rise and fall of the pulse are very sudden, and the amplitude may also be higher. It is seen in aortic regurgitation.

b. **Slow rising or anacrotic pulse:** The pulse wave is slow to rise and occurs when the ventricular ejection is prolonged as in aortic stenosis.

c. **Pulsus alternans:** The pulse beats though regular are alternately small and large in amplitude. Severe damage to the left ventricle may cause this type of pulse.

d. **Thready pulse:** Thin, thready pulse is a feature of shock and is due to decrease in the stroke volume.

(Consult Chart 5-1 for the other types of arterial pulse).

4. **Volume.** The "volume" of the pulse refers to the **amplitude of the movement or expansion of the artery during the passage of pulse wave.** It is a rough guide to the pulse pressure. Experience is necessary before a student can distinguish a low volume pulse (thin, thready pulse) of low stroke output from a bounding pulse of hyperkinetic circulation, as in fever, pregnancy, anemia, thyrotoxicosis, etc.

5. **Tension.** The amount of tension (or pressure) applied **to best feel the artery** can give only a very rough idea about the diastolic blood pressure; and **the amount of pressure required to obliterate the artery gives** a rough estimate of systolic pressure.

6. **Condition of the vessel wall.** The radial artery is **emptied out** by pressing on it with the finger toward the heart, and an attempt is made to roll the vessel against the bone, by the other two fingers. In most young persons, the "empty" artery is so compliant that it cannot be felt as a separate structure. However, the vessel becomes palpable in middle age, and is felt as a cord-like structure in old age due to atherosclerosis and calcification. (The surface may show irregularities, and the vessel may be tortuous.)

Another way to note the condition of the vessel wall (when emptied out of blood) is to compress the brachial artery with a thumb and then palpate the radial artery by rolling it against the bone. (A "full" radial artery is normally palpable in many thin individuals).

7. **Delay.** When the left femoral artery and the right radial artery are palpated simultaneously the two pulses normally beat together. A delay in the femoral artery is seen in coarctation of the aorta.

8. *Equality on the two sides.* The arterial pulse of one side is always compared with that of the other side for all of its features described above. Normally, there is no difference between the two.

Examine all Other Arterial Pulses. The examination of other pulses is important: brachial—at the elbow; carotids—in the neck; femoral—in the groin; posterior tibial—behind medial malleolus; and dorsalis pedis—on the dorsum of the foot at the midpoint between medial and lateral malleoli, at the base of the first metatarsal bone.

Q. 3 What is tachycardia and what are its causes?

Tachycardia. An increase in heart rate above 100/min is called tachycardia.

Physiological tachycardia is seen in:

1. **Emotional excitement, nervousness, and apprehension:** For example, at the time of an interview.

2. Muscular exercise.

3. **In the newborns:** The heart rate may be 120-150/min; it gradually decreases during infancy and childhood.

4. **Sex:** The rate is comparatively higher in females; there may be tachycardia during pregnancy.

5. **Diurnal variations:** Higher rates are seen in the evening and may exceed 100/min.

Pathological tachycardia is seen in—

1. **Fever due to any cause:** For every 1°C rise in temperature, the heart rate increases by about 10-14 beats/min. The raised temperature acts directly on the SA node and generates more action potentials per unit time.

2. **Thyrotoxicosis:** Increased metabolism of SA node generates more action potentials.

3. **Atrial flutter and fibrillation:** The pulse is fast and irregular.

4. **Paroxysmal atrial tachycardia:** Sudden onset and as sudden an offset are characteristic features.

5. **Circulatory shock:** The pulse is fast and weak (thready pulse).

Q. 4 What is bradycardia and what are its causes?

Bradycardia.   A decrease in heart rate below 60/min is called bradycardia.

Physiological bradycardia is seen in—
1. **Athletes:** The resting heart rate may be 50-55/min; it is due to increased vagal tone.
2. **Sleep and meditation:** The rate may be below 55 during deep meditation.
3. The rate may be below 60/min under **basal conditions**, i.e., before a person gets out of bed after a good night's sleep.

Pathological bradycardia is seen in—
1. **Myxedema:** Hyposecretion of thyroid hormone is commonly associated with low pulse rates.
2. **Heart block:** The rate depends on the degree of heart block. In complete heart block, the ventricular rate may be 30-40/min (idio-ventricular rhythm).
3. **General weakness and debility** following prolonged illness.
4. **Drugs:** Treatment with drugs such as digitalis and sympatholytics (e.g., propranolol).

Q. 5 What is apex-pulse deficit?

Normally the pulse rate and the ventricular rate (as determined by auscultation at the heart) are identical. However, in the case of extrasystoles (premature beats) and atrial fibrillation, some of the ventricular beats are too weak to be felt at the radial artery so that the heart rate is higher than the radial pulse rate—a condition called **pulse deficit or apex-pulse deficit.**

Q. 6 Examine the neck veins of the subject provided for jugular venous pressure.

Pulsations in the neck. Both arterial and venous pulsations may be seen in the neck, especially in thin persons. However, venous pulsations can be easily occluded by pressure with a finger above the clavicle. Arterial pulsations are stronger, increase with heart rate on mild exertion, and cannot be easily occluded.

Examination of venous pressure. The venous pressure can usually be estimated by watching the degree of distension of peripheral veins, especially the neck veins. For example, **in normal, resting, sitting individuals, the neck veins are not distended**. However, when the right atrial pressure rises, as in congestive heart failure, the veins become distended.

(Consult Chart 5-2 on Jugular Venous Pulse Tracing).

Jugular Venous Pressure

The **external jugular vein,** a superficial vein, begins in the parotid gland near the angle of the jaw, descends through the neck across the sterno-mastoid muscle to empty into the subclavian vein.

The **internal jugular vein** passes down the neck, lateral to internal and common carotid arteries to unite with the subclavian vein.

Since both jugular veins connect with the right atrium (the right external jugular vein being almost in line with this chamber), they can act as a manometer for the right atrium, reflecting all its pressure changes, thus providing valuable information about right aterial pressure (normally, a few mm of Hg), which represents the **"central venous pressure"**. (Consult Chart 5-2 for details).

Procedure

The subject is made to lie on his back, with the upper part of the body supported at an angle of 45 degrees to the horizontal **(Figure 3-2)**, with the chin pointing slightly to the left. The neck veins are then inspected carefully. Normally, slight pulsations in the neck veins are seen just above the clavicle. This level is the same as the sternal angle (angle of Lewis) whatever the position of the thorax. The vertical distance between the right atrium and the sternal angle indicates the mean hydrostatic pressure, which is normally 2-3 cm of water (1-2 mm Hg). The veins are then inspected in the upright position. Normally, no pulsations are visible. In right heart failure, however, the right

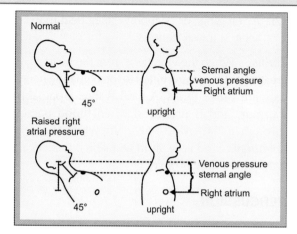

Figure 3-2. Jugular venous pressure. See text for details

atrial pressure, and thus the jugular venous pressure is raised, the veins are full and show pulsations even in the upright position.

EXAMINATION OF THE HEART

Inspection

Q. 7 Inspect the precordium in the subject provided and give your findings.
Precordium is the area of the chest wall lying in front of the heart. The subject should be examined in the recumbent and sitting position, and in good light. The following observations are made:
A. It is noted if there is any **deformity**, such as kyphosis (forward bending of spine), scoliosis (sideward bending of spine), or **bulging** of the precordium (enlargement of heart).
B. Inspection for **cardiac pulsation and apex beat.** The precordium is inspected from all angles to see if any pulsations are visible—any pulsation in this region is called **cardiac impulse** or **cardiac pulsation**, which is due to a forward systolic thrust of the apex of the left ventricle. Normally, the area of cardiac pulsation is well outlined and covers an area of about 2 cm and no other pulsation is visible over the precordium, including the base of the heart.

Apex beat

It is the **lowest and the outermost point of definite cardiac pulsation.** It is usually visible and palpable, and is located 8-10 cm (about 3½-4 inches; according to body build) from the mid-sternal line, in the left 5th intercostal space. Normally, it is almost always within the mid-clavicular line (or nipple line in the male).

The apex beat may not be visible in some normal persons because:
  i. It may be located behind a rib.
 ii. The chest wall may be thick due to fat or muscle.
iii. The emphysematous lung may cover part of the heart.
 iv. The breast may be pendulous.
C. Inspection for **other pulsations.** It is done in the precordium and nearby regions.
  i. Arterial pulsations in the neck may be visible in hyperdynamic circulation, as in—anxiety, hyperthyroidism, aortic regurgitation, and hypertension.
 ii. Pulsations to the right or left of the upper sternum may be due to aortic aneurysm.
iii. Enlargement of the right ventricle, or enlarged left atrium due to severe mitral regurgitation may cause pulsations in the left upper parasternal region.
 iv. Pulsations in the epigastrium are most commonly due to pulsations of abdominal aorta increased by emotional excitement in thin individuals, or enlargement of the right ventricle, or due to hepatic pulsations from tricuspid regurgitation.
  v. Pulsations in the superficial arteries of thorax may be visible in coarctation of aorta.

PALPATION

Q. 8 Palpate the chest of the subject provided for apex beat. What is its significance?
For locating the position of the apex beat by palpation, the flat of the hand is placed over the

heart, base of the palm over the base of the heart, and the fingers pointing towards the apex. Once the cardiac pulsation is felt, the ulnar border of the hand and then the tip of the index finger is used to locate and confirm the point of apex beat already defined by inspection. The apex beat should then be marked by a marker pen.

Position.   The apex beat is located 8-10 cm from the midsternal line, in the left 5th intercostal space. To locate the 5th space, the sternal angle (angle of Lewis)—the junction between manubrium sterni and body of sternum—is first located. The second costal cartilage articulates with sternum at this level; the 2nd intercostal space is below the 2nd rib. The 5th space can now easily be counted downwards and located.

If the apex beat is not palpable, the patient is then turned over to the left side, or sits up and bends forward. However, despite all efforts the apex beat may still not be palpable for the reasons already mentioned.

Note
One should always make it a habit, especially if the apex beat is not palpable in its usual place, to palpate the chest on both sides, with hands placed on either side, so as not to miss dextrocardia.

Character.   In normal persons, the apex beat gently raises the palpating finger. The strength of this thrust increases after exercise, in nervousness, in hyperthyroidism, or in left ventricular hypertrophy.

Significance of Palpating the Apex Beat
  a. Enlargement of the heart due to hypertrophy or dilatation may shift the apex beat.
  b. Pulling or pushing of the mediastinum due to lung disease may shift the position of the apex beat.
  c. Diffuse, sustained and more forceful thrust indicates left ventricular hypertrophy or hyperkinetic circulation.

  d. A "tapping" or "slapping" apex beat may be seen in mitral stenosis.

Thrills.   When the vibrations from the heart or its great vessels are transmitted to the palpating hand, they are called thrills. A thrill is thus a palpable murmur, and is produced when blood passes through a narrowed valve, or when there is abnormal blood flow, as in congenital defects, or if the blood flow is rapid.

PERCUSSION

Q. 9 Demarcate the borders of the heart by percussion.
The *upper border of the liver* is first demarcated by starting the percussion downward along the midclavicular line till the resonance changes to dullness. Then, starting in the midaxillary line, 2 or 3 spaces above the liver dullness, percussion is carried out toward the right sternal margin. Normally the *right border of the heart*, which is formed by the *right atrium*, lies behind the sternum.

Left border of the heart: The position of the apex beat is first located. Percussion is done in the 5th, 4th, and 3rd intercostal spaces, starting in the left midaxillary line and going towards the heart till the notes change from resonance to dullness. Each point where dullness appears is marked with ink, and when these points are joined, the left border is marked.

The area of cardiac dullness increases in pleural effusion, while it may be decreased in emphysema.

AUSCULTATION

Q. 10 Auscultate the heart sounds over the mitral, tricuspid, aortic, and pulmonary areas.
Heart sounds
It is good practice to palpate the carotid artery while listening to the heart sounds because the carotid pulse coincides with the first sound. As a routine, the four cardiac areas, named according to the valves from which sounds arise (**Figure 3-3**), are auscultated first. This is followed by

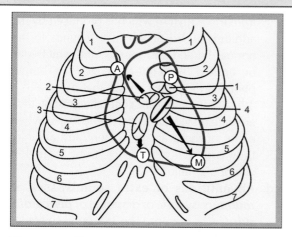

Figure 3-3. Diagram showing the projection of heart valves and the auscultatory areas. (1) Pulmonary artery valve, P—Pulmonary area, (2) Aortic valve, A—Aortic area, (3) Tricuspid valve, T—Tricuspid area, (4) Mitral valve, M—Mitral area. The ribs are numbered from 1 to 7 on each side

auscultation in between these areas. The different areas are:

Mitral area. The mitral area corresponds to the apex beat, i.e., 5th intercostal space about 8-10 cm from the midsternal line.

Tricuspid area. This area lies just to the left of the lower end of the sternum.

Aortic area. It lies to the right of the sternum in the 2nd intercostal space.

Pulmonary area. It lies to the left of the sternum in the 2nd intercostal space.

Note
The corresponding valves of the heart do not lie under these areas; only the sounds produced by these valves are heard best over these areas.

Over all these areas of auscultation, both the first and the second heart sounds are heard clearly, though the first sound is heard better in mitral and tricuspid areas while the second sound is heard better in aortic and pulmonay areas.

Differentiation between First and Second Heart Sounds:

1. The heart sounds are always timed with the simultaneous palpation of carotid artery pulsation. The **1st sound coincides with the carotid pulse**. The 2nd sound follows a little later.

2. The **1st heart sound**, which is due to the simultaneous closure of the atrioventricular valves, is prolonged (0.1-0.17 sec), of low pitch (20-40 Hz) and booming in character. Phonetically, it is likened to the syllable *"LUB"*. It coincides with the R-wave of the ECG (see Chart 5-4) and is best heard over the mitral area.

   The **2nd heart sound**, which is due to the closure of aortic and pulmonary valves, is shorter, abrupt and clear, and of high pitch. Phonetically, it resembles the spoken sound *"DUP"*. It may precede, coincide, or follow the T-wave of the ECG, and is best heard over aortic and pulmonay areas.

3. The time interval between the 1st and the 2nd heart sounds is shorter than the time interval between the 2nd sound and the next 1st sound. The sequence is thus: LUB-DUP-pause, LUB-DUP-pause, and so on as shown in **Figure 3-4**.

Note
The opening of the heart valves does not produce any sounds; only their closure produces sounds; e.g., clapping of the hands produces a sound, opening the palms does not.

Deviations of Heart Sounds from the Normal:
  a. **The intensity of the sounds** may be different.
  b. **The sounds may be split**, the two elements being very close together, which is a very important feature of split sounds. Splitting may be imitated by the syllables—*"L-LUB"* and *"D-DUB"*. Split sounds may be audible in some normal young persons, though in the elderly, they may be pathologic as in bundle branch block.

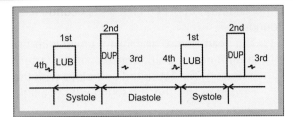

Figure 3-4. Diagrammatic representation of heart sounds. LUB and DUP—phonetic representation of 1st and 2nd heart sounds respectively. The diagrammatic representation of 3rd and 4th heart sounds is to indicate that they have a lower frequency than the 1st and 2nd sounds

c. **A triple rhythm** (gallop rhythm when the heart rate is above 100/min) may be present. Splitting of heart sounds must be differentiated from triple rhythm which is produced by the addition of 3rd or 4th heart sounds to the normal 1st and 2nd sounds, and which may be limited by *"LUB-DUP-DUP"*. (Though phonocardiography shows that a 3rd and a 4th (atrial) sounds are generally present, they are difficult to hear with a stethoscope. When either of these are prominent and audible, they produce a triple rhythm, as in left ventricular failure).

d. **Adventitious or extra sounds**, such as *murmurs* (systolic or diastolic) or *pericardial rub* may be present. (The 3rd sound coincides with rapid ventricular filling and is due to vibrations set up by the sudden inrushing of blood. The 4th heart sound is due to atrial systole).

3-4

Clinical Examination of the Gastrointestinal Tract (GIT) and Abdomen

Disorders of GIT are quite common in our country. Loss of appetite, indigestion, diarrhea, abdominal pains etc are the common complaints. The underlying causes of these complaints are easy to identify if proper history has been taken and physical examination carried out. The examination of the abdomen constitutes a major part of the clinical examination of GIT (alimentary system).

Since the location of abdominal viscera is more or less anatomically exact, it is easy to identify the viscera involved in a particular patient.

IMPORTANT SIGNS AND SYMPTOMS OF GIT DISEASE

These include: loss of appetite (dyspepsia), difficulty in swallowing, burning sensation behind the sternum or in the epigastrium, eructations, abdominal swelling, distension and pain, nausea and vomiting, diarrhea, constipation, hematemesis (vomiting of blood), dark stools, jaundice (present, or past history), loss of weight, fever, etc.

History of Illness. Some leading questions may be required to be asked (if not already mentioned by the patient), particularly loss of appetite, flatulence, nausea and vomiting, abdominal pain etc. as mentioned above.

General Physical Examination. Note the build and nutrition, and look for anemia, jaundice, clubbing of fingers. Record the vital signs. **Oral cavity** should always be checked for the health of the teeth and gums, tongue tonsils, and oropharynx.

EXAMINATION OF ABDOMEN

It is customary to divide the abdomen into nine regions by two horizontal (B,C) and two lateral vertical lines (A, A'). Each vertical line is taken from midclavicle to midinguinal point. The upper horizontal line passes across the abdomen at the lowest points on the costal margin (10th costal arch). The lower horizontal line joins the tubercles of iliac crests.

Abdominal Regions. The regions marked by these lines are shown in **Figure 3-5.**

In the upper abdomen: (1): right hypochondrium; (2): epigastrium; (3): left hypochondrium.

In the middle abdomen: (4): right lumbar; (5): umbilical; (6): left lumbar.

In the lower abdomen: (7): right iliac fossa; (8): hypogastrium; (9): left iliac fossa.

The value of these regions in clinical practice is to describe the position of pain, tenderness, rigidity, tumors, and so on. Since some of the viscera are mobile and constantly change position, these zones are **not** used as anatomical landmarks for them.

The subject should be lying flat on his back, arms by the sides, on a firm bed. Relaxation of the abdominal wall is very essential. The subject is examined from the right side.

INSPECTION

Q. 1 Inspect the abdomen in the subject provided and give your findings.

The following are observed:

1. **State of the skin.** Whether stretched; presence of scars (previous operations) and striae (due to gross stretching); and pigmentation. Presence of prominent veins on the abdomen which is abnormal and is seen in obstruction of vena cava.

2. **Contour or shape.** There are three main types of abdominal contours:
   a. **Flat abdomen:** The rib margins and the abdominal wall are at about the same level.
   b. **Globular or round abdomen:** A generalized and symmetrical fullness (i.e., a forward convexity) may be due to fat (obesity), fluid (ascites), flatus (gas), fetus (pregnancy), or feces (chronic constipation)—the five classical features. There may be sagging of the abdominal wall due to loss of muscle tone.
   c. **Scaphoid abdomen:** The scaphoid, boat-shaped, or sunken abdomen shows a forward concavity. It is seen in extreme starvation, wasting diseases, carcinoma, especially of esophagus and stomach, and sometimes in very thin individuals.

3. **Abdominal asymmetry.** The normal abdomen is symmetrical. Asymmetric localized distention or bulging may be due to gross enlargement of liver, spleen, or ovary or due to tumors.

4. **State of umbilicus.** Normally the umbilicus is slightly retracted and inverted or level with the skin surface. It may be everted or ballooned out in umbilical hernia, raised intra-abdominal pressure, or it may be transversely stretched in ascites (fluid in the peritoneal cavity).

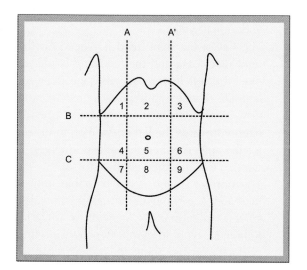

Figure 3-5. Abdominal regions. (See text for details)

5. **Movements with respiration.** The abdomen moves freely with respiration, rising gently during inspiration, and falling during expiration. (In females, the respiratory movements are mainly thoracic). The abdominal movements may be restricted in generalized peritonitis, inflammation of diaphragm, or injury to the abdominal muscles, and in tense ascites.

6. **Visible pulsations.** Epigastric pulsations of abdominal aorta are frequently visible in nervous, thin individuals. Pulsations from a pulsating liver or from right ventricle may also be seen in the epigastrium.

7. **Visible peristalsis.** Peristalsis may be visible as movement of a shadow on the abdomen in persons with thin abdominal wall, in malnourished children, and cachexia. Except for these examples, visible peristalsis may be an indication of pyloric, and small and large intestinal obstruction. One has to observe the abdomen from several angles to detect peristalsis. It may be induced by gentle kneading of the abdomen, or by applying a cold stimulus to the skin.

8. **Hernial sites.** The hernial sites in the groin should be checked for any swelling with straining or coughing.

PALPATION

Q. 2 Palpate the abdomen for liver.

Note
Before palpating the abdomen, the patient is asked about any pain or tenderness (pain on pressure), and such areas are the **last to be palpated.**
    The subject should be relaxed, with hips and knees flexed, and head turned to one side. The subject is asked to take deep breaths through the mouth. Palpation is generally started in the left iliac fossa, and worked anticlockwise to end in the suprapubic region.

Protocol
The right hand is placed flat on the abdomen, with the wrist and the forearm in the same horizontal plane (one may have to bend down or kneel). The relaxed hand is "moulded" to the abdomen, not held rigidly, with the fingers almost straight with slight flexion at the metacarpophalangeal joints (Fingers are never "poked" in the abdomen).

Palpation for liver
The palpation for the liver starts in the right iliac fossa and then gradually worked up to the right costal margin. As the patient inspires deeply, the fingers are pressed firmly inwards and upwards. If the liver is palpable, it meets the radial aspect of the index finger as a sharp regular border. It is sometimes palpable in children and adults, but generally it is palpable only when it is enlarged.

    If palpable, the character of its surface is noted—whether soft and smooth, very firm, or hard and irregular. The liver is enlarged in congestive heart failure, amebic hepatitis, liver abscess, viral hepatitis, malignancy, leukemias, and so on.

Q. 3 Palpate the spleen in the subject provided. Palpation of spleen.

1. The subject is relaxed, with the arms by the side, and hips and knees flexed to relax the abdominal wall.

2. The flat of the right hand is placed on the right iliac fossa and the left hand is placed over the left lowermost rib cage postero-laterally. The left hand presses medially and downwards while the right hand presses deeply towards the left costal margin to feel for the spleen (when the spleen enlarges, it does so towards the right iliac fossa).

3. The normal spleen is not palpable until it increases 2 or 3 times its normal size. Enlarged spleen (splenomegaly) is seen in: malaria, Kala-azar, typhoid, portal hypertension and portal cirrhosis, acute leukemias, chronic myeloid leukemia, and some anemias.

Q. 4 Palpate the kidneys in the subject provided.
Since both kidneys are located behind the peritoneum, the examiner employs both hands for their palpation.

Palpation of Left Kidney.
1. The subject should be relaxed, with both knees and hips flexed.
2. The right hand is placed anteriorly in the left lumbar region while the left hand is placed posteriorly under the costal margin. As the subject takes a deep breath, the left hand presses forwards, and the right hand presses backwards, upwards, and inwards; and an attempt is made to feel for the kidney between the pulps of the fingers of the two hands.
3. The left kidney is not usually palpable unless enlarged or low in position.

Palpation of Right Kidney.
1. The right hand is placed anteriorly in the right lumbar region with the left hand placed posteriorly in the right loin. As the subject takes a deep breath, the left hand presses forwards and the right hand pushes inwards and upwards; and an attempt is made to feel for the kidney between the fingers of the two hands.
2. The lower pole of the right kidney is commonly palpable in thin subjects as a smooth, rounded swelling which descends on inspiration.

PERCUSSION

Q. 5 Percuss the abdomen and give your findings.
Using light percussion, all the nine regions of the abdomen are percussed systematically. A resonant (tympanitic) note is heard all over the abdomen except over the liver where the note is dull. The percussion note varies depending on the amount of gas in the intestines. Ascites, tumors, enlarged liver or spleen, enlarged glands, etc. give a dull note.

Q. 6 Test for the presence of free fluid in the abdominal cavity.
The collection of free fluid in the peritoneal cavity is called ascites. Over 1500 ml of fluid must accumulate before it can be detected by physical examination.

Ascites has to be differentiated from two other common causes of diffuse enlargement of the abdomen, namely, a massive ovarian cyst, and obstruction of distal small bowel, large bowel, or both.

Tests for detection of fluid
1. Shifting dullness. Since a fluid gravitates to the dependent parts, it flows into the flanks and the intestines float in the umbilical region when the patient lies on his back. The abdomen is percussed first with the patient lying on his back, when both flanks show dullness, while the umbilical region shows a tympanitic note. The subject is then rolled on to his left side; a resonant note is now obtained from the right flank while the left flank sounds a dull note due to shifting of fluid to the left flank and the intestines floating up to the right flank. A similar procedure is repeated with the patient rolled on to his right side, when the left flank will now give a resonant note.

The shift of the fluid and the accompanying dullness is called "shifting dullness", i.e., dullness due to shifting of fluid with a change in the position of the subject.

2. Fluid thrill. The patient lies supine. One hand is placed over the lumbar region of one side and a sharp tap or flick is given over the opposite lumbar region. A *wave* or *fluid thrill* is felt by the detecting hand. A similar sensation may be felt if the abdominal wall is very fat. To avoid this, the subject is asked to place the edge of his hand firmly along the midline; this damps any vibrations in the abdominal wall.

3. Horse shoe-shaped dullness. When the amount of ascitic fluid is moderate, the fluid collects in the flanks and the hypogastric region, while the intestines float up in the upper umbilical and epigastric regions. On percussion, the flanks and hypogastric regions produce dullness, whereas the epigastric and upper umbilical regions remain tympanitic.

In the case of *intestinal obstruction*, the percussion note is tympanitic all over. In the case of a large ovarian cyst, the percussion note is resonant in the flanks, and dullness with convexity upwards, over the pelvis.

AUSCULTATION

Q. 7 Auscultate the abdomen of the subject provided.
Auscultation of the abdomen is done to listen for bowel sounds and whether they are normal, increased or absent, and for detecting bruits in the aorta and other abdominal vessels.

The stethoscope is to be placed on one site—usually just to the right of the umbilicus—and kept there until bowel sounds are heard. *It should not be moved from site to site*, and of course, there is no question of comparing the sounds on the two sides.

Normal bowel sounds are heard as intermittent gurgles, low- or medium-pitched, with an occasional high-pitched noise or tinkle. In *gastrointestinal obstruction*, these sounds may be greatly exaggerated, increasing in intensity with waves of pain. On the other hand, in *paralytic ileus* (intestinal paralysis) due to peritonitis or other causes, the sounds are absent—a condition called "silent abdomen".

3-5

Clinical Examination of the Nervous System

Student Objectives
After completing this clinical examination, you should be able to: 1. Realize the importance of knowing the anatomy and physiology of the nervous system. 2. Name the various cranial nerves, their functions, and the subjective and objective features of their lesions. 3. Classify sensory receptors and sensations. 4. Trace the sensory pathways. 5. Name the motor pathways, their origin, course, termination and functions. 6. Elicit various superficial and deep reflexes and indicate their clinical significance. 7. Test the motor and sensory functions. 8. Enumerate the differences between upper and lower motor neuron lesions.

History Taking

Taking a careful history of illness is of great importance (as in other systems) and frequently requires as much or more skill than in later physical examination in a case of neurological disease. Impatience, boredom, disbelief, embarrassment and reproach usually act as a barrier to communication with a patient of low level of intelligence, or when she/he is confused, or not fully conscious. In such cases, help has to be taken from the patient's attendants.

In a neurology patient, the *history of progress of disease* will provide valuable leads to the parts of the nervous system involved and the nature of underlying pathology. As knowledge increases, more information may be obtained by asking leading questions.

Common Signs and Symptoms of Neurological Disease

These include: speech and language defects, partial unconsciousness with restlessness, sleep disorders and altered behavior; motor defects such as weakness, paralysis, fits (convulsions), rigidity, tremors, involuntary movements; sensory disturbances; and effects of involvement of cranial nerve.

The major causes of these signs and symptoms include: vascular insults (hemorrhage, ischemic strokes), head and spinal injuries, degenerative diseases, infections (bacterial and viral) and so on.

Diagnosis of Nervous System Diseases

The diagnosis of a neurology patient depends primarily on correlating the signs and symptoms to the underlying disease process. The anatomical diagnosis depends on the assessment of changes in motor and sensory functions, alteration in reflexes, and subjective and objective features of lesions of cranial nerves.

Clinical Examination of Nervous System

This should proceed along the following lines: Examination of higher functions; speech functions; cranial nerves; motor functions; reflexes; sensory functions; and evidence of trophic changes.

I. EXAMINATION OF HIGHER FUNCTIONS

Apart from motor and sensory functions and maintenance of vital signs, the brain is concerned with the higher functions of consciousness, intellect, and mentation. Note the following:

1. **Appearance and behavior.** Is the patient well-groomed or unkempt; disturbed or agitated; whether the attention wanders; any flight of ideas. Note personal hygiene – nails, hands, hair.
2. **Emotional state.** Note if the mood is elevated or depressed, or if there is flattening of emotions. Does he appear confused, or does he live in a world of his own. Enquire about sleep and dreams.
3. **Delusions and hallucinations.** Delusions are false beliefs which continue to be held despite evidence to the contrary (e.g., believing that someone is out to kill me"). Hallucinations are false impressions (visual, or auditory; e.g., taking a rope to be a snake).
4. **Level of consciousness.** Is there any clouding of consciousness? Ask him about events around him. Is there dementia (loss of memory), or coma (a deep state of unconsciousness from which the patient cannot be roused).
5. **Orientation in place and time.** Ask the patient about the date, month and year, and whether he is in a hospital or at his home. Disorientation is an important sign of organic diseases of the brain and in psychiatric disorders.
6. **Memory.** Test for recent and past memory by asking pointed questions. In brain injuries, for example, recent memory is affected much more than past memory.
7. **General intelligence.** This will be evident during history taking. Ask for educational history and work record. One simple test is to ask her/him to continue deducting 7 from 100. Tests for reasoning and "absurdities" test can give a fair idea of the intelligence.

II. SPEECH (LANGUAGE) FUNCTIONS

While animals can express their feelings by sounds, gestures and postures (e.g., an angry dog), only man can express his feelings, ideas, thoughts by using symbols (i.e., words) representing ideas, things, etc.

Thus, true speech, i.e., the ability to understand and express in symbols, is one of the highest functions of the human brain. For normal speech, not only the cerebral cortex must be intact but the motor mechanisms that control articulation (uttering of words) must also be perfect.

Speech has two components: a *receiving* or *sensory part* (*vision, hearing*), and *expressing or motor part* (*spoken* and *written* speech). Thus, the disorders of speech may be aphasias or dysarthria.

Aphasias, i.e., loss of the ability to understand and use symbols, may be *sensory* (or *fluent*) that are due to lesions in the Wernicke's area (area for understanding), or *motor* (or *non-fluent*) that are due to lesions in the Broca's area (area 44). The third type of aphasia is called *global aphasia* that is due to lesions involving both Wernicke's and Broca's areas.

Dysarthria is simply the inability to utter words though the patient knows what to say.

Tests

Look for defects of articulation. Test the patient for various types of aphasias. Give him various common objects and ask him to name them, and the purpose for which they are used.

III. THE CRANIAL NERVES

There are 12 pairs of cranial nerves. Some of them are purely sensory (afferent), others are motor (efferent), while still others are mixed, i.e., they contain both sensory and motor fibers.

A sound knowledge of the anatomy and physiology of cranial nerves is essential in order to understand the logic of methods employed in testing them, and the clinical significance of any abnormalities that may be detected.

The 1st or Olfactory Nerve (Sensory)

Q. 1 Test the sense of smell in the subject provided. What is the pathway for smell?
Consult Expt 27 Section 2.

The 2nd or Optic Nerve (Sensory)

The following aspects of optic nerve function are tested:
A. Visual acuity. (Distant and near vision)
B. Field of vision.

C. Color vision
D. Examination of fundus

A. Visual Acuity

Q. 1 Test the visual acuity of the subject provided.
Visual acuity, i.e., the ability to see subjects clearly, is tested for distant as well as for near vision.

Testing for distant vision.   For testing distant vision, special types (consult Expt 5-11 for Snellen chart) of print varying in size are used. Each eye is tested separately. The subject is seated at a distance of 6 m (20 feet) from a well-lighted chart and the central visual acuity is recorded as a fraction as that of a person with normal vision, as described in Expt 5-11.

Testing for near vision.   The subject holds the Jaeger chart (consult Expt 5-12 for the description of this chart) at the ordinary reading distance and reads the printed material of varying sizes down the chart. The result is expressed as J1, J2, J3, etc. A person with normal vision can read the smallest test type at a distance of about 15 inches.

B. Color Vision

Q. 2 Test the color vision of the subject provided.
The color vision is tested with Ishihara charts (consult Expt 5-13 for description of these color plates). The other methods for testing color vision are Holmgren wools, and the Edridge-Green lantern, as described in Experiment 5-13.

C. Field of Vision

Q. 3 Test the peripheral field of vision of the subject provided, using the confrontation test.
It is a rough test to compare a person's visual fields with the examiner's own (presuming his own to be normal). The subject and the examiner sit facing each other about 3 feet apart. When testing the subject's left eye, he places his cupped right hand over his right eye, and with the left eye he fixes his

gaze on the examiner's right eye, while the examiner closes his left eye. The subject is instructed not to move his left eye in any direction. The examiner then holds out his right arm to its full extent, midway between himself and the subject, and asks the subject to say "yes" when he sees any movement of the examiner's finger. If no movement is perceived, the hand is moved in, kept still and the finger moved once again. In this way, the examiner compares his own *first sighting* of the movement with that of the subject.

Using this procedure, the peripheral field is tested in all the four quadrants—temporal, upper, lower and nasal. The subject's right eye is tested in a similar manner. The normal peripheral field of vision extends beyond 90° on the temporal side, about 50° in the vertical direction, about 55° on the nasal side, and about 65° downwards. Only gross changes in the field of vision can be detected with this method. Scotomas (blind areas within the field of vision) are impossible to locate, for which a perimeter is employed (see Expt 2-15).

When testing vision for color and visual fields, it is essential to ensure that any refractive error is corrected and that no other disease affecting acuity of vision or visual fields is present.

Oculomotor and Pupillary Innervation—The 3rd (Oculomotor), 4th (Trochlear), 6th (Abducent) and Sympathetic Nerves

The 3rd, 4th, and 6th cranial nerves are usually considered together because they function as a physiological unit in the control of the eye movements. The 6th nerve supplies the lateral rectus, the 4th nerve innervates the superior oblique, and the 3rd nerve supplies all the other external ocular muscles. It also sends fibers to the levator palpebrae superioris and through the ciliary ganglion, it supplies parasympathetic fibers to the sphincter pupillae and the muscle of accommodation, the ciliary muscle (contraction for near vision).

The sympathetic fibers emerge along the 1st and 2nd thoracic nerves, synapse in the superior cervical ganglion, from where postganglionic fibers pass upward along the internal carotid artery to supply dilator pupillae, the involuntary fibers in levator palpebrae superioris, and ciliary muscle contraction for far vision.

Before testing these nerves, observe—
1. If there is any squint—the patient should also be asked if he/she sees double (diplopia).
2. The condition of the pupils—whether they are equal in size and regular in outline, whether they are abnormally dilated or contracted, and their reaction to light and accommodation.

Q. 1 Test the conjugate movements of the eyes in the subject provided.
Normally the movement of the eyes are simultaneous, and symmetrical so that the visual axes meet at a point at which the eyes are directed. This is called **conjugate movements** of the eyes.

To test the eye movements, the head of the patient must be fixed with the left hand and he/she must be asked to follow the examiner's index finger to the right, to the left, upwards and downwards as far as possible in each direction. Normally, the eyes move 50° outwards, 50° downwards, 50° inwards, and 33° upwards. The rotatory movements should also be tested. It is observed if there is any limitation of movement in any direction.

(The brain stem centers of 3rd, 4th, and 6th cranial nerves probably control reflex movements of the eyes, while conjugate movements of voluntary origin are under the control of higher cortical centers via the corticonuclear tracts).

Q. 2 Demonstrate the light reflex in the subject provided. What is the pathway of this reflex?
Direct light reflex. Each eye is tested separately in a shady place. The subject is asked to look at a distance. A bright light from a torch, **brought from the side of the eye**, is shined into the eye—the result is a prompt constriction of the pupil. When the light is switched off, the pupil quickly dilates to its previous size.

Indirect or consensual light reflex. A hand is placed between the two eyes, and light is shined into one eye, observing the effect on the pupil of the unstimulated side. There is a constriction of the pupil in the other eye—a response called the indirect or consensual light reflex. Thus, the pupils of both eyes constrict when light is thrown into any eye.

Pathway of direct light reflex. Retinal receptors → Optic nerve → Optic chiasma → Optic tract → Pretectum of midbrain → Edinger-Westphal nuclei of both sides → Oculomotor nerve → Ciliary ganglion → Ciliary nerves → Sphincter muscle of iris → Constriction of pupil.

Q. 3 What is the cause of consensual light reflex?
When the retinal receptors of one eye are stimulated by light, nerve impulses pass along optic nerve, optic chiasma, optic tract, and reach the pretectal region of midbrain. Here, some of the fibers from each side terminate on the Edinger-Westphal nuclei of both sides. As a result, when light falls on the retina, the pupils on both sides constrict.

Q. 4 Demonstrate the reaction of the pupil to accommodation for near vision.
The subject is asked to look at the far wall of the room. The observer then suddenly brings his finger, holding it vertically, about 15 cm in front of the subject's nose, and the subject is asked to look at it. The response is convergence of the eyes and pupillary constriction as he accommodates for the finger. The pupils dilate as the finger is moved away.

Q. 5 What is the pathway for accommodation reflex?
Pathway for accommodation reflex. The pathway for the accommodation reflex is as follows: Retina → Optic nerve → Optic tract → Lateral geniculate body → Geniculocalcarine tract (Optic radiation) → Visual cortex (area 17) → Frontal eye-field area (area 8 αβδ) → Edinger-Westphal nucleus of opposite side → Oculomotor

nerve → Ciliary ganglion → Ciliary nerves → Constrictor pupillae muscle. (Sympathetic system plays almost no role in accommodation).

Q. 6 What is Argyll-Robertson pupil?
A pupil in which the accommodation reflex is present but the light reflex, both direct and consensual, is absent, is called the **Argyll-Robertson pupil.** The lesion, usually neurosyphilis, is located in the pretectum of the midbrain behind the optic tract and the 3rd nerve nucleus, thus interrupting the pathway of light reflex while leaving the accommodation pathway intact.

Comments
Changes in the pupil in cases of head injury and cardiac arrest provide important diagnostic and prognostic information. Inequality of the pupils may indicate a rising intracranial tension due to hematoma. Dilated and fixed pupils, non-reacting to light, may suggest serious and irreversible brain damage. Pupillary responses to light are also watched during anesthesia.

The 5th or Trigeminal Nerve (Sensory and Motor)

A. Sensory Functions

Q. 1 Demonstrate the corneal reflex.
Light wisp of absorbent cotton is twisted to a fine hair. The subject is asked to look at the far wall and, approaching from the side, the lateral edge of the cornea is lightly touched with the cotton. (The cornea should never be wiped with the cotton and the central cornea should never be touched, because ulceration may occur if there is corneal anesthesia). The response is bilateral blinking; and the two sides should be compared. The afferent path of this reflex is ophthalmic division of the 5th nerve, the efferent path is 7th nerve, while the center is in the nuclei of these nerves in the pons.

The **conjunctival reflex**, also a superficial reflex, is elicited in the same manner as corneal reflex. Touching the conjunctiva with a wisp of cotton causes bilateral blinking. (The conjunctiva of the lower lid is supplied by maxillary division of the 5th nerve).

The **nasal or sneeze reflex,** i.e., sneezing when the nasal mucosa is irritated, also employs 5th nerve as its afferent path, while the motor path employs motor components of 5th to 10th cranial and upper cervical nerves.

Q. 2 Test the general sensory functions of the trigeminal nerve.

In addition to the corneal and palpebral conjunctiva, the 5th nerve supplies greater part of the face, forehead, temporal and parietal regions, and nasal and buccal mucosa. The sensory fibers arise from unipolar cells in the semilunar or gasserian ganglion and supply the skin and mucosa described above. The nerve also contains **sensory proprioceptive fibers** which innervate muscle spindles in the muscles of mastication, and possibly also in the external ocular muscles. The motor components supply the muscles of mastication.

The sensations of touch, pain, and temperature over the face are tested, as elsewhere on the body as described later, with a wisp of cotton, pin pricks, and warm and cold objects.

B. Motor Functions

Q. 3 Test the motor functions of the trigeminal nerve in the subject provided.

The motor fibers of the 5th nerve, (its nucleus lies at the mid-pontine level) innervate the muscles of mastication—masseter, temporalis, and medial and lateral pterygoids—and the tensor tympani of middle ear.

1. The subject is asked to open his mouth and show the teeth. Normally, the jaw is symmetrical. If there is paralysis on one side, the jaw deviates to the side of paralysis, the healthy pterygoids pushing it to that side.
2. The subject is asked to clench his teeth—the temporalis and masseter muscles contract and become equally prominent on the two sides. The muscles can be palpated to note if there is any difference in the strength of contraction.
3. The subject is asked to open his mouth and move the mandible from side to side.

4. The jaw jerk (maxillary reflex) is tested by placing a finger on the chin below the lower lip, with the mouth open, and striking it with a percussion hammer. The response is closure of the mouth. Normally this jerk is hardly detectable, but it is exaggerated in upper motor neuron lesions (as are other deep reflexes). Both the afferent and efferent paths are along 5th nerve and the center is in the pons.

(The mandibular division of 5th nerve also supplies parasympathetic fibers to the salivary glands).

The 7th or Facial Nerve (Almost Purely Motor)

The facial nerve supplies all the superficial muscles of the face and scalp (except levator palpebrae superioris which is supplied by 3rd nerve), external ear, and the stapedius in the middle ear. The chorda tympani runs with this nerve for part of its course. The parsympathetic fibers from the superior salivatory nucleus innervate the blood vessels and glandular cells of sublingual and submaxillary glands, and glands in the mucosa of pharynx, palate, nasal cavity, and paranasal sinuses.

Q. 1 Test the motor functions of the facial nerve in the subject provided.
Testing the upper face

1. The subject is asked to look up and wrinkle the skin on his forehead (occipitofrontalis muscle tested). Normally, the wrinkling of the skin is symmetrical on the two sides. By asking the subject to frown, the corrugator supercilii can be tested.
2. He is asked to shut his eyes as tightly as possible. (The corners of the mouth also get drawn up). The examiner then tries to open one and then the other eye. Normally, it is impossible to do so against the subject's wishes. (Orbicularis oculi muscles tested).

When one tries to shut the eyes tightly, the eyeballs roll upwards, a normal response called *Bell's phenomenon.* In Bell's palsy (see below), when the patient closes his eyes, the upward movement of the eyeball becomes obvious because closure of the affected eye is not possible.

Testing the lower face

1. The nasolabial folds on both sides are observed, which are normally symmetrical. Paralysis on one side causes flattening of the folds on that side; it also affects facial symmetry at rest or during voluntary facial movements.

2. The subject is asked to smile or show his upper teeth, or to whistle. Normally, the face remains symmetrical (Levator angularis muscle tested). Paralysis of one side causes the angle of the mouth to be drawn towards the healthy side, while that on the paralysed side remains stationary. The buccinator is also involved in whistling.

3. The subject is asked to inflate his mouth with air and blow out his cheeks (Buccinator tested). Each inflated cheek is then tapped with a finger. If there is paralysis, the air escapes easily through the angle of the mouth on the paralysed side.

4. The subject is asked to depress the lower lip (Depressor labii inferioris and quadratus labii inferioris tested). In case of paralysis, the asymmetry is obvious.

Facial paralysis results quite commonly from lesions of upper or lower motor neurons. To differentiate between these two, it is important to remember that 7th nerve nuclei innervating muscles of *upper* face are under bilateral cortical motor control, while the facial nuclei supplying the lower face are controlled from the opposite motor cortex only.

Therefore, in **supranuclear lesion** (upper neuron paralysis; e.g., capsular hemiplegia), only the muscles of lower part of face are paralysed, i.e., the forehead can be wrinkled and the eyes closed. In **infranuclear lesion** (lower motor neuron paralysis, i.e., lesion of facial nucleus or facial nerve—as in Bell's palsy), both the upper as well as the lower parts of the face are equally affected (paralysed). If paralysis is complete, the whole side

of the face is smooth and free from wrinkles. The lower eyelid droops, the angle of the mouth sags, and saliva may dribble. The Bell's phenomenon is present. The taste sensation from the anterior two-thirds is lost, and sounds seem unusually loud (hyperacusis) due to paralysis of stapedius which normally attenuates loud sounds. Listening to a shrill whistle will test the stapedius.

Since the 7th nerve is related to many cranial nerves and other structures during its course, involvement of some of these helps in localizing the site of lesion.

Q. 2 Test the taste function of the facial nerve.
Consult Experiment 26 Section 2.

The patient should always be asked about any abnormal taste sensations or hallucinations of taste, which may form the aura of an epileptic fit, particularly in temporal lobe epilepsy.

The 8th or Vestibulocochlear Nerve (Composite Sensory Nerve)

The 8th cranial nerve has two components: the cochlear nerve and the vestibular nerve. The cochlear nerve supplies the cochlea and subserves hearing, while the vestibular nerve supplies the semicircular canals (SCC; for dynamic equilibrium) and the labyrinth (otolith organ, utricle and saccule; for static equilibrium) and subserves equilibrium, balance, and sensation of bodily displacement.

The symptoms of cochlear nerve involvement include tinnitus (ringing, buzzing, hissing, singing, or roaring noises in the ear); deafness; hearing scotomas (selective deafness to certain pitches and noises); and sensory aphasia in supranuclear lesions.

The symptoms of vestibular nerve damage include vertigo (a feeling of giddiness); nystagmus (a rhythmic to and fro movement of the eyes); and some general symptoms like nausea, vomiting, tachycardia, and low blood pressure.

Q. 1 Perform the Rinne test on the subject provided.

Q. 2 Perform the Weber test on the subject provided.

Q. 3 Demonstrate the Schwabach test of hearing.

Consult Experiment 23 Section 2 for answers to these questions.

Q. 4 Perform the whisper test in the subject provided.

The simplest way of testing for hearing loss is the use of human voice. A conversational voice is generally heard at a distance of 10-12 feet in each ear, separately. The whisper test is the simplest test for assessing gross defects in hearing.

The examiner stands on one side of the subject and closes the subject's opposite ear with his own finger. He then asks the subject's name, nature of his work, etc by gently whispering into his ear from a distance of 12-14 inches. The procedure is repeated on the other side.

A ticking watch may be gradually brought towards each ear of the subject, separately. The examiner can then compare the subject's hearing with his own.

Q. 5 How will you test the vestibular function in the subject provided?

In the **Barany caloric test,** the subject's head is tilted back 60°, and his external auditory meatus is irrigated with 250 ml of water at 30°C (7° below body temperature) for 40 seconds. The test is repeated with water at 44°C (7° above normal). The endolymph in the horizontal canal (which becomes vertical with head tilt) moves due to convection currents, thus stimulating the receptors in the crista ampullaris.

The normal response to caloric stimulation is nausea, horizontal nystagmus, past pointing, and falling to stimulated side. In vestibular dysfunction, these reactions to stimulation are diminished.

In the **Barany chair test,** the subject is seated in a special chair which can be rotated at a definite speed, with the subject's head tilted to specified positions to stimulate a particular pair of semicircular canals. The effects of acceleration and deceleration, i.e., nystagmus, vomiting, past pointing, and tendency to fall, can then be observed.

The 9th or Glossopharyngeal Nerve (Mixed Nerve)

The 9th nerve is motor to the middle constrictor of pharynx and stylopharyngeus, and sensory for the posterior third of the tongue (both general and taste sensations), and mucous membrane of the pharynx. Parasympathetic fibers from inferior salivatory nucleus, after relaying in the otic ganglion, innervate parotid gland. This nerve is rarely involved alone, but generally with the 10th and 11th nerves.

Q. 1 How will you test the 9th cranial nerve?
Tests for 9th nerve
1. The sensation of taste over the posterior third of the tongue is tested.
2. Each side of the pharynx is touched lightly with a wooden spatula. The response is constriction of the pharynx. The afferent path is 9th nerve; the center is in medulla; and the efferent path is 10th nerve. Thus, this *pharyngeal (or gag) reflex* tests vagus as well.
3. A soft touch is applied on the soft palate; the response is elevation of the soft palate. The reflex arc is the same as in the gag reflex described above.

The 10th or Vagus Nerve (Mixed Nerve)

The vagus nerve is motor for soft palate, pharynx, and intrinsic muscles of the larynx. *Somatic sensory fibers* from unipolar cells in jugular ganglion supply external auditory meatus and part of the ear. The *visceral sensory fibers* of unipolar cells in ganglion nodosum innervate pharynx, larynx, trachea, and thoracic and abdominal viscera. The **parasympathetic fibers** arise from nucleus ambiguous and supply the heart (inhibitory), bronchial muscle and glands, glands and the smooth muscle of most of the gastrointesinal tract, and suprarenal gland.

Q. 1 How will you test the vagus nerve in the subject provided?

1. The *pharyngeal and palate reflexes* are tested as described for 9th nerve.
2. Using a tongue depressor, the subject is asked to open his mouth wide and say "ah". The response is constriction of posterior pharyngeal wall (Vernet's rideau phenomenon), and movement of the uvula backwards in the midline. But in vagal paralysis, the uvula is deflected to the normal side.
3. The subject is asked for history of regurgitation of food through the nose, which is due to total paralysis of vagus; a nasal voice may also be noted.
4. Laryngoscopy is done to note the position and movement of the true vocal cords.

The 11th or Accessory Nerve (Motor Nerve)

This purely motor nerve innervates some muscles in the pharynx and larynx (internal or medullary branch, arising from nucleus ambiguus), as well as sternomastoid and the trapezius (external or spinal branch arising from the anterior horn cells of upper 5 or 6 spinal cord segments).

Q. 1 Test the spinal part of the accessory nerve in the subject provided.

1. The examiner presses on the shoulders from behind and asks the subject to shrug his shoulders (this tests the upper part of trapezius). If the 11th nerve is damaged, shrugging is weaker on that side; the shoulder also droops. The subject is asked to approximate his shoulder blades against examiner's resistance (this tests the lower part of the muscle).
2. A hand is placed against the right side of the subject's face and he is asked to rotate the head to the right. The left sternomastoid is seen to become prominent. The procedure is repeated on the left side also. In case of a unilateral lesion, the head cannot be rotated to the healthy side.

3. The examiner places a hand on the subject's forehead and asks him to bend his head forwards against resistance. Normally, both sternomastoids become prominent.

The 12th or Hypoglossal Nerve (Motor Nerve)

The motor fibers arise from the hypoglossal nucleus in the lower part of the floor of the 4th ventricle. The fibers innervate the muscles of the tongue and depressors of the hyoid bone. A few proprioceptive fibers from the tongue probably run in this nerve.

Q. 1 Test the hypoglossal nerve in the subject provided.

1. The subject is asked to push out his tongue as far as possible. Normally, it remains in the midline (genioglossus tested). If the 12th nerve is paralysed, the tongue is pushed over to the side of the lesion by the healthy muscles on the opposite side. The affected side is also wasted, wrinkled, and may show fasciculation, which indicates lower motor neuron lesion.
2. The subject is asked to move the tongue from side to side over the lips and against the walls of the cheeks (extrinsic and intrinsic muscles of the tongue tested). A finger is placed against the cheek while the subject is asked to press against it with his tongue through the wall of the cheek. The strength of contraction is compared on the two sides.
3. The subject is asked to touch the tongue to the palate (palatoglossus tested), and to depress the tongue in the floor of the mouth (hypoglossus tested).

IV. THE MOTOR FUNCTIONS

Types of Motor Activities
  i. Muscle tone and reflexes; mostly spinal mechanisms (involuntary).
 ii. Gross and fine, skilled movement (voluntary).
iii. Semiautomatic movements (e.g., chewing, swallowing, swinging of arms while walking)

There is, however, no clear cut demarcation between voluntary and involuntary movements, one activity often merging into another.

COMPONENTS OF THE MOTOR SYSTEM

The motor system consists of: motor areas of cerebral cortex, subcortical structures (basal ganglia, cerebellum, reticular formation, vestibular nuclei etc), descending motor tracts (the so-called upper motor neurons (UMN), lower motor neurons (LMN), and the skeletal muscles. **Figure 3-6** shows the components of the motor system.

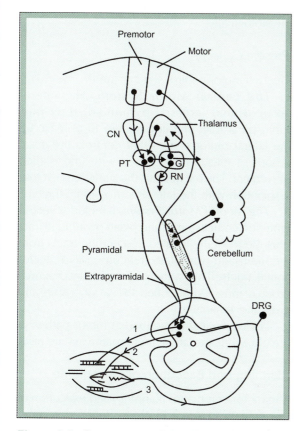

Figure 3-6. Components of the motor system. CN: Caudate nucleus; PT: putamen; G: globus pallidus; RN: red nucleus; 1: alpha motor neuron supplying extrafusal muscle fibers; 2: gamma motor neuron supplying intrafusal muscle fibers; 3: afferent fiber from muscle spindle

A. Muscles. The skeletal muscles can contract only in response to signals received from their motor nerves. The input to the motor neurons is through two sources:

i. Dorsal nerve root fibers for muscle tone and reflexes.

ii. Descending motor tracts for voluntary movements and postural reflexes.

During any movement, when the agonists contract, the antagonists relax at the same time. This is achieved by reciprocal innervation which is a spinal segmental mechanism.

The role of a stable posture is very essential in every movement. Every movement begins in a certain posture and ends in another posture. There is thus a continuous adjustment of posture by changes in muscle tone as movements progress.

Proximal Group of Muscles. The axial muscles (hip, trunk, shoulders) and the proximal muscles of the limbs make up this group. They are mainly concerned in maintenance of posture, equilibrium, and gross movements.

Distal Group of Muscles. This group includes the muscles of the distal parts of the limbs (fingers, hands, wrists). They are not involved in posture and equilibrium but in voluntary, fine and skilled movements such as those during writing, typing, playing on a musical instruments etc (i.e., manipulative behavior).

B. Lower Motor Neurons (LMN). The anterior horn cells of spinal cord and the motor cranial nuclei in the brainstem that directly innervate the skeletal muscle fibers are called LMN. Their axons leave the CNS via ventral roots (or motor cranial nerves) and eventually become the motor supply to the muscles.

In the spinal cord, the most medially located motor neurons *(the medial motor system)* innervate the proximal group of muscles (for posture), while the laterally located neurons *(the lateral motor system)* innervate the distal group of muscles (for fine skilled movements).

The lower motor neurons constitute the "final common pathway" for all motor signals that leave the CNS on their way to skeletal muscles.

C. Upper Motor Neurons (UMN).

The unqualified term UMN is applicable to those cerebral cortical neurons that directly or indirectly (i.e., via subcortical structures: cerebellum, basal ganglia, vestibular nuclei etc) activate lower motor neurons.

The term UMN has traditionally been used for the corticospinal tracts **(Figure 3-7)** that form the pyramids in the medulla, i.e., *direct (crossed) corticospinal-pyramidal system.*

While the *lesions of LMN* cause flaccid paralysis, muscle atrophy and absence of deep (stretch) reflexes, the *lesions of UMN* cause spastic paralysis and exaggerated deep reflexes without muscle atrophy. This leads us to believe that 3 types of UMN need to be considered because:

i. Lesions in posture regulating pathways produce spastic paralysis.

ii. Lesions in corticospinal and corticobulbar fibers cause weakness rather than paralysis.

iii. Cerebellar lesions cause incoordination.

D. "Extrapyramidal" System.

It is a widely used term for those tracts (from basal ganglia etc) that indirectly control LMN but are not part of direct cortico-spinal-pyramidal system. This term is now being less frequently used clinically and physiologically.

Present Concept

The two motor control systems are:

1. *The Lateral Motor System.* The lateral corticospinal (crossed pyramidal) tract plus rubrospinal tract that lies anterior to it, make up the lateral motor system that controls the distal groups of muscles concerned with fine, skilled movement. The red nucleus thus functions in close association with the lateral corticospinal tract.

2. *The Medial Motor System.* It includes ventral (anterior) corticospinal (uncrossed pyramidal) tract plus the medially-located descending tracts from the brainstem (vestibulo-, reticulo-, olivo-, tecto-spinal tracts). This system controls the proximal group of muscles (described above) for posture and gross movements.

Phylogenetically, the medial motor pathways are old, while the lateral motor pathways are new.

Planning and Execution of Movements

The motor command, planning, and execution of movements **(Figure 3-8)** is now believed to occur in the following manner:

Commands: Motor commands originate in cortical association areas.

Planning: Planning occurs in cerebral cortex, basal ganglia, and in lateral cerebellum, and possibly in thalamus

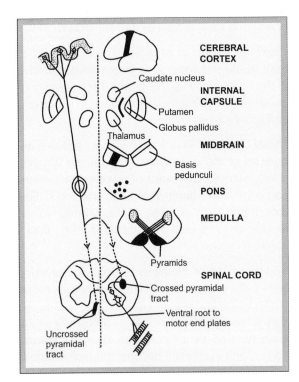

Figure 3-7. Diagram showing the origin, course and termination of corticospinal-pyramidal system. The location of the tract at each level is shown on the right. The majority of fibers cross to opposite side in lower medulla to descend as lateral corticospinal tract. Along with rubrospinal tract that lies in front of it, it forms the lateral motor control system that controls distal group of muscles

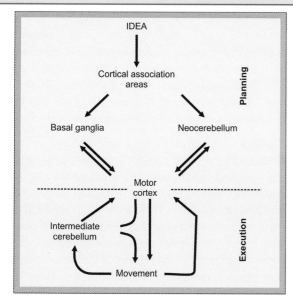

Figure 3-8. Diagram to show the planning and execution of voluntary movements

Execution: Motor commands go from cortical and premotor areas to the LMN for execution.

Feedback information about the status of a movement is sent back from proprioceptors to cerebellum which compares actual performance with intended movement and adjusts signals from cortical areas to smoothen out errors, if any.

Testing The Motor Functions

1. Nutrition or bulk
2. Muscle tone
3. Power or strength
4. Coordination of muscular activity
5. Reflexes
6. Presence of abnormal movements
7. Gait.

1. Nutritional or Bulk

Q. 1 Test the state of nutrition in the upper and lower limbs of the subject provided.
State of nutrition or bulk of muscles. This can be easily estimated by inspection, palpation, and by measuring the circumference of the limbs with a tape measure at certain points, and comparing them on the two sides.

In *upper limbs*, the circumference is measured 5 inches above the elbow and 4 inches below it.

In *lower limbs*, the circumference is measured 9 inches above the knee and 6 inches below it.

The *muscle mass decreases* in muscular atrophy (the muscles are smaller and softer), which may be generalized or localized. It may result from cachexia, disuse (prolonged confinement to bed, or when a limb is kept in a plaster cast), or as a consequence of lower motor neuron disease.

The *muscle mass increases* (hypertrophy) with physical exercise, and in certain occupations requiring excessive workload. In certain diseases of muscles—dystrophy and pseudohypertrophy, though the muscle bulk is increased, they are weak.

2. Muscle Tone

Q. 2 Test the tone of the muscles in the upper limbs.
Muscle (or muscular) tone. This term refers to the continuously maintained state of slight tension or tautness in the healthy muscles even when they appear to be at rest. An increase in tone is called *hypertonia*, while a decrease in tone is called *hypotonia*.

Muscle tone is tested by noting the resistance offered to passive movements done by the examiner on various joints of the subject/patient. The examiner holds the limb on either side of a joint to be tested, and passively moves the joint through the full range of its movements. The ease or difficulty with which a joint can thus be moved is noted and compared with the similar joint on the opposite side.

Test. The examiner holds the forearm of the subject with one hand, and alternately flexes and extends the wrist with the other hand. Tone at the fingers, elbow, and shoulder is tested in a similar manner. In the lower limbs, passive movements are done at the ankle, knee and hip comparing these on the two sides.

In hypertonia, the patient's muscles resist the passive movements, while in hypotonia the movements become free and the joints can be hyperextended.

Muscle Tone.   Muscle tone, i.e., the slight tautness in a muscle, implies the contraction of a small number of motor units scattered throughout the muscle, but a number which is not enough to cause movement at a joint. (If the tendon of a muscle, say biceps, is cut from its insertion, the muscle shortens—a proof of tone).

Muscle tone is a spinal stretch reflex (static reflex) phenomenon, which results from a slight stretch of the muscle spindles scattered in between the ordinary (extrafusal) muscle fibers. Afferent impulses from the stretch receptors of the spindles enter the spinal cord where they reflexly excite anterior horn cells (alpha neurons). These neurons, in turn, discharge *out of step and at a low rate,* which leads to contraction of a certain number of muscle fibers; and this is manifested as muscle tone. Damage to any part of the reflex arc abolishes muscle tone.

Muscle tone does not produce fatigue because only a small number of muscle fibers contract at a time; these fibers relax and another group takes up activity. This process of rotation of activity prevents the occurrence of fatigue.

But what is the cause of stretching of the muscle spindles to start with? From the time of early growth, the bones grow longer at a rate faster than that of muscles. This maintains a slight stretch on the muscles, and therefore, on the spindles, throughout the lifetime of an individual, so that the muscles remain in a state of tone.

Though muscle tone is a spinal reflex mechanism, it is mainly regulated by supraspinal pathways—the pyramidal (corticospinal) and extrapyramidal tracts. The anterior cerebellum, via the subcortical structures, has a facilitatory effect on muscle tone.

Hypertonia. This occurs in lesions of upper motor neuron (corticospinal) and extrapyramidal systems.

Spasticity. The term refers to hypertonia resulting from *lesions of the corticospinal system.* The

increased tone is of *clasp-knife type,* i.e., when the limb is moved, maximum resistance is offered at once, but it suddenly gives way after some effort on the part of the examiner. Spasticity is therefore a form of rigidity which is sensitive to stretch, i.e., it is *"stretch-sensitive".* It is usually maximum in flexors of the arms and extensors of the legs.

Rigidity.   The hypertonia of rigidity results from *diseases of the basal ganglia* (e.g., Parkinsonism), and is called extrapyramidal rigidity. It may be of *cog-wheel* type in which the resistance to passive movement decreases in jerky steps (probably a combination of tremor and rigidity), or of *lead-pipe* type in which resistance is felt throughout the passive movement. The rigidity of Parkinsonism is commonly accompanied by akinesia, i.e., poverty of movement.

Hypotonia is seen in lower motor neuron disease and cerebellar lesions. Passive movement is unusually free and frequently through a greater range than normal.

3. Power or Strength

Q. 3 Test the muscle strength in the upper limbs of the subject provided.
A preliminary observation of how a subject, (but especially a patient), walks, or stands up from the sitting or supine position, shakes hands, or performs other everyday movements such as buttoning a shirt or combing the hair, can provide a quick and reliable means for assessing muscle weakness, or paralysis, if any.

The muscle power at big and small joints is then tested by asking the subject first to move parts of the body, and then against resistance of the examiner's hand, and compared with similar muscles on the opposite limb.

  i. **Abductor pollicis brevis.** The subject is asked to abduct his thumb in a plane at right angles to the palmar aspect of the index finger, against the resistance of the examiner's own thumb. The muscle can be seen and felt to contract. This muscle is supplied by the median nerve which is sometimes damaged by compression in the carpal tunnel at the wrist (carpal tunnel syndrome).

ii. **Opponens pollicis.** The subject is asked to touch the tips of all his fingers with the tip of his thumb. The examiner opposes each movement with his index finger or thumb.

iii. **First dorsal interosseous.** The subject is asked to abduct his index finger against resistance.

iv. **Interossei and lumbricals.** The subject's ability to flex his metacarpo-phalangeal joints and to extend the distal interphalangeal joints is tested. The interossei also adduct and abduct the fingers.

v. **Flexors of fingers.** The subject is asked to squeeze the examiner's index and middle fingers to assess the force of grip.

vi. **Flexors of the wrist.** The subject is asked to bring his fingers towards the front of the forearm, while the examiner opposes this movement with his fingers.

vii. **Extensors of the wrist.** The subject is asked to make a fist (both flexors and extensors contract), while the examiner tries to flex the wrist against the subject's effort to maintain that position.

viii. **Brachioradialis.** The subject's arm is placed midway between pronation and supination, and then asked to bend the forearm up, while the examiner opposes this movement by grasping the subject's hand. The muscle can be seen and felt to stand out in its upper part.

ix. **Biceps.** The subject is asked to bend up the forearm against resistance in full supination. The muscle stands out clearly.

x. **Triceps.** The subject is asked to straighten out his forearm against resistance.

xi. **Supraspinatus.** The subject is asked to lift his arm straight out at right angles to his side. The first 30° of this movement is brought about by supraspinatus and the rest 60° is carried out by the deltoid.

xii. **Deltoid.** The arm is held out, in abduction, straight out. The subject offers resistance while the examiner tries to depress the elbow. The anterior and posterior fibers help to draw the abducted arm forwards and backwards which can also be tested against resistance.

xiii. **Infraspinatus.** With the forearm flexed to a right angle, the subject is asked to tuck his elbow into his side. Then he is asked to rotate the limb outward against resistance.

xiv. **Pectorals.** The subject is asked to stretch the arms out in front of him and then to clasp his hands while the examiner tries to hold them apart.

xv. **Serratus anterior.** The subject is asked to push forward with his hands against resistance, such as a wall. When this muscle is paralysed, the scapula is "winged".

xvi. **Latissimus dorsi.** The subject is asked to clasp his hands behind his back while the examiner, standing behind the subject offers resistance to downwards and backwards movement. When the subject is asked to cough, the two posterior axillary folds can be felt by the examiner.

Q. 4 Test the muscle strength in the lower limbs.

i. **Plantar flexion and dorsiflexion of the toes and the ankle.** These are tested by asking the subject to perform these movements against resistance.

ii. **Extensors of the knee.** The subject's knee is bent and while the examiner presses against his shin, the subject is asked to straighten out the leg again.

iii. **Flexors of the knee.** The subject's leg is raised up from the bed, and while the examiner supports the thigh with one hand and holding the ankle with the other hand, the subject is asked to flex the knee joint.

iv. **Extensors of the hip.** With his knee extended, the subject lifts the foot from the bed, and is asked to push it down against resistance.

v. **Flexors of the thigh.** With his leg extended, the subject is asked to raise the leg off the bed against resistance.

vi. **Abductors of the thigh.** The subject's legs are placed together and he is asked to separate them against resistance.

vii. **Adductors of the thigh.** The limb is abducted and then the subject is asked to bring it back towards the midline against resistance.

viii. **Rotators of the thigh.** With the limb extended and resting on the bed, the subject is asked to roll it outward or inward against resistance.

Testing the Muscles of the Trunk

i. The subject is asked to sit up in bed from the supine position without the help of his arms (abdominal muscles tested).

ii. The subject lies on his face and tries to raise his head by extending the neck and back. The muscles can be seen to become prominent (extensors of the back tested).

Q. 5 How is muscle strength graded?
Grading of muscle power (or weakness) The muscle strength is graded as follows:

Grade 0   Complete paralysis.
Grade 1   A flicker of contraction only.
Grade 2   Muscle power is detected only when gravity is excluded by suitable postural adjustment.
Grade 3   The limb can be held against the force of gravity, but not against resistance.
Grade 4   Some degree of weakness is there which is commonly described as poor, moderate or fair strength, i.e., movements are possible against the examiner's resistance but are weak.
Grade 5   The muscle power is normal both without load and with the examiner's resistance.

4. Coordination of Muscular Activity

Q. 6 Test the musclar coordination in the upper limbs of the subject provided.
Coordination of movements. This term refers to the smooth interaction and cooperation of groups of muscles in order to perform a definite motor task. Coordination of movements depends on afferent impulses coming from muscle and joint receptors, integrity of dorsal columns of the cord, cerebellum and its tracts, and the state of muscle tone. Though vision can control and direct a motor act to some extent, it is not concerned in the coordination of most normal movements.

If coordination of movements becomes impaired *(ataxia)*, the carrying out of motor activities becomes difficult and sometimes even impossible.

1. *"Finger-nose" test.* The subject is asked to extend his arm to the side and then touch the tip of his nose with the tip of his index finger, first with the eyes open and then with the eyes closed. The other limb is tested similarly. A normal subject is able to perform these acts accurately, both slowly and rapidly.

2. The subject is asked to touch his each finger in turn with the tip of the thumb.

3. The subject is asked to draw a large circle in the air with his forefinger.

4. The subject is asked to make fists, flex the forearm to right angles, tuck the elbows into his sides, and then to alternately pronate and supinate his forearms as rapidly as possible. An inability to perform such rapid movements is called **dysdiadochokinesia**. It is an important sign of cerebellar disease where the movements on the affected side become very clumsy or even impossible to carry out.

Watching a patient dressing or undressing, picking up pins from a table, handling a book, etc can provide useful information about muscle coordination.

Q. 7 Test the muscle coordination in the lower limbs.

1. The subject is asked to walk along a straight line. The examiner watches carefully as the subject turns to walk back. The subject may also be asked to walk along a line, placing the heel of one foot immediately adjacent to the toes of the foot behind (tandem walking). If incoordination is present, the subject soon

deviates to one or the other side and takes a zigzag course like that of a drunk.

2. **"Heel-knee" test.** The subject lies on his back, and is asked to lift one foot high in the air, to place its heel on the opposite knee, and then to slide the heel down the leg towards the ankle. The test is done first with the eyes open and then with eyes closed, and it is repeated on the other side.

3. The subject is asked to draw a large circle in the air with his toe.

Q. 8 Test the subject provided for Romberg's sign.

Romberg's sign. This sign is a test for the **loss of position sense** (sensory ataxia) in the legs. It is not a test for cerebellar function.

The subject is asked to stand with the feet as close together as possible, and if he can do it, which a normal person can, he is asked to close his eyes. A normal person can do so with ease.

However, if the Romberg's sign is present, the patient starts to sway from side to side as soon as he closes his eye. Thus, the patient is more unsteady when his eyes are closed than when his eyes are open. In *sensory ataxia* (lesion of dorsal columns of cord or dorsal roots, as in tabes dorsalis) the sensory information from the legs is lacking; therefore the patient becomes unsteady without the help of vision. In *cerebellar ataxia*, the patient is unsteady on his feet whether the eyes are open or closed.

Q. 9 Perform any three cerebellar function tests in the subject provided.

1. Test the "finger-nose test" in the upper limbs. In cerebellar disease, as the finger approaches the nose, it shows tremor (called "intention" tremor, i.e., tremor appears when a movement is performed and is not present at rest) and may undershoot or overshoot the mark.

2. Test the coordination in the lower limbs by asking the subject to walk along a straight line.

3. Test the muscle tone in the upper and lower limbs. There is hypotonia in cerebellar

disease. (Hypotonia also explains the pendular or swinging response when the knee jerk is elicited with the legs hanging freely over the edge of a chair).

5. Reflexes

Definition. A **reflex,** or **reflex action,** is an involuntary contraction of a muscle or a group of muscles (or secretion of a gland) in response to a specific stimulus, and which involves some part of the central nervous system (brain and spinal cord).

Clinically tested reflexes. These include: *superficial reflexes* (from skin and mucous membranes) and *deep reflexes* or *tendon reflexes.* In health, these reflexes should be present and equal on the two sides of the body.

A. **Superficial reflexes** from the skin and mucous membranes.

B. **Deep reflexes or tendon reflexes.**

C. **Visceral reflexes.**

For each reflex, the student should know:

i. The method of its elicitation.

ii. The response (normal and abnormal).

iii. The receptors and the afferent (sensory) path.

iv. The center.

v. The efferent (motor) path, and

vi. The clinical significance of the reflex or reflexes, i.e., their value in localization of the site of lesion, assessing the integrity of the sensory and motor pathways, the influence of higher centers, and in differentiating between the upper and lower motor neuron lesions.

A. SUPERFICIAL REFLEXES

These include the plantar response; the epigastric and abdominal reflexes; cremasteric, gluteal, and anal reflexes; the ciliospinal reflex; and the various mucous membrane reflexes described earlier with cranial nerves.

Response. In all the skin reflexes, there is contraction of the underlying muscles when a particular area of the skin is stimulated by scratching, stroking, or pinching.

Reflex Arcs. The reflex arcs for the skin reflexes appear to be long and complex, and include a number of interneurons between the sensory and the motor neurons of the reflex arc. The afferent impulses appear to be carried up by dorsal columns and spinothalamic tracts and end somewhere in the midbrain, thalamus or cerebral cortex. From here, impulses are carried by corticospinal and extrapyramidal tracts to the anterior horn cells innervating the muscles involved in the reflex. This is the reason why the skin reflexes are absent in the upper motor neuron lesions.

Q. 1 Elicit the flexor plantar reflex in the subject provided.
Flexor Plantar Reflex (Plantar Flexor Reflex).
The subject is asked to relax the muscles of the legs. A light scratch is given with a thumbnail (it should always be tried first), a key, or the blunt point of the patellar hammer, along the **outer edge of the sole of the foot, from the heel toward the little toe, and then medially along the base of the toes up to the 2nd toe.** The response to this stimulation of the skin in healthy adults is: plantar flexion and drawing together of the toes, often including the big toe, dorsiflexion and inversion of the ankle, and sometimes, contraction of the tensor fascia lata. With stronger stimuli, the limb may be withdrawn (flexed at the knee and hip) and adducted at the hip. This is the normal response in the adults, and is called the flexor plantar reflex (or the plantar flexor reflex). It is never completely absent in healthy individuals. Afferent (tibial nerve): L-5, S-1,2; Center: S-1,2; Efferent (tibial nerve): L-4,5 segments of the spinal cord.

Extensor Plantar Reflex (Plantar Extensor Reflex).
In infants, the response is a dorsiflexion of the big toe and retraction of the foot and occasionally dorsiflexion and fan-like spreading of the other toes. In adults, such a response (first described by

Babinski in 1896) is seen in lesions of corticospinal system. This abnormal response is called the *extensor plantar reflex* or the *Babinski sign* (Babinski toe sign; positive Babinski; or "upgoing toe"). In this response the dorsiflexion of the toes (the big toe dorsiflexes first) is followed by dorsiflexion of the ankle and flexion of the knee and the hip. (The stimulus must be applied over the lateral region of the sole because the medial region may give a normal response).

In some cases of positive Babinski, the reflexogenic area (i.e., the region from which it is obtained), spreads out over a large area so that the same response is obtained by squeezing the calf muscles, by a firm downward movement over anterior tibia (Oppenheim's sign), by pinching the Achilles tendon (Gordon's reflex), or by stroking the lateral malleolus (Chaddok's sign). [The clawing movement of the fingers and the thumb upon flicking the terminal phalanx of the index finger is called the **Hoffmann's sign** (the equivalent of Babinski in the upper limb)].

The Babinski sign is perhaps the most important single physical sign in clinical neurology. It has great significance in differentiating between an organic lesion and a functional disorder (e.g., psychoneurosis) because it never occurs in the latter conditions.

Babinski sign is seen in the following:
1. Infants below the age of 1 year, i.e., until the corticospinal tracts get myelinated and become functional. The plantar response becomes flexor in the next 6-8 months when the child learns to walk.
2. Upper motor neuron (UMN; corticospinal or pyramidal) lesions such as cerebral vascular disease (e.g., capsular hemiplegia), disseminated sclerosis, etc.
3. Spinal cord tumors—the pyramidal fibers are very sensitive to pressure, hence their early involvement in such cases.
4. Deep narcosis, coma due to any cause, and following an attack of grandmal epilepsy when the patient becomes unconscious. (It is

temporary in some forms of coma and after epileptic fits).

5. Biochemical disturbances, such as hypoglycemia, in which convulsions may occur.

Q. 2 Why does Babinski sign appear in corticospinal tract lesions?

Any movement of a limb or part of a limb which increases the length of the limb is physiologically an *extension* movement, and any movement which decreases the length of the limb is a *flexion* movement.

The normal plantar response to stimulation is plantar flexion (downward movement) of the toes, which is physiologically an extensor response though brought about by muscles which are called flexors in anatomical terms. The Babinski response, i.e., extensor plantar reflex, was named extensor because the upward movement of the big toe is caused by a muscle which the anatomists call extensor hallucis longus, though physiologically it is a flexor muscle.

The older extrapyramidal system is concerned with controlling primitive spinal cord activities such as flexion (like an animal crawling into a hole), and the protective *nociceptive flexor withdrawal reflex* described by Sherrington in a decerebrate animal (application of a painful stimulus to a paw leads to withdrawal of that limb as a whole; this **mass flexor withdrawal reflex** can be better shown in a spinal animal or spinal man, because "isolated" spinal cord favors flexor activity).

The newer control system, controls higher order of motor activity including the downward movement of the toes in response to a scratch on the sole of the foot—a response which helps us to walk (e.g., when an infant learns to walk, the contact with the ground acts as a stimulus and the resulting plantar flexion of the toes helps to propel the body forward).

Therefore, as long as the corticospinal system is intact, it keeps the primitive activities under check; but when it is damaged, the older activities

are released from its inhibitory effect, and this is expressed as the nociceptive flexor withdrawal reflex, a part of which is the Babinski response. Thus, the Babinski sign is a release phenomenon.

Q. 3 Demonstrate abdominal reflexes in the subject provided.

The subject should be relaxed and in supine position with the abdomen uncovered.

A light scratch, with a key or blunt point, is given across the abdominal skin, directed toward the umbilicus, in the upper, middle, and lower regions. The response is a brisk ripple of contraction of the underlying muscles. The centers for these reflexes are: Upper abdominal: Th-8,9,10; Middle: Th-9,10,11, and Lower abdominal: Th-10,11,12 segments of the spinal cord.

These reflexes are absent in UMN lesions above their segmental level in the spinal cord. They may indicate the segmental level of thoracic spinal cord lesion by their absence.

The abdominal reflexes are sometimes difficult to elicit in obese or elderly, in anxious subjects, and after repeated pregnancies due to loss of muscle tone.

Q. 4 Elicit the ciliospinal reflex.

The skin of the neck of the subject is pinched; the response is dilatation of the pupil. The pathways in the spinal cord and the sympathetic trunk must be intact. Afferent path: Skin of the neck region; Centre: Th-1,2; Efferent: Cervical sympathetic. Loss of ciliospinal reflex is used as a measure of depth of coma; it is also one of the criteria of brain death.

Q. 5 Demonstrate any three superficial reflexes.

The student should elicit one mucous membrane reflex (e.g., corneal), one abdominal reflex, and the plantar response.

The *epigastric reflex* can be demonstrated in the males by giving a scratch downwards from the nipple on the front of the chest; the response is a drawing of the epigastrium on that side. The center is in Th-7,8 segments.

B. DEEP REFLEXES

The deep reflexes are also called the *tendon reflexes*, or *tendon jerks* or simply *"jerks"* because when the tendon of a lightly stretched muscle is given a single, sharp blow with a rubber hammer (patellar or percussion hammer), the muscle contracts briefly and then relaxes, i.e., it gives a "jerky" response.

Stimulus

The stimulus that initiates a deep reflex is the sudden *stretching of the muscle spindles*, which sends a synchronous volley of impulses from the primary sensory endings into the spinal cord. In the cord, these impulses directly (monosynaptically) stimulate the anterior horn cells which innervate the stretched muscle (**Figure 3-9**). Thus, these reflexes are monosynaptic stretch reflexes.

> **Important**
>
> It may be noted that it is the *spindle receptors and not the tendon receptors* which are stimulated though the hammer is struck on the tendon and not on the muscle belly. All muscles are somewhat excitable to direct mechanical stimulation, which is a direct response and not a stretch reflex. (The tendon receptors respond to excessive stretch—as in inverse stretch reflex, when the muscle relaxes suddenly).

Q. 6 Demonstrate the knee jerk in the subject provided.

Supine position. The subject is asked to relax his legs, and is reassured that the patellar hammer will not cause injury. His legs are semiflexed, and the observer supports both knees by placing a hand behind them. The patellar tendon is then struck midway between the patella and the insertion of the tendon on the tibial tuberosity. (The tendon is located by palpation before striking it. The hammer should be held between the fingers and thumb, and the swing should be at the wrist and not at the elbow or shoulder). The response is extension of the knee due to contraction of the quadriceps femoris muscle. Afferent and efferent paths:

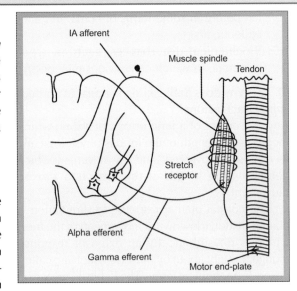

Figure 3-9. Diagram showing the monosynaptic reflex arc for stretch reflexes. Stretching the muscle (as by a tap on its tendon) excites muscle spindle receptors which, in turn, stimulate alpha motor neuron to cause a brief muscle contraction

Femoral nerve; Centre: Lumbar 3,4 segments.

Sitting position.   The subject is seated in a chair and is asked to cross one leg over the other, and then the reflex is elicited. The leg can be seen to kick forwards; the muscle can also be felt to contract if the observer places his hand on the lower front of the thigh.

A better way to elicit this reflex is to ask the subject to sit with both legs dangling loosely over the edge of the chair. It permits a more rapid comparison of the two knee jerks.

The knee jerk may be pendular in acute cerebellar disease and present on the side of the lesion. It may be sustained in chorea. In hypothyroidism, there may be delayed return of the leg to the resting position. In hyperthyroidism, the jerks are brisk.

Q. 7 Elicit the ankle jerk.

The subject lies supine, the knee is semiflexed, and the hip externally rotated. Then with one hand, the examiner slightly dorsiflexes the foot so as to stretch the Achilles tendon (tendo-calcaneous), and with the other hand, the tendon is struck on its posterior surface. The response is plantar flexion of the foot due to contraction of the calf muscles.

Another method is to ask the subject to kneel over a chair so that he faces the back of the chair and his ankles lie, over its edge. The ankle jerks are then tested as described above. Afferent and efferent: Tibial nerve; Center: Sacral 1,2 segments.

Q. 8 Test the biceps jerk in the subject provided.

The subject's elbow is flexed to a right angle and the forearm semipronated and supported on the examiner's arm. The examiner then places his thumb on the biceps tendon and strikes it with the hammer. The response is contraction of the biceps causing flexion and slight pronation of the forearm (If the patient is in bed, his forearm may rest across his chest). The afferent and efferent paths are musculocutaneous nerve and the center is in 5th and 6th cervical segments.

Q. 9 Elicit the triceps reflex.

The arm is flexed to a right angle and is supported on the examiner's arm. The triceps tendon is then struck just proximal to the point of the elbow. The response is extension at the elbow. Afferent and efferent paths: Radial nerve; Center: C-6,7.

Q. 10 Test the radial supinator and wrist reflexes.

The arm is placed to a right angle and the forearm placed midway between pronation and supination. Upon striking the styloid process of the radius, there is supination at the elbow. Afferent and efferent paths: Radial nerve; Center: C-6,7,8.

In **wrist reflexes,** there is flexion or extension at the wrist when the corresponding tendons are struck with the percussion hammer. For flexion, the afferent and efferent paths are median nerve, and center is C-6,7,8. For extension, the afferent and efferent paths are along the radial nerve, and the center is C-7,8.

Q. 11 What is reinforcement of reflexes and when is it required?

The briskness of knee jerk (and other deep reflexes) varies greatly from person to person but it is hardly ever absent in health. Occasionally, it may be very weak or even appear to be absent. In such cases, *reinforcement* (Jendrassik maneuver) is employed. This is done by asking the subject to perform some strong muscular effort, such as clenching the teeth, or locking the fingers of both hands as hard as possible and then trying to pull them apart while the examiner strikes the patellar tendon. The reflex generally becomes evident.

Reinforcement acts by increasing the excitability of the anterior horn cells due to "spilling" over of impulses from the neurons involved in reinforcement effort to the motor neurons of the reflex. In addition, gamma motor neuron activity increases the sensitivity of the spindle receptors to stretch. It also, perhaps, acts by distracting the subject's attention.

Q. 12 When are the deep reflexes diminished or absent?

The **tendon reflexes are diminished or absent,** on one or both sides, in lesions involving the afferent pathways (e.g., tabes dorsalis), the anterior horn cells themselves (e.g., poliomyelitis), or the efferent pathways. In peripheral neuropathies or peripheral nerve injuries, both sensory and motor fibers are affected.

The tendon jerks are also abolished by spinal shock, e.g., severe injury to the cord. (In fact, all motor and sensory functions are lost below the site of lesion for the duration of the spinal shock). Tendon reflexes are also lost bilaterally in coma.

As mentioned earlier, the deep reflexes may be sluggish or appear to be abolished in some healthy individuals; reinforcement is employed in these cases.

Q. 13 When are the deep reflexes exaggerated?

The **deep reflexes are exaggerated (hyperreflexia)** in the following conditions:

1. Upper motor neuron lesions above the anterior horn cells, especially when the hyperreflexia is unilateral, or accompanied by other signs of UMN disease.
2. Anxiety or nervousness.
3. Hyperexcitability of the nervous system, as in hyperthyroidism, and tetanus.

The cause of exaggeration of deep reflexes in lesions of corticospinal system is the hypertonia (spasticity) resulting from overactivity of the stretch reflexes; this system keeps these reflexes under check. When this inhibition is lost, the deep reflexes are more easily elicited. Exaggeration of reflexes is thus a "release" phenomenon—as is the Babinski response.

Q. 14 What is clonus? Demonstrate this phenomenon in the subject provided.

Clonus.   It is a series of involuntary contractions of certain muscles in response to stretch. This phenomenon is closely allied to deep reflexes and can often be demonstrated at the ankle when these reflexes are exaggerated. It is of greater importance when it is increased by maintaining and increasing the stretch on the muscle.

Ankle clonus.   The subject's knee is slightly flexed and the leg is held up by supporting it with a hand placed behind the knee. The examiner then suddenly dorsiflexes the foot after grasping its forepart. The sudden stretch of calf muscles results in their alternate contraction and relaxation. There may be 2 or 3 oscillations ("pseudo", "spurious", or "exhaustible" clonus) in normal persons who are very tense or anxious, but "true", "sustained", or "inexhaustible" clonus is present only in UMN lesions (The plantar reflexes are flexor in normal persons).

Patellar clonus.   The subject's leg is placed in extension. The examiner holds the patella from its sides with his thumb and fingers and then presses it sharply and firmly downwards. If clonus is present, the patella shows a rapid up and down movement, which continues as long as the stretch is maintained.

C. VISCERAL REFLEXES

The visceral reflexes include: pupillary reflexes, reflexes from the heart and lungs (sino-aortic, Hering-Breuer, etc), deglutition, vomiting, defecation, micturition, and sexual reflexes. Those which are tested clinically are: pupillary,

oculocardiac, carotid sinus reflex, bulbocavernosus, and sphincter reflexes. The tests employed for assessing autonomic function are based on some visceral reflexes.

Q. 15 Demonstrate some visceral reflexes in the subject provided.

1. Pupillary reflexes.   The light reflex, accommodation reflex, and ciliospinal reflexes may be demonstrated.

2. Oculocardiac reflex.   While the examiner feels the pulse of the subject with one hand, a gentle pressure is applied on the eyeball with the thumb of the other hand. The response is a slowing of the heart. Afferent: Trigeminal nerve; Center: Medulla; Efferent: Vagus nerve.

3. Carotid sinus reflex.   Pressure with the thumb on the carotid sinus in the neck (on one side only, never on both sides) causes slowing of the heart. Afferent: Glossopharyngeal; Center: Medulla; Efferent: Vagus. This reflex is hyperactive in some persons with marked vasomotor instability; slight stimulation of this type may cause fainting (carotid sinus syncope).

MOTOR NEURON LESIONS

Q. 16 What is meant by the terms upper motor neurons and lower motor neurons? What are the chief distinguishing features of the lesions of these neurons?

- See above for the definitions of upper and lower motor neurons.

Lesions of Lower Motor Neurons.   The lower motor neurons may be interrupted by lesions in the anterior horns (e.g., poliomyelitis; effects purely motor), in the anterior nerve roots (trauma; compression), in the peripheral nerves (trauma; neuropathies), or at their terminations in the muscles (motor end plates). The trophic changes often associated in diseases involving LMN are mainly due to associated damage to sensory nerves and autonomic systems.

The main features of LMN lesions are: complete loss of power (paralysis) of individual muscles or groups of muscles, hypotonia and flaccidity, diminished or absent deep reflexes, loss of affected superficial reflexes, pronounced muscle wasting and trophic changes (skin often cold, blue and shiny, ulcers). Partial or complete reaction of degeneration can be demonstrated in the affected muscles.

Lesions of Upper Motor Neurons. These neurons may be damaged anywhere along their course from the cerebral motor cortex to their termination in the brain stem and spinal cord. Lesions restricted purely to pyramidal tracts cause muscle weakness, while lesions of extrapyramidal system alone cause spastic paralysis, tremors and abnormal movements or posture. Clinically, the typically UMN lesion in the internal capsule involves both pyramidal and extrapyramidal fibers and causes hemiplegia. Lesions of UMN in the brain stem usually involve various cranial nerves which helps in the localization of the lesion. Thus, used unqualified, the term upper motor neuron lesion may sometimes be confusing.

The main features of UMN lesions (capsular hemiplegia) are: paralysis of movements rather than muscles, incomplete loss of muscle power, hypertonia and spasticity of 'clasp-knife' type, increased tendon (deep) reflexes, diminished or absent abdominal reflexes, Babinski's sign, generalized muscle wasting due to disuse; there are no trophic changes. The reactions of the muscles to Galvanic and Faradic currents are normal.

Presence of Involuntary Movements

The abnormal movements that may be seen in neurological diseases consist of various types of muscle contractions. First note whether the abnormal movements are *localized* or *widespread*. Also they may be present *at rest* or *during motor activity*. The term *spasm* refers to any exaggerated and involuntary muscle contraction. If the contraction is continuous, it is called *tonic*. If there is a series of short contractions with partial or compete relaxations in between, it is called *clonic*.

A. Localized involuntary movements. These include:

1. *Fibrillation.* They are due to contraction of a single muscle fiber. Usually, they cannot be seen though they can be recorded as EMG.
2. *Fasciculation.* These are due to contraction of one or more motor units and are visible on the skin.
3. *Myoclonus.* It is a sudden shock-like contraction of a single muscle or a group of muscles.
4. *Tremor.* It is an involuntary, regular, rhythmic and purposeless movement due to alternate contraction and relaxation of agonists and antagonists. Fine tremor is seen in anxiety and hyperthyroidism. Coarse tremor is seen in Parkinson's disease, cerebellar lesions, alcoholism, barbiturate and heavy metal poisoning.

B. Generalized involuntary movements

1. *Chorea.* These involuntary movements, seen in degeneration of caudate nucleus, are jerky, rapid, irregular and unpredictable.
2. *Athetosis.* These involuntary movements are relatively slow, writhing contractions of arms. They are sometimes combined with choreiform movements.
3. *Ballism.* These movements are flinging, intense, and violent, usually involving peripheral parts of limbs. The lesion is in the nucleus of Luys.
4. *Tics.* These are sudden, rapid, repeated movements, usually in the form of blinking of eyes, or wriggling of shoulders.

Gait

The term gait refers to the manner, style, or pattern of walking. To examine the gait, exclude diseases of the bones and joints, and the legs and feet should be exposed. Some common forms of abnormal gaits are:

1. *Spastic (hemiplegic) Gait.* The patient walks on a narrow base. Since the knee cannot be flexed and the foot properly lifted off the ground, he drags his foot on the ground and

tends to describe a semicircle with the affected leg the toes scraping the ground.

2. *Stamping Gait.* The patient raises each foot suddenly and brings it down on the ground with a thump. It is seen in sensory ataxia (e.g., tabes dorsalis). He may be quite steady as long as he can see the ground and the position of his feet.

3. *Drunken or reeling gait.* This ataxic gait is seen in cerebellar lesions, the patient walks on a broad base, with the feet apart. The gait is clumsy and zigzagging like the gait of a drunkard. The ataxia is equally severe whether the eyes are closed or open.

4. *Festinant Gait.* This is seen in Parkinson's disease. Walking is usually slow and the patient takes short, shuffling steps. Sometimes there is an uncontrolled acceleration while walking, a process called festinant gait. When gently pushed forward, the patient may be unable to stop as he chases his own center of gravity (propulsion). Similarly, when pushed back, he is unable to stop (retropulsion).

V. SENSORY FUNCTIONS

PHYSIOLOGICAL AND ANATOMICAL CONSIDERATIONS

Definition

When the process of response of a sensory apparatus reaches our consciousness (awareness), it is called a sensation. Thus, sensations or senses are conscious experiences or feelings aroused by stimuli.

Classification of Sensations

The sensations are classified into the following groups and subgroups:

I.   **General Sensations.** These further divided into 3 groups:

  a. *Cutaneous Sensations*: touch, cold, warmth, pain and possibly itch.

  b. *Deep Sensations:* proprioceptive, pressure-pain from bones, joints, tendons and muscles.

  c. *Visceral Sensations:* sensation of distension, tightness, and pain from the viscera.

The term **somesthetic (somatic)** sensations refers to those from somatic structures, such as skin, muscles, bones, joint, etc (as opposed to those from visceral structures).

II. **Special Sensations.** Vision, hearing, taste, smell, and equilibrium senses are traditionally grouped together as special sensations.

  • Testing of special sensations is discussed in Section 2 UNIT III.

Components of Sensory System

Every sensation has the following components, as shown in **Figure 3-10**.

1. **Receptors.** A sensory receptor may be formed by the naked, bare or free (non-medullated) terminal part of an afferent nerve fiber, or the nerve endings may be associated with non-neural cells, the two together making up organized receptors called *sense organs.*

The sensory receptors possess a very important property called *functional specificity*, i.e., each type of receptor responds best only to one particular type of stimulus (the adequate stimulus) for which it has the lowest threshold.

Sensory receptors act as *peripheral analyzers* or *biological transducers*. They transduct (convert) a given form of energy (e.g., electromagnetic (light), mechanical, thermal, chemical, etc) into electrical potentials (APs; signals).

2. **Peripheral Pathways.** All afferent or sensory information (APs) concerned with sensory (and motor) functions is carried to the CNS via the unipolar primary afferent neurons (the main sensory neurons) that have their cell bodies in the dorsal root ganglia (DRG) of the spinal cord or the equivalent ganglia of sensory cranial nerves.

3. **Central Pathways.** The afferent information is then carried to the higher parts of the CNS through a chain of neurons (one synapsing on the next), which may be called 1st-order, 2nd- order, and

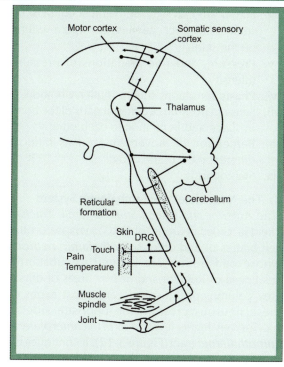

Figure 3-10. The components of the sensory system

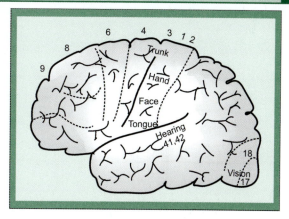

Figure 3-11. Diagram showing the cortical receiving areas for sensations

3rd- order neurons, though one or more neurons may be interposed between them.

4. Thalamus. It is an important relay station for all sensations, except smell, on their way to the cerebral cortex.

5. Cerebellum, Reticular Formation etc. These structures, though not directly concerned with our conscious perception of senses, do receive afferent information that is concerned with coordination of movements.

6. Sensory Areas of Cerebral Cortex. There is a functional localization of sensations, each being represented in a specific *primary area.*, as shown in **Figure 3- 11.** Thus, there are areas for general somatic sensations (areas 3, 1, 2), vision (area 17), hearing (areas 41, 42), taste (lower part of 3, 1, 2), and smell (uncus).

The cortical areas around these primary areas are called *association areas* where sensory signals are further analyzed.

"Labeled Line Principle"

This principle, also called *'Muller's law of specific nerve energies"*, forms the cornerstone of sensory physiology. It states that the pathways for each sensation, from the receptors to the cerebral cortex are clear-cut and fixed. Thus, whether a touch stimulus is applied to touch receptors, or its pathway is stimulated anywhere along its course, the sensation produced is always touch.

This principle also answers the question that if all sensory signals are carried as APs, then how do we experience different modalities of sensations. It appears that this is still an unknown cognitive function of the cerebral cortex.

Pathways for General Sensations

Sensory information that reaches our consciousness is carried by 2 main ascending tracts: *Dorsal column-Medial Lemniscal System (DC-MLS)*, and the *Anterolateral Spinothalamic System.*

Non-conscious afferent information is carried to subcortical structures by various ascending tracts, as already mentioned.

I. Dorsal Column-Medial Lemniscal System

The two wholly myelinated tracts—the fasciculi gracilis and cuneatus (tracts of Goll and Burdach) in the dorsal white columns of the spinal cord **(Figure 3-12)** are formed by the central processes

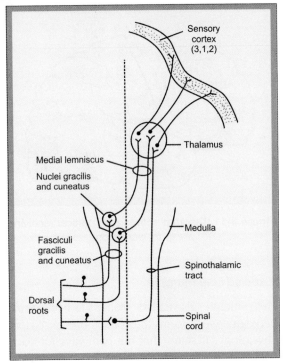

Sensory cortex (3,1,2)

Thalamus

Medial lemniscus

Nuclei gracilis and cuneatus

Medulla

Fasciculi gracilis and cuneatus

Spinothalamic tract

Dorsal roots

Spinal cord

Figure 3-12. The dorsal-column medial-lemniscal system and the anterolateral spinothalamic system for the general sensations

of 1st- order DRG neurons. These tracts ascend to lower medulla where they synapse on 2nd-order neurons in the nuclei gracilis and cuneatus. The axons of 2nd-order neurons cross to the opposite side in the medial lemnisci (sensory decussation), reach the thalamus, relay in the nucleus ventralis posterolateralis, from where 3rd-order neurons project to somatic sensory areas 3, 1, 2.

Functions. This system carries mechanoreceptive sensations only and performs the following functions:

i. Appreciation of fine touch, such as movement of a hair.

ii. Touch localization and two-point discrimination.

iii. Appreciation of gradation of intensity of touch stimuli.

iv. Sensations that signal movement on the skin, such as an insect crawling, and figure-writing on the skin.

v. Pressure, and fine gradations of pressure intensity.

vi. Phasic sensations such as flutter-vibration.

vii. Sense of position of different parts of the body in space and in relation to each other.

viii. Perception of movement (and its rate) of different parts of the body.

ix. Stereognosis.

II. The Anterolateral Spinothalamic System

(The Anterior and Lateral Spinothalamic Tracts)
The 1st- order neurons (of DRG) synapse on the cell bodies of 2nd-order *spinothalamic neurons* whose cell bodies are located in substantia gelatinosa of Rolandi and nearby areas of dorsal grey columns of the spinal cord. Most axons of these neurons cross to the opposite side at successively higher levels to form the *anterolateral spinothalamic tract* (Figure 3-12). It continues up through the brainstem as the spinal lemniscus to join the medial lemniscus in upper pons, the two lemnisci terminate in the thalamus from where 3rd-order neurons project to somatic sensory cortex.

Functions

The *anterior spinothalamic tract* carries crude touch and pressure, the localization of which is poor.
The *lateral spinothalamic* tract carries:

i. Pain from skin, muscles, bones and joints (somatic pain).

ii. Pain from the viscera (visceral pain).

iii. Temperature sensation, both warm and cold.

iv. Tickle and itch.

v. Sexual sensations.

Terminology

Hypoalgesia means decrease of cutaneous sensations, especially pain sensation. The term *analgesia* refers to loss of pain sensation. *Hyperalgesia* is exaggerated sensitivity to pain so that a mild stimulus that was painless before now evokes pain. *Hyperesthesia* refers to increased sensitivity to cutaneous sensations. *Paresthesia* refers to abnormal sensations, e.g., pricking, numbness, sense of insects crawling on the skin.

Clinical Testing of General Sensations

The clinically tested general sensations include:
1. Touch. It includes: light touch, pressure, touch localization, and two-point discrimination.
2. Proprioception.
3. Flutter vibration.
4. Pain.
5. Temperature: cold and warmth.
6. Stereognosis.

For each sensation the student should know: the receptors involved, and the peripheral and central pathways, i.e. the chains of neurons which carry the sensory signals from the receptors to the thalamus, and thence to the somatic sensory cortex.

Equipment required. Pins, cotton, compass, hot and cold water in test tubes.

Touch (Tactile) Sensation

The sensation of touch is aroused by a mechanical deformation (indentation, stretching) of the skin. The stimulus is not pressure but *non-uniform change in pressure with time* which deforms the skin or deeper somatic tissues. The receptors include: Type I and type II cutaneous mechano-receptors (Merkel discs and Ruffini corpuscles), and naked nerve endings. (See Expt 2-28 also).

Touch is a very rapidly-adapting sensation, ie, it persists for only a very little longer than the stimulus. (Were it not for rapid adaptation of touch, it would be impossible to wear clothes). In contrast, the sensation of pain does not show adaptation.

Fine Touch and Crude Touch. Fine touch (epicritic), a more critical type of sensation, helps to localize the stimulus. It is also concerned with fine gradations of intensity. These aspects of touch are carried by $A\beta$ and $A\gamma$ fibers into the CNS and then by the D-C Medial-Lemniscal system. Crude touch (protopathic), concerned with poorly-localized diffuse pressure, is carried by $A\delta$ and C fibers into the CNS and then by the anterior spinothalamic tract.

Q. 1 Test the sensation of light touch, touch localization and two-point discrimination in the upper limbs of the subject provided.

The subject should be alert and attentive, and the procedure should be explained to him. The subject is asked to close or cover his eyes. A wisp of cotton wool is used to gently touch the skin on the fingertips, palms, back of the fingers, and hand (non-hairy areas; movement of a single hair with a pin can arouse this sensation), and arms. The examiner asks "now?" and the subject responds with a "yes" or "no". The response is occasionally checked without the stimulus. If an area of anesthesia is found in the patient, it should be carefully compared with the corresponding area on the opposite side.

Touch Localization. Stroke a wisp of cotton lightly over the palm, back of hand, and over the arm and ask the subject to indicate the area touched. (Consult Expt 2-28 also).

Tactile discrimination (or two-point discrimination. Test this with a pair of dividers as described in Expt 2-28.

Touch-pressure. Test this by applying pressure over the skin with a finger tip or the blunt end of a pencil.

Proprioception

The proprioceptive sensations arise from the stimulation of receptors within the body tissues (proprius= self) and include sense of position and movement. While *static proprioception* is concerned with awareness of location of different parts of the body (body image), *kinesthetic sensation* (kin- = motion; -esthesia = perception) is concerned with perception of the rate of movement of different parts of the body.

Conscious and Non-conscious Proprioception. Part of the proprioceptive information reaches consciousness at primary and association somatic sensory areas via the DC-ML system. Non-conscious proprioceptive information from muscle spindles, Golgi tendon organs and nerve endings around joints (joint kinesthetic receptors) is carried via spinocerebellar, spinoreticular, spinovestibular and other similar tracts, and is meant for subcortical structures where it aids in the coordination of motor activity.

Q. 2 Test the proprioceptive sensation in the subject provided.
Position sense.   The subject is told that his finger (or toe or elbow, ankle, etc) will be moved up or down and he is asked to indicate in which direction it has been moved. He is asked to close or shield his eyes. Then the examiner gently moves the terminal phalanx or the finger or toe in one or the other direction. A normal person is able to appreciate displacement of only a few degrees at various joints.

When a limb is placed in a certain position, the subject should be able to place his opposite limb in a similar position.

Sense of movement.   (Kinesthetic sense; Kinema = movement): A digit, finger, toe, or other joint is gradually moved to a new position, and the subject is asked to say "yes" as soon as he perceives the movement.

Part of proprioceptive information reaches consciousness (conscious kinesthetic) while the rest reaches the cerebellum where it aids it in coordinating muscular activity.

Vibration

Flutter-vibration is a phasic sensation caused by repeated mechanical simulation of touch receptors and pacinian corpuscles, the frequency for the two being 6-40/sec and 40-400/sec respectively.

Q. 3 Test the sense of vibration.
The foot of a low frequency tuning fork is placed over bony prominences, such as knuckles, head of radius, elbow, patella, malleoli, iliac crest, etc. The subject is normally conscious of a vibratory tremor, and not just the sensation of touch. The

subject is asked to tell when the feeling of vibration stops; the examiner then confirms it on his own knuckles.

Pain

The stimulus for pain is actual or potential damage to the tissues. Though pain is an unpleasant sensation, it is said to be a "cry for help" as it is commonly the first symptom that brings a patient to the doctor.

The receptors are naked nerve terminals of Aδ and C fibers, and the APs are carried up the CNS by spinothalamic tract, as described above.

Pain has both *epicritic* and *protopathic* components, and there is no adaptation to pain sensation (otherwise it would lose its protective function).

Stimuli of Pain. Intense chemical, thermal, or mechanical stimuli can stimulate pain receptors. Injury to tissues releases kinins, prostaglandins, and potassium ions that stimulate pain endings.

Q. 4 Test the sensations of pain in the upper limbs of the subject provided.
This sensibility may be tested either with a *cutaneous stimulus*, such as the prick of a pin, or by *pressure* on deeper tissues, such as muscles and bones.

The procedure is explained to the subject/patient. He is asked to close his eyes, and corresponding points on the nailbed, pulp of fingers (this is less sensitive to pain), palms and back of the hands, and arms are tested with an ordinary pin.

Pressure pain is tested by squeezing the arm muscles, or a pressure applied on the wrist bones (calf muscles and Achilles tendon in the lower limbs). Loss of pain sensation is called analgesia. There may be analgesia without loss of touch sensation (anesthesia) in a patient.

Temperature

Q. 5 Test the sensation of temperature in the upper limbs of the subject provided.
This sensation is tested by using two test tubes containing cold and warm (not hot) water. The

tubes should be interchanged at random. The patient is asked to report "cold" or "warm".

Stereognosis

Q. 6 Test the sensation of stereognosis in the subject provided.

Stereognosis, ie, the ability to identify common objects by feeling them, with eyes closed, is a complex sensation based on the synthesis of many sensations, such as touch, pressure, temperature, etc. Certain features of an object—its size, shape, form, weight softness or hardness, roughness or smoothness (e.g., the milled edge of a coin), dryness or wetness—help us to identify an object.

The subject is asked to close his eyes, and common objects like a coin, pencil, key, matchstick, etc are placed in his hand, one after the other. He has to name each object and the purpose for which it is used. (If a patient cannot name them, he is asked to describe these).

Experimental Physiology

(Amphibian and Mammalian Experiments)

**It is both a privilege and a responsibility to work on experimental animals.
Treat it as such, with full awareness.**

The student usually begins the experimental work on the amphibian nerve and muscle tissues after removing them from the frog's body. The great advantage of these tissues is that they can function as isolated preparations for many hours when handled carefully and kept moist with a suitable solution. These tissues get their oxygen from the atmospheric air.

Frog nerve-muscle preparation. The Frog's *gastrocnemius muscle-sciatic nerve preparation*, first employed by Jan Swammerdam, a Dutch physiologist, in the later half of 17th century, is a simple preparation for the study of many features of skeletal muscle contraction and nerve function. Frog's *sartorius* is another muscle employed for such studies. However, the gastrocnemius muscle has a much greater cross-sectional area than that of sartorius and hence develops much greater force required for moving the lever system during isotonic contractions.

Within the body, the skeletal muscles are activated by trains of action potentials in their motor nerves. In the isolated preparation, the muscle can be made to contract by either stimulating its nerve, or by directly stimulating its belly.

Frog heart. Many properties of cardiac muscle can be demonstrated on the frog's heart either within or outside the animal's body. Since the cause of heart beat lies within the heart itself, it continues to beat outside the animal's body, in isolation from the nervous system.

Mammalian experiments. Dog, rabbit, and rat are the commonly used animals for student experiments. A variety of physiological functions can be demonstrated in these animals.

> **CAUTION**
> You are a Biological Preparation. The Mains Current—220 Volts AC 50 Hz—is Potentially Lethal. Handle the Electric Kymograph with Utmost Caution. Ensure that it is Properly Earthed. Un-Insulated Wires or Improperly Earthed Kymograph and Other Apparatuses may Produce a Burn and/or Severe Shock. If in Doubt, Call the Electrician on Duty in the Laboratory.

Study of Apparatus

Excitability. It is the property or faculty of living cells due to which they respond to stimuli. Though all cells are excitable, this property is best developed and demonstrable in nerve and muscle cells, called "excitable tissues". Thus, muscle cells respond by contracting, nerve cells (neurons) respond by generating and transmitting action potentials, and gland cells respond by producing a secretion.

Stimulus. A stimulus is a change in the environment of an excitable tissue which causes the tissue to respond in its own particular fashion.

Types of Stimuli. The different types of stimuli are:
1. **Physical:** Drying, cooling, warming.
2. **Mechanical:** Tapping, pinching, cutting, crushing.
3. **Chemical:** Dilute acids and alkalis, and other chemicals.
4. **Osmotic:** Strong salt solutions, glycerine (it is hygroscopic).
5. **Electrical:** The different types of electrical stimuli are: Galvanic current (continuous, or direct current, DC); Faradic or induced current; rectilinear (rectangular), and sine wave (AC, or alternating current).

Choice of Stimulus: Of all the types of stimuli mentioned above, electrical stimuli are chosen for experimental work for the following reasons:
1. Their strength (in volts), and duration (in msec) can be easily controlled.
2. Since their duration is very short, they do not cause any damage to the tissues. Thus, they can be applied repeatedly, if required, without producing any harmful effects.
3. They resemble the natural mode of excitation of the tissues, i.e., the phenomena of resting

potentials, and action potentials are electrical in nature.

Type of electrical stimuli employed. Of the different types of electrical stimuli, the **induced** or **Faradic current** is generally employed for student work; it is very short-lived, does not cause damage, and can be applied repeatedly. **Rectilinear** (rectangular) current is obtained from an electronic stimulator. The voltage rises immediately to the desired level and is maintained there for the desired duration (measured in milliseconds). Thus, the strength (volts) and the duration (msec) can be pre-selected. The **Galvanic current** is the usual form of electrical stimulus which is employed for neuro-physiological studies, and in clinical situations (e.g., in testing for reaction of degeneration). The usual household electric supply, alternating current, AC, 220 volts, 50 Hz is lethal as such, and is never employed without modifying it, such as converting it to DC-low volts.

Degrees of stimuli. A **threshold** (minimal, or liminal) stimulus is the minimum strength of stimulus that is just sufficient to produce a response. A **subthreshold** (subminimal, or subliminal) stimulus is weaker than a threshold stimulus and is unable to produce a response. A **maximal** stimulus produces a maximum response and **submaximal** and **supramaximal** stimuli are weaker or stronger than a maximal stimulus, respectively.

APPARATUSES

The different apparatuses the students will be using include the following:

1. Source of current.
In order to get induced current, a constant current of low voltage is fed into the primary coil of the induction coil. Low volts (3-6 volts) are obtained

either from dry battery cells (each of 1.5 volts) connected in series, or from a "central low-voltage unit". The latter combines a rectifier unit and a step-down transformer to convert the mains AC current into DC current and to step-down its voltage to a few volts. This constant current is then supplied to all the work benches.

2. The keys.

A key is used as a switch to complete ("make") or interrupt ("break") an electrical circuit. The different types of keys are:

i. **Simple key.** An ordinary electrical "on-off" switch is mounted on a wooden or vulcanite base. The two poles of the switch are connected to two adjustable screw terminals. Other types of simple keys include metal blocks, morse key, and unspillable mercury key. The simple key is included in the primary circuit, as shown in **Figure 4-1**.

ii. **Short-circuiting key.** It is included in the secondary circuit (**Figure 4-1**) to prevent accidental passage of current into the tissues. It also prevents unipolar induction. Various types are available: Du-Bois Reymond,

Sherrington, and switch type. It has 4 terminals, the two left and the two right hand terminals are permanently connected. The two poles of the switch are connected to the two inner terminals. When the switch is "closed", it will short-circuit the induced current. When the switch is "opened", the current will pass into the stimulating electrodes.

3. Induction coil
(Du-Bois Reymond Inductorium, 1849).

It is a simple device to convert Galvanic current into the exciting form of Faradic (induced) current.

Principle. A flow of current in a wire (or a coil) produces a magnetic field in the space around it, which, in turn, can induce a current in another wire or coil placed nearby. In other words, a change in the magnetic field around a wire or a coil induces an electric current in it.

Consider two thick iron wires, "P" (primary) and "S" (secondary) placed near to, and parallel with each other. When Galvanic current (e.g., from a dry battery cell) starts or stops in wire "P", or

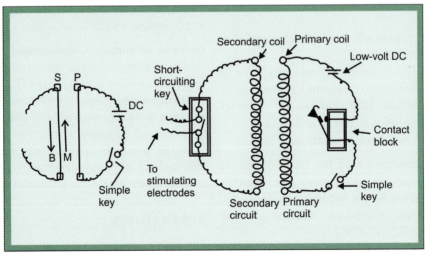

Figure 4-1. Left: Genesis of induced current. Flow of direct current (DC) in wire P causes induced (Faradic) current in a nearby wire (S, secondary) only at make or break of DC. Arrows show the direction of induced current at make (M) and break (B) of direct current. **Right:** Circuit for electrical stimulation of frog's nerve or muscle. The contact block makes and breaks the primary circuit by the striker of the rotating drum. The circuit can also be completed by tapping the spring with a finger

when its strength is changed, a momentary current is induced in the wire "S". The induced current in "S" is in the opposite direction at make, and in the same direction at break of the primary circuit (**Figure 4-1**). When current flows steadily in wire "P", there is no induced current in "S".

The primary coil consists of 250-300 turns of relatively thick, cotton covered, copper wire wound round a wooden reel which contains a bundle of soft iron wire pieces in its core (they increase the induction effects by their magnetization). The secondary coil has 7000 to 8000 turns of thin enamelled, copper wire wound round another wooden reel which is hollow. There is no connection between the two coils. However, the distance between the two coils can be increased or decreased, i.e., the secondary coil may lie, over the primary, or be moved away from it.

Factors affecting strength of induced current: The following factors are involved:
1. The number of turns of wire in the two coils—this is, of course, fixed.
2. The strength of direct current fed into the primary coil—it can be increased or decreased.
3. The distance between the primary coil and the secondary coil—greater the distance, weaker the induced current.
4. The angle between the two coils—when the secondary coil is at right angle to the primary, there is no induced current; as the angle is decreased, the strength increases.

"Break-induced" current versus "make-induced" current.
The strength of the induced current depends not only on the voltage in the primary coil, but also on the rate of change of current in this coil—whether from zero to a certain level (at "make") or from that level to zero (at "break"). When the Galvanic current starts to flow in the primary coil, it induces current not only in the secondary coil, it also induces current in the adjacent turns of wire in the primary coil itself, but in a direction opposite to the original current.

This self-induction effect impedes and slows down the rate of rise of the original Galvanic current from zero to the preselected level. However, at "break", the rate of change of Galvanic current (fall to zero) is sudden, as there is no self-induction effect. As a result, the change in the magnetic field is greater at "break" than at "make". Therefore, the "break-induced" current is stronger than the "make-induced" current.

Neef's hammer. It is fitted on the side of the induction coil (**Figure 4-2**) and is included in the primary circuit when multiple, repeated stimuli are required. It consists of an electromagnet and a horizontally mounted T-shaped iron bar with a spring. When the current is switched on, the iron bar vibrates up and down, thus repeatedly "making" and "breaking" the primary circuit at a rate of 30-40 to over 100 per second. Platinum points are provided on the iron bar and the contact screw to withstand sparking.

4. Electric kymograph ("drum").
The Sherrington-Starling kymograph is a machine for obtaining and displaying graphically the time course of events in tissues manifesting movement (i.e., muscle contractions). It runs on the mains 220 volts AC current. The speed is selected by means of a calibrated **speed setting lever** (**Figure 4-3**). The two prongs of this lever have to be pressed together to move it up or down for engaging at a particular speed slot. There is one slot marked "N" (neutral) where the gears get disengaged from the motor. A **variable speed lever** permits speeds (fast and slow) between 0.12/0.25 mm/sec and 320/640 mm/sec (not revolutions per minute, RPM). Two switches operate as ON/OFF switches: (i) the **mains switch** labeled ON/OFF—this should always be left "ON", (ii) a **clutch lever**, which engages or disengages the gears. This is used as ON/OFF switch to prevent damage to the gears. The cylinder may be rotated easily by hand when the clutch lever is in the horizontal (OFF) position.

A **spindle** projects up from the top of the kymograph for holding the cylinder on which the

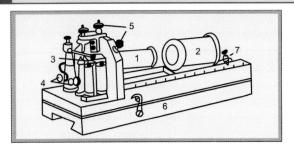

Figure 4-2. The Du Bois–Reymond induction coil. (1) Primary coil, (2) Secondary coil, (3) Neef's hammer assembly, (4) Terminals for Neef's hammer, (5) Input terminals for primary coil (the output terminals of the secondary coil are not shown), (6) Wooden base with scale, (7) Pointer, for indicating distance between primary and secondary coils

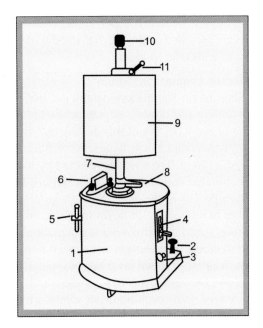

Figure 4-3. Electric kymograph: (1) Kymograph body containing electric motor and gear system, (2) Leveling screw, (3) On-off switch for mains current, (4) Calibrated speed setting system, (5) Clutch lever, (6) Electric contact block, (7) Spindle, (8) Dual electric contact arms, (9) Cylinder, (10) Screw lift for cylinder, (11) Lever for fixing cylinder on the spindle (The variable speed setting lever is not visible in this view)

record is obtained. **Dual electric contact arms** (also called the **"striker"**) are fitted, one over the other, at the base of the spindle, and rotate along with it. The two arms of the striker can be drawn apart when two stimuli, one after the other, are required. **A contact block** is fitted on the top of the kymograph body, at the level of the striker. It has a "spring contact" bearing a plastic button, and two electrical terminals. When these terminals are included in the primary circuit, this circuit will be completed only when the striker pushes the spring contact in to bring the two platinum points into contact with each other. Thus, the contact block terminals function as a simple key in the primary circuit, their purpose being to mark the point of stimulation on the recording surface. The circuit will also be completed when the spring contact is pushed in with a finger. A 6" x 6" cylinder, with a glazed paper wrapped around it, is firmly fixed on the spindle with the locking lever, because a loosely-fixed cylinder will shift its position on the spindle, thus invalidating the result. Two leveling screws are provided at the base of the drum for adjusting the tilt of the cylinder towards or away from the writing lever (**Figure 4-3**).

Clockwork and mechanical (pulley driven) kymographs. These are also used in some laboratories.

Effective stimulus. As the spindle rotates at a fast speed, each time the striker touches the contact spring (thus completing the primary circuit), there is an instantaneous "make" followed immediately by a "break" of the circuit. The two "make" and "break" induced current shocks thus produced act as a single stimulus, because the second shock (at "break") falls within the refractory period of the first shock (at "make"). Therefore, **it is the "make-induced current" which is the effective (stimulating) stimulus**. With slower speeds of the drum, the "make" shock can be eliminated by moving the secondary coil to a distance at which it becomes ineffective.

5. Frog muscle chamber
(Luca's moist chamber; muscle trough)

It is a transparent perspex bath, 6" × 4" × 2", with a clamp and drain pipe, in which the muscle can be immersed in the Ringer's solution. The trough is carried on an upright stand (QTVT stand) which has a quick stop at its base. Ordinary adjustable stands may also be used.

6. Writing Lever

A L-shaped writing lever is employed for magnifying and recording muscle contraction. It has a horizontal arm which bears a writing point at its end, and on which a weight can be hung near the fulcrum. The vertical arm of the lever has a hook which descends into the trough, and to which the tendon of the muscle is tied via a thread. (When properly set up, there should be no laxity in the thread). The two arms of the lever must remain firmly fixed to the spindle, and at right angle to each other to get maximum leverage. An **after-load screw** fitted in the frame supports the vertical arm (for after-loading), or it can be withdrawn away from it (for free-loading), as described later.

Ink-writing lever. An ink-writing stylus (filled with ink) can be fitted on the writing lever. It can then directly inscribe on the glazed paper without the need of "smoking" its surface.

7. Starling heart lever

It is used for recording the mechanical events of the frog's heart. The frame of the lever carries a light, flat lever arm with a finely-adjustable tension spring which supports the writing lever in the horizontal position. A piece of thread tied to the writing lever carries a bent pin which can be hooked through the apex of the ventricle when its contractions are to be recorded. When the heart contracts, it pulls the lever down; when it relaxes, the spring pulls the lever back to its horizontal position.

8. Isometric lever

It consists of a holder which carries a steel tension spring and a flat writing lever. This lever is used for recording isometric contractions.

9. Variable interrupter

It works on the same principle as the Neef's hammer. By adjusting the arc of vibration of the pendulum with the help of a stop screw, a variable number (6-80/sec) of induction shocks can be given.

10. Time marking

A time marking, or a time tracing, is required on the recording surface in most experiments. The following types of time markers are employed:

a. **Tuning fork.** A tuning fork of 100 or 256 Hz is used for fast events such as muscle contraction. The tuning fork, carrying a stylus on one of its prongs, is set into vibration, and the stylus is gently touched to the smoked surface, below the graph obtained. The time interval between two crests (or two troughs) represents 0.01 sec (n=100), or 0.0039 sec (n=256). Electrically vibrated tuning forks are also available.

b. **Spring time marker.** A heavily weighted and calibrated vibrating spring, in which an occasional tap with a finger maintains its vibrations may also be used. Two adjustments of 1/2 and 1/5 sec per complete cycle are provided.

c. **Electromagnetic time marker.** It is used along with the central low-voltage unit, and can provide "make-break" contacts at intervals of 1,2,5 and 10 seconds.

11. Stimulating electrodes

These are employed for delivering electrical stimuli to the tissues. The usual type supplied with the muscle chamber consist of ball-and-socket-mounted silver electrodes fitted over one side of the chamber. Wooden electrodes, which consist of two copper wires fitted in a thumb-sized block of wood or vulcanite block, are quite simple to use.

12. Student stimulator

Electronic stimulators with a DC output of 0-15 volts are now available. Each of the main stimulus parameters, i.e., volts, pulse duration, pulse frequency, mode of operation (single; repetitive,

1-100/sec; or an external trigger) are controlled by knobs provided for the purpose. The "external trigger" is for use with the contact block of the kymograph.

13. Smoking
The cylinder with the glazed paper is slipped over the horizontal spindle of the smoking stand and the paper is smoked with an intensely black flame obtained by passing coal gas through benzene or kerosene placed in the handle of the burner. The cylinder is rotated by hand while smoking it to obtain a thin and uniformly black layer of soot. The paper will get burnt if it does not fit evenly and tightly around the cylinder, or if the flame is played on a stationary cylinder.

14. Varnishing
A 2% solution of shellac or resin in methylated spirit is used as a varnishing and fixing medium. After getting a record, the paper is cut through with scissors and the paper, with the graph side up, is passed once through the solution taken in a tray. After draining the excess solution, the paper is put on the pegs of the drying board and allowed to dry at room temperature. After it dries, a fine coat of shellac or resin remains on the paper, making it a permanent record.

ELECTRICAL CONNECTIONS

Figure 4-1 illustrates the connections required for obtaining induced current stimuli (induction shocks). Low-resistance cotton-covered copper wire, or ordinary flex wire, is wound round a pencil to give coiled wire pieces.

a. **Circuit for single "make" and "break" stimuli.** *Primary circuit:* low volts (battery, etc), simple key, and primary coil connected in series. *Secondary circuit:* secondary coil, short-circuiting key and stimulating electrodes are connected as shown in **Figure 4-1**.

b. **Taking kymograph in circuit.** *Primary circuit:* low volts, simple key, primary coil, and contact block of drum are connected in series. *Secondary circuit:* as above. The drum terminals are taken in the primary circuit

when one wants to mark the point of stimulation, or when two successive stimuli are needed.

c. **Taking Neef's hammer, variable interrupter, or vibrating reed in circuit.** *Primary circuit:* low volts, simple key, Neef's hammer of induction coil, or vibrating reed or variable interrupter, and primary coil. *Secondary circuit* is as above. This circuit is used for getting repeated stimuli, such as for producing tetanus, or for stimulating the vagus nerve.

Arranging The Apparatus

Place the induction coil just in front of you, the kymograph just beyond it, the simple key on the right side, and the short-circuiting key on the left.

The muscle trough should be placed to the left of the induction coil so that the writing lever is at a tangent to the surface of the cylinder. This will allow you to see the writing point and the graph being obtained without unnecessary bending and twisting.

Trouble Shooting

If, after making the required connections, there is no response, try to locate the fault in a step-by-step fashion.

1. Check the Galvanic current by holding one end of a piece of wire on one terminal and brushing its free end on the other terminal. Sparking indicates good current. A voltmeter will indicate the voltage.

2. Check the simple key, and the contact block terminals in a similar fashion. Switch on the drum; each time the striker touches the contact spring, there is sparking. This checks out the primary circuit.

3. **Secondary circuit:** Place the severed leg from the frog on the secondary coil terminals; if it twitches with each induction shock (as the spindle rotates), the fault lies beyond this point. "Open" (i.e., switch off) the short-

circuiting key and place the "leg" on the electrodes, and switch on the drum. If the leg muscles twitch with each shock, the stimuli are, evidently, reaching the electrodes. If the stimulation of the nerve does not give a response, put the electrodes directly on the muscle belly; if the muscle contracts with each shock, the nerve has been damaged. Replace the preparation with the one kept in reserve for such a contingency. If all efforts fail, seek the help of the electrician and your tutor.

Ringer's Solution

This solution is isotonic with the frog's tissues and has optimal ionic constituents. The isotonic saline for frog is 0.6% NaCl, while for mammals it is 0.9% NaCl solution. The composition of Ringer is as follows:

Sodium chloride	= 0.6 g
Calcium chloride	= 0.01 g
Potassium chloride	= 0.0075 g
Sodium bicarbonate	= 0.01 g
Distilled water	to 100 ml.

4-2

Dissection of Gastrocnemius Muscle-Sciatic Nerve Preparation

Your tutor will demonstrate the dissection steps for obtaining the nerve-muscle preparation. Keep the preparation moist with Ringer during and after dissection. Do not use a scalpel during dissection.

> **CAUTION**
> The frog must be properly "stunned" and "pithed", otherwise it is likely to "wake up" during the dissection.

1. Stunning.   The animal is stunned to render it unconscious (anethesia is not suitable). Hold the frog, gently but firmly, by its waist, in a duster cloth. Give a good blow on its head with a wooden mallet; one or two blows should suffice; repeated blows look neither humane and decent, nor are they required.

2. Pithing.   The purpose of pithing is to destroy the brain and the spinal cord so that the animal feels neither pain, nor there are any reflex or voluntary movements during the dissection (Girl students may be provided with pithed animals).

Hold the animal in your left hand, and flex its head with your index finger. With the other hand, push a long and sharp-pointed *pithing needle* firmly through the skin and bone into the spinal canal, at a point where a line joining the posterior borders of tympanic membranes cuts the middle line. Push the needle anteriorly into the skull and rotate it to destroy the brain. Withdraw the needle and direct it backwards into the spinal canal to destroy the spinal cord. As the cord is being destroyed, the muscles of the limbs are thrown into convulsions due to irritation of the spinal motor neurons. Once the cord has been properly destroyed, the limbs will hang down loosely and limply, and pinching a toe with a forceps will not cause reflex withdrawal of that limb.

The animal is now "dead" in the sense that it is no longer conscious, does not "feel" any pain, and there are no voluntary or reflex movements. But the various organs, such as heart, muscles, etc are still "alive" and can be used for experimental work.

3. Cut through the skin with scissors completely all around the trunk just below the forelimbs. Seize the skin in a duster and strip this "trouser" of skin right down to the toes. Place the skin and other waste tissue in the tray.

4. Place the frog on its abdomen, pick up the urostyle with a forceps, and give a cut under it with a scissors. Cut through the muscles on its either side, taking care not to injure the underlying nerves. Extend these lateral cuts forwards, and using a bone forceps, cut through the hip girdle on either side. Lift up the urostyle and see the sciatic and other nerves emerging from the vertebral column and running parallel to the urostyle. Cut the vertebrae above and below the exit of sciatic nerves. Do not attempt to separate these nerves at this time.

5. Now you have a piece of vertebral column, and the three trunks of sciatic nerves still attached to it on either side. Using a bone foreceps, and a slightly oblique cut, divide this piece into two pieces. Lift each piece with forceps and snip away the nerves going to nearby tissues, taking care not to injure the sciatic nerves which can be seen disappearing into the thigh muscles.

6. Cut through the fascia covering the thigh muscles, and gently separate them with a blunt glass probe. The sciatic nerves will now becomes visible on both sides. Holding the vertebral piece with a forceps, free the nerves to about 2 cm above the knee joints. As you snip their branches, the thigh muscles show twitch-like contractions due to mechanical stimulation of the motor fibers.

Note

Do not directly pick up a nerve with forceps but lift it up by the vertebral piece. Once the nerve is damaged by mishandling, the muscle may continue to twitch occasionally, thus making it difficult to carry out any experiment.

7. Separate the tendon of the gastrocnemius from its insertion with a scissors and strip the muscle from the bones right up to knee joint. Tie, a stout thread around the tendon just above the sesamoid bone (which is buried in the tendon). Repeat on the other side.

8. With a bone forceps, cut off the tibio-fibula below the knee joint and the thigh bone just above the point to which the sciatic nerve has been freed. Trim away any excess muscle tissue from around the knee joint.

9. The dissection is now complete and you have two nerve-muscle perparations. Pass a stout all-pin through each knee joint (in between the bones and not through the muscle tissue). The pin will be required to fix one end of the muscle firmly while the other end pulls on the hook of the writing lever. Carefully lift up the preparations and transfer them to a container of Ringer solution, taking care not to let the nerve hang down in the process.

Mounting the preparation in the muscle chamber. Push the pin firmly into the cork fitted in the bottom of the chamber, and tie the thread to the hook of the lever. Adjust the lever along the edge of the muscle trough so that the writing lever is horizontal and there is no slag in the thread. Apply a weight hanger and 10 g weight on the lever about 3 cm from the fulcrum.

4-3

Simple Muscle Twitch
(Effect of a Single Stimulus)

PRINCIPLE

A single stimulus applied to the sciatic nerve results in a sharp, momentary contraction of the muscle, followed immediately by its relaxation—a response called the *muscle twitch*. The upward movement of the lever is recorded in the form of a curve. A time tracing recorded below the graph allows the calculation of various time periods.

APPARATUS

1. Source of galvanic current (dry cell, accumulator, low-voltage unit) •Low-resistance wire for connections •Simple and short-circuiting keys •Induction coil.
2. Kymograph (drum); cylinder with smoked paper, or glazed paper for ink-writing stylus.
3. Muscle chamber, with stimulating electrodes weight hanger of 5 g mass, with a 10 g weight hung near the fulcrum.
4. Tuning fork (n = 100 or 256) •Dividers •Stout pins •Stout thread •Frog Ringer.

PROCEDURES

1. Set up the primary and secondary circuits. Include the drum in the primary circuit to obtain single induction shocks with every revolution of the cylinder.
2. Mount the preparation in the muscle chamber and tie its thread to the hook. Adjust the lever so that it is horizontal, and has a weight hung on it about 3 cm from the fulcrum. Support the vertical arm of the lever with the after-load screw. (This screw will support the load until the activated muscle exerts a force sufficient to lift the load).
3. Reposition the cylinder so that the record will be obtained about 4 cm above its lower edge, and just ahead of the overlapping part of the paper. Keep the writing point 2-3 cm away from the cylinder.
4. Set the clutch on the OFF (horizontal) position, engage the gear lever at the fastest speed (640 mm/sec), and place the nerve on the electrodes. Switch on the mains current. Switch OFF the simple key, and switch ON the short-circuiting key.
5. Put the clutch ON, close the simple key and open the short-circuiting key. Every time the striker touches the spring contact, thus completing the circuit, the muscle contracts. Watch 2-3 contractions to verify the suitability of the height of lever movement. Adjust if necessary.

Stop the drum with the clutch, close the short-circuiting key, and open the simple key.

6. When ready to record, bring the writing point (or the ink-writing stylus) in contact with the paper, at a tangent; and rotate the cylinder *by hand* to draw a base line all around the paper.

7. **Marking the point of stimulus.** Bring the striker in contact with the contact spring (the induction shock will pass at this point) and, steadying its position with the left hand, raise the writing point, with a finger, 5-6 cm above the base line, as shown in **Figure 4-4**.

8. Release the clutch, and let the drum speed become uniform. Switch on the simple key. The moment the striker passes the contact block, "open" the short-circuiting key but close it as soon as the muscle has contracted. Stop the drum, put the gear lever at "N" (neutral), switch off the simple key, and move the lever away from the cylinder.

9. You now have a record (graph) of a single muscle contraction. In order to divide the base line into contraction and relaxation periods, take the writing point to the summit of the

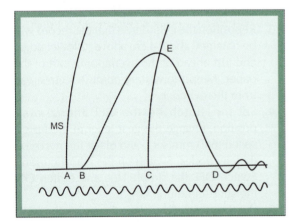

Figure 4-4. Simple muscle twitch. MS: moment of stimulation, AB: latent period, BC: contraction period, CD: relaxation period, BE: contraction phase, ED: relaxation phase. Tuning fork = 100 Hz. The waves at the end of the response are due to bouncing of the lever on the afterload screw and have no significance

curve with your hand and draw a line from this point to the base line in one continuous smooth motion. Do not attempt to draw a vertical line from the summit to the base line, because the writing point does not move vertically up and down but in an arc-like fashion.

10. **Recording the time trace.** Set a tuning fork into vibration by striking one of its prongs on the heel of your hand (both prongs will vibrate). Holding the fork from its base, and keeping it horizontal (so that the stylus vibrates up and down), bring the stylus in gentle contact with the revolving cylinder, below the base line, moving the stylus slightly downwards to avoid overlapping of the waves being recorded (The time tracing must be recorded at the same speed at which the muscle contraction was recorded).

11. Remove the cylinder from the spindle, discuss your graph with your tutor, and if it is okayed, get it signed. Cut along the overlapping part of the paper with scissors (always avoid recording your graph on this part of the paper), and remove it carefully without smudging the smoked surface. Lay the paper flat, face up, on a table and enter the following data:
    a. The title of the experiment (e.g., Simple Muscle Twitch).
    b. Preparation used (Frog's gastrocnemius muscle-sciatic nerve preparation).
    c. Frequency of the tuning fork (n = 100, or n = 256, as the case may be).
    d. Your name, and the date on which the experiment was done.
    e. Label the various parts of the graph.

12. Fix your graph as described earlier and allow it to dry at room temperature. Cut out and trim your graph neatly; then paste it in your workbook.

Note
Since this is your first experiment, the procedures have been described in details. In subsequent experiments, only the relevant procedural details will be described.

OBSERVATIONS AND RESULTS

Observe your own graph and compare it with those obtained by your work partners. Is there anything unusual? Are there any small waves after the twitch is over? Is there a single base line or more than one? Is any part of the tracing missing?

Note that the contraction does not begin immediately upon application of the stimulus. The brief interval between the moment of stimulation and the start of contraction is called the **latent period**. It is followed by the **contraction and the relaxation periods** as shown in **Figure 4-4**. In order to calculate the duration of these periods, do not draw vertical lines from the points A, B, C and D on to the time tracing. Instead, use a pair of dividers; open up its points as required, place these on the time trace, and count the number of waves for each period. For example, if there is one wave for latent period, its duration will be 0.01 second (with n = 100). The two phases of the muscle curve are called **contraction phase** (BE) and **relaxation phase** (ED). The calculated durations of various periods in this experiment are:

Latent period (AB)	= 0.01 sec
Contraction period (BC)	= 0.04 sec
Relaxation period (CD)	= 0.05 sec
Total twitch duration in the frog's gastrocnemius muscle	= 0.1 sec

Compare your results with the expected durations of the twitch, and its various periods, and if these vary greatly, try to find out the reason.

QUESTIONS

Q. 1 What type of nerve is the sciatic nerve? Why does its stimulation cause muscle contraction? Is the muscle twitch recorded by you a normal physiological event?

The sciatic nerve is a mixed nerve carrying motor or efferent fibers (axons of anterior horn cells; lower motor neurons) to the muscle fibers, and sensory or afferent fibers from the sensory receptors, such as muscle spindles, joint, and tendon receptors, etc. to the spinal cord. Experimentally, a single supramaximal stimulus applied to the nerve simultaneously activates all the motor fibers, and action potentials (APs; nerve impulses) so generated travel to the neuromuscular junctions of all the muscle fibers where they release acetyl choline. This transmitter generates muscle action potentials in almost all the muscle fibers, which is followed by near-simultaneous, short-lived contraction of the muscle fibers called a muscle twitch. A twitch of all the muscle fibers can also be produced by direct stimulation, provided the muscle is reasonably small, because in large muscles it is rather difficult to apply sufficient current. The sensory fibers of the sciatic nerve are also stimulated, but they have no effect on the twitch.

The twitch recorded in this experiment is almost certainly not a physiological event, because the nervous system never stimulates all the motor neurons supplying a muscle simultaneously, except perhaps in the case of a tic. The usual repetitive stimuli come sufficiently close together so that the muscle does not relax between APs, and each fiber produces a sustained contraction called tetanus. The twitch, however, is much simpler to study especially in an isolated preparation since it is less likely to undergo fatigue.

Q. 2 Why is the kymograph included in the primary circuit?

The drum is taken in the primary circuit for two reasons: firstly, to obtain a single induction shock (the "make" induced current is the effective stimulus), and, secondly, to mark the point of stimulation.

Q. 3 What is the cause of latent period? How can this period be increased or decreased? What is 'true' latent period?

Cause of latent period. The latent period is due to a chain of events, including:

1. The time taken by the APs to travel from the point of stimulation to the motor end-plates.
2. Release of acetylcholine, sodium influx, and generation of muscle action potential which leads to contraction.

3. Viscosity of the muscle.
4. Inertia of the lever system which has to be overcome before contraction can be recorded.

The latent period can be increased by:
1. Stimulating the nerve near its vertebral end.
2. Immersing the muscle in cold Ringer at about 5°C, which slows down various electro-chemical events; it also increases the viscosity of the muscle.
3. Applying more load on the lever which makes the lever "heavier", thus increasing its inertia.

The latent period can be decreased by—
1. Stimulating the nerve as close to the muscle as possible.
2. Immersing the muscle in warm Ringer at about 45°C, which speeds up various chemical processes; it also decreases the viscosity of the muscle.
3. Decreasing the load on the muscle, which decreases its inertia.

True latent period. If the muscle is directly stimulated (to exclude the time spent in conduction of APs in the motor fibers), and if an optical recording system is employed (to exclude the inertia of the mechanical lever), the latent period is much reduced, which is called the true latent period.

Q. 4 What is meant by the terms "tension" and "load"?

Contraction is the active process of shortening of a muscle during which force is generated. **Tension** is the force exerted by a contracting muscle on an object. **Load** is the force exerted by the weight of an object on a contracting muscle, i.e., it is the resistance offered to muscle shortening. Thus, *muscle tension and load are opposing forces*. To lift a load, the muscle tension must exceed the load. If the load is greater than the muscle tension, the load will not be lifted and no external work will be done.

Note
It is important to note that the muscles show only two types of mechanical responses—shortening

and development of force or tension, and both usually occur together.

Q. 5 What type of muscle contraction is recorded in this experiment?

The muscle contraction recorded in this experiment is the *isotonic* (same tension) type. The distance the lever moves indicates the degree of shortening, i.e., the strength of contraction. The muscle does external work since it moves the load a certain distance, the tension remaining the same.

Comments

Since a load is moved, it involves the phenomenon of inertia and momentum. In the beginning, the inertia of the lever slightly delays its upward movement (though the tension is rising), but then the muscle contracts and the lever starts to move up and continues to move (or jerk up) due to momentum, even after the contraction has ended. Therefore, an *isotonic contraction tends to last longer.* Furthermore, the height of the recorded tracing is not a true indicator of the strength of contraction because of the "jerking up" of the lever. For these reasons, *isometric* recordings are preferred for studying various features of muscle contraction, such as length-tension relation, and force-velocity and work-velocity relations.

Q. 6 What is isometric contraction? Do such contractions occur in the body?

Muscles consist not only of *contractile components* (contractile proteins) but also *elastic* and *viscous elements* (elastic fibers, tendons, connective tissue sheaths, blood vessels, etc), which are arranged *in series* with the contractile components. Therefore, if both the ends of a muscle are rigidly fixed, it is possible for the muscle fibers to contract without an appreciable shortening of the *muscle as a whole*, though there is development of tension. Such a contraction is called *isometric* ("same measure" or length). (The myofibrils do contract and shorten, and in doing so, they stretch the in-series elastic elements. There are "parallel" elastic elements also in the muscle).

A recording system in which one end of the muscle is attached to a force transducer, and the other to an isotonic lever, will record both tension and shortening.

Note
Even during isotonic recording of an after-loaded muscle, there is an *initial period of isometric contraction* during which the tension is rising, until it exceeds the load and shortening of the muscle occurs and the load is lifted.

Both isotonic and isometric contractions occur in the body, and even in the same muscles. For example, in attempting to lift a car, muscles generate great tension or force but they cannot shorten. However, the same muscles can lift a lighter load. Similarly, antigravity muscles (i.e., muscles which maintain our posture against gravity), such as extensors of the back, hips, and knees contract isometrically to maintain the erect posture, but they can shorten to cause movements at these joints.

Q. 7   What is meant by "after-loaded" and "free-loaded" contractions?
See Expt. 4-10.

Q. 8   How would you ascertain whether a twitch has been recorded in the "after-loaded" or "free-loaded" condition?
After the muscle twitch is over, a few waves or oscillations are recorded. These are not a part of muscle contraction, but a result of muscle elasticity and jerking of the lever on the "stop screw" due to its momentum. These waves are called *physiological* or *shatter waves*. If the muscle is in the after-loaded state, the shatter waves appear mainly above the base line, but if it is free-loaded (or preloaded), the waves are recorded mainly below the base line.

Q. 9   What are the factors which determine the height of the simple muscle curve?
1. Strength of stimulus.
2. Initial length of muscle fibers (preload).
3. Type of loading.

4. Temperature.
5. Type of muscle fibers in the muscle.
6. **Inertia of the lever system:** Greater is the instrumental inertia, lower is the height of the twitch curve.
7. **Magnification of the lever:** The magnification by the lever depends on the ratio of the lengths of the vertical and horizontal arms. This is, of course, fixed in a given lever. A longer horizontal arm will cause greater magnification.

Note
The frequency of stimulation, whether two or more successive stimuli, determines the force of contraction. In the present context, however, we have employed a single stimulus.

Q. 10   Which properties of muscle are demonstrated in this experiment?
The important properties demonstrated in this experiment include excitability, contractility, relaxation, and conductivity (the sarcolemma conducts action potential in both directions from the motor end-plate which is usually located about the middle of the fiber).

Q. 11   What is excitation-contraction coupling? What is the sliding filament theory of muscle contraction?
Excitation-contraction coupling.   It is the process by which excitation, which is an electrical event, leads to contraction of the muscle, which is a mechanical phenomenon. Usually, one does not occur without the other. What is the link between excitation and contraction? The linking or the coupling agent is calcium which, as a result of depolarization, is released from a highly specialized system of internal membranes, as described below.

The arrival of action potential at the motor end-plate leads to depolarization of the sarcolemma, which is transmitted, via the T-tubules, into the very interior of the muscle fiber to all the myofibrils. This releases large amounts of calcium from the terminal cisterns (lateral sacs) of the triads into the sarcoplasm. The calcium ions bind to troponin C

(TnC), cause a change in its shape which, in turn, physically pushes the tropomyosin strands laterally, thereby exposing the "active" sites ("binding" sites for myosin heads) on the actin filaments. The ATP is then split. The knob-like heads (cross bridges) of myosin filaments now immediately bind to the active sites, and tilt back (i.e., they straighten out; this is called the *"power stroke"*), thus resulting in sliding of thin (actin) filaments over the thick (myosin) filaments. (Seven myosin binding sites are uncovered for each molecule of TnC that binds a calcium ion). Since the myosin heads attach to, tilt, and detach from successive binding sites on the thin filaments, this process has been called the *"walk along"* mechanism of muscle contraction.

Q. 12 Which factors are responsible for muscle relaxation?

The following factors are involved in relaxation:
1. After the contraction is over the calcium is actively pumped back into the sarcoplasmic reticulum by a pump called the Ca^{2+}–Mg^{2+} ATPase. Once the concentration of Ca^{2+} in the sarcoplasm has fallen sufficiently low and Ca^{2+} is removed from troponin, the chemical interaction between actin and myosin ends, and the muscle relaxes.
2. In resting muscle, the troponin-tropomyosin complex functions as a relaxing protein that prevents interaction between myosin and actin filaments.
3. Finally, it may be pointed out that ATP provides the energy both for contraction as well as relaxation.

Q. 13 Can you get an idea about the speed of muscle contraction from your graph?

Since the muscle curve shows displacement of the writing point (or pen) against time, a tangent drawn to the curve at the point of maximum slope can give an idea about the velocity of muscle shortening, i.e., steeper the slope, faster the speed of shortening.

4-4

Effect of Changing the Strength of Stimulus

Single "make" and "break" stimuli of successively increasing strength, from subthreshold to supramaximal, are applied to the sciatic nerve and their effect on force of muscle contraction is recorded separately on a stationary drum.

PROCEDURES

1. Set up a nerve-muscle preparation and a stimulation unit for obtaining single "make" and "break" stimuli. **Exclude the drum from the primary circuit**, and do not connect it to the mains AC supply.

2. Engage the gear at the "N" position, and, with the writing point clear of the cylinder, move the secondary coil away from the primary to a point just beyond the threshold level, by testing with "make" and "break" stimuli.

3. Draw a base line, and start with subthreshold stimuli (**Figure 4-5**). Shift the secondary coil towards the primary, in steps of 3 cm, and pass "make" and "break" stimuli at each position of the coil. Record the responses, in pairs, at each position, after rotating the cylinder by hand, and noting the distance of the secondary coil until it slips over the primary coil.

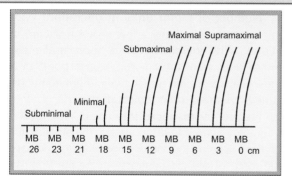

Figure 4-5. Effect of increasing the strength of stimulus on the force of contraction of skeletal muscle. The points of stimulation of subthreshold stimuli are marked below the base line. The first response appeared with a break stimulus, with the secondary coil 21 cm away from the primary coil

4. With subthreshold stimuli, mark the point of stimulation *below* the base line, otherwise it will be mistaken for a weak contraction, as shown in **Figure 4-5**.

5. Summation of subminimal stimuli: Move the secondary coil to just beyond the threshold position, then rapidly switch the simple key ON and OFF a few times until the effects of these stimuli are summated and a contraction results. (This is not shown in **Figure 4-5**).

6. Label the response "M" (for "make" stimulus) and "B" (for "break" stimulus), and the position of the secondary coil, in cm, under each pair of responses.

Precautions

1. The writing point should not be removed from the cylinder during the experiment so that it presses on the paper with the same force each time a stimulus is applied.
2. The tilt of the cylinder should be so adjusted that the writing point remains in contact with the paper throughout its upward movement.

QUESTIONS

Q. 1 What is a motor unit?
A single anterior horn cell (alpha motor neuron), its axon and all its branches, and all the muscle fibers innervated by this neuron is called a *motor unit.*

Q. 2 What are the different grades or degrees (in terms of strength) of stimuli?
Refer to Experiment 4-1 for definitions.

Q. 3 Which stimulus is the threshold stimulus in your experiment?
The "break" induced shock with the secondary coil at 21 cm is the threshold stimulus, i.e., the minimum intensity of stimulation that would activate enough motor units to cause contraction of the muscle. It is also obvious that this stimulus is stronger than the "make" induced shock for reasons already discussed.

Q. 4 Why does the force of contraction increase when the strength of stimuli, in the submaximal range, is gradually increased?
The sciatic nerve contains motor fibers of varying excitability. Subthreshold stimuli fail to excite any, while a threshold stimulus excites a few motor units and the muscle gives a weak contraction. As the strength of the stimuli is increased, more and more fibers are recruited into activity and the force of contraction goes on increasing. This phenomenon is called *quantal* or *multifiber summation.*

Q. 5 Why does the force of contraction not increase after the strength of stimulus is increased beyond the maximal level?
A maximal stimulus is that which excites all the motor fibers, and therefore all the motor units are already contracting to their maximum extent (all or none law; see below). As a result, any further increase in the strength of the stimuli (supramaximal stimuli) has no effect in increasing the force of contraction.

Q. 6 What is "all-or-none" law? How is it applicable to excitable tissues?
The *"all-or-none" law* (or "all-or-nothing") refers to the relatioship between the *strength of a stimulus* and the *extent of response of a single unit* of excitable tissue (*unit tissue*), be it a *nerve fiber, a motor unit, a single skeletal muscle fiber,* or *the heart as a whole.* The law states that under the

same experimental conditions, a "unit tissue" responds to its maximum possible extent, (or does not respond at all, if the stimulus is subthreshold) whatever the strength of stimulus as long as it is at or above the threshold level. In the case of a nerve fiber, the height of action potential and its other features, remain unchanged even when the strength of stimulus is increased. Similarly, a motor unit, a single skeletal muscle fiber, or the heart as a whole (because it is a functional syncytium) contract maximally, if they respond at all; an increase in the strength of stimulus does not increase the force of contraction. However, the skeletal muscle as a whole does not obey the "all-or-none" law.

The "all-or-none" law does not mean that the force of contraction of a unit muscle tissue cannot be increased in any way; the law only means that *this cannot be achieved by increasing the strength of stimulus.* For example, increase in the initial length of muscle fibers (called the "preload"), or increase in the frequency of stimulation increases their force of contraction (this does not go against the "all or none" law). Thus, the law applies to the strength of stimulus only.

Q. 7 How is the force of muscle contraction graded (varied) in the intact body? How are skeletal muscles inhibited?

Voluntary movements, which depend on the activity of many different efferent pathways (pyramidal and extrapyramidal) converging on the anterior horn cells, are very weak at times and very powerful at other times. This *gradation of muscular activity* is brought about in the following ways:

1. **Number of motor units in operation:** With minimum activity, only a few motor units are in action. With increasing effort, more and more motor units from the "motor neuron pool" of a muscle are recruited into activity, a phenomenon called *"multiple motor unit summation"*.

2. **Frequency of nerve impulses:** Varying the frequency of muscle stimulation is the other major method used by the motor control system to vary the force of muscle contraction. As the impulse frequency increases, its effects are summated (wave summation), and the muscle tension increases. Though the sarcoplasmic Ca^{2+} concentration does not increase beyond a certain limit, the *duration of the active state* is increased due to the repetitive release of Ca^{2+} from the terminal cisterns.

3. **Synchronization of impulses:** Different motor units are, at any one time, in different phases of activity—some contracting and others relaxing; algebric summation occurs and the muscle gives a steady but weak pull. With increasing synchronization, the force increases.

4. **Initial length of muscle fibers:** Up to an optimal limit, greater the initial length of muscle fibers (i.e., before they contract), greater is the force of contraction. This, however, is not the usual method of varying the force of contraction in the body.

5. **Warming up:** It is a complex mechanism which increases muscle performance.

There is no inhibitory nerve supply to the sketetal muscles and no inhibitory potentials are generated in these fibers. The only response is an end-plate potential (called an EPSP in the CNS). Each time a motor neuron fires an impulse, enough acetyl choline is released to bring the muscle fibers to threshold.

Effect of Temperature on Muscle Contraction

Keeping the point of stimulation unchanged, single contractions are recorded, first at room temperature, then at about 40°C, and finally at about 5°C. The effect of temperature on the amplitude of contraction, and on various periods is noted.

EXPERIMENTAL PROCEDURES

1. With the muscle immersed in Ringer at room temperature (note the temperature with a thermometer), record a simple muscle twitch.
2. Replace the solution with Ringer at 40°C, wait for about half a minute, and record another contraction, taking care to keep the point of stimulation unchanged.
3. Replace the hot Ringer with cold Ringer at 5°C, and record another twitch after waiting for about a minute.
4. Remove the cold Ringer and replace it with Ringer at about 50°. Record the irregular twitches of the muscle on a stationary drum ahead of the previous tracings.
5. Using the writing point of the lever, draw lines from the summit of each curve to the base line. Record a time tracing with a tuning fork below the graph.
6. Remove the paper, label your graph appropriately indicating the temperature for each twitch. Tabulate your results, indicating the height of each curve in cm, and the durations of various periods. Enter these data in your workbook.

QUESTIONS

Q. 1 What is the effect of moderately high temperature on the muscle twitch?
Warm Ringer (up to, say, 40°C) increases the excitability and hastens various metabolic processes in the muscle; it also decreases the viscosity. The total twitch duration decreases, with all the three periods reduced. The *speed of contraction* increases, as is evident from the steep slope of the contraction phase; relaxation is also faster. The higher amplitude of the muscle curve is a lever artifact, due to jerking up of the lever as a result of decreased viscosity, i.e., it does not mean an increased force of contraction (Isometric recording would give a true indication of the force of contraction).

High temperature, (say, 45 to 50°C and above) causes coagulation of muscle proteins, the muscle shortens, and goes into an irreversible state called "heat rigor". Heat rigor does not occur in the body as such a high temperature is incompatible with life, though another type of rigor, called rigor mortis, is seen after death.

Q. 2 What is the effect of low temperature on muscle contraction?
Cold has opposite effects due to slowing down of chemical processes and increase in viscosity. If the temperature is reduced to 0°C or below, the excitability is lost. However, if the muscle is gradually re-warmed, excitability is regained.

In hibernating mammals, the body temperature falls *naturally* to around 15°C without any ill effects on arousal. *Induced hypothermia* produced by cooling the skin or blood, where the core temperture can be reduced to about 25°C, is frequently employed in patients during operations on the brain or heart. Rats can be cooled to 0-1°C for short periods and then revived. But formation of ice crystals damages the tissues by dehydration if such hypothermia is prolonged.

Q. 3 What is rigor mortis and what is its importance?

Rigor mortis, in which there is shortening and rigidity of muscles, occurs some hours after death. The rigidity is due to loss of all the ATP which is required for detachment of cross-bridges which are fixed to actin filaments in an abnormal and resistant manner. Depending on the environmental temperature and other factors, the rigidity disappears after some hours due to destruction of muscle proteins by enzymes released from cellular lysosomes. The appearance and disappearance of rigidity and other factors help a forensic expert in fixing the time of death.

4-6

Velocity of Nerve Impulse

Keeping the point of stimulation unchanged, the sciatic nerve is stimulated first near the knee joint, and then at its vertebral end. The difference in the two latent periods, and the length of the nerve allow calculation of the velocity of nerve impulses.

EXPERIMENTAL PROCEDURES

1. Set up the nerve-muscle preparation of a large frog, and a stimulating unit to provide maximal stimuli. Include the drum in the primary circuit.

2. Draw a base line, and mark the point of stimulation. Place the electrodes on the nerve as near the knee joint as possible and record a simple muscle twitch.

3. Shift the electrodes to the vertebral end of the nerve and, keeping the point of stimulation unchanged, record another contraction. Run a time trace, preferably with a tuning-fork of high frequency (256 Hz). Measure the length of the nerve between the two points that were stimulated.

4. Remove the paper and enter the relevant data. Use a pair of dividers to measure the two latent periods.

Calculation of Velocity

For example, the length of the nerve = 6 cm, and the difference between the two latent periods = 1/256 sec (i.e., 1 wave). Thus, the nerve impulses have taken 1/256 sec to travel 6 cm. Therefore, the velocity would be = 6 × 256 = 1536 cm = 15.36 m/sec (consult Expt 2-29).

QUESTIONS

Q. 1 What conclusions would you draw from this experiment?
One can conclude that the conduction of nerve impulses is not an instantaneous phenomenon (unlike conduction of electricity which is almost instantaneous, about 300,000 km/sec). Considering that the electrical and chemical changes in the muscle are identical in the two contractions, the difference in the latent periods must be due to transmission of the impulses from the vertebral end of the nerve to the other.

Q. 2 What are the factors which affect the velocity of conduction of nerve impulses?
  1. **Species differences:** Compared to mammals, the velocity is lower in amphibia.
  2. **Diameter of nerve fiber:** The conduction velocity is about 5 m/μm diameter of the fiber.
  3. **Presence of myelin sheath:** In myelinated fibers, the nerve impulse jumps from one node of Ranvier to the next, a process called saltatory (jumping) conduction. (Ionic fluxes occur only at the nodes).

4. **Temperature:** It also affects the conduction velocity, warming increasing it and cooling decreasing the velocity.

Q. 3 What is a nerve impulse (action potential)?

How is it transmitted?
Consult Chart 5-8 for answer.

Q. 4 How are nerve fibers classified?
See Expt. 2-30.

4-7

Effect of Two Successive Stimuli

When two successive stimuli ("paired" stimuli) are applied to the sciatic nerve, the response of the muscle to the first stimulus affects its response to the second stimulus. The interval between the two stimuli can be varied by appropriately separating the two prongs of the "striker" as described below.

Dual electric contact arm ("striker"). The dual electric contact arm, or the striker, fitted at the bottom of the spindle, has two prongs; the lower prong is firmly screwed to the spindle, while the upper prong can be moved back as much as desired. Thus, two successive stimuli can be applied *during one complete revolution of the cylinder*; the first stimulus (with the lower prong) arriving at the same point of stimulation, while the second stimulus (with the upper prong) can be made to fall during the latent, contraction, or the relaxation periods of the twitch resulting from the first stimulus, or after the first twitch is over.

Note
Each contraction resulting from two successive stimuli may be recorded on the same location of the paper as shown in **Figure 4-6**, or in the form of separate graphs after repositioning the cylinder on the spindle after each response.

EXPERIMENTAL PROCEDURES

1. Set up a nerve-muscle preparation, and a stimulation unit to supply supramaximal stimuli

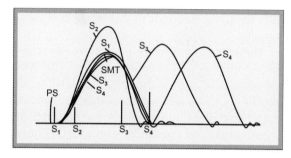

Figure 4-6. The effect of two successive stimuli on muscle contraction. Five responses are shown. The first stimulus in each case falls at PS, the second stimulus arriving at S_1, S_2, S_3, and S_4. See text for details

(to avoid quantal summation); include the drum in the primary circuit.
2. Draw a base line, mark the point of stimulation (PS), and record a single twitch, and label it SMT.
3. Move the upper prong of the striker back by 0.5-1 cm so that the 2nd stimuli would fall during the first or second half of the latent period of the first twitch (your point of stimulation will show this). Record another contraction and label the point of 2nd stimulus and the contraction obtained as S_1.
4. Move the upper prong further back, in steps, so that the second stimulus will fall during the contraction phase, then during relaxation phase, and finally, after the first twitch is over. Label the points of stimulation and the three contractions

obtained S_2, S_3, and S_4, respectively, as shown in **Figure 4-6**.

QUESTIONS

Q. 1 What is refractory period? Is it the same in all the excitable tissues?
After a tissue has responded to an effective stimulus, there is a very brief interval of time, called the *refractory period*, during which the tissue loses its excitability, i.e., it does not respond to a second stimulus. It is divided into *absolute refractory period (ARP)* and *relative refractory period (RRP)*. During ARP, the tissue does not respond to another stimulus howsoever strong it may be; while during RRP, the tissue responds to a stronger than usual stimulus.

The muscle and nerve tissues are refractory during their action potentials (APs). The ARP corresponds to most of the spike potential, while the RRP coincides with its later part (activation and inactivation of sodium channels; see **Figure 5-8**). The AP in skeletal muscle lasts only for 3-5 msec (i.e., early half of latent period of a twitch), but the mechanical response, which starts just before the end of AP, lasts much longer (300-400 msec). Since the contractile machinery has no refractoriness, the effect of two or more stimuli can be added up.

In contrast, the cardiac muscle is refractory throughout its contraction phase which lasts almost as long as its action potential (i.e., 200-300 msec). A second stimulus applied during contraction phase is, therefore, ineffective. The muscle must start relaxing before it can respond to another stimulus (consult **Figure 5-9** for details).

In nerve fibers, the refractory period, which corresponds to the spike potential, lasts for 0.3 to 0.4 msec (consult Chart 5-8 for details).

Q. 2 Describe the graphs obtained when the second stimulus is applied during different phases of the simple muscle twitch resulting from the first stimulus.
  a. **Latent period:** As the early half of this correspond to ARP, a second stimulus applied during this period has no effect. The muscle

responds only to the first stimulus and the graph obtained is similar to that obtained with a single stimulus. If the second stimulus falls during the later half of latent period, the effects of the two are added up and the graph obtained is of higher amplitude.
  b. **Contraction phase:** When the second stimulus is applied during the contraction phase, the muscle continues its contraction and the graph obtained shows an increase in the force of contraction—an effect called *"summation of contractions"* or *"wave summation"*, which is due to beneficial effect. Also, the response starts from a 'higher' base line.
  c. **Relaxation phase:** When the second stimulus arrives during relaxation phase, the relaxation is arrested and another contraction results, the force of contraction being more due to beneficial effect. This phenomenon is sometimes called *"superposition"* or *"imposition"* of waves.
  d. **After the first twitch:** When the second stimulus is applied after the relaxation is complete, there is another response and two twitches are obtained, the second being more forceful. The increase in the height of the second curve is due to beneficial effect.

Q. 3 What is beneficial effect and what is its cause?
Beneficial effect.   The effects of two successive stimuli described above mean that the contraction produced by the first stimulus is somehow beneficial for the second contraction, due to which the muscle contracts with greater force. The causes of this effect are—
  1. In a single twitch, the Ca^{2+} released from the terminal cisterns into the sarcoplasm is rapidly mopped up during relaxation. When there is no relaxation, or incomplete relaxation, some Ca^{2+} remains in the sarcoplasm for a longer time, and this, together with additional Ca^{2+} released by the second stimulus, increases the *duration of the active state*. The prolonged active state increases the amount of stretch on the series elastic elements of the muscle

so that more force is transmitted to the recording system (or to the bones in the intact animal), thus increasing the height of the curve.

2. Decrease in the viscosity of the muscle resulting from the first contraction decreases the elastic inertia of the muscle, which may contribute to beneficial effect.

3. Some increase in H^+ ion concentration may be contributing to the beneficial effect.

4. A sight increase in temperature also contributes to the beneficial effect.

Q. 4 Why are supramaximal stimuli employed for this experiment?

Supramaximal stimuli are employed to avoid quantal summation, because with such a stimulus, all the motor fibers in the sciatic nerve are stimulated. Thus, the second stimulus cannot bring more motor fibers into action and thereby increase the force of contraction.

4-8

Genesis of Tetanus (Effect of Many Successive Stimuli)

If instead of applying two successive stimuli (as was done in the last experiment), many successive stimuli are applied, the response of the muscle depends on the frequency of stimulation. At low rates of stimulations, the muscle gives jerky or tremulous contractions called **subtetanus**. At high frequencies, the muscle remains in a state of smooth, sustained, and forceful contraction called **tetanus**.

EXPERIMENTAL PROCEDURES

1. Exclude the drum from the primary circuit, but include, in its place, either a vibrating reed or a variable interrupter to provide 5-30 stimuli/sec, or the Neef's hammer to provide 40 or more stimuli/sec, as required. Engage the gear lever at 25 mm/sec speed (medium speed).

2. Set up a nerve-muscle preparation and stimulate it with gradually increasing frequencies, *for a few seconds each time.* Note the following effects:

a. *5 stimuli per second:* Each contraction starts after complete relaxation of the previous twitch, and succeeding contractions, with brief intervals between them, show a progressive increase in force. This phenomenon, called the "staircase effect", is due to beneficial effect.

b. *10 stimuli per second:* Successive contractions begin immediately after the lever touches the base line (duration of one twitch is 0.1 sec). The contractions are also more forceful due to beneficial effect, as shown in **Figure 4-7**.

c. *15-25 stimuli per second:* Since the interval between the stimuli is less than 0.1 sec, successive contractions begin before the relaxations are completed. The graph shows a progressive increase in amplitude up to a certain level beyond which there is no further increase a phenomenon called "treppe" or "staircase effect". On stoppage of stimulation, the lever returns to the base line. The series

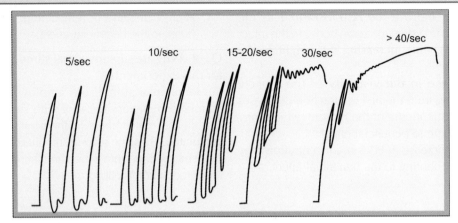

Figure 4-7. Genesis of tetanus. The approximate rate of stimulation is indicated above each set of recording. At lower rates, single contractions occur, while with increasing rates, subtetanus (clonus) and then tetanus (sustained contraction of the muscle) occur. Fatigue sets in if tetanic stimulation is continued

of jerky contractions of the muscle is called *subtetanus, incomplete tetanus,* or *clonus* (**Figure 4-7**).

d. *More than 30-40 stimuli per second:* With such high rates (obtained with Neef's hammer), successive stimuli arrive before the muscle begins to relax, so that it remains in a state of sustained, smooth, and forceful contraction called *tetanus.* The graph shows an increasing slope of the uninterrupted tracing, which exceeds the peaks of single twitches. When the stimulation is stopped, the muscle relaxes immediately; but if it is continued, the plateau is maintained until the muscle begins to fatigue, after which it relaxes gradually.

QUESTIONS

Q. 1 What is "tetanizing" or "fusion" frequency?

The *"tetanizing"* or *"fusion"* frequency is that rate of stimulation at which there is complete fusion of individual contractions to produce tetanus. In amphibian muscle and in "slow" muscle fibers,

the tetanizing frequency is about 30/sec, while in mammalian muscle and in "fast" fibers, it is 60 or more stimuli per second.

Q. 2 What is "treppe" or "staircase effect"?

When a skeletal muscle is stimulated with a series of stimuli *just below the tetanizing frequency,* there is a progressive increase in the tension (force) developed during each twitch until, after a number of contractions, there is no further increase in tension. Treppe (German word for staircase) can also be demonstrated in cardiac muscle, which, however, cannot be tetanized due to its refractoriness during the contraction phase. Treppe should not be confused with summation of contractions and tetanus.

Q. 3 Why does a tetanically contracting muscle develop more tension than that developed during a single twitch?

How much tension is *developed* by a muscle depends on the active state of the contractile components; and how much tension is *transmitted* to the recording system (or to the bone) depends on the amount of stretch (laxity or tautness) exerted on the series elastic components (SEC) of the muscle, as already explained.

During one twitch contraction, enough Ca^{2+} is released to engage all the myosin heads to the actin sites, but it is removed quickly from the cytoplasm and relaxation occurs. With repeated stimuli, Ca^{2+} remains longer in the cytoplasm, increasing the *duration of the active state* (due to continuous recycling of myosin heads). This increases the amount of stretch on the SEC and the tension developed rises. Up to a certain point, greater the frequency of stimulation, greater is the tension developed, the maximum being 3 to 4 times that of a twitch.

Q. 4 What is meant by the term "genesis of tetanus" ? Can you demonstrate tetanus in your body?

The term refers to the "generation" or production, of tetanus by gradually increasing the frequency of stimulation of the nerve-muscle preparation until tetanus results.

By definition, tetanus is a smooth and sustained contraction of a muscle, without reference to the frequency of stimulation. If you make a strong fist, your forearm muscles will contract tetanically.

The term tetanus should not be confused with a disease called tetanus. In this condition, there are widespread convulsions in the body due to tetanus toxin released by the infecting bacteria. Vaccination is a common practice to provide immunity against this disease.

Q. 5 What is the nature of muscle contractions in the body? Are they simple twitches, subtetanic, or tetanic contractions?

The results of this experiment are of great practical importance, because the character of voluntary and reflex movements depends on the *nature of discharge from the motoneurons* (motor neurons)— the *number* of activated neurons, the *frequency* of their firing, and their *synchrony*. The firing rate varies from 5-10/sec (during weak contractions) to over 100/sec (during strong contractions). Basically, all contractions are tetanic in nature. Weak contractions result from low frequency firing, but the expected jerkiness and the disadvantage of incomplete tetanus is overcome by the asynchronous discharge (out of step firing) of groups of motor units. When one group is firing, the others are silent, and vice versa. Algebric summation occurs, the individual variations are evened out, and a smooth contraction results. The degree to which the motoneuron discharge is asynchronous, is related both to the force and duration of contraction. (In the subtetanus experiment, the muscle fibers contract and relax at the same time in response to the low frequency stimulation. Such a situation does not occur in the body). With increasing firing rates and, of course, with more recruitment of motor neurons, contractions become stronger until, at and beyond the tetanizing rate, sustained and powerful contractions result.

As already mentioned, the simple muscle twitch is not a physiological event except perhaps in the case of a tic (Expt 4-3).

Phenomenon of Fatigue and its Site (Effect of Continued Stimulation)

When the muscle is stimulated repeatedly for a prolonged period of time, it loses its physiological property of contraction—a phenomenon called fatigue. However, it regains its property of contraction after some time.

PROCEDURES

1. Set up a nerve-muscle preparation, and stimulation and recording systems as for a "Simple muscle twitch". Draw a base line and mark the point of stimulation. Record a single contraction and label it as 1.

2. Switch on the drum and record all the subsequent contractions until the muscle fails to contract.

3. Stop the drum, and place the stimulating electrodes directly on the muscle. Rotate the cylinder by hand so that the stylus touches the paper just ahead of the graph obtained by you. Tap the contact spring with a finger so that a single induction shock is delivered directly to the muscle. Label this contraction DS (direct stimulation) as shown in **Figure 4-8**.

4. Stimulate the sciatic nerve, once each time, at intervals of 3 or 4 minutes to determine if there is any recovery from fatigue via stimulation of nerve. Note the time for recovery.

> **Note**
> Another method is to record one contraction after every 20 contractions, with the lever off the cylinder in between the recordings. Still another method is to record the excursions of the lever on a second cylinder rotating at a slow speed of 2.5 mm/sec.

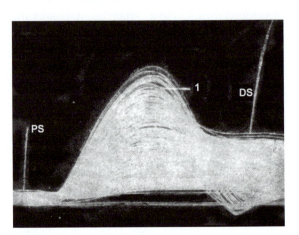

Figure 4-8. The phenomenon of fatigue. PS: point of stimulation. The record shows repeated contractions of the muscle through stimulation of its nerve. PS: point of stimulation, 1: first contraction, the following few contractions show beneficial effect. DS: direct stimulation of the muscle with electrodes placed on it

QUESTIONS

Q. 1 Comment on the graph obtained by you.
The first few contractions increase in amplitude due to beneficial effect. As stimulation is continued, there is a progressive increase in latent period, and a decrease in amplitude. The rise of tension is slower, and relaxation is more gradual and incomplete. Finally, the muscle fails to contract altogether, and the lever does not return to the base line, i.e., the muscle remains in a state of partial contraction called *contraction remainder*.

After the muscle undergoes fatigue through stimulation of its nerve, it responds briskly to direct stimulation. After a variable period, the muscle responds once again to stimulation of its nerve.

Q. 2 What is the site and cause of fatigue in the nerve-muscle preparation?

Site of fatigue.   The only 3 possible sites are: the nerve fibers, the neuromuscular junctions, and the muscle fibers. The fact that the nerve is practically unfatiguable, and that direct stimulation of muscle causes contraction, indicates, by exclusion, that neuromuscular junction is the seat of fatigue in this very artificial preparation which has no blood supply. The **cause of fatigue** is depletion of acetylcholine from the motor nerve endings and interference with neuromuscular transmission by substances like pyruvic and lactic acids, and breakdown products of ATP.

It can be shown that nerve is not the site of fatigue by bringing the nerve of a fresh preparation in contact with the nerve of the fatigued preparation. The second muscle responds to every induction shock while the first one does not—the first nerve merely acting as an electrical conductor. Recording of action potentials from the first nerve can also show that it is not the seat of fatigue. (If direct stimulation of muscle is continued, fatigue occurs due to exhaustion of glycogen. There is no recovery from fatigue in this case).

Q. 3 How is fatigue studied in man and what is its cause?

Fatigue in man is studied by using a *Mosso's ergograph* in which work is performed by a finger or thumb in lifting a weight. The effect of stimulation of median nerve, and of occlusion of branchial artery can also be studied (See Expt. 2-35).

Q. 4 What is contraction remainder and what is its cause?

A delay in the relaxation period is an early sign of fatigue. When fatigue sets in, the muscle is unable to relax fully and remains in a state of partial contraction called *contraction remainder.* Since ATP, by removing Ca^{2+} ions from the cytoplasm, is responsible for relaxation, a decrease of ATP and accumulation of metabolites appear to be responsible for the inability of all the myosin heads to disengage from the active sites on actin filaments (Compare with rigor mortis).

4-10

Effect of Load and Length on Muscle Contraction (Free-and After-Loading)

A load can act on a muscle either before it starts to contract (free-loading) or after the contraction has started (after-loading). Using successively increasing loads (weights), muscle contractions are recorded in these two conditions. The work done by the muscle for each weight can then be calculated.

PROCEDURES

1. Set up your experiment as for simple muscle twitch. Draw a base line and mark the point of stimulation. Put a weight hanger on the lever about an inch from the fulcrum.

2.   After-loading: Ensure that the after-load screw is in firm contact with, and supports, the vertical arm of the lever, so that the weight does not stretch the muscle. Record a single contraction (with only the weight hanger) and label it 0 (no load). Using 10 g weights, record another 5 contractions with 10, 20, 30, 40, and 50 g loads; and label the curves, accordingly.

3.   Free-loading (preloading or foreloading): Remove all the weights from the hanger, and withdraw the after-load screw right up to the frame of the lever so that it will no longer support the vertical arm of the lever. Record 6 contractions using 0, 10, 20, 30, 40, and 50 g loads. Each time a 10 g weight is added on the hanger, the lever sags down more and more, thus stretching the muscle more and more. Lift the muscle trough each time to bring the writing point to the original base line.

Note

The free- and after-loaded contractions may be recorded separately on two locations on the paper, but on the same base line.

The contractions can also be recorded on a stationary drum by rotating the cylinder forwards by hand through 2 cm after each increase of load, as shown in **Figure 4-9**. In this case, only the height of contraction can be noted. On a rotating cylinder, however, one can record the height, the speed of shortening, and various periods of each contraction curve.

OBSERVATIONS AND RESULTS

After-loading. As the load increases, the latent period increases due to lever inertia. The height decreases because the muscle has to lift greater loads. The contraction period decreases due to decrease in the duration of active state, while the relaxation period decreases because the load hastens the return of the lever to the base line.

Free-loading. The latent period decreases for a few contractions, then it may increase a little or remain unchanged. The height (force) of contraction increases for the first few contractions (up to a physiological limit), then it starts decreasing. The speed of contraction also increases as can be seen from the slope of the curve. Since the duration of the active state does not change, the contraction time does not change. The relaxation period decreases because the load hastens the return of the lever.

Calculation of work done. The following data are needed for calculation of the work done for

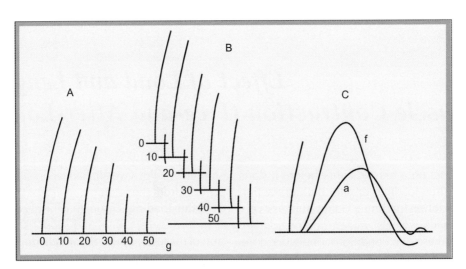

Figure 4-9. Effect of load and length on muscle contraction. A: After-loading, B: Free-loading. All contractions were recorded on a stationary drum, the free-loaded contractions being recorded from successively lower levels. C: Two contractions recorded with 20 g weight each, on a rotating drum. a: muscle after-loaded; f: muscle free-loaded

each weight (load) in both free-loaded and after-loaded contractions.

a. Height of contraction curve for each weight, (H).
b. Long arm of the lever, from fulcrum to the stylus, (L).
c. Short arm of the lever, from fulcrum to the point where weight is hung, (l).
d. The actual height through which the weight has been lifted, (h).

$$\text{Magnification of the lever (magnification factor)} = \frac{L}{l}$$

$$h = H/\text{magnification factor} = \frac{H}{L/l} = \frac{lH}{L}$$

Work done = W (g) × h (cm), where
W = weight in g, and h = actual height in cm.

Multiply with 981 to express the result in ergs. Plot your results on a graph paper indicating the weight on the abscissa and the work done on the ordinate.

QUESTIONS

Q. 1 What is meant by the terms "tension" and "load"?

See Q/A 4 Expt. 4-3.

Q. 2 Why does a free-loaded muscle contract more forcefully and work more efficiently than an after-loaded muscle? What is optimum load?

When a muscle is removed from the body, it shortens, because muscles in the body are in a state of slight stretch. This length of the muscles is called the "resting length", at which the tension generated is maximum. The gradual stretching of the gastrocnemius during free-loading increases the initial length of the muscle fibers, which increases its force of contraction and work efficiency. When the muscle is after-loaded, the initial phase of contraction is isometric contraction and, therefore, the work done is less than that

of free-loaded contraction. As the load increases, the work efficiency decreases.

Q. 3 What is Starling's law and what is its basis? Can it be demonstrated in your experiment?

The **Starling's law** (or Frank-Starling law) states that "the force (or energy) of contraction, however measured, is a function of the initial length of the muscle fibers". Up to a physiological limit, *greater the initial length, greater is the force of contraction.* Though originally described for the heart, it is also applicable to the skeletal muscle. [In the case of heart, the diastolic filling determines the initial length (preload) of muscle].

The length of the muscle fibers determines the degree of overlap between myosin and actin filaments. There is an optimal sarcomere length (2.2 µm) at which every myosin head is opposite an active site on the actin filament. Therefore, maximum force is obtained when the preload (initial length) it set at this sarcomere length of 2.2 µm. At shorter lengths, actin filaments bump into each other and decrease the overlap. When overstretched, the thin filaments are pulled out, thus decreasing the overlap. In both cases, force obtained is decreased.

The Starling's law can be demonstrated by recording a free-loaded and an after-loaded contraction with the same load, say, 30 g. The free-loaded contraction is more forceful.

Q. 4 Do free-loaded and after-loaded contraction occur in the body?

Varying the preload (i.e., the initial length) is not an important method of varying the force of contraction of muscles because the muscle lengths generally depend on the type of motor activity being performed. But if it is possible to stretch the muscles, more force can be obtained, as is done by weight lifters who allow the weight to stretch their muscles before they lift the weight with a sudden effort. Stretching and warm-ups by athletes probably serve the same purpose. Throwing a stone may be considered as associated with free-loading. Lifting an object from the ground involves after-loaded contractions.

Exposure of Frog's Heart and Normal Cardiogram

Exposure of the Frog's Heart

1. Stun and pith a frog and lay it on its back in a dissection tray. Using a scissors, incise the skin in the midline from xiphisternum to the jaw. Extend the lower end of this cut laterally and remove both pieces of skin. The anterior chest wall is now exposed.

2. Give a horizontal cut in the muscles at the level of xiphisternum. (Do not cut through the abdominal wall, otherwise the viscera will spill out). Using bone forceps and scissors, cut through the pectoral girdles and remove the chest wall in one piece. The heart will now be revealed beating in its pericardial sac. Note its size. Slit through the pericardium and remove it right up to the base of the heart. The size of the heart will be seen to increase.

OBSERVATIONS

Examine the heart carefully and note that it differs structurally from the mammalian heart.

1. There is **one ventricle**, separated from the **two atria** by the atrioventricular groove, and the **bulbus arteriosus** which arises from the ventricle and divides into two aortae. Lift the ventricle up and find behind it the **sinus venosus** with the two venae cavae emptying into it.

2. A careful observation will reveal the **white crescentic line** between the sinus and the right atrium. This is the site of the Remak's and Bidder's ganglia of the vagus nerves.

3. The color of the ventricle becomes pale during systole as blood is forced out of it. Feel the hardening of the ventricle when it contracts. There are no valves in the frog's heart.

4. **Sequence of heart beats.**   The contractions of the **four units** of the heart are progressive. The sinus leads off, followed by the atria, ventricle and the bulbus, in that order. The rate of the heart depend on the frequency of the sinus, as it is the pacemaker. Pour cold Ringer on the heart to slow it down in order to appreciate the pauses between the contractions of the cardiac chambers.

NORMAL CARDIOGRAM

The cardiogram is a record of the mechanical activity of the heart, while electrocardiogram is a record of the electrical activity of the heart. In this and the following experiments, the mechanical events of the heart will be recorded with a Starling's heart lever.

Procedures

1. Transfer the frog to the frog board or trough. Fit the Starling heart lever on the vertical rod of the stand directly above the heart, and pass the sharp hook of the bent pin through the apex of the ventricle, taking care not to puncture its cavity.

2. Lift the heart gently by raising the lever, and adjust its position so that its movements are satisfactory, and its mean position is horizontal. Note that during systole, the lever is pulled down, while during diastole the spring of the lever pulls it back to its former position.

3. Move the stand carrying the preparation and the lever so that the lever is at a tangent to the cylinder, and the writing point is lightly touching

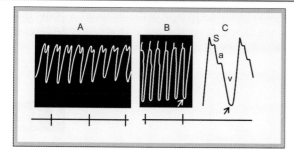

Figure 4-10. Record of spontaneously beating heart of frog. (A): In this trace only the atrial and ventricular events are seen. (B): In this trace, recorded from another frog, contractions of sinus (S), atria (a) and ventricle (v), followed by relaxations, can be seen as shown in the diagram (C): Contraction of truncus arteriosus occurs just before the beginning of ventricular diastole (arrow)

the cylinder surface. Record the cardiac activity for about 15 cm on the paper, with the drum moving at the slow speed of 1.2 mm/sec, and then at 2.5 mm/sec.

4.   Record a time tracing of 5 sec with the time signal marker below the graph obtained. Compare your graph with that shown in **Figure 4-10**, and note how many peaks have been recorded. Note the rhythm of the heart, and calculate the rate of the heart. (The frog's heart rate varies from 30 to 50 per minute, depending on the atmospheric temperature).

Note

Do not handle your preparation more than is absolutely essential, as excessive handling will give poor results. It is important to remember that contraction of a particular part of the heart may not produce a definite peak, because peaks can result from temporal overlapping of contractions of two regions. Two peaks, one for the atria and one for ventricle are commonly recorded, and three peaks are not uncommon; the record may also be quite complex. Try to identify the heart movement which is responsible for a particular peak. Intelligent use of event marker, along with careful observation, can provide useful information for this purpose.

QUESTIONS

Q. 1 Why is frog's heart used for the study of properties of heart?

The frog heart is a convenient preparation because it will continue to beat after the chest is opened. It obtains an adequate supply of oxygen directly from the blood in its chambers and from the atmosphere. (It has no coronary circulation). Its rate is sufficiently slow to allow observation of its sequence. Also it continues to function over a wide range of temperatures. The properties which can be studied include excitability, automaticity, rhythmicity, contractility, conductivity, refractoriness, and all-or-none law.

Q. 2 Describe the graph obtained by you.

The downstroke of the tracing represents systole, and the upstroke diastole. There is atrial systole followed by atrial diastole, then ventricular systole (this is the strongest of the four contracting units) is followed by diastole. (Contraction of sinus may also be recorded if a large frog has been used. The heart rate is...../min and the rhythm is regular).

Q. 3 What is the cause of the heart beat? Can it continue to beat outside the body?

The cause of the heart beat lies within the heart inself, i.e., in the pacemaker which lies within the wall of the sinus venosus. The pacemaker spontaneously and rhythmically generates action potentials (cardiac impulses) which pass quickly to atria, ventricle, and bulbus from muscle cell to muscle cell. There is no definite fibrous ring between the atria and the ventricle. The muscle fibers in this region run circularly around the heart and not directly from atria to ventricle. This may account for the normal delay between the atria and the ventricle. There is no impulse generating and conducting system such as that found in the mammalian heart.

When removed from the frog's body and kept in Ringer placed in a Petridish, the heart will continue to beat. If the sinus, atria, and the ventricle are cut and separated from each other, each unit, in due course, will be seen to beat at its own inherent rate, the sinus rate being the fastest, and ventricle slowest (idioventricular rhythm). (Heart transplantation is a life-saving procedure as the

heart continues to beat in the recipient's body. But since there is no nerve supply, the heart rate cannot increase much during exercise).

Effect of Temperature on Frog's Heart

PROCEDURES

1. Set up your experiment for recording frog's cardiogram. Pour Ringer at room temperature on the heart to keep it moist; note the temperature of the Ringer. With the drum running at slow speed, pour Ringer solution warmed to about 40°C on the heart, drop by drop, until there is obvious increase in its rate and force.
2. Stop the kymograph, and pour Ringer at room temperature on the heart till it resumes the previous rate and force. Then record the effect of cold Ringer at about 5°C in the same manner.
3. Record a 5-sec time tracing below the graph obtained. Label your tracing, indicating with

arrows, the points where hot and cold Ringer was applied. Calculate the heart rate at these temperatures and enter the data in your workbook.

Effect of Temperature on the Heart

At high temperature, there is an increase in the metabolic activity of the pacemaker cells, which generate more cardiac impulses per unit time (due to increase in the slope of phase 4 of the AP), thus increasing the heart rate. Increased metabolic activity of the working cells of the atria and ventricle increases the force of contraction. Cold has the opposite effects due to decrease in the metabolic activity. Tachycardia due to fever is due to the effect of high temperature on the SA node, which is the pacemaker.

Effect of Adrenalin, Acetylcholine, and Atropine on Heart

Adrenalin. It is a neurotransmitter in the brain. A sympathomimetic agent, it is also released by the adrenal medulla. Acting directly on the cardiac muscle cells, it increases their permeability mainly to Ca^{2+} ions and, to some extent, to Na^+ ions. Influx

of Na^+ in the pacemaker cells increases the slope of phase 4 of the AP (they reach firing level soon) and hence the increase in heart rate. The large influx of Ca^{2+} in the working cells increases their force of contraction (positive inotropic effect).

Acetylcholine (ACh). It is also a neurotransmitter and is released at many sites in the nervous system. Acting directly on the pacemaker cells, it increases their permeability to K^+ ions, which causes more of these ions to move out. The resulting hyperpolarization (more negativity inside) decreases the slope of phase 4 of the AP, which increases the time interval between the APs, thus decreasing the heart rate. Acting directly on the working cells (atria and ventricle), ACh increases their permeability to K^+ ions; the K^+ efflux shortens phase 2 of AP, which decreases the Ca^{2+} influx and, therefore, the force of contraction (negative inotropic effect) (see Chart 5-9 for details of APs).

PROCEDURES

1. Record some normal beats. Stop the drum and pour a few drops of 1 in 10,000 solution of adrenalin on the heart. Record the increased rate and the force. Stop the drum and wash the heart with Ringer.

2. Record a few normal beats, then pour a few drops of 1 in 100,000 solution of acetylcholine. Record the decrease in rate and force. As the heart is beating, apply 0.5% atropine solution. There will be no effect, i.e., the heart will remain inhibited.

3. Stop the drum, wash with Ringer, and study the effect of acetylcholine *after* applying atropine solution on the heart—the heart will not be inhibited this time. Label the graph appropriately.

Atropine. It is a parasympatholytic agent and blocks the action of ACh by attaching itself to the membrane receptors of cardiac muscle cells. Therefore, when applied on the heart after ACh, it has no effect, but when applied *before* ACh, atropine blocks the inhibitory action of ACh. (There are no impulses coming in the vagi or sympathetic nerves, because the frog's brain has already been destroyed. Therefore, when applied on the heart, atropine does not increase its rate).

QUESTIONS

Q. 1 What is meant by the terms adrenergic, noradrenergic, and cholinergic fibers?
Adrenergic fibers (neurons) are those which release adrenalin at their nerve terminals; noradrenergic fibers release noradrenalin (all postganglionic sympathetic neurons, excepting a few, are noradrenergic; see below); while cholinergic fibers release acetylcholine at their endings.

Q. 2 What are catecholamines and how are they inactivated in the body?
Catecholamines are a group of substances which are synthesized from tyrosine by hydroxylation and decarboxylation. These include adrenalin (methylnoradrenalin), noradrenalin, and dopamine (also a neurotransmitter). They are mostly taken up by the nerve endings which secrete them, and the rest are degraded by the enzymes monoamine oxidase (MAO) and catechol-O-methyl transferase (COMT) into vanillylmandelic acid (VMA) and others, which are excreted in the urine.

Q. 3 What are the locations in the body where acetylcholine is released? How is it synthesized in the body?
Synthesis of ACh from choline and acetyl-CoA is catalyzed by the enzyme choline acetyltransferase.

Sites where acetylcholine is released. Acetylcholine is released at the following sites:
  a. Preganglionic sympathetic nerve endings (in the ganglia).
  b. Preganglionic and postganglionic parasympathetic nerve endings.
  c. Postganglionic sympathetic fibers supplying the sweat glands, pilomotor muscles, and those supplying the blood vessels of skeletal muscles are cholinergic (all others are noradrenergic).
  d. Neuromuscular junctions of all skeletal muscle fibers (the anterior horn cells of spinal cord and the equivalent motor neurons of cranial nerves are thus cholinergic).
  e. Many synapses in the central nervous system, and some amacrine cells in the retina.

Q. 4 What are the different types of actions of acetylcholine in the body?

Acetylcholine has two main types of actions— **muscarinic** (muscarine is an alkaloid of a poisonous mushroom), and **nicotinic** (nicotine is an alkaloid of tobacco) actions.

Muscarinic actions. These are the actions of ACh on cardiac muscle (inhibition), smooth muscle, and exocrine glands, including sweat glands. These actions are blocked by the drug atropine.

Nicotinic actions. These are the actions of ACh on motor end-plates (blocked by curare, etc) and on postganglionic neurons in autonomic ganglia (blocked by hexamethonium, and other drugs).

Q. 5 How is acetylcholine inactivated in the body? What are anticholinesterases?

ACh must be rapidly removed from the site of its action if repolarization is to occur. The enzyme *acetylcholinesterase (AChE)* catalyzes the hydrolysis of ACh to choline and acetate, which are reused. *Anticholinesterases* are drugs which inhibit the action of AChE so that ACh is preserved at the site for a longer time. These drugs include physostigmine (eserine), neostigmine, and di-isopropylfluorophosphate (DFP), an ingredient of some pesticides and nerve gases. Neostigmine is used in the treatment of myesthenia gravis.

4-14

Effect of Stimulation of Vagosympathetic Trunk and Crescent; Vagal Escape; Effect of Nicotine and Atropine

EXPERIMENTAL PROCEDURES

1. **Exposure of vagosympathetic trunk.** Expose the heart as before. Identify the narrow strip of petrohyoid muscle which runs from the base of the skull to the hyoid bone as it crosses a very shiny tendon. Lift up the lower border of the muscle and you will find the vago-sympathetic trunk and carotid vessels crossing the shiny tendon. Expose the other trunk also. Put loose ligatures around them so that they can be lifted up for stimulation.

   Include the Neef's hammer (for repeated stimuli) and an event marker in the primary circuit.

2. **Stimulation of vagosympathetic trunk.** Record a few normal beats, then stimulate the vagosympathetic trunk for 4-5 seconds.

Note the stoppage of the heart during diastole (**Figure 4-11**).

3. **Stimulation of crescent.** After normal beats are restored, stimulate the white crescentic line for a few seconds and note cardiac inhibition as above. Repeat steps 2 and 3 on the other side.

4. **Vagal escape.** Stimulate the vagus once again, but continue the stimulation until the heart starts to beat again, i.e., it escapes the vagal effect. Test the other side as well.

5. **Nicotine.** After normal beats are restored, pour a few drops of nicotine solution on the heart. Note that there is no effect. Now perform the following experiments:
   a. Stimulate the vagosympathetic trunk— there is no inhibition of the heart.
   b. Stimulate the crescent—the heart is inhibited, as shown in **Figure 4-11**.

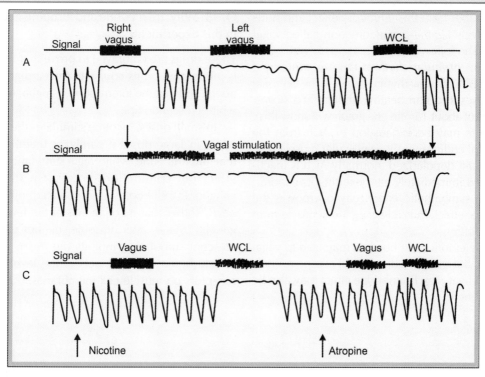

Figure 4-11. A—Effect of electrical stimulation of vagosympathetic trunk and white crescentic line (WCL: crescent). B—Phenomenon of vagal escape. C—Frog's heart treated with nicotine and atropine followed by stimulation of vagus and white crescentic line (WCL) after each drug. (Using these procedures, an unknown drug (eg, nicotine, atropine, adrenalin, acetylcholine can be identified by the student)

6. **Atropine.**   Wash the heart with Ringer. When normal beats are restored, pour atropine on the heart. Note that there is no effect on the heart. Now perform the following experiments:
   a. Stimulate the vagosympathetic trunk—the heart is not inhibited (**Figure 4-11**).
   b. Stimulate the crescent—the heart is not inhibited.

QUESTIONS

Q. 1 What type of nerve fibers are present in the vagosympathetic trunk?

The vagosympathetic trunk contains preganglionic parasympathetic nerve fibers, and postganglionic sympathetic fibers (in mammals the two systems run separately), but there are many more vagal fibers than sympathetic. Therefore, vagal effects usually predominate. As in other locations, parasympathetic ganglia (where preganglionic fibers end and synapse on the postganglionic neurons) are situated in or near the organs supplied by this system. The ganglia, called Bidder's and Remak's, are situated in the crescentic area. The inhibitory effects of vagal and crescent stimulation are due to release of acetylcholine which increases cardiac cell permeability to K^+ ions, as described in the last experiment.

Q. 2 What is vagal escape, and what is its cause?

Vagal escape.   When the vagus (it supplies the ventricle in amphibia) is stimulated, the heart at first stops, but as the stimulation is continued, the heart escapes from this inhibitory effect and starts to beat once again—a phenomenon called vagal escape. The following factors are involved:

1. *Idioventricular rhythm*: Due to prolonged inhibition a new rhythm center in the ventricle causes it to start beating, though at a slower rate of about 15/min (the graph will show this).
2. There may be exhaustion of ACh from the vagal endings, or the ventricular muscle may remain depolarized (normally ACh is inactivated immediately after exerting its action).
3. The sympathetic effect may overpower the vagal effect, thus releasing the ventricle from inhibition.

Strong emotions in humans may lead to vagal syncope, but the immediate vagal escape restores the heart beat (The Brainbridge effect may also be involved here).

Q. 3 Why are nicotine and atropine employed in this experiment?

These drugs are employed to prove that the vagus is interrupted on its course to the cardiac muscle fibers, and that the interruption (ganglia) lies at the white crescentic line.

In small doses, nicotine stimulates the ganglia, while in large doses it paralyzes them. The fact that, after nicotine, while vagal stimulation has no effect but stimulation of crescent (the post-ganglionic cell bodies are stimulated) inhibits the heart, shows that incotine acts at the level of the ganglia. Since, after atropine, neither vagal nor crescent stimulation inhibits the heart, one can conclude that atropine acts at the level of ACh receptors on muscle cell membranes.

4-15

Properties of Cardiac Muscle (Stannius Ligatures)

The conduction of activity from the sinus to the atria (and from atria to sinus), and from atria to the ventricle, can usually be blocked by tying ligatures between these chambers. This usually leaves the ventricle quiescent or inactive (not contracting). Under these conditions, **ventricular excitability** (stimulus-response relation), **autorhythmicity, conductivity, refractory period, all-or-none law, staircase,** and **response to repetitive stimuli** can be demonstrated.

PROCEDURES

Refractoriness in the Beating Heart: Extrasystole and Compensatory Pause

1. Arrange to obtain single "make" and "break" induction stimuli. Include an event marker in the primary circuit to indicate the exact moment in the cardiac cycle at which a stimulus will fall.
2. Expose the heart and transfer the frog to the trough; attach the heart to the Starling heart lever. Adjust the event (signal) marker so that it will write about 2 cm above and in the same vertical line as the writing point.
3. Bring the stimulaing electrodes in gentle contact with the ventricle. While watching the heart and the tracing, pass single stimuli during early, middle, and late phases of systole and diastole, with a few normal beats in between each stimulation.

Note that when the stimulus falls during any part of systole, it has no effect (**Figure 4-12**); the heart continues to beat as before. But when the

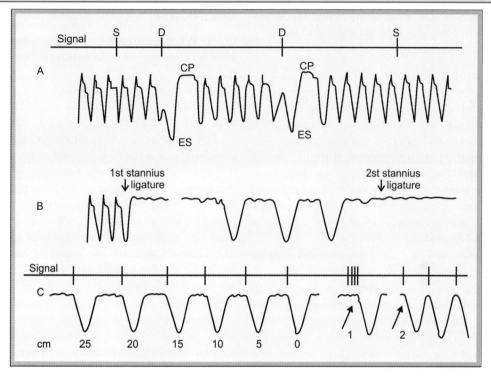

Figure 4-12. A—Refractoriness of cardiac muscle. The signal trace indicates the moment of stimulation of the ventricle during the cardiac cycle. Outside stimulation of ventricle during systole (S) has no effect; stimulation during diastole (D) produces an extrasystole (ES) followed by a compensatory pause (CP). B—Stannius ligatures, showing the hierarchy of pacemaking in the heart. After 1st ligature, the sinus and the rest of the heart beat at different rhythms. The ventricle stops beating after 2nd ligature and remains inactive for many minutes. C—The inactive ventricle is employed for showing all-or-none law; summation of subminimal stimuli (arrow 1) and staircase phenomenon (arrow 2). The distance between primary and secondary coils, in cm, is shown for all-or-none law

stimulus falls during diastole, the heart contracts immediately. This extra contraction called **extrasystole**, or **premature beat**, is followed by a pause called the **"compensatory pause"**. This experiment also shows the properties of **excitability, contractility, autorhythmicity** and **conductivity** (stimulation of any part causes contraction of the rest of the heart).

Stannius Ligatures

These are employed to make the heart inactive or quiescent (non-contracting) during which some properties of the heart can be demonstrated.

lst Stannius ligature. Using a fine forceps, pass a stout ligature thread under the truncus arteriosus, and bring its ends to the dorsum of the heart. Check that the tie will lie, between the sinus and the atria. Record some normal beats, then tie the thread with a single knot over the crescent. If the whole heart continues to beat at its previous rate, the ligature must be in the wrong place and should be removed. If it has been applied properly, the sinus will continue to beat as before, while the atria and the ventricle will stop during diastole after one or two beats (**Figure 4-12**). In most cases, these begin to beat after a variable period of 10-20 minutes, though at a slower atrial rate (pacemaker in the atria); record this activity and tie the 2nd Stannius ligature.

2nd Stannius ligature.   Tie a tight ligature between the atria and the ventricle; the ventricle immediately stops contracting while the sinus and atria continue to beat at their own different rates. (The 1st Stannius ligature is still in place).

a. Summation of subniminal stimuli.   Select "make" and "break" stimuli that are just below the threshold level. Pass a number of these subniminal stimuli rapidly, one after the other, till the ventricle responds due to summation of these stimuli, as shown in **Figure 4-12**.

b. All-or-none law. Starting with subthreshold stimuli, increase the strength of stimuli until there is a contraction (threshold response). Continue to apply single stimuli of increasing strength, allowing at least 10-sec intervals between each response. Note that though the strength of each stimulus is successively increased, the force of contraction remains the same.

c. Staircase effect.   Watching the tracing carefully, pass 3 or 4 stimuli, one after the other, so that a fresh contraction occurs immediately after the previous relaxation is over. Note the successive increase in the force of contraction of the ventricle due to beneficial effect (consult Expt 4-7 for explanation).

d. Refractory period.   This can also be shown on a quiescent heart by applying pairs of stimuli with an interval of about 1 sec (with an electronic stimulator, or by switching the simple key ON and OFF). Repeat the stimulation, after increasing or decreasing the interval between the two stimuli as required, until you obtain the transition from one response to two responses. The interval between the two deflections of the event marker can provide an estimate of the refractory period.

e. Stimulate the heart with a tentanizing frequency (30/sec or more); note that the tracing shows irregular deflections but there is no sustained contraction of the ventricle, as was seen in the skeletal muscle. The heart must begin to relax before it can respond to another stimulus.

QUESTIONS

Q. 1 What is the cause of compensatory pause after an extrasystole? Do extrasystoles occur in humans?

Cause of compensatory pause.   The pause that follows an extrasystole is due to the following reason:

During the extrasystole, when the usual cardiac impulse from the pacemaker reaches the ventricle, it finds that it is already contracting (due to extrasystole) and in the absolute refractory period, so it has no effect. The ventricle has, therefore, to wait for the next impulse from the sinus to arrive before it can contract—hence the brief pause. The first contraction after the pause is often more forceful than the usual beat, due to Ca^{2+} being made available for a longer period (Ca^{2+}–induced Ca^{2+} release).

Extrasystoles are commonly seen in medical practice, the common causes being smoking, excessive worry, myocardial damage, digitalis overdose, etc. Some ectopic focus (other than the normal site) in the atria or the ventricles generates an impulse which causes a premature beat. It is the strong beats (due to added stroke volume) following the pauses which are felt by the patient as palpitation.

Q. 2 What is the cause of the long refractory period of the heart muscle and what is its advantage?

The long refractory period is due to the prolonged action potential of the working cardiac muscle fibers (200-300 msec) which is almost as long as the contraction phase. The advantage of this is that the cardiac muscle cannot be put into tetanus. If the heart were to remain contracted, it would lose its only function, as that of a pump.

Q. 3 What is all-or-none law? Which tissues obey this law? Are all-or-none law and the Starling's law of the heart incompatible?

Consult Expt 4-4 for answer.

Q. 4 What is staircase phenomenon and what is its cause?

Consult Expt 4-8 for explanation.

Q. 5 Why cannot Stannius ligatures be employed in mammalian heart?

The Stannius ligatures cannot be employed in mammalian hearts because they would cut off the blood flow through the coronary arteries, thus depriving the musculature of oxygen and other nutrients. When the blood supply is shut off, the muscle soon undergoes necrosis (death).

4-16

Perfusion of Isolated Heart of Frog

Composition of Ringer-Locke solution. The fluid required for perfusing the isolated heart of frog has the following composition:

NaCl	0.60 g
$CaCl_2$	0.010 g
KCl	0.0075 g
$NaHCO_3$	0.01 g ($NaHCO_3$ must be completely
Na_2HPO_4	0.001 g dissolved before $CaCl_2$ is added)
Glucose	0.1 g (to be added just before use)
Distilled water	. . . . . .to 100 ml

PROCEDURES

1. Expose the frog's heart and pass a thread around the sinus and tie, a loose knot. Make a small slit in the sinus, introduce a Syme's cannula into it, and tie, a tight knot around it.
2. Cut the aorta and other vessels and lift the cannula along with the heart. Fit a Starling heart lever, upside down, on a stand, and fix the cannula in a clamp directly above the heart. Connect the side arm of the cannula to a reservoir containing Ringer-Locke solution; and raise the reservoir about 30 cm above the heart to provide a pressure head.
3. Push the bent pin of the lever through the apex of the ventricle, make necessary adjustments and record a few beats. Note that, in this case, the upstroke is systole and the downstroke diastole. After the tracing has stabilized, raise the reservoir to increase the perfusion pressure. If done properly, the force of contraction will increase, thus demonstrating the Starling's law of the heart.
4. Add 1.0% NaCl solution via the side tube of the cannula, and record its effects. Wash the heart with the perfusion fluid, and study the effects of 1% KCl and 1% $CaCl_2$ solutions.
5. Wash the heart well with Ringer-Locke solution and study the effects of adrenalin and acetylcholine.

Effect of sodium ions. Perfusion of the heart with a high concentration of Na^+ alone causes weakening and finally failure of contraction of the heart, which stops in diastole. Increased ECF sodium interferes with the action of calcium which is the link between excitation and contraction.

Effect of potassium ions. Excess K^+ decreases the rate and force of contraction, the heart finally stopping in diastole. A high ECF K^+ decreases the resting membrane potential of the muscle cells (because of reduction in the concentration gradient across the cell membrane), and the intensity of the action potential. As a result, the force of contraction gradually decreases and the heart stops beating.

Effect of calcium ions. Excess of Ca^{2+} increases the force of contraction, and the heart ultimately stops in systole (calcium rigor). Part of the excess Ca^{2+} ions in the EFC of the T-tubules are added to the Ca^{2+} released from the terminal cisterns. As a result more Ca^{2+} is made available to the contractile machinery, and the force increases. The heart stops in systole because diastole does not occur.

342   A Textbook of Practical Physiology

Study of Reflexes in Spinal and Decerebrate Frogs

Observe a frog placed on a frog board. The head is well raised on the forelimbs, the hind limbs are flexed, and respiratory movements are present. The frog responds to various stimuli (e.g., a prick) by jumping or crawling away. When put on its back, it quickly rights itself. When put in a basin of water, it swims. This indicates the presence of *righting reflexes.*

SPINAL FROG

Using a bone cutter or stout scissors, cut off the frog's head just behind the tympanic membranes, thus separating the spinal cord from the brain. Put the frog back on the board. Immediately after the cut, all functions are suspended below the level of the cut. There is complete paralysis of the limbs, i.e., there are no spontaneous (voluntary) movements. Prick the skin of a limb with a needle—there are no reflex responses. This state of depression of the spinal functions is called **spinal shock**. It lasts for a variable period; a few minutes in the frog, a few hours in the dog; and a few weeks in man.

When the stage of spinal shock disappears the stage of **reflex activity** is seen. Though respiratory movements are absent, the limbs are now drawn well up to the body; but the *voluntary movements (jumping, crawling)* are absent: Draw down one limb—it is quickly drawn up. Pinch one limb—the stimulated limb is withdrawn (flexor reflex). Pinch with greater force; all the limbs are flexed (irradiation of impulses). Put the animal on its back—the frog cannot right itself. Put it in water—it cannot swim and sinks to the bottom, i.e., the *righting reflexes are absent.* Now destroy the spinal

cord with a pithing needle—no reflex can be demonstrated now.

DECEREBRATE FROG

Take another frog; cut off its head just behind the level of the eyes. This section separates the olfactory lobes and cerebral hemispheres from the optic lobes and the spinal cord. This means that the body is now controlled by the spinal cord plus posterior part of the brain, and not by spinal cord alone, as is the case in a spinal animal.

After the shock passes off, note the following: the sitting posture is normal; the respiration almost so. However, the animal remains motionless, i.e., *there are no voluntary movements.* Put the frog on its back—it immediately rights itself, i.e., righting reflexes are present, (due to intact vestibular apparatus). Pinch a limb—the animal makes complex movements (i.e., more than a simple reflex) and jumps or crawls away. Place it on one end of the board and tilt it—the frog climbs up the inclined board. Tilt the board the other way—the frog turns and crawls back.

QUESTIONS

Q. 1 What is meant by encephalization of function? What is the cause of spinal shock?
During the course of evolution, controls of more and more functions have shifted headward, i.e., the lower parts of the nervous system (spinal cord, brain stem, etc) have become dependent on the higher centers for the performance of their functions—a process called **encephalization of function**. Thus, the functioning of spinal cord neurons depends to a large extent on continuous

(tonic) facilitatory discharges in the descending pathways, especially corticospinal, reticulospinal, and vestibulospinal tracts. When the cord is suddenly deprived of these higher influences, it temporarily loses its reflex functions—a state called spinal shock. The higher the animal is on the ladder of evolution, the longer the duration of spinal shock.

Q. 2 How does a decerebrate frog differ from a decerebrate higher animal?

A decerebrate frog differs from a decerebrate higher animal, say, a cat, in the following ways: in a *decerebrate frog,* the muscle tone and posture are almost normal, righting reflexes are present, and the animal can perform complex movements on stimulation. On the other hand, in a *decerebrate cat,* there is extensive rigidity (neck extended, back arched, all limbs extended), the righting reflexes are absent, and the animal cannot perform complex reflex movements. The voluntary movements are absent in both.

Q. 3 What is classical decerebrate rigidity?

When Sherrington, in 1906, transacted the brain stem in the upper pons between the superior and inferior colliculi (between red nuclei and vestibular nuclei), the cat, as soon as it came out of anesthesia, showed a marked increase in muscle tone, especially the antigravity muscles. This is called *classical decerebrate rigidity.* The cut blocks the normal inhibitory signals from the cortex and caudate nucleus to the descending inhibitory reticular formation of the brain stem. The descending facilitatory reticular formation being tonically active now, increases the activity of the spinal stretch reflexes by stimulating the gamma efferents. As a result, the muscle tone, which is a reflex phenomenon, increases. Thus, decerebrate rigidity is a release phenomenon.

4-18

Experiments on Anesthetized Dog

The rabbit and the dog are the usual mammals employed for practical class work. The dog (7-10 kg) must be quarantined for 10 days. Never frighten, annoy, or give pain to the animal. If scratched or bitten by the dog, thoroughly scrub the area with soap and water, then wash with alcohol and apply carbolic acid.

INSTRUMENTATION

1. **Brodie-Starling long-paper electric kymograph.** It is fitted with assemblies for a manometer for recording blood pressure (BP), a Brodie, or Marey tambour for recording respiratory movements, an event marker, a time marker, a stimulating unit, and tuning knobs for speed control.

2. **Manometer.** It is a U-shaped glass tube containing mercury. One limb carries a float with a curved undersurface and a light-weight steel capillary bearing a writing point. The other limb has a side tube for connecting the manometer to an arterial cannula, and a vertical tube for connecting to a pressure bottle containing an anticoagulant. A manometric slide-adjustable scale is fitted between the two limbs for noting the blood pressure.

3. **Pressure bottle.** It has two tight-fitting rubber corks bearing glass tubes, one at the top for air entry, and the other near the bottom for connecting to the manometer. The bottle contains 3.8% sodium citrate solution. A pressure is created in the pressure recording system by raising the bottle.

This prevents coagulation of blood and entry of blood into the manometer.

4. **Francis-Francois arterial cannula.** It has a nozzle, a bulb, and a side-arm bearing a short piece of rubber tube and a clamp. A clot, if any, can be removed through the side-arm.

5. **Operation table.** The stainless steel top has two halves, with a removable drain pipe between and under them. The surface can be heated with electric lamps. Cleats are provided on the table edges for fastening the animal. A steel upright carries the instrument tray.

6. **Instrument tray.** The instruments required include scalpels, scissors, artery forceps, bulldog clamps, retractors, tracheal cannula (Y-shaped or Z-shaped), venous cannula, arterial cannula, gauze pieces and cotton swabs wetted with normal saline, and various drugs.

EXPERIMENTAL PROTOCOL

1. Calibrate the recording surface, in mm Hg, with the help of manometric scale and the writing point.
2. Anesthetize the animal with nembutal [pentobarbitone sodium; 35 mg/kg body weight injected in a leg vein (marginal vein of the ear in rabbit)]. Make a 7-8 cm midline cut in the neck, expose the trachea by blunt dissection, insert the tracheal cannula and tie it in position with stout thread. Connect the cannula to the tambour. (The respiratory movements may also be recorded by tying a stethograph around the animal's chest).
3. Create a pressure of about 100 mm Hg in the manometer by raising the bottle.
4. Expose the femoral artery for about 4 cm in one thigh and tightly ligate it away from the heart. Place a bulldog clamp away from the ligature. Lift up the swollen segment of the artery, give a small nick in its wall, insert the arterial cannula and tie it in position.
5. Insert a venous cannula in the femoral vein in the other thigh, and connect it to a burette containing 0.9% sodium chloride solution.

This route will be employed for injecting drugs.

6. Using blunt dissection on either side of the trachea, expose 3 cm of both common carotid arteries in the middle of the neck. Place loose thread ties around the arteries. Lift up the vagus. Place two loose ties around it.
7. Identify the smaller nerve, which is the cervical sympathetic trunk. Place a loose tie, around it, lift it up, and place it on the electrodes of the stimulating probe. If it has been correctly identified, its stimulation will cause dilation of the pupil on that side. (In the rabbit, the nerve fibers from the stretch receptors in the aortic arch run as a separate nerve—the aortic depressor nerve—which also runs in the carotid sheath. In other mammals, these fibers run in the vagus).

The Blood Pressure Tracing

In 1733, the Rev Stephen Hales, an English clergyman, inserted a brass cannula into the femoral artery of a mare and connected it to a 9 feet long glass tube. On releasing the ligature on the artery, the blood rose to a height of 8 feet 3 inches, and oscillated above and below this level. When he inserted the cannula in the femoral vein, the blood column rose only 12 inches. This was the first instance of a quantitative determination of the blood pressure.

The mercury manometer cannot record the systolic and diastolic pressures, because mercury has a high inertia and a low natural frequency. It dampens the fluctuations; the high values are less and the low values are high. As a result, the oscillations of the mercury with each beat of the heart are small. The recorded tracing, therefore, represents fluctuations around the *mean arterial pressure*. Usually, three types of fluctuations in pressure are recorded:

i. **Cardiac waves.** These small waves are caused by successive cardiac contractions, and are superimposed on the respiratory waves.

ii. **Respiratory waves (Traube-Hering waves).** These waves, which are composed of cardiac waves, represent fluctuations in blood pressure synchronous with the movements of respiration. The waves show a rise of pressure during inspiration and a fall during expiration. The waves may be quite large if the respiration is slow and deep. The blood pressure rises during inspiration due to: (a) irradiation of impulses from the inspiratory centre to the vasomotor center which lies nearby, (b) the increase in intrathoracic negativity causes increased venous return and therefore cardiac output, and (c) the rise in heart rate also increases the cardiac output and hence the blood pressure.

iii. **Meyer waves.** The Meyer waves, also called *vasomotor waves*, are small changes in blood pressure over long periods of time, encompassing a number of respiratory waves. These waves result primarily from baroreceptor activity, as well as of vasomotor center. When the blood pressure is low (50-80 mm Hg), chemoreceptors contribute mostly to generate these waves, as the influence of baroreceptors becomes very weak.

EXPERIMENTS

Note the general features of the BP tracing and identify the cardiac and respiratory waves. Note the rate and rhythm of breathing. Then perform the following experiments and note the results:

1. **Carotid occlusion.** Clamp both the carotid arteries, pressing on the event marker at the same time. Note the rise in blood pressure. When the pressure has stabilized at the new level, remove the clamps from the arteries and the finger pressure from the event marker.

Carotid occlusion lowers the pressure in the carotid sinuses, which increases the BP due to stoppage of inhibitory discharges from them (consult Expt 2-9 on carotid occlusion). Since the aortic baroreceptors are sill functioning, the rise in pressure is not excessive. Stimulation of carotid

bodies by ischemia also contributes to the rise in blood pressure.

2. **Vagal stimulation.** The first example of inhibition discovered in physiology was in 1845 when Weber brothers found that weak stimulation of vagus decreased the heart rate and force while strong stimulation stopped the heart.

The cervical vagus contains afferent fibers from aortic body chemoreceptors, aortic arch mechanoreceptors, mechanoreceptors from heart, chemoreceptors from coronary and pulmonary chemoreceptors, and stretch receptors in small airways (for Hering-Breuer reflex). The efferent fibers for the heart arise form nucleus ambiguus, and terminate on clusters of neurons (nervous nuclei of Dogel, Remak, Bidder, and Ludwig) located in the SA node (mainly right vagus) and AV node (mainly left vagus). The postganglionic fibers form these ganglia innervate the atria, the nodes, and the AV bundle. There are very few fibers, if any, supplying the basal parts of the ventricles, which is the reason why the ventricles escape the inhibitory effect of continued vagal stimulation.

a. **Stimulate one vagus and then the other,** with weaker and stronger stimuli. In both cases, there is slowing of the heart and fall in blood pressure, and stoppage of the heart with stronger stimuli. The respiration is usually arrested.

With slower beating of the ventricles, the diastolic period is prolonged, ventricular filling is more, and the stroke volume is increased. These are reflected in wide swings in the oscillations of the mercury column. If stimulation is continued after stoppage of heart, the ventricles usually "escape" and start to beat at the slower idioventricular rhythm of 20 to 30 beats/min (pacemaker in the ventricles). Vagal escape perhaps also suggests that the vagus has very little direct effect on the ventricular activity (consult Expt 4-14 on vagal escape in Frog heart).

b. **Section of vagi:** Cut first one vagus and then the other between the two ties. There is an increase of heart rate due to loss of vagal tone. The respiration becomes slower and deeper.

Vagal tone.   A prolonged excitation which is not accompanied by fatigue is called tone. There is appreciable vagal tone and a moderate sympathetic tone in man. If vagal tone in humans is blocked with atropine, the heart rate increases from the resting value of about 70/min to 150-170 beats/min. If both cholinergic and noradrenergic system are blocked with drugs (pharmacologic denervation), the heart rate is about 100/min.

   c.   *Stimulate the peripheral ends of the cut vagi,* first one then the other. There is inhibition of the heart as before. There is no effect on respiration.

   d.   *Stimulate the central ends of the cut vagi,* first on one side and then on the other. There is stoppage of respiration due to excitation of afferent fibers coming from the stretch receptors of the lungs (These fibers are involved in the Hering-Breuer reflex). There is no effect on the heart.

3.   *Inject 5 µg of adrenalin* (1 in 10,000 solution; 1 ml = 10 µg) intravenously. There is an immediate but small and transient fall in BP (due to slight fall in total peripheral resistance), which is at once followed by a rise, due mainly to increase in cardiac output. The baroreceptor signals which inhibit the vasomotor center also inhibit the respiratory center located nearby. Thus, a rise in blood pressure may depress the respiration, or even cause a temprorary stoppage of respiration—a condition called *adrenalin apnea.*

4.   *Inject 5 µg of noradrenalin* into the vein. There is no initial fall in the blood pressure, and the rise in pressure is much greater and more sustained. The mean pressure rises in spite of reduction in cardiac output by the baroreceptor mechanism. This drug causes intense vasoconstriction of almost all the systemic arterioles via alpha-1 receptors.

5.   When the blood pressure has returned to control levels, inject 2 µg of *acetylcholine* (1 in 100,000; 1 ml = 1 µg) intravenously. There is a marked decrease in heart rate and blood pressure due to inhibition of the heart. When the pressure has returned to control level, repeat the dose after first injecting atropine. There will be no inhibition of heart now (consult Expt 4-13 for details).

6.   Effect of asphyxia.   Close the tracheal cannula to produce asphyxia, i.e., hypoxia plus hypercarbia. There is a gradual increase in the rate and depth of respiration, and a rise in blood pressure. As the asphyxia progresses, the animal makes violent respiratory efforts. Increased PCO_2 stimulates the vasomotor center, thus increasing the BP. Acting on the respiratory center via medullary chemoreceptors, and reflexly via carotid and aortic bodies, a high PCO_2 stimulates breathing. A low PO_2 stimulates respiration reflexly, but its action on the medullary neurons is depressant (consult Expt 2-2 for details).

   The animal may be revived at this time, but if the asphyxia is continued, the toxic effects of CO_2 on the heart and the brain result in fall of BP and depression of breathing. There is generalized muscle twitching and failure of respiration. Ventricular fibrillation and cardiac arrest occur in 4 to 5 minutes.

7.   Effect of raised intrathoracic pressure on systemic arterial pressure.   After the blood pressure returns to control level, simultaneously place a fingertip over the tracheal cannula and, with the other hand, squeeze the thoracic cage just below the ribs to prevent the descent of diaphragm. There is a fall in blood pressure due to decrease in venous return resulting from raised intrathoracic pressure.

8.   Effect of hemorrhage. It depends on the *amount of blood removed* and the *rapidity of bleeding.* Cannulate the other femoral artery and remove blood equivalent to 10 ml/kg body weight into a measuring cylinder (normal blood volume = 80 ml/kg body weight). Note the fall in blood pressure, which is due to decrease in venous return, and thus of cardiac output. The breathing may show an increase in rate (tachypnea), which is due to poor perfusion of carotid bodies (aortic bodies are ineffective because the vagus nerves have been cut).

About 50% of the blood is present in the veins at any one moment. Therefore, constriction of veins is an important compensatory mechanism which tends to restore circulating blood volume after hemorrhage; the other compensatory processes for restoring blood volume and pressure being arteriolar constriction and decreased formation and increased reabsorption of tissue fluid in the capillaries. (The receptors primarily responsible for monitoring the "fullness" of the cardiovascular system and for regulating the blood volume are the low pressure stretch receptors in the atria).

Charts

This section includes idealized normal charts, figures, and graphs on which the students are quizzed/tested during their class tests and university examination. Of course, the charts on which the students are tested are not labeled.

The students should, however, note that the questions/answers mentioned here are not exhaustive. It will be a good practice if they make up other related questions and try to answer them during discussions with their classfellows.

5-1

Arterial Pulse Tracing (Figure 5-1)

Q. 1 What is arterial pulse?

With each systolic ejection of blood from the left ventricle, the aorta expands and then recoils, thus setting up a *pressure wave* or pulse wave. This rhythmic pulsatile phenomenon which is transmitted from segment to segment of the systemic arteries, and which can be felt, is called the arterial pulse.

(The transmission of the arterial pulse, which has a velocity of 6-10 meters/sec, should not be confused with the passage of blood which moves at a velocity of about 0.5 m/sec).

Q. 2 How is an arterial pulse tracing obtained?

A *sphygmograph* is employed to make a graphic representation of the radial artery at the wrist. The apparatus is kept in position with straps, and its padded knob is adjusted over the artery. The movements of the knob are amplified by a lever system and recorded on a moving strip of paper via a hinged surface-writing lever. Electronic transducers and recorders are employed these days.

Q. 3 What are the various waves of the arterial pulse tracing?

The steep upstroke is called the *anacrotic limb,* or the *percussion wave.* It is due to expansion of the artery resulting from ventricular systole, and corresponds to the maximum ejection phase. The leisurely downstroke is called the *catacrotic limb.* In the descending limb, there is a negative wave— the *dicrotic notch* which is followed by a positive wave—the *dicrotic wave.* A small wave, called the tidal wave is sometimes recorded soon after the peak of the tracing.

Q. 4 What is the cause of the dicrotic notch and the dicrotic wave?

At the end of ventricular systole, the pressure within it falls below that in the aorta. The elastic aorta now recoils, causing the blood column to momentarily sweep back toward the heart, thus setting up the dicrotic notch. This reverse flow of blood closes the aortic valve, the blood column rebounds from the closed aortic valve, and this is

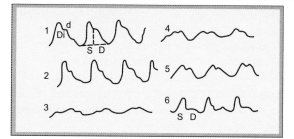

Figure 5-1. Forms of arterial pulse. (1) Normal pulse, Di–dicrotic notch, d–dicrotic wave, S–systole, D–diastole, (2) Corrigans (water-hammer), (3) Plateau, (4) Parvus, (5) Bisferiens, (6) Dicrotic, S–systolic, D–diastolic

recorded as the dicrotic wave, as shown in Figure 5-1.

Q. 5 Can you indicate the systolic and diastolic phases of the ventricle on the arterial pulse tracing?

The maximum ejection phase lasts from the start of the upstroke to the peak of the percussion wave while the reduced ejection phase lasts from the peak to the dicrotic notch. The rest of the time period, i.e., from the dicrotic notch to the start of the next upstroke, represents diastole.

Q. 6 What is collapsing, water-hammer, or corrigans pulse?

A *collapsing pulse* is characterized by an abrupt rise and a sudden descent of the pulse wave. It is seen most commonly in aortic regurgitation, in which the incompetent valve cannot close properly to prevent backflow of blood from the aorta back into the left ventricle. The rapid upstroke is due to the greatly increased stroke volume while the collapsing character is caused by two factors: The diastolic "run-off" of blood back into the ventricle, and the rapid "run-off" of blood toward the periphery because of a low systemic vascular resistance (due to arteriolar dilatation). There is no dicrotic notch or the dicrotic wave. This type of pulse is also found in patent ductus arteriosus, or a large arteriovenous communication.

Q. 7 What is a 'slow rising' pulse, or pulsus parvus?

Pulsus parvus (parvus = small) is a small, weak pulse which rises slowly and has a late systolic phase. The weak upstroke is due to decreased stroke volume. It is seen in conditions with diminished left ventricular stroke volume and a narrow pulse pressure, especially in aortic or mitral stenosis, left ventricular failure and hypovolemia. (The term anacrotic pulse was formerly used to describe this slow rising pulse).

Q. 8 What is Bisferiens pulse?

It is a combination of slow rising and collapsing pulse, and is seen when aortic stenosis and aortic regurgitation are both present.

Q. 9 What is dicrotic pulse?

There are two palpable waves, one in systole, and the other in diastole. It is encountered most frequently in patients with a very low stroke volume, especially in those with dilated (congestive) cardiomyopathy (infarction).

Q. 10 What is plateau pulse?

The pulse wave rises slowly, there is a delayed and sustained peak, and the pulse fades away slowly. Such a pulse is sometimes seen in aortic stenosis.

Q. 11 What is pulsus alternans?

The pulse beats are regular, but alternately large and small in amplitude. This type of pulse can be palpated and is encountered in left ventricular failure. When the left ventricle is severely diseased, it characteristically develops alternate strong and weak beats. This variation in strength, which can be detected clinically, should not be confused with an arrhythmia.

Q. 12 What is pulsus paradoxus?

The term describes the marked decrease in pulse volume (and blood pressure) which occurs on deep inspiration in patients with a large pericardial effusion or severe asthma (Thus, it is an accentuation of the normal physiological fall in blood pressure by 8-10 mm Hg). The paradox is that while the pulse may not be felt at the wrist, heart sounds may still be heard at the precordium.

Comments

Since the arteries are not perfectly elastic, the pulse wave is gradually dampened as it progresses along the vessels. With the great reduction of pressure in the arterioles, the damping effect is great and little pulsations may be seen in the capillaries. However, if the arterioles dilate, as they do in hot weather and after exercise, the pulsations reaching the capillaries are greater and may be transmitted to the venules. Similarly, when the pulse pressure is greatly increased as in aortic regurgitation, the pulsations are seen in the capillaries. Properly applied pressure on a nail-bed, or on the mucosa of the lip (with a glass slide) will show alternate flushing of the blanched margin.

5-2

Jugular Venous Pulse Tracing (Figure 5-2)

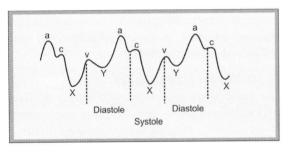

Figure 5-2. The normal jugular venous pulse tracing, showing three positive waves—a, c and v and two negative waves or descents–**X** and **Y**

Q. 1 What is meant by jugular venous pulse? How is a record of this event obtained?

Jugular venous pulse (JVP). The term jugular venous pulse refers to the pulsations observed in the jugular veins in the neck. These venous pulsations are due to the pressure changes in the right atrium that are reflected back into the large veins near the heart.

The JVP tracing is obtained by placing a suitable transducer over the vein and recording the pressure changes on the electronic polygraph. Before the days of ECG, this cardiac event used to be recorded with the Mackenzie, ink polygraph, by placing the neck receiver over the vein and connecting it to the recording system.

Q. 2 Name the various waves recorded in the JVP tracing?

The JVP record shows three positive waves—**a, c,** and **v**, and two negative waves or descents—**X** and **Y** (The letters *a, c,* and *v* stand for: *a* = atrial wave; *c* = carotid (or ventricular wave), and *v* = "venous stasis" wave).

Q. 3 What is the cause of 'a' wave?

The *a* wave is due to atrial systole (duration = 0.1 sec). During atrial systole, the pressure inside, which was rising gradually, now rises suddenly and is reflected back as the *a* wave in the JVP tracing (the contracting atrium also holds back blood in the vein). It corresponds with the last phase of ventricular filling (last rapid filling). The *a* wave is followed by the **X** descent which shows the *c* wave.

(Most of the ventricular filling occurs passively, the atrial systole contributing only about 30% to it. At rapid rates, the atrial contribution becomes important).

Q. 4 How is the *c* wave caused?

The **c** wave is due to the bulging of the tricuspid valve (atrioventricular or AV valve) towards the atrium at the beginning of isovolumetric (isometric) phase of ventricular systole (see Figure 5-4 also).

At the end of atrial systole, the ventricle starts contracting isovolumetrically as a closed chamber (the pulmonary valve is still closed and will not open till the pressure in the ventricle exceeds the diastolic pressure in the pulmonary artery, and causes the valve to bulge back into the atrium which is recorded as the upstroke of the **c** wave).

At the end of isovolumetric contraction, the pulmonary valve opens and the ventricle ejects blood into the pulmonary artery. This pulls the AV ring downwards, the atrial pressure decreases, and the downstroke of the **c** wave is inscribed . (The *c* wave is thus a *mechanical artifact of the valve motion*. A cardiac valve opens or closes due to a pressure gradient across it).

Q. 5 What is the cause of *v* wave?

The **v** wave represents the passive rise of atrial pressure and venous stasis in the jugular vein as venous return continues before the tricuspid valve opens at the end of isovolumetric relaxation of the right ventricle (Ventricular systole continues between the *c* and the *v* waves).

As the tricuspid valve opens, and blood rapidly enters the ventricle, the fall in atrial pressure causes the **Y** descent.

(Once the tricuspid valve opens, the atrium and the ventricle are a common chamber, and pressure in both cavities falls as ventricular relaxation continues. Thus, most of the ventricular filling occurs before atrial systole).

Q. 6 What is the clinical significance of the JVP tracing?

The recording of the JVP tracing is not a routine clinical procedure, because a simple clinical examination of the neck veins (see Expt 3-3) can provide important information about some cardiac conditions.

However, the procedure is non-invasive and the JVP tracing shows some characteristic changes in certain heart diseases. For example, there is a prominent *a* wave in right ventricular hypertrophy and tricuspid stenosis, while this wave is absent in atrial fibrillation. There is a sudden fall in the **Y** descent when right atrial pressure is elevated. The interval between the *a* and *c* waves is increased in heart block.

5-3

Electrocardiogram (ECG) (Figure 5-3)

Q. 1 What is ECG and what is its basis?

Electrocardiogram (ECG). The ECG is a record of the electrical activity of the heart during the cardiac cycle.

During diastole, the cardiac muscle cells are positively charged on the outside and negatively charged on the inside (as are the other cells of the body), but electrodes placed on the skin do not detect any voltage changes, i.e., the tracing is on the isoelectric line. However, excitation of a portion of the heart reverses the potential in this area, and the outside of the cells becomes negatively charged with respect to the ground. Thus a potential difference exists between the depolarized and the non-excited cells. This potential difference, after suitable amplification, can be recorded from the surface electrodes and is referred to as the electrocardiogram.

Q. 2 What is meant by the term lead?

Lead. The term lead is employed for the *specific points of electrical contact* (electrode positions) on the limbs and on the chest in front of the heart, as well as to the *record* obtained from any two

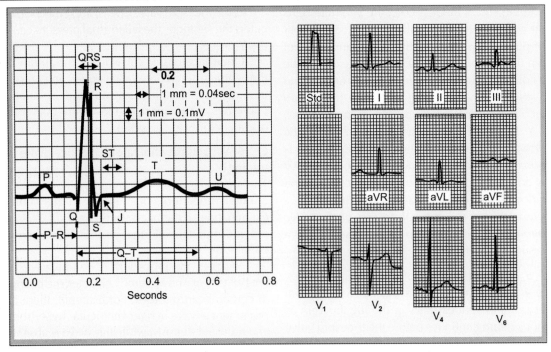

Figure 5-3. The diagram of normal ECG (left), showing the various waves, segments, times, and voltages. The normal sequence of PQRS and T in an actual ECG record; leads I, II, III aVR, aVL, aVF, V_1, V_2, V_4 and V_6 are shown on the right

electrodes. For example, right arm and left arm constitute lead I; right arm-left leg is lead II; and left arm-left leg is lead III. Similarly, chest leads are V_1, V_2, V_3 and so on.

(The ECG is recorded by using two active electrodes (bipolar limb, and chest leads), or by using an active or exploring electrode to an indifferent electrode that is kept at zero potential).

Q. 3 What do the lines on the ECG paper indicate?

The paper is divided into 1 mm squares by thin lines, every 5th line being thicker, both horizontally and vertically. The time duration is measured *horizontally*, 1 mm representing 0.04 sec (0.2 sec between two adjacent thick lines), while the amplitude of a wave is measured *vertically*, 10 mm representing 1 millivolt. The ECG is recorded at a standard paper speed (25 mm/sec) and amplification (1 mV causes a deflection of 10 mm).

Q. 4 What are the various waves recorded in a normal ECG and what do they represent?

The deflections or waves recorded in an ECG are: P, Q, R, S, and T. A small wave—the U wave—is sometimes recorded after the T wave. These waves represent depolarizations and repolarizations of the atria and the ventricles.

Q. 5 What is the P wave due to and what is its duration?

The P *wave*, commonly called the "atrial complex", represents the start of depolarization in the SA node (site of origin of cardiac impulse and the first part of the heart to be depolarized) and depolarization of the atria. Normally, it is an upward deflection (i.e., above the isoelectric line), except in lead aVR where it is inverted. It is less than 0.11 sec in duration, and measures less than 2.5 mm in amplitude. The P wave is replaced by F (flutter or fibrillation) waves in atrial fibrillation where there is no coordinated electrical or mechanical activity of the atria.

Q. 6 What is PR segment?
PR segment. The PR segment extends from the end of P wave to the start of QRS complex, and is normally isoelectric.

Q. 7 What is PR interval and what is its cause and normal duration?
PR interval. The PR or PQ interval, if Q wave is present, is a measure of the **atrioventricular (AV) conduction time,** i.e., the time taken by the excitatory wave to pass from the atria to the ventricles, including the delay at the AV node. Thus, it indicates the conduction time of the AV node and the bundle of His which connects the atria and the ventricles. The AV node is reached at the top of the P wave.

The PR interval is measured from the beginning of P wave to the onset of QRS complex (ventricular depolarization). Its normal duration is 0.12 to 0.2 sec, depending on the heart rate. The PR interval is prolonged in various types of heart block.

Q. 8 Which wave represents atrial repolarization?
Atrial repolarization. It is associated with very small electrical changes (atrial T wave) which are not recorded on the conventional surface ECG because they are almost always completely obscured by the larger QRS waves.

Q. 9 What is the cause of QRS complex?
QRS complex. The QRS represents **ventricular depolarization** and lasts less than 0.08 sec (maximum, 0.12 sec), i.e., two small squares. The ventricular depolarization spreads from the endocardium to epicardium through the walls of the ventricles.

The **Q wave** is the first negative wave after *P* and represents excitation of upper interventricular septum. It is often inconspicuous.

The **R wave** is the first prominent positive wave after *P*. It represents excitation of anteroseptum and major part of myocardium.

The **S wave,** the negative wave after *R*, represents activation of posterior basal part of ventricles (These waves represent three instantaneous vectors).
QS complex. If the entire QRS complex is negative, it is called QS complex.

Q. 10 What is the cause of T wave? What is vulnerable period?
T wave. The T wave is due to ventricular repolarization. Normally, it is in the same direction as the QRS complex because repolarization follows a path that is opposite to that of depolariztion, i.e., it occurs from epicardium to endocardium (One of the reasons for this is that the endocardial areas have a longer period of contraction and are thus slower to repolarize).

A *vulnerable period* occurs during the downslope of the *T* wave, when the ventricle is partially repolarized and the cardiac muscle fibers are in a state of relative refractoriness. An ectopic stimulus in the ventricles due to myocardial damage may bring on extrasystoles or fibrillation.

Q. 11 What is *J* point and what is its significance?
J point. The *J* point occurs at the end of QRS complex; at this time the entire ventricular muscle is depolarized. Normally, the *J* point is on the isoelectric line but it is displaced up or down by the current of injury resulting from myocardial ischemia or infarction.

Q. 12 What is ST segment?
ST segment. This segment extends from the *J* point to the onset of *T* wave. Normally, it is isoelectric, but may vary from + 0.5 to +2.0 mm in chest leads. Elevation or depression of ST segment, (due to current of injury), indicates myocardial damage.

(Since the current of injury continues to flow during *diastole* of the heart (*TP interval*), it shifts the zero potential line (drawn through the *J* point) up or down, giving the impression of elevation or depression of the ST segment).

During the ST segment interval, the entire ventricular myocardium is depolarized.

Q. 13 What is the cause of *U* wave? Is it always present?

The U wave is seen just after the T wave in some individuals. It is possibly due to a slow repolarization of the intraventricular contracting system (papillary muscles).

Q. 14 How can you determine the heart rate from an ECG tracing?

When the heart rhythm is regular, the heart rate can be determined in any of the following two ways:

1. By dividing 1500 by the number of small squares between two successive *R* waves (RR interval). The reason for this is that 1500 small squares represent 1 minute (1 small square = 0.04 sec) and RR interval represents one cardiac cycle.

   For example:
   Number of small squares between
      2 *R* waves = 21
      Heart rate = 1500 ÷ 21 = 71 per minute
2. By dividing 60 by the RR interval in seconds.
   For example:
   Number of small squares between 2 R waves = 20
   RR interval = 20 × 0.04 = 0.80
   Heart rate = 60 ÷ 0.80 = 75 per minute.

Q. 15 What is the clinical importance of ECG?

The main areas in which ECG can provide useful diagnostic and prognostic information are: abnormal rhythms including various degrees of heart block; the detection and localization of changes in cardiac muscle in ischemic heart disease (coronary artery disease; angina, infarction); hypertrophy of atria and ventricles; detection of changes in electrical activity due to pericardial disease; and changes in electrical activity resulting from general metabolic and electrolyte changes.

ECG has a special importance in exercise tests employed for detecting ischemia of the myocardium resulting from narrowing of coronary arteries. At rest, the ECG may be normal, but with increasing level of work on a treadmill (according to a definite protocol), the ST segment may reveal ischemia. The treadmill test (TMT) is often combined with special imaging methods which use radioactive tracer elements.

Q. 16 What is complete heart block? Is this condition compatible with life?

In this condition, the conduction of cardiac impulses from the atria to the ventricles is completely blocked due to a disease of the AV node, or the bundle of His, which is the only pathway of conduction from atria to ventricles. There is complete dissociation between atria and ventricles, the two beating at entirely different rates. Also, the *P* waves and QRS complexes bear no relation to each other. The atria usually beat at their usual rate while the ventricles beat at rates of 35 to 45/min (idioventricular rhythm) depending on the location of the new pacemaker for the ventricles (the new site is generally distant to the site of lesion).

Though heart block is compatible with life, a serious emergency may arise when the rate is 15-20/min. In some of these cases, there are prolonged periods, lasting a minute or more, during which ventricles do not contract at all (asystole). As a result of cerebral ischemia, there is dizziness and fainting (Stokes-Adams syndrome). It is in such cases that artificial pacemakers are inserted.

Comments

Einthoven's triangle: The two shoulders and the left leg (i.e., the region where the thigh connects electrically with the fluids around the heart) form the apices of an equilateral triangle—the Einthoven's triangle which surrounds the heart. Thus, the heart is placed approximately in the middle of a volume conductor. Lines that bisect each side of the triangle (i.e., at the zero axis of each side, where the potential is zero at all times) meet the center of the triangle at the heart.

The *Einthoven's law* states that if the potentials of any two of the three bipolar limb ECG leads are known at any instant, the third can be determined mathematically.

Vectorcardiography deals with the analysis of the contours of various waves in different ECG leads in relation to changes in the electrical axis of the heart with reference to the planes of the body. Limb leads provide ECG in the frontal plane of the body, and chest leads provide ECG in the horizontal plane. Vector loops can also be inscribed on a persistence oscilloscope.

In normal hearts, the average direction of the vector of the heart during ventricular depolarization (the mean QRS vector) is about +59 degrees. This means that during most of the ventricular depolarization, the apex of the heart remains positive with respect to the base of the heart.

5-4

Cardiac Cycle (Figure 5-4)

Q. 1 What is the cause of contraction of the heart?
The cause of cardiac contraction lies within the heart itself (the autonomic nerves only modify this activity). The SA node spontaneously generates action potentials (cardiac impulses) which spread over the atria and then to the ventricles via the AV node and the bundle of His (The atrial muscle of the SA node is the first part of the heart to depolarize and repolarize).

Q. 2 What is cardiac cycle and what are its main events? What are the durations of atrial and ventricular systole and diastole?
The sequence of changes that occur in the heart from one beat to the next is called a **cardiac cycle**. During one cycle, there are changes in pressures, volumes, electrical potentials, opening and closure of valves, and sound production due to closure of valves. The durations of atrial and ventricular systole and diastole are:
Atrial systole = 0.1 sec, diastole = 0.7 sec;
Ventricular systole = 0.3 sec, diastole = 0.5 sec.

Q. 3 What is ventricular end-diastolic volume? How much is the contribution of atria to ventricular filling?
The *ventricular end-diastolic volume (VEDV)* is the amount of blood present in each ventricle at the end of diastole; it amounts to about 120-130 ml. The atrial contraction contributes 20 to 30% towards ventricular filling (Atrial contribution becomes important at high cardiac rate because it is mainly the diastolic period that is cut down).

Q. 4 What is ventricular end-diastolic pressure and what is its significance?
The ventricular end-diastolic pressure (VEDP) is the pressure in each ventricle at the end of diastole; normally it is near zero or a few (3-5) mm Hg. The VEDV and VEDP are interrelated and change together, setting the pre-load for the next ventricular contraction, i.e., the initial length of the muscle fibers.

Q. 5 What is stroke volume?
The **stroke volume**, or **stroke output** is the volume of blood ejected by **each ventricle separately** per beat. Normally, the stroke volume amounts to about 70-80 ml. Cardiac output is the amount of blood ejected per minute, i.e., stroke volume x heart rate; at rest, it amounts to about 5 to 6 liters/min.

Q. 6 What is ventricular end-systolic volume and what is ejection fraction?
The ventricular end-systolic volume (VESV) is the amount of blood that remains in each ventricle at the end of systole. At rest, it amounts to about 50-

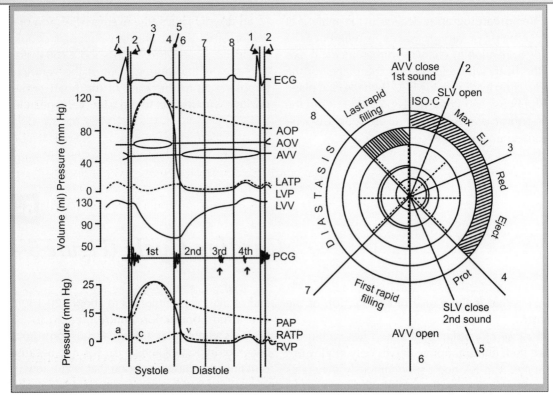

Figure 5-4. Left: Events of the cardiac cycle showing pressure changes in aorta (AOP), left ventricle (LVP), left atrium (LATP), right atrium (RATP), right ventricle (RVP) and pulmonary artery pressure (PAP). Electrical changes (ECG), sound production (PCG) are shown. The opening and closing of atrioventricular valve (AVV) and aortic valve (AOV), and changes in left ventricular volume (LVV) are also shown. Right: Cardiac cycle time = 0.8 sec. Outer circle: ventricular events, Inner circle: atrial events. Dotted lines indicate the circles divided into 8 equal segments, each 0.1 sec. Solid lines separate various phases of the cardiac cycle. Shaded segments: systole, unshaded: diastole. Note that for half the cycle, all four chambers are in diastole (relaxing).

Numbers 1 to 8 represent events in both diagrams. (1): start of isovolumetric systole, closure of AVV and 1st heart sound, (1-2): isovolumetric systole (0.05 sec), (2-3): maximum ejection (0.1 sec), (3-4): reduced ejection (0.15 sec), (4-5): protodiastole (0.05 sec), (5-6): isovolumetric relaxation (0.1 sec); (1-8): atrial diastole (0.7 sec), (1-4): ventricular systole (0.3 sec), (4-1): ventricular diastole (0.5 sec)

60 ml. The *ejection fraction*, i.e., the percent of VEDV that is expelled, is about 65%. Thus, the ventricles do not empty out completely when they contract.

(When heart contracts forcefully, the VESV can fall to as low as 10-20 ml. But when there is a large venous return, the VEDV can be as high as 150-180 ml in the normal heart. Thus, by increasing the VEDV and decreasing the VESV,

the stroke volume can be increased to nearly double its resting value, as happens during muscular exercise, during which the heart rate also increases).

Q. 7 What are the maximum and minimum pressures in the left and right ventricles?
The maximum pressure in the left ventricle is just above 120 mm Hg, when the aortic systolic

pressure is 120 mm Hg. The minimum pressure is a few mm Hg.

The maximum pressure in the right ventricle is just above 25 mm Hg, when the pulmonary artery systolic pressure is 25 mm Hg. The minimum pressure is a few mm Hg.

Q. 8 During which phase of ventricular systole is the rise in pressure maximum?

The maximum rise in ventricular pressure occurs during *isovolumetric contraction* (the length of muscle fibers remains approximately constant) when the pressure rises from 0 to 80 mm Hg (minimum pressure in aorta). The ventricle contracts as a closed chamber (blood is incompressible) because blood cannot leave it until the aortic valve opens. In the right ventricle, the pressure rises from near 0 to 10 mm Hg when the pulmonary valve opens.

Q. 9 During which phase of cardiac cycle does the maximum fall in ventricular pressure occur?

The maximum fall in ventricular pressure occurs during the *isovolumetric relaxation* phase when the pressure falls from about 80 mm Hg to near zero. During this phase, the ventricle is a closed, isolated chamber. This phase lasts 0.04 sec and ends at the peak of atrial pressure *v* wave as ventricular pressure falls below atrial pressure and the bicuspid (mitral) valve opens.

Q. 10 What is protodiastole? Is it part of systole or of diastole?

During this very brief (0.02 sec) phase of *protodiastole* (before diastole), the ventricular systole has ceased but relaxation has not yet started. When the already falling ventricular pressure (i.e., during reduced ejection) falls below that in the aorta, the transient reversal of blood flow in the root of the aorta causes the aortic valve first to float away from aortic walls and then to close abruptly. Thus, protodiastole ends with closure of semilunar valves and production of second heart sound.

Some workers consider protodiastole as part of diastole because muscle contraction has stopped; others consider it as part of systole because muscle relaxation has not yet started.

OTHER QUESTIONS

Q. 11 What are the pressures in the aorta?

Q. 12 What are the pressures in the right ventricle and the pulmonary artery?

Q. 13 What is phonocardiography. When do the heart sounds occur during the cardiac cycle and what is their cause?

5-5

Oxygen Dissociation Curve (Figure 5-5)

Q. 1 What are the gas concentrations and pressures in the arterial and venous bloods?

The arterial blood (Hb = 15 g %) contains about 20 ml/100 ml of oxygen (15 × 1.34; 1 g Hb combines with 1.34 ml O_2), at a partial pressure of about 100 mm Hg (actually a little less; this PO_2 is due solely to 0.3 ml O_2 dissolved in plasma).

The CO_2 content is 48%, at a PCO_2 of about 40 mm Hg.

The venous blood contains about 15% oxygen at a PO_2 of 40 mm Hg (this PO_2 is due to 0.1 ml % of O_2 dissolved in plasma). The CO_2 content is 52 ml %, at partial pressure of 45 mm Hg.

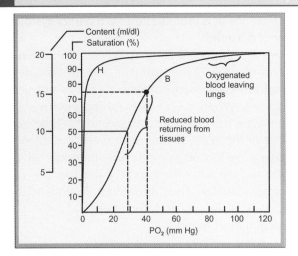

Figure 5-5. Oxygen dissociation curve. The inner (saturation) vertical scale expresses (content ÷ capacity × 100). The next scale (content) gives the O_2 content (ml/dl) of blood, assuming a normal Hb concentration (15 g/dl) and combining power (1.34 ml O_2/g Hb) B: Dissociation curve of whole blood, H: Dissociation curve of simple Hb solution in water

The rest of the gas pressure (760 minus O_2 and CO_2 pressures) is due to nitrogen dissolved in plasma (0.98%). Nitrogen is not present in any combined form.

Q. 2 What is the difference between oxygen content and oxygen capacity?

The term *oxygen content* refers to the amount of O_2 actually present in a given sample of blood, while *oxygen capacity* refers to the total amount of oxygen that can be carried by blood when the Hb is fully saturated with O_2.

The term *percentage saturation* refers to the percent of Hb that is saturated with O_2. For example, arterial blood is nearly 100% saturated, while venous blood is 75% saturated, i.e., 75% of the Hb molecules are carrying oxygen.

Q. 3 What are the special features of reactions of hemoglobin and oxygen?

The Hb molecule has 4 subunits and the heme of each subunit contains one atom of the metal iron.

It is this iron (ferrous) which is the binding site for O_2, and can combine with one molecule of oxygen (a reversible reaction).

The oxygenation of Hb occurs in 4 separate steps. At first, one molecule of O_2 is taken up by Hb; this increases its affinity for the second molecule of O_2 and so on, the affinity being maximum when the third molecule of O_2 has been taken up. This *shifting affinity of Hb for O_2* is responsible for the upper part of oxyhemoglobin dissociation curve being flat.

Q. 4 What does the oxyhemoglobin dissociation curve represent?

The *oxyhemoglobin dissociation curve*, or *oxygen dissociation curve*, represents the relationship between partial pressures of oxygen and the percentage saturation of Hb with oxygen.

Q. 5 How is oxyhemoglobin dissociation curve obtained?

About 5 ml of blood is exposed to gas mixtures (O_2, CO_2, and N_2) of varying, but known composition (and thus partial pressures), in each of the 10 tonometers (these are cylindrical glass vessels, of 250 ml capacity, with nozzles and stop-cocks). The blood samples are allowed to equilibrate with O_2 at the same tension as that present in each tonometer. The O_2 content, and thus the percent saturation, of each sample is then determined. The results are plotted in the form of a curve with PO_2 along the abscissa (X-axis) and percentage saturation (or O_2 concentration) in the ordinate (Y-axis). The graph that is obtained is called oxyhemoglobin dissociation curve of the blood. Such a curve can be obtained under different conditions of temperature, PCO_2 and H^+ ion concentrations, not only for blood, but also for myoglobin and a simple solution of Hb.

Q. 6 What is P_{50} and what is its importance?

The P_{50} is the partial pressure of O_2 at which the blood is 50% saturated, i.e., when it has given up half of its oxygen. The normal P_{50} is 25-30 mm Hg. It serves as an index for shifts in the curve that occur under different conditions.

Q. 7 What is the significance of the sigmoid or 'S' shape of the dissociation curve?

The **'flat top' of the curve,** which is due to increased affinity of the fourth oxygenation reaction, means that the alveolar PO_2 (and therefore, arterial PO_2) may fall, say, from 100 to 60 mm Hg, without greatly reducing the degree of saturation of blood with O_2, the saturation decreasing from 97 to 90%. On the other hand, if PO_2 increases from 97 mm Hg to, say, 400 mm Hg, the saturation increases from 97 to 100% (though dissolved O_2 will increase). Thus, at moderately high altitudes, an individual would suffer little from impairment of O_2 uptake from the alveoli.

The **steep part of the curve** shows that large amounts of O_2 can be given out with relatively minor falls of tissue fluid PO_2. That is, tissue fluid PO_2 does not have to fall very much for O_2 to be released from Hb. In heavy exercise, extra amounts of O_2 are released with little further fall in tissue PO_2 than down to 20-25 mm Hg.

Because of the sigmoid shape of the curve, the dissociation of oxyHb acts as a buffer for tissue PO_2. When this PO_2 falls below 40 mm Hg, extra amount of O_2 are given up; when this PO_2 tends to rise (as when one enters areas of compressed air) above 40 mm Hg, less O_2 is released from the Hb to the tissues (the curve above 60 mm Hg is flat). Thus, Hb automatically delivers O_2 to tissues at a PO_2 that is held rather tightly between 20 mm Hg and 40 mm Hg (high PO_2 can be damaging to the tissues, as is low PO_2).

Q. 8 What does a shift of the dissociation curve to the right signify? Name the factors that cause the 'right shift'.

A shift of the curve to the right (as indicated by shift of P_{50}) indicates a decreased affinity of Hb for oxygen, i.e., the unloading of O_2 is facilitated (more O_2 is released at the same PO_2, though actually, the pressure gradient is increased).

Shift of the oxyHb curve to the right. The shift of the curve to the right is caused by the following:

1. **Increase in CO_2:** When tissues become active, their own CO_2 production increases, and this lowers the affinity of Hb for oxygen. The resulting right shift increases the pressure gradient between capillary blood PO_2 and tissue PO_2. The CO_2 not only lowers the pH, it also causes vasodilation in active tissues.

2. **Increase in H^+ ion concentration:** This also causes a right shift. There are other sources of hydrogen ions besides CO_2. A change in pH from 7.4 to 7.2 causes a right shift by 15%.

3. **Increase in temperature:** A rise in temperature causes a right shift, i.e., more O_2 is released. The rise in temperature by itself causes vasodilation in the active tissues.

4. **Increase in concentration of 2-3, biphosphoglycerate (2-3, BPG):** There are high concentrations of 2-3, BPG, a byproduct of glycolysis, in the red blood cells. It acts as a highly charged polyanion which decreases the affinity of Hb for oxygen by binding to the beta chains of reduced Hb but not to those of oxyhemoglobin. Thus, the presence of DPG favors dissociation of O_2 from the Hb. The concentration of BPG rises within 40-60 minutes of exercise, at high altitudes, in anemia, and under the influence of androgens and thyroid hormones.

Q. 9 What does a shift of the dissociation curve to the left signify? Name the factors that cause a left shift.

Shift of the curve to the left. It indicates increased affinity of the Hb for oxygen, i.e., the oxygen remains tenaciously bound to Hb and is less readily given up. The factors that cause a shift to the left and upwards are: a fall in PCO_2, rise of pH (i.e., decreased hydrogen ion concentration), decrease in the concentration of 2-3, BPG, and the presence of large amounts of fetal Hb and abnormal hemoglobins. The fetal Hb has greater affinity for O_2 due to poor binding of BPG by the gamma chains (HbF causes increased O_2 release to fetal tissues under hypoxic conditions in which the fetus exists).

Q. 10 What is Bohr's effect and what is its importance?

The shifts in the oxyhemoglobin dissociation curve that occur due to changes in PCO_2 and hydrogen ions is called *Bohr's effect.* This effect enhances release of O_2 in the tissues, and then again, in the lungs, it significantly enhances the oxygenation of blood in the lungs. In the lungs, the CO_2 diffuses out and the blood PCO_2 and H^+ ion concentration fall (because of resulting decrease in blood H_2CO_3).

The reverse of Bohr's effect, called *Haldane's effect,* is also true. Binding of O_2 with Hb in the lungs tends to displace CO_2 from the blood.

Q. 11   What is coefficient of utilization?

The percent of blood that gives up its oxygen as it passes through the tissue capillaries is called the *coefficient of utilization.* At rest, it is about 25%, while during heavy exercise, the coefficient of utilization of the whole body can increase to 75-80% (in local areas of active tissues, it may be 100%, i.e., almost all of the oxygen may be extracted by the tissues).

Q. 12   What are the features of oxygen dissociation curves of a simple solution of hemoglobin and of solution of myoglobin in water?

The **oxygen dissociation curve of a simple solution of Hb** is a rectangular hyperbola (see Figure 5-5). It means that this Hb will not give up its O_2 until the PO_2 falls to 2-3 mm Hg, and even then little O_2 is given up. Also, this curve does not show Bohr effect. Thus, the Hb in simple solution would not function as a suitable supplier of O_2 to the tissues.

The dissociation curve of blood, as we have seen, is S-shaped. The dissimilarity between the curves of Hb solution and blood is due to the presence of CO_2 and hydrogen ions, 2-3, BPG, and electrolytes and inorganic salts in the blood, and of course the fact that Hb in the blood is confined to the red cells.

The **dissociation curve of unimolecular myoglobin** (Mgb; it has one iron atom) is also rectangular hyperbola; it also does not show Bohr effect. Myoglobin, present in the muscles takes up O_2 from blood at low pressures much more readily than blood. Even at a PO_2 of 40 mm Hg, the Mgb is still 95% saturated with O_2. It does not give up O_2 until the PO_2 falls to below 5 mm Hg. Thus, it acts as a temporary store of O_2 in the muscles, supplying O_2 during muscle contractions when their blood flow ceases (blood flow is restored when they relax).

5-6

Lung Volumes and Capacities (Figure 5-6)

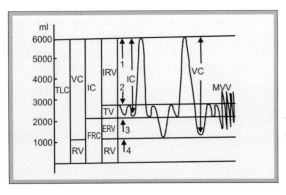

The student should go through experiment 2-3 on "Spirometry" and study Figure 5-6 carefully, considering it as an unlabelled chart. The related questions are given at the end of experiment 2-3.

Figure 5-6: Lung volumes and capacities. The volumes do not overlap; the capacities are made up of two or more volumes. Arrows: (1) Maximum inspiratory level; (2) Resting inspiratory level; (3) Resting expiratory level; and (4) Maximum expiratory level. Standard abbreviations used

Strength-duration Curve (Figure 5-7)

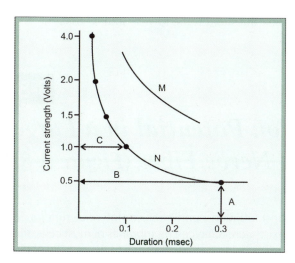

Figure 5-7. Strength-duration curve. (A) Rheobase, (B) Utilization time, (C) Chronaxie, (N) Nerve, and (M) Muscle

Q. 1 What does the strength-duration curve represent? How is this curve obtained?

Strength-duration curve (Chronaxie, curve). The chronaxie, curve represents the relationship between the *strength of a stimulating current* and the *time duration for which it must be applied* to produce an action potential in an excitable tissue. (The strength of a stimulus must rise to its effective level within a very short time to be effective; if it rises slowly, it is ineffective; the fiber tends to 'accommodate' to the presence of the current—perhaps due to semi-permanent inactivation of the sodium channels. Further, for a stimulus to be effective, it must be passed for a certain minimum time, i.e., for an adequate time).

A stimulating and a recording unit are set up where both **strength (voltage)** of a stimulus as well as its **duration (msec)** can be pre-selected (in the stimulating unit) before it is applied to the tissue

under study. Starting with a weak stimulus of a long duration, various combinations of the two are applied till a stimulus of **minimum strength** and of **adequate duration** is found that is effective. For example, in the record shown in Figure 5-7, a stimulus of 0.3 or 0.4 volt was ineffective even when it was passed for more than 0.5 msec. A stimulus of 0.5 v was found to be effective when it was passed for 0.3 msec (it was ineffective when it was applied for 0.1 or 0.2 msec). Similarly, when the stimulus intensity was increased to 1 v, it had to be applied for 0.1 msec before it became effective. With further increases in strength, the duration of the stimulus decreased, but only upto a limit above which there was no further decrease in the duration of a stimulus.

Q. 2 What is rheobase?

Rheobase. It is the minimum strength of stimulus current (0.5 v in this case) which when passed for an adequate time (measured in msec) will produce an action potential. The time for which the rheobase is passed is called the *utilization time* (0.3 msec in this case). The utilization time decreases as strength of stimulus increases.

Q. 3 What is chronaxie, and what is its significance?

Chronaxie. It is the minimum duration of time for which a current twice the rheobase (0.5 × 2 = 1 volt in this case) must be passed to elicit a response. Thus, the chronaxie, is 0.1 msec in the case cited here. Chronaxie, is an indicator of the excitability of a tissue; shorter the chronaxie, greater is the excitability, and vice versa. Chronaxie, curves are charted in lesions of nerves or muscles to assess the degree of damage and to follow the progress of recovery.

Q. 4 What are the chronaxie values of different excitable tissues?

The chronaxie, values of excitable tissues are:

Tissue	Chronaxie, (msec)
Large myelinated nerve fibers	0.1
Small myelinated nerve fibers	0.2
Non-myelinated nerve fibers	0.5
Skeletal muscle fibers	0.5-1
Cardiac muscle fibers	1-3

It is obvious that the large myelinated nerve fibers are the most excitable of the tissues, i.e., their threshold is the lowest of these tissues.

5-8

Action Potential in a Large Myelinated Nerve Fiber (Figure 5-8)

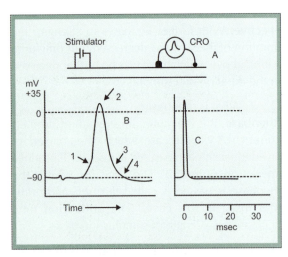

Figure 5-8. Diagram of action potential in a thick mammalian myelinated nerve fiber. (A) Method of recording monophasic action potential. (B) Action potential drawn with time distortion to show its various components. Arrows 1—Firing level, 2—Overshoot and start of repolarization (positive part of action potential), 3—Repolarization slows down, 4—Beginning of after-depolarization. (C) Action potential drawn without time distortion, showing the typical spike

Q. 1 What is resting membrane potential, and what is its cause? How is this potential recorded?

Resting membrane potential (RMP). Under resting unstimulated conditions, a potential difference exists across the cell membranes of most cells, the inside being negative relative to the outside of the cell. By convention, this resting membrane potential (RMP) is indicated with a negative sign. The RMP varies from tissue to tissue, ranging from –6 to –100 mV. In the excitable tissues, nerve and muscle cells, the RMP is usually between –70 and –90 mV.

The cell membranes are selectively permeable to various ions due to the presence of ion channels, which are transmembrane proteins embedded in the bilipid cell membrane. A portion of the protein molecule functions as a sort of 'lid' or 'gate' over the outer (ECF) or inner (ICF) side of the aqueous pore of the ion channel. The movements of these gates are controlled by *changes in the membrane potential,* i.e., these gates open or close at specific membrane potentials. Such channels are called *"voltage-gated" channels* (There are *"ligand-gated" channels* also which open when a chemical agent attaches to the ion channel).

Cause of resting potential. The Na$^+$-K$^+$ pump (an ATPase) located in the cell membrane maintains a high concentration of K$^+$ ions inside the cell (ICF), and a high concentration of Na$^+$ ions outside the cell (ECF). As a result of this concentration gradient, the K$^+$ ions passively diffuse out of the cell through the *continuously open K$^+$ leak channels* (they are only slightly permeable to Na$^+$ ions, hence they are also called K$^+$ -Na$^+$ leak channels). However, the K$^+$ ions that move out of the cell do not enter the ECF, but instead they stick to the outside of the membrane where they are balanced by the negatively charged impermeant anions (mainly proteins, also organic phosphates and sulfates) sticking to the inside of the membrane. When the amount of K$^+$ bound to the outside of the membrane is sufficient to cause a membrane potential (MP) that can prevent any net increase in K$^+$ efflux, a state of equilibrium is reached. In this state, the MP is equal to the Nernst potential for K$^+$ (E$_K$), which is -90 mV.

Recording of RMP. The RMP can be recorded by placing one electrode on the outside of the fiber while a glass capillary micro-electrode (tip diameter less than 0.5 µm) is inserted (pierced) into the interior of the fiber. When the electrodes are connected, through a suitable amplifier to a CRO, the RMP is recorded.

Another method of recording RMP is to crush a small segment of the nerve fiber so that the outside of the fiber in this region becomes equally negative as is the inside. One electrode placed on the injured part, and the other on the nearby uninjured region will record a potential difference—the so-called *injury potential* (a micro-electrode is thus not required).

Q. 2 What is an action potential and how is it recorded? What is its practical application?
Action potential (AP). An action potential is the rapid and sequential change in the membrane potential of a nerve (or muscle) fiber when it is conducting an impulse. The AP is the 'signal' that is transmitted along the cell membrane, without decrement, and is the only proof of conduction of activity. The AP in a nerve fiber is called a *nerve impulse* (nerve AP), while an AP in a muscle fiber is called the *muscle action potential* (muscle impulse).

An action potential has two phases—the **upstroke** or **depolarization (excitation)** which is due to sodium influx, and a **downstroke** or **depolarization (recovery)** which is due to efflux of potassium ions.

Recording of action potential. The AP can be recorded by using either extracellular or intra-cellular electrodes. The intracellular electrodes record the RMP and action potential which is monophasic, i.e., in one direction. Extracellular electrodes, where both the electrodes are placed on or near a nerve or muscle, record a biphasic AP, but not the resting potential.

Clinical application. Extracellular recordings are useful in recording the electrical activity of the excitable tissues in clinical situations, such as electrocardiogram (ECG), electroencephalogram (EEG), electromyogram (EMG; recordings from nerves and muscles), electroretinogram (ERG), and so on.

Q. 3 What are the components of an action potential and what is their ionic basis?
The record of an action potential shown in the Figure 5-8 shows the following components.

The stimulus artifact. This is due to leakage of current from the stimulating to the recording electrodes, and though undesirable, it marks the point of stimulation. The **latent period** (isopotential interval) extends from this point to the start of depolarization and is due to the conduction of the impulse. [The slower and partial depolarization from –90 mV to about –75 mV produced by a marginal stimulus is called the **local response** which is a graded response (this is not shown in the figure above)]. The rapid depolarization from the firing level of -75 mV to the overshoot (i.e., reversal of potential to +40 mV), and the quick fall of potential to about –75 mV constitutes the **spike potential** (its shape resembles that of spike; duration = 0.4 msec). [The overshoot and reversed potential above the zero potential is called the positive part of the action potential]. The repolarization from –75 mV to the resting potential is termed **after-depolarization (negative after potential).** After the RMP is reached the membrane remains slightly hyperpolarized for 40-50 msec, a phase called **after-hyperpolarization (positive after potential).**

In addition to potassium leak channels, which are responsible for the resting potential, the cell membrane also contains *voltage-gated Na+ channels* (fast channels) and *voltage-gated K+ channels.* The outer gate (**m** gate) of Na+ channel is called the *activation gate,* while its inner gate (**h** gate) is called *inactivation gate.* The K+ channel has only one gate—the outer or **n** gate. These gates open and/or close in response to changes in the membrane potential.

Spike potential. At rest, both voltage-gated Na+ and K+ channels are closed (**m** and **n** gates closed, **h** gates open). A slight decrease in membrane potential causes a few Na+ channels to open, but the increased efflux of K+ restores the RMP. However, if the depolarization causes more Na+ channels to open, there is greater influxes of Na+ and greater depolarization (an example of positive feedback). When the firing level is reached, a large number of Na+ channels open rapidly (*Na+ channel activation;* **m** gates open) and the membrane permeability to Na+ ions rises by 500 to 5000 times. As a result of this, there is a massive influx of positively charged Na+ ions, the potential rises to zero and then overshoots to about + 40 mV. The E_{Na} of + 60 mV is not reached because the Na+ channels rapidly begin to close (*Na+ channel inactivation,* closure of **h** gates) during the later part of the upstroke. Increasing positivity inside also restricts Na influx.

The rapid repolarization from +40 mV to about –75 is due to K+ efflux resulting from the opening of voltage-gated K+ channels (**m** gates open); these channels open slowly, remain open for a longer time, and close slowly. Thus, it is the time sequence of the opening and closing of these two types of channels which is responsible for the shape of the spike (It may be pointed out that the number of ions involved in RMP and AP is very small, only a fraction of the total number of ions).

After depolarization. The slowing down of repolarization from –75 mV to –90 mV is due to the slow return of K+ channels to their closed state. The net movement of positive charges (K+ ions) restores the resting potential.

After hyperpolarization. The slight increase in negativity is recorded because a few K+ ions continue to diffuse out before all the K+ channels close (closure of **n** gates). Activation of the Na+ – K+ pump by the Na+ ions gained during the AP also contributes to this phase. The number of ions involved is very small relative to their total numbers. Significant gains and losses of these ions can only be shown after repeated and prolonged stimulation.

Q. 4 What are electrotonic potentials?
Subthreshold stimuli, though not able to produce an action potential, do cause small, localized, short-lived changes in membrane potential (MP). Cathodal stimuli cause *catelectrotonus* (less negativity) while anodal stimuli cause *anelectronus* (more negativity). (These potential changes can be seen by placing recording electrodes within a few mm of stimulating electrodes). When the strength of stimulus is increased (**the cathode is usually the stimulating electrode since it moves the potential towards the firing level**), the resulting local response leads to Na+ channel activation, and thus an AP. Anodal stimuli are hyperpolarizing.

The electrotonic potentials are passive changes in potential as a result of subtraction or addition of charges.

Q. 5 What is refractory period?
For a very brief period of time after a tissue has responded to a stimulus, the tissue is unable to respond to a second stimulus. This property of a tissue is called the refractory period.

Q. 6 What is absolute refractory period and what is its cause?
The **absolute refractory period (ARP)** corresponds to the period of time from the point of firing level to about one-third of repolarization. During ARP, an extra stimulus, howsoever strong it may be, will not produce a second AP.

The refractoriness is due to the closure of **h** gates of Na$^+$ channels, and these gates will not start to open until repolarization is about one-third complete. The ARP decides the number of impulses (APs) that can be transmitted along a nerve fiber. For example, if the ARP is 1 msec, the fiber can transmit about 1000 impulses/sec.

Q. 7 What is relative refractory period?

The **relative refractory period (RRP)** lasts from the end of ARP to the start of after depolarization. During this period, stimuli stronger than normal can cause excitation.

The excitability of the nerve is increased during after depolarization, while it is decreased during after hyperpolarization. Thus, refractory period lasts during action potential.

Q. 8 What is a compound action potential?

In a mixed nerve containing fibers of different diameters, recordings made at some distance from the point of stimulation show a complex AP showing many spikes. This multi-peaked AP is called compound action potential. The first spike to arrive belongs to the fastest conducting Aa fibers; this is followed by Ab and Ad spikes. If group B and C fibers are also present, their spikes will also be seen.

To record this potential, a part of the nerve is crushed so that this region remains in a depolarized state. One electrode placed on this injured region and the other on a nearby uninjured part will record injury potential. When the nerve is stimulated at a distance, the arrival of APs will cause the injury potential to disappear, thus producing many peaks.

Q. 9 How is an action potential propagated?

The propagation of an action potential involves the generation of APs on contiguous patches of the membrane along the nerve fiber. The depolarized area of the membrane acts as a "current sink" which draws positive charges from the adjacent polarized regions and this results in passive current flow. Because "new" APs are being generated constantly, the magnitude of the APs does not change as it is being propagated. The speed of conduction of the AP is proportional to the square root of the fiber diameter.

In a myelinated fiber, the AP propagates at a fast speed due to *saltatory conduction*, the AP jumping from one node of Ranvier to the next, because the cell membrane is exposed to the EFC only at the nodes.

5-9

Action Potentials in Cardiac Muscle Fibers (Figure 5-9)

Q. 1 What type of action potentials are recorded from the cardiac muscle cells?

There are two types of cardiac muscle fibers: those present in the **cardiac impulse generating and conducting system** (SA and AV nodes, bundle of His, and its branches) and the normal **"working"** or **contracting cells** which make up the bulk of the atria and the ventricles, including the subendocardial plexus of Purkinje fibers. The pacemaker

(P) cells of the SA and AV nodes are *slow (or slow response)* fibers having a slow speed of conduction, while the rest of the fibers are *fast (or fast response)* fibers. Under abnormal conditions (e.g., hypoxia due to ischemia), the fast fibers can become slow fibers and generate action potentials.

The pacemaker cells (p cells) of SA and AV nodes have *unsteady "resting" potential* and show *pacemaker potentials*, while the working cells are

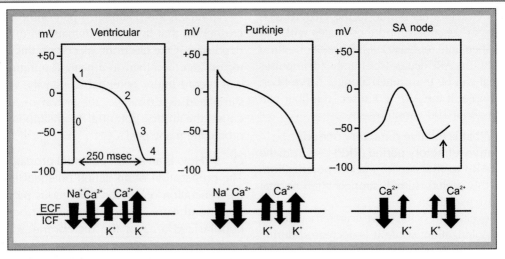

Figure 5-9. Diagram showing action potentials in cardiac muscle fibers showing the duration, strength, and period of flow of ions (ionic currents) underlying the potentials. Phase 4 in SA node fiber is unsteady (arrow). EFC and ICF: Extracellular and intracellular fluids.

characterized by a *steady resting potential* and, when excited, a 4-phase action potential that shows a plateau (Figure 5-9).

Q. 2 What is the cause of the plateau in the action potential of working myocardial cell? What is the significance of the plateau?

a. The sharp depolarization (upstroke) is due to the activation (opening) of the fast Na^+ channels and the rapid Na^+ influx (the Na^+ current, I_{Na} ; as in nerve, Na^+ influx is favored by the electrostatic charges across the cell membrane, i.e., positivity outside and negativity inside).

b. The initial rapid repolarization is due to increased conductance of Cl^- and K^+ ions and inactivation of Na^+ channels. This is followed by the plateau.

c. The plateau (the flat part of AP; sustained depolarization) is due to Ca^{2+} influx through the more slowly opening *voltage-gated Ca^{2+} channels* (the Ca^{2+} current, I_{Ca}; channels start to open at a potential of about -50 mV). The slow opening and the still slower closing of the Ca^{2+} channels results in a sustained depolarization — the plateau.

The significance of the plateau is the following: calcium enters the cell during the plateau (phase 2), and is added to the Ca^{2+} released from the terminal cisterns. The prolonged availability of the activator Ca^{2+} to the contractile machinery of the cell causes a prolonged contraction phase of the cardiac muscle. Since the AP and the period of Ca^{2+} removal from the cytoplasm are nearly equal, summation and tetanus are not possible (The force of contraction can vary with the amount of calcium entering the cell).

d. The final rapid repolarization (phase 3) is due to inactivation of calcium channels, and a relatively rapid increase in K^+ permeability; the resulting K^+ efflux completes the repolarization.

In between the action potentials (phase 4) the working cells show a steady resting potential of -90 mV. In the heart, these cells are excited by cardiac impulses originating in the SA node.

Purkinje cells. The Purkinje fibers, which are barely contractile, lead from the AV node, through the bundle of His and its branches, and into the ventricles where they become continuous with the ventricular muscle fibers. Compared to ventricular muscle fibers which have a conduction velocity of 0.3-0.5 m/sec, the Purkinje fibers conduct APs at a speed of 2-4 m/sec. The Purkinje fibers also exhibit the longest plateau phase of any cardiac fibers, which also provides them with the longest refractory period (this prevents a backward conduction of depolarization). The various parts of the conductive system and, under abnormal conditions (e.g., ischemia), parts of the myocardium are capable of spontaneous discharges.

Q. 3 Describe the electrical activity of pacemaker cells.

Pacemaker potentials. The rhythmically discharging cells (normally present only in SA and AV nodes) have a membrane potential of about -55 to -60 mV. After each action potential, this potential slowly declines to the firing (threshold) level. This slow diastolic deporlarization (it occurs during diastole of heart), also called "pacemaker potential" or "prepotential", is the cause of automaticity.

The action potentials in pacemaker cells are largely due to Ca^{2+} influx through the L (long-lasting) Ca^{2+} channels, with hardly any contribution by Na^+ influx. Because of this, there is no rapid depolarization, hardly any overshoot, or a sharp spike. At the peak of each AP, K^+ efflux brings about repolarization; then K^+ efflux decreases and the membrane begins to depolarize (early part of prepotential). The later part of prepotential is due to Ca^{2+} influx through the T (for transient) Ca^{2+} channels.

Q. 4 How much is the absolute refractory period of cardiac muscle? What is the advantage of this period?

The cardiac muscle fiber is absolutely refractory to a second stimulus during most of its action potential, i.e., throughout the contractile response of 0.3 second. It means that cardiac muscle fiber must begin to relax before it can respond to another stimulus, i.e., the cardiac muscle cannot be tetanized. Refractoriness is therefore, a safety mechanism for the pumping action of the heart. This muscle fiber is relatively refractory during the last part of the action potential (This is in sharp contrast to skeletal muscle which has a short AP of 2-3 msec and repetitive stimuli produce tetanus).

5-10

Dye Dilution Curve (Figure 5-10)

Q. 1 What is meant by the terms cardiac output and cardiac index? How is cardiac output measured?

Cardiac output. This is the amount of blood ejected by each ventricle separately per minute. Thus, if the stroke volume (stroke output, output per beat) is 75 ml, and the heart rate is 70/min, the cardiac output would be $75 \times 70 = 5250$ ml/min. Normal cardiac output (CO) in healthy adults is 4.5-6 liters/min (10% lower in females). **Cardiac index** is the cardiac output per m^2 body surface area. Normal: 2.4-3.5 l/min, slightly higher in males and considerably higher in children.

Methods for determination of cardiac output The various methods for the estimation of CO are:

Direct methods include mechanical flow meter, electromagnetic flow meter, ultrasonic flow meter, cardiometry and electromagnetic catheter tip velocity meter.

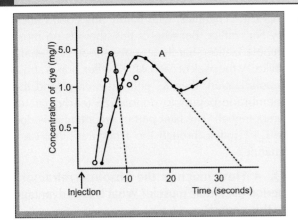

Figure 5-10. Indicator dye (Evans blue) concentration curves plotted on semilog paper. (A) subject at rest, (B) subject during exercise.

Indirect methods include indicator-dilution methods, Fick method, inhalation of inert gas, ballistocardiography, echocardiography, and radiographic methods.

Q. 2 What is the basis of indicator dilution methods for determining cardiac output? Describe the dye dilution method and compare it with thermal dilution method.
Basis of indicator dilution methods. If a suitable indicator (I = amount injected) is added to an unknown volume of fluid (V), the volume of the fluid can be estimated from the resulting concentration of the indicator (C) with the equation V = I/C (using Evans blue dye, this method is employed for estimation of the blood volume).

Similarly, the flow (F) of a fluid can be measured if the mean concentration of the indicator (C) is determined for the time (T) required for that indicator to pass a given site. The flow (F) is measured from the equation: F/C.T

Indicators employed. Some of the indicators are: Evans blue (T-1824), cardio-green, hypotonic and hypertonic saline, ascorbate, cold saline, and radioactive isotopes.

Hamilton's dye dilution method. A known amount of the dye Evans blue is rapidly injected into the arm vein and its mean concentration in a series of samples of brachial arterial blood, collected at 1-2 sec intervals, is determined photoelectrically. (Brachial artery puncture can be avoided by measuring the rise and fall of dye concentration in plasma by shining a light through the vasodilated ear lobe on to a photocell). Usually, re-circulation of the dye occurs before the passage of dye is complete, i.e., the concentration starts to rise, as shown above in the Figure 5-10. After the peak concentration is reached, the exponential decrease in dye concentration is extrapolated to zero concentration, and the mean concentration of the dye during the time period calculated.

Cardiac output (F) = 60.I/C.T, where I is the amount of dye injected, C is the mean concentration of dye during first circulation in mg/liter, and T is the time taken for first circulation in seconds.
In the resting state example shown in Figure 5-10:

$$\text{Cardiac output} = \frac{60 \times 5}{35 \times 1.5} = 5.6 \text{ liters/min.}$$
(Dye injected = 5 mg; mean concentration in (35 seconds = 1.5 mg/liter)

For the exercise example:

$$\text{Cardiac output} = \frac{60 \times 5}{10 \times 1.4} = 21.4 \text{ liters/min}$$
(Dye injected = 5 mg; mean concentration in 10 seconds = 1.4 mg/liter)

Thermodilution method. A double-lumen catheter with a thermistor at its tip is inserted into the arm vein and floated into the pulmonary artery. Cold saline is injected through a proximal opening which lies within the right ventricle. The temperature change of blood measured by the thermistor which lies downstream, is inversely proportionate to the amount of blood flowing through the pulmonary artery. It is a preferred method because the saline is harmless, there is little change in temperature of surrounding tissues, and no recirculation occurs.

Q. 3 What is Fick principle and what is its application in physiology?

Fick principle. The Fick principle states that the amount of substance (X) taken up (or removed) by an organ (or by whole body) is equal to the rate of blood flow (Q) multiplied by the difference between the concentration of the substance before (C_1) and after (C_2) passing through the organ, i.e., $X = Q \, (C_1-C_2)$

$$Q = \frac{X}{C_1 \times C_2}$$

The Fick principle (Adolf Fick, 1870) is an important concept which is used to measure the cardiac output as well as the blood flow through any organ (kidney, brain, liver, etc). This is also the standard method against which all other methods of estimating cardiac output are checked.

Determination of cardiac output by Fick method.

By measuring the amount of O_2 taken up per minute by the venous blood as it passes through the lungs, and the O_2 concentration difference between the arterial blood and mixed venous blood, the blood flow through the lungs can be calculated.

$$\text{Cardiac output} = \frac{\text{Oxygen consumption per minute}}{\text{Arterio venous } O_2 \text{ difference}}$$

Since the cardiac output of the two ventricles is identical, Figure 5-10 also gives the output of the left ventricle.

(Consult Q. No. 18 in Section 6 on Calculations for an example of Fick method).

Indirect Fick method

In this method where CO_2 excretion by the lungs is used, arterial puncture and cardiac catheterization are avoided. Arterial CO_2 is determined from alveolar air sample, while mixed venous blood CO_2 is estimated by rebreathing into a closed bag. The CO_2 in the bag comes into equilibrium with venous blood in the lungs. The rebreathing is done in an interrupted manner so that blood CO_2 is not increased.

Q. 4 How is cardiac output regulated?

Factors affecting cardiac output. Changes in heart rate and/or stroke volume can cause changes in the cardiac output. The heart rate is primarily controlled by the cardiac nerves—the sympathetic stimuli increasing it (chronotropic effect), while vagus has opposite effect. The stroke volume, which depends on the strength, speed, and extent of contraction of ventricular muscle (and, of course, on VEDV) is determined partly by neural signals—sympathetic stimuli increasing the force of contraction (inotropic effect) at any given fiber length [homometric (same length) or extrinsic regulation]. The force of cardiac contraction is also dependent on its preload, i.e., the degree to which the cardiac fibers are stretched by the blood [Frank-Starling, heterometric (different lengths), or intrinsic mechanism], as well as on the afterload, i.e., the aortic pressure.

If the heart rate alone is increased (without increasing the force), as by an artificial pacemaker, the stroke volume decreases in proportion to the increase in heart rate (as rate increases, the diastolic period is cut down). However, during muscular exercise, sympathetic stimulation markedly increases the rate, and moderately increases the stroke volume (VESV decreases). But at very high rates, the stroke volume also decreases.

Thus, cardiac output is controlled by (a) Cardiac factors—homometric and hetermetric mechanisms, and (b) Peripheral factors, i.e., venous return. The factors which increase the venous return include skeletal muscle pump, respiratory pump, pressure gradient, and the volume of blood.

Snellen's Chart (Figure 5-11)

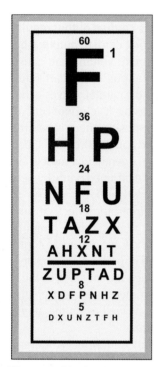

Figure 5-11. Snellen's test types. Reduced in size from standard chart seen at 6 meters

arranged in eight lines. The top letter, the largest, is visible to the normal eye at a distance, of 60 meters, and the subsequent lines at distances of 36, 24, 18, 12, 9, 6, and 5 meters, respectively. The distances for each line are indicated above each line. The letters are so designed that, from a specified distance, the letter as a whole subtends an angle of 5 minutes (5') of arc at the nodal point of the eye. Further, the breadth of each line or stroke, and the breadth of spaces or gaps between two lines or two curves subtend an angle of one minute (1') of arc at the nodal point of the eye. (The nodal point of the eye, which lies at about the middle of the lens, is the optical center of the eye. A ray passing through this point does not suffer refraction).

In the *Landolt ring chart,* the gap in the ring is positioned at random in the 8 lines of the chart. The subject identifies the location of the gap down the chart. The width of the gap subtends an angle of 1 minute of arc at the nodal point, from the respective distances.

In the *"E" test chart,* the letter *E* is printed in 8 lines, the "legs" of the letters pointing in different directions. Beginning with the top letter, the subject (e.g., a child who cannot read) has to indicate the direction in which the legs of each letter are pointing.

Q. 1 What is Snellen's chart and what is it used for?

The *Snellen's chart* (or Snellen's types) is a especially constructed chart of test types. It is used, for clinical purposes, to measure the acuity (acuteness) of vision of a subject for distant vision, i.e., the ability to see distant objects clearly, a phenomenon called spatial discrimination.

Q. 2 Describe the Snellen's chart.

A Snellen's chart has a series of printed letters, black on a white background, of varying sizes,

Q. 3 How is visual acuity measured with the Snellen's chart?

The subject is normally seated at a distance of 6 meters (20 feet) from a well-lighted chart, and each eye is tested separately, with or without glasses as the case may be. The subject reads the letters down the chart as far as he or she can read. The visual acuity (VA) is recorded according to the formula, VA = d/D, where d is the distance at which the letters are read, and D is the distance at which the letters should be read by a person with normal vision, i.e., it is the ratio of the patient's acuity to that of a normal person's acuity. Thus, if only the top letter is visible, the visual acuity is 6/60. If the subject can read only the first 4 lines, then the VA is 6/18, and so on. A normal person should read at least the 7th line, i.e., have a visual acuity of 6/6 (20/20 in terms of feet; commonly pronounced "twenty-twenty" vision.

If the visual acuity is less than 6/60, the patient is moved towards the chart until he can read the top letter. For example, if it is visible at 2 meters, the VA is 2/60. Visual acuities less than 1/60 are tested/recorded as *'counting fingers'* (CF; patient correctly counts fingers when held in front of his or her face); *'hand movements'* (HM), *'perception of light'* (PL), or *'no perception of light'* (no PL).

Q. 4 What is meant by the term visual acuity?
The term **visual acuity** refers to the ability of the eye to resolve or recognize two point sources of light (or two point objects) as separate. The VA is expressed as *minimum separable*, i.e., the minimum distance between two point sources of light when they can be recognized as two points instead of one. This means that if the distance between two points is less than the minimum separable, they will be seen as one. The two points when perceived as two, subtend an angle of 1 minute at the nodal point; this corresponds to distance of 4.5 μm between the retinal images of the two points. Since the diameter of a foveal cone is about 1.5 μm one unstimulated cone separates the two images. Some people can separate the two images even when the visual angle is only 25 seconds (retinal distance between images = 2 μm).

Q. 5 What are the factors that affect visual acuity?
Factors affecting visual acuity. The visual acuity, which is a complex retinal and visual cortical mechanism, is affected by the following factors:

1. **Illumination of the surface.** Bright illumination causes *edge enhancement,* i.e., the boundary between a bright field and a dark field is enhanced or emphasized.
2. **Brightness contrast.** It depends on the luminances of the dark and the darker regions of the pattern.
3. **The time of exposure.** A light flash of very short duration may not be preceived.
4. **Errors of refraction.** Obviously, the VA is reduced by any error of refraction because the images on the retina are blurred. In such cases, the VA will be raised by making the patient look through a small aperture, which increases the depth of focus and reduces the amount of blurring caused by any error in focusing or by aberrations.
5. **Wavelength of light.** The chromatic aberrations of the optical system tend to reduce VA for mixed light sources, while monochromatic light increases visual acuity.
6. **Region of the retina stimulated.** The VA is maximum at the fovea centralis and decreases away from it.

5-12
Jaeger's Chart

Q. 1 What is Jaeger's chart and what is it used for?
The **Jaeger's chart** is made up of test types of reading material of various sizes, with the smallest size at the bottom. The notation (size of letters) used in the chart is based on the printer's point system, the smallest being N5.

The chart is used for testing the near vision. The subject holds the chart at the ordinary reading distance, and reads down the chart. The near vision is recorded as the smallest type which the subject can read comfortably. The result is expressed as J1, J2, J3, etc, for each eye separately. J1 (smallest size) indicates normal near vision.

These days, a modification of the original Jaeger system chart is used, the results being expressed in terms of printers' point system—N36, N18, N8, N6 and N5, instead of J1, J2, etc. A **Landolt ring chart** for near vision is also available. Charts with pictures are used for testing near vision in children.

Q. 2 How does the eye accommodate for near vision?

Accommodation for near vision. The eye accommodates (adjusts) for near vision by increasing the refractive power of the lens, i.e., *the lens becomes more convex*, mainly on the anterior surface.

At rest, i.e., when the eye is looking at a distant object and the ciliary muscle is relaxed, the maleable and elastic lens is held under tension by its suspensory ligament and is pulled into a flattened shape. In this state, parallel rays of light coming from the distant object are brought to focus on the retina and the object is seen clearly. However, when the eye looks at a near object (closer than 6 m), the divergent rays are brought to a focus 'behind' the retina so that the image on the retina is blurred, i.e., out of focus. This *blurring of the image on the retina acts as a stimulus* for the reflex contraction of ciliary muscle, which pulls the ciliary body forwards and inwards. As a result, the lens ligament becomes lax, the tension on the lens capsule decreases, and the lens, due to its elasticity, bulges forwards. The increase in refractive power of the lens brings the image forwards onto the retina and the image becomes clearly visible. When the gaze is shifted to a distant object, the ciliary muscle relaxes and the lens becomes less convex. (The ciliary muscle is the most frequently used muscle in the body as we shift our gaze from distant to mid-distance and near objects, and then in the reverse order as we scan the environment).

Q. 3 What is near response?

During accommodation for near vision, the eyes converge and the pupils constrict, in addition to increase in the convexity of the lens. This 3-part response—accommodation, convergence of eyes, and pupillary constriction, is called *the near response* or *the accommodation reflex* (consult Expt 2-18).

Q. 4 What is the range of accommodation?

Range of accommodation. It is the distance between the far point and the near point of the eye.

Far point. It is the farthest point from the eye at which an object is seen clearly. This point is infinity in the normal eye. A distance of 6 meters from the eye is considered as the practical far point because light rays from this distance are parallel.

Near point. It is the nearest distance from the eye at which an object can be seen clearly. It is 9-10 cm at age 10 years.

Q. 5 What is the amplitude of accommodation?

The difference in the refractive power of the lens in the two states of *complete relaxation* and *maximal accommodation* is called the *amplitude of accommodation.*

The total refractive power of the eye is about 60 diopters (66 D in some cases). Of this 60 D, the cornea contributes 44 D, while the refractive power of the lens is 16 D in a young person. During maximal accommodation, the refractive power of the lens can add another 14 D to its refractive power. Thus, the amplitude of accommodation is 14 diopters (30-16 = 14 D).

Q. 6 What is presbyopia and what is its cause?

Presbyopia. It is a refractive error of the eye in which the amplitude of accommodation is decreased (Presbyopia: Greek for "old man's eyes").

As age advances, the lens becomes less elastic (due to denaturation of lens proteins, etc) and the ability to accommodate for near vision declines, the near point moving away from the eye. Close work and reading become more and more difficult

Plate   1

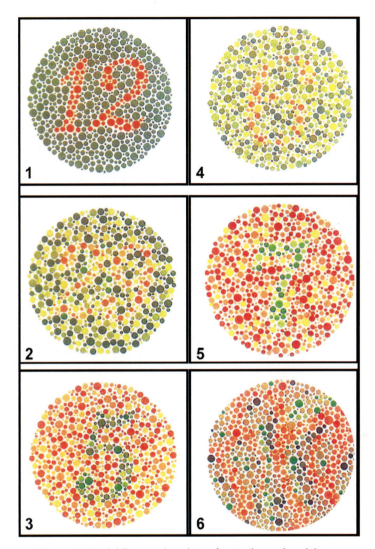

Figure 5-12. Ishihara color plates for testing color vision

and the reading material is held farther and farther away from the eyes. This condition of presbyopia appears by mid-forties, when convex lenses are needed for near work. The amplitude of accommodation which was about 12-14 D in younger age, may only be 1 D by age 70 years.

5-13

Ishihara Charts

The Ishihara charts are used for testing the color vision in a susbject.

COLOR VISION

The human eye is sensitive to all wavelengths of light from 350 to 700 nm, which constitute the visible part of the electromagnetic spectrum. The color sense is perceived by 3 types of cones in the retina, each cone containing a specific photo-pigment that is maximally sensitive to one of the three primary colors—red, green, and blue. The sense of white and any spectral or even extra-spectral color (e.g., purple) is due to the varying degrees of stimulation of red-sensitive or long-wave pigment (723-647 nm), green-sensitive or middle-wave pigment (575-452 nm), and blue-sensitive or short-wave pigment (492-417 nm).

Mechanism of Color Vision. Two mechanisms—retinal and cortical—are involved in color vision. The *retinal* mechanism is based on the Young-Helmholtz trichromatic theory of color vision that depends on 3 types of cones, each with a specific photopigment that is maximally sensitive to one color. The ganglion cells contribute to color vision by adding or subtracting inputs from one or the other area.

The *cortical* mechanism involves projections from the retina to the parvocllular part of lateral geniculate nucleus of thalamus, from where fibers project to clusters of cells (blobs) arranged in a mosaic in layer IV of the visual cortex (area 17). The primary visual area, along with visual association area (area 18), is involved in color perception.

Q. 1 What are Ishihara charts and what are they used for?

The Ishihara charts consist of a series of litho-graphic color plates available in book form. The plates are so constructed that numbers and wavy lines made up of spots of confusing colors are printed against backgrounds of differently colored spots of identical size (**Figure 5-12, Plate 1**).

Procedure for testing color vision.

1. Seat the subject in a room which is adequately lit by daylight. Direct sunlight or use of electric light may cause a discrepancy in the result due to changes in the shades of colors.

2. Ask the subject to read the numbers or trace the wavy lines on successive plates. The correct answers are given at the end of the book to exclude the possibility of the examiner being color blind.

The person with normal color vision will read, for example, **plate 1** in **Figure 5-12** as 5, while a person with defective color vision will read it as 2. The results with other color plates are given below in table 5.1:

TABLE 5.1			
Results of Ishihara test			
Plate	Person with Normal color vision	Person with red-green deficiency	Person with blindness
1.	12	12	12
2.	29	70	X
3.	5	2	X
4.	6	X	X
5.	7	X	X
6.	X	5	X

The mark X shows that the plate cannot be read.

Q. 2 What is deuteranopia?
The prefix *deuter-* refers to the green color (green cone system), and the suffix-*anopia* refers to blindness. Thus deuteranopia is color blindness for green color. These patients cannot distinguish colors in the red-green portion of the spectrum.

Q. 3 What is tritanopia?
The prefix *trit-* refers to the blue color. So, tritanopia is color blindness to blue color. This condition is very rare.

Q. 4 What is protanopia?
The prefix *prot-* refers to the red color. Protanopes lack the red-sensitive cone system and confuse the colors in the red-green part of the spectrum.

Q. 5 What is red-green blindness?
The green, yellow, orange, and red colors between the wavelengths of 525 and 700 nm are normally distinguished from each other entirely by the red and green cones. If either one or both of these cone systems are missing, the person cannot distinguish red from green. The person is not color blind in the sense that he or she cannot see these colors, but the individual does not see the colors in the way a normal person does. Thus the person may not be able to distinguish the deep green of a leaf from the red of sealing wax.

Q. 6 What is meant by the terms deuteranomaly, protanomaly, and tritanomaly?
The suffix *anomaly* refers to color weakness. Thus these terms refer to weakness for green, red and blue colors, respectively.

Protanomaly, protanopia, deuteranomaly and deuteranopia are sex-linked inherited disorders, the abnormal gene being located on the X-chromosome.

Q. 7 What are the other tests employed for testing color vision?
The two other commonly used tests for color vision are the following:
1. **Edridge-Green lantern.** In this electric apparatus, different colored glass pieces can be brought in front of a small illuminated area, the size of which can be varied. The subject identifies the colors one after the other. The effects of rain and fog can be added to the colors by bringing appropriate lenses in front of the colors.
2. **Holmgren's wools.** In this test, small pieces of woollen threads of different colors and hues (a hue is a mixture of a color with white) are placed in a heap on a table. The subject is given a test skein and is asked to pick out matching wool pieces. The subject only matches colors and does not name them.

Q. 8 In which groups of people is color vision of vital importance?
Color vision is of particular importance in the following groups of people:
1. Drivers of air, sea and road transport vehicles, e.g., railway engine drivers, bus and truck drivers, pilots, etc.
2. Workers in textile industry, where dyeing of cloth requires a high degree of color perception.
3. Paint and printing industries.
4. Interior decorators and visual artists.

Oral Glucose Tolerance Test (OGTT)
(Figure 5-13)

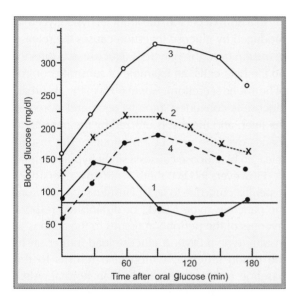

Figure 5-13. Oral glucose tolerance curves. (1) Normal, (2) Mild diabetes mellitus, (3) Severe diabetes mellitus, and (4) Liver disease

Q. 1 How is oral glucose tolerance test curve obtained?

Oral glucose tolerance test (OGTT). This test is carried out according to the following protocol:

The patient is placed on a diet which includes 200-300 g of carbohydrates per day for 3 days prior to the test (starvation produces a diabetic type of response). The subject fasts for 15 hours before the test which is generally done in the morning. Urine and fasting venous blood samples are collected for their glucose concentrations. The patient then drinks 75 grams of glucose (50 grams in children under 14 years of age) in 300 ml water over 5 minutes. Venous blood samples are then collected after 30, 60, 90, 120, and sometimes, after 150 and 180 minutes. Urine is collected after 60 and 120 minutes.

The glucose concentrations of the blood samples are determined and plotted against time. (Intravenous glucose, 0.5 g per kg body weight, is sometimes used, particularly in cases of abnormalities of intestinal absorption of glucose).

Q. 2 Describe the normal glucose tolerance curve.

Normally, the fasting venous plasma glucose level varies between 80 and 90 mg % (4.4-4.9 mmol/l), the upper limit of the normal being 110 mg % (6/mmol/l). [A fasting level less than 110 mg % excludes diabetes mellitus, DM]. After ingesting glucose, the peak level of 130-140 mg % is reached in about 30-40 minutes. The glucose level starts decreasing and falls back to fasting value, and then to below fasting level in about 120-150 minutes. The 120 minute value is less than 140 mg % (7.8 mmol/l), and no value exceeds the renal threshold of glucose of 180 mg % (9.9 mmol/l). No sample of urine contains glucose.

Q. 3 What is the renal threshold for glucose?

Renal threshold for glucose. It is the *plasma level of glucose* at which glucose first appears in the urine in more than the normal minute amounts (Normal urine contains a few mg of glucose which are undetectable with the usual tests).

The renal threshold for glucose is 180 mg %. As long as blood glucose level is below this level, all the filtered glucose is reabsorbed in the proximal tubules, but when the level exceeds 180 mg %, all the excess glucose is excreted in the urine.

Q. 4 Describe the glucose tolerance curve in diabetes mellitus.

The shape of the OGTT curve is quite different in a patient of DM as compared to that of a normal person. The fasting blood glucose level is almost always above 110 mg %, and generally above 145 mg %; it may exceed 200 mg % (Two fasting levels $\geq$ 145 mg % confirm the diagnosis of DM). The glucose levels after ingestion of glucose, and the peak value, depend on whether the patient is *prediabetic* or has *mild* or *severe diabetes*. The peak value, which may cross 300 mg %, is reached only after about 90 minutes, and the fasting level is reached only after 4-5 hours. Also, the glucose level fails to fall below the fasting level. The urine samples show the presence of glucose if the renal threshold is crossed.

Prolonged OGTT is found in the following:
1. Diabetes mellitus.
2. **Pituitary diabetes** (due to excess growth hormone), and **adrenal diabetes** (due to excess of cortisol, the chief glucocorticoid of adrenal cortex).
3. **Liver disease.** The liver is unable to handle the glucose load. The curve resembles that of prediabetes or mild diabetes mellitus, except that the fasting blood glucose level is *below* the normal fasting level.

Comments
Glucose is too large a molecule to diffuse through the cell membrane channels into the cells. However, it is transported into all cells by *facilitated diffusion*, which is a carrier-mediated process. In muscle, adipose, and connective tissues (they form the bulk of the body weight), the cells depend on insulin for glucose entry into them. Insulin facilitates this process by increasing the number of **glucose transporters** (GLUT 4; there is a family of GLUTs, numbered 1 to 5). These GLUTs are different from the **sodium-dependent glucose transporters** (SGLT 1, sodium-glucose cotransporters) responsible for the secondary active transport of glucose out of the intestinal and renal tubules (the Na^+ concentration gradient and its transport provides the energy for glucose transport). Thus, glucose entry into muscle, adipose and connective tissue cells requires insulin, while intestine, kidneys, liver, RBCs, and most of the brain do not require insulin for glucose entry.

In a normal person, the artificial hyperglycemia produced by glucose ingestion causes the release of insulin from the pancreas (glucose acts directly on the beta cells, an example of substrate control of hormone secretion). About 60% of the absorbed glucose is converted into glycogen and stored in the liver, and the rest is utilized by the peripheral tissues over the next 60-90 minutes. The insulin released by glucose causes a slight hypoglycemia.

However, in DM, there is already a persistent hyperglycemia due to lack of insulin secretion from the pancreas (type I DM), or diminished responsiveness of the peripheral tissues to the actions of insulin (type II DM). A glucose load further raises the blood glucose, which also returns to baseline much more slowly than normal. Also, there is no hypoglycemia following the return of blood glucose to the fasting level.

Q. 5 What is tubular load? How much is it for glucose?
The *tubular load*, or the *filtration load*, is the amount of a substance delivered to the renal tubules, per minute, due to the process of filtration. It depends on the plasma level of that substance and the glomerular filtration rate (GFR).

With a blood glucose level of 80 mg %, and a GFR of 125 ml/min, the tubular load is about 100 mg/min ($80 \times 125/100$). When the glucose level is 180 mg % (renal threshold for glucose), the tubular load is 225 mg % ($180 \times 125/100$).

Q. 6 What is meant by transport maximum? How much is the transport maximum for glucose?
The *transport maximum (Tm)* is the maximal rate at which substances that are actively reabsorbed (e.g., glucose, some amino acids, uric acid,

phosphates, and possibly albumin) or secreted (e.g., creatinine, PAH, penicillin, etc) can be transported across the tubular epithelial cells. This maximum limit is due to the saturation of the specific carrier systems—proteins or enzymes — involved in the process.

The transport maximum for glucose (Tm_G) in the adult individual is about 320 mg per minute (350 in males and 300 in females). This means that a maximum of 320 mg of glucose can be transported (reabsorbed), per minute, from the tubular fluid of both kidneys into the blood. Tm_G is nearly constant and depends on the number of functioning tubules. Tm is therefore, used clinically to assess renal function.

Substances absorbed passively do not have a transport maximum.

Some solutes have no definite upper limit for unidirectional transport and, hence, have no Tm. The reabsorption of Na^+ along the nephron has no Tm, and secretion of K^+ by the distal tubules has no Tm.

Comments

As mentioned earlier, glucose and Na^+ bind to a common carrier SGLT 1 in the luminal membrane and as Na^+ moves down its concentration and electrical gradients, glucose is also carried into the cells. The Na^+ is then pumped out of the cell by the Na^+-K^+ pump into the lateral intercellular spaces and glucose is transported by GLUT 2 into the interstitial spaces via the basal cell membrane, and thence into the peritubular capillaries by simple diffusion. As in the intestine, it is the difference in the luminal and basolateral GLUTs that makes it possible for a net movement of glucose across these epithelial cells. Renal tubular transport of glucose, as also of intestinal, is *not* facilitated by insulin.

Q. 7 If Tm_G is 320 mg/min, why does glucose appear in the urine when the plasma glucose level is 180 mg %, at which the tubular load is 225 mg/minute?

With a Tm_G of 320 mg/min, and a GFR of 125 ml/min, one would predict that the renal threshold

for glucose would be 256 mg % ($320/125 \times 100 = 256$). That is, glucose would first appear in the urine at a plasma glucose level of 256 mg %. However, the actual renal threshold is 180 mg %, at which the tubular load is 225 mg/minute. The reason for this discrepancy is the following: The renal tubules show considerable variability in their length, and filtration and reasorptive capacities. Some tubules have a much lower Tm_G than others. In these tubules, some glucose remains unabsorbed (after saturation of the carrier system) even at a lower plasma glucose level, and is excreted in urine. This phenomenon, called *splay*, refers to the curved portion observed in glucose reabsorption and excretion graphs.

Though the affinity of the transport system is high, a finite concentration of glucose must remain in the tubular fluid to fully saturate the transport system. Some glucose may remain unabsorbed before saturation occurs.

Q. 8 What are the causes of hyperglycemia and what are its effects?

Diabetes mellitus is the major cause of hyperglycemia. Secondary forms of diabetes occur in **chronic pancreatitis, pheochromocytoma** (excess adrenalin from adrenal medulla), acromegaly (excess growth hormone), and Cushing's syndrome (excess cortisol). It is also present when there is excessively rapid absorption of glucose after meals, especially after gastrectomy, etc. It may also be encountered after meals in liver disease.

The **effects of hyperglycemia** are due to an increase in the osmolality (osmotic pressure) of the blood. As tubular load exceeds Tm_G, glucose appears in the urine (*glycosuria*). The presence of large amounts of osmotically active glucose particles in the filtrate causes loss of large amounts of water (**polyuria** due to osmotic diuresis); there is also loss of large amounts of Na^+ and K^+ as well. The resulting dehydration leads to excessive water drinking (**polydipsia**) via the thirst center of the hypothalamus. The intracellular deficiency of glucose in the neurons of the feeding center of the hypothalamus causes excessive eating (**polyphagia**).

Comments

The *long-term damaging effects of DM* are primarily due not to hyperglycemia, but to **abnormal lipid metabolism;** the major tissues of the body switching over from the carbohydrate to fat metabolism in the absence of insulin. Excessive breakdown of fats causes *hyperlipidemia, ketosis,* and *ketoacidosis. Atherosclerosis* of retinal arteries may cause blindness, while in the coronary, cerebral, and renal arteries, it may lead to myocardial infarction, cerebral hemorrhage (stroke), or renal failure. There is *loss of body weight* due to the depletion of fat and protein stores. In fact, DM has been called more a disease of fat metabolism than of carbohydrate metabolism.

Q. 9 What is hypoglycemia and what are its effects?

A plasma glucose level of less than about 45 mg% is called **hypoglycemia**. However, the level at which symptoms appear varies markedly from person to person, especially in diabetics. Hypoglycemia may be fasting (no food taken), or postprandial (or reactive; after meals). The commonest cause of *fasting hypoglycemia* is overzealous treatment (overdosage) of DM with insulin injection (in type II DM), or sulphonylurea (which is taken orally, in type II DM). It may also occur in islet cell tumors, liver failure, and pituitary insufficiency. Alcoholics on a drinking binge may forget to ingest food.

Hypoglycemia after meals occurs after gastric surgery or vagotomy (done in cases of peptic ulcer),

where rapid gastric emptying and rapid glucose absorption cause excessive release of insulin. Plasma glucose falls more rapidly than the insulin level, and hypoglycemia results.

The **symptoms of hypoglycemia** include: sweating, tremors, anxiety, and hunger, which are due to sympathetic stimulation and release of adrenalin from adrenal medulla. The CNS symptoms include dizziness, diminished mental activity, personality changes, convulsions, and coma.

Comments

The maintenance of plasma glucose within narrow limits is essential for health. Hypoglycemia is dangerous, more serious in the short-run than hyperglycemia, because glucose is the primary energy source of the brain. In contrast to other tissues, brain cannot utilize free fatty acids (FFA) as energy source. Though, short-chain metabolites of FFA, such as acetoacetic acid and beta hydroxybutyric acid, can be efficiently oxidized by the brain, ketosis requires many hours to develop. Therefore, absence of glucose, like that of O_2, produces deranged function, tissue damage or even death if the deficit is prolonged.

Q. 10 What is renal glycosuria?

The presence of glucose in the urine even when the renal threshold for glucose of 180 mg % is not exceeded is called *renal glycosuria*, i.e., glycosuria due to renal disease. It is a congenital disorder associated with a low renal threshold for glucose.

Calculations

Calculations are another method of assessing the students' understanding of the subject. The calculations included in this section are based on idealized 'given' data. However, when students are tested on these, the teacher often 'manipulates' the given data. A student should be able to explain and reason out why the results are at variance with the expected normal values.

Q. 1 Calculate the velocity of nerve impulse in the frog's nerve-muscle preparation from the data given below.

Data

(a) Latent period with stimulation
    of spinal end of the nerve   = 0.01 sec
(b) Latent period with stimulation
    of muscle end of the nerve   = 0.005 sec
(c) Length of the nerve between
    the two stimulated points   = 7.5 cm.

- -

Difference in the two latent periods
                = 0.0 1 – 0.005 sec = 0.005 sec
Distance travelled by the nerve
        impulses in 0.005 sec = 7.5 cm
Distance travelled by the nerve impulses in 1 sec

$$= \frac{7.5 \cdot 1000}{5} = 1500 \, cm$$

The velocity of the nerve impulse = 15 m/sec.

Q. 2 Calculate the work done by the muscle from the following data.

Data

(a) Height of recorded contraction (H) = 5 cm
(b) Long arm of the lever
    (L, from fulcrum to writing point)   = 15 cm
(c) Short arm of the lever
    (l, from fulcrum to point of load)   = 2.5 cm
(d) Weight (load) lifted   = 15 g.

- -

$$Magnification \, factor = \frac{L}{l} = \frac{15}{2.5} = 6$$

Load lifted = 15 g
Actual height through which load was lifted (h)

$$= \frac{Height \, of \, contraction}{Magnification \, factor} = \frac{5}{6} = 0.83 \, cm$$

Work done = Load x Height (h)
              = 15 × 0.83 = 12.45 g cm

Q. 3 Determine the absolute counts of neutrophils, eosinophils, and basophils from the data given below.

Data

(a) Total leucocyte count   = 7800/mm^3
(b) Neutrophil count   = 65%
(c) Eosinophil count   = 3.5%
(d) Basophil count   = 0.5%

- -

Absolute neutrophil count   = 7800/100 x 65
                                              = 4875/mm^3

Absolute eosinophil count   = 7800/100 x 3.5
                                              = 273/mm^3

Absolute basophil count   = 7800/100 x 0.5
                                              = 39/mm^3

Q. 4 Determine the mean corpuscular hemo-globin (MCH) from the data given below.

  Data

(a) Hemoglobin concentration=14.5 g/dl
(b) RBC count   = 4.8 million mm^3
(c) Packed cell volume   = 42%

- -

$$MCH = \frac{Hb\ g/dl \cdot\ 10}{RBC\ count\ in\ millions/mm^3}$$

$$= \frac{14.5 \cdot\ 10}{4.8} = 30\ pg\ (30\ \mu\mu g)$$

Q. 5 Calculate the mean corpuscular volume (MCV) from the data given below.

  Data

(a) RBC count   = 4.5 million/mm^3
(b) Packed cell volume (PCV) = 40%
(c) Hb concentration   = 14 g/dl

- -

$$MCV = \frac{PCV \cdot\ 10}{RBC\ count\ in\ millions/mm^3}$$

$$= \frac{40 \cdot\ 10}{4.5} = 88\ \mu m^3\ (cubic\ micrometers)$$

Q. 6 Calculate the mean corpuscular hemo-globin concentration from the data given below.

  Data

(a) Hemoglobin concentration = 9 g/dl
(b) Packed cell volume (PCV)   = 36%
(c) RBC count   = 3.4 million/mm$^{3.}$

- -

$$MCHC = \frac{Hb\ g\%}{PCV}\times 100 = \frac{9}{36}\times 100 = 25\%$$

Q. 7 Determine the color index from the data given below.

  Data

(a) Hb concentration   = 16 g/dl
(b) RBC count   = 6 million/mm^3
      (Normal 100% RBC count = 5.0 million/mm^3)
      (Normal 100% Hb   = 15 g/dl)

- -

1. 5.0 million/mm^3 RBC   = 100%
     count 6.0 million/mm^3
     RBC count will be
     6/5 × 100   = 120%
2. 15.0 g% hemoglobin   = 100%
     16.0 g% Hb will be
     16/15 x 100   = 107%

$$Color\ index = \frac{Hb\ percent\ of\ normal}{RBC\ count\ percent\ of\ normal} = \frac{120}{107} = 0.89$$

Q. 8 Calculate the platelet count from the data given below.

  Data

(a) Number of platelets in
      80 smallest squares   = 34
(b) Dilution of blood employed = 1 in 200
                                                  (1:200)

- -

Number of platelets in
   80 smallest squares   = 34
Volume of these 80 squares = 1/50 mm^3
(volume of 1 smallest square = 1/4000 mm^3)
Thus, 1/50 mm^3 contains   = 34 platelets
∴ 1 mm^3 contains 34 x 50   = 1700 platelets
Dilution employed is 1 in 200
Number of platelets in
   undiluted blood = 1700 x 200 = 340,000/mm^3
The platelet count is 3.4 lacs/mm^3.

Q. 9 Determine the reticulocyte count from the data given below.

  Data

(a) Number of RBCs in
      50 oil-immersion fields   = 1500
(b) Number of reticulocytes in
      100 oil-immersion fields   = 45

- -

Number of RBCs in
   50 oil-immersion fields   = 1500
∴ Number of cells in
   100 oil-immersion fields   = 3000
Number of reticulocytes in
   100 oil-immersion field   = 45 (data)

Thus, per 3000 RBCs, there are 45 reticulocytes

∴ Per 100 RBCs, there are

$45/3000 \times 100 = 1.5$ reticulocytes

The reticulocyte count is 1.5% of red cells.

Q. 10 Find out the physiological dead space from the data provided below.

Data
(a) Tidal volume $= 450$ ml
(b) Alveolar air PCO_2 $= 40$ mm Hg
(c) Expired air PCO_2 $= 26$ mm Hg

- -

Physiological dead space

$$= \frac{Alveolar\ air\ PCO_2 - expired\ air\ PCO_2}{Alveolar\ air\ PCO_2} \cdot Tidal\ volume$$

$$= \frac{40-26}{40} \cdot 450 = 157\ ml.$$

Q. 11 Find out the expiratory reserve volume (ERV); residual volume (RV); inspiratory reserve volume (IRV); and functional residual capacity (FRC) from the given data.

Data
(a) Total lung capacity $= 5200$ ml
(b) Tidal volume $= 450$ ml
(c) Inspiratory capacity $= 3000$ ml
(d) Vital capacity $= 4000$ ml

- -

ERV = VC – IC $= 4000 - 3000 = 1000$ ml
RV = TLC – VC $= 5200 - 4000 = 1200$ ml
IRV = IC – TV $= 3000 - 450 = 2550$ ml
FRC = RV + ERV $= 1200 + 1000 = 2200$ ml

Note
Consult Figure 2-2 on lung volumes and capacities.

Q. 12 Determine the oxygen carrying capacity and oxygen content of arterial and venous blood samples from the data provided below.

Data
(a) Percentage saturation of arterial blood with oxygen $= 97\%$
(b) Percentage saturation of venous blood with oxygen $= 75\%$

(c) Hemoglobin concentration $= 14.5$ g/dl

- -

Oxygen carrying capacity of blood (ml/100 ml)
$=$ Hb g% $\times 1.34$ $= 14.5 \times 1.34$
$= 19.43$ ml/dl

$$Formula\ for\ O_2\ content\ of\ blood = \frac{Percentage\ saturation \cdot Capacity}{100}$$

$$Oxygen\ content\ of\ arterial\ blood = \frac{97 \cdot 19.43}{100} = 18.84\ ml/100\ ml$$

$$Oxygen\ content\ of\ venous\ blood = \frac{75 \cdot 19.43}{100} = 14.57\ ml/100\ ml$$

Q. 13 Find out the breathing reserve and the dyspnea index from the data provided below.

Data
(a) Respiratory rate $= 12$/min
(b) Tidal volume $= 500$ ml
(c) Maximal voluntary ventilation (MVV) $= 130$ liters
(Syn: maximal ventilatory volume)

- -

Respiratory minute volume (RMV; volume of gas expired per minute)$= 500 \times 12$
$= 6000$ ml

Breathing reserve $=$ MVV– RMV
$= 130-6$
$= 124$ liters.

(It means that the ventilation can be increased from 6 l/min to 130 l/min with maximum effort).

Dyspnea index (Breathing reserve percent)

$$= \frac{MVV - RMV}{MVV} \cdot 100 = \frac{130-6}{130} \cdot 100 = 95\%$$

(When the dyspnea index falls below 70% (dyspnea point), dyspnea is present. We are not conscious of breathing until ventilation is doubled. Breathing is not uncomfortable (i.e., dyspnea point is not reached) until ventilation increases 3 or 4 times the resting level).

Q.14 Calculate the respiratory quotient from the data given below.

Data
(a) Volume of expired air in 6 minutes = 30 liters
(b) Percentage of CO_2 in expired air　= 4.2%
(c) Oxygen consumption in 6 minutes = 1470 ml

- -

Volume of expired air in 6 minutes　　= 30 liters
Volume of expired air in 1 minute　　= 5 liters
Percentage of CO_2 in expired air　　= 4.2%
∴ 5000 ml of expired air in 1 minute
　　contain = 5000 × 4.2 = 210 ml of CO_2
Oxygen consumed in 6 minutes　　= 1470 ml
∴ Oxygen consumed in 1 minute　　= 1470/6
　　　　　　　　　　　　　　　　= 245 ml

$$Respiratory\ quotient\ (RQ) = \frac{CO_2\ output/min}{O_2\ consumed/min}$$

$$= \frac{210}{245} = 0.85$$

Q.15 Find out the basal metabolic rate (BMR) of the subject from the data given below.

Data
(a) Oxygen consumption
　　in 6 minutes　　= 1470 ml
(b) Body surface area
　　(BSA) of the subject = 1.6 m²
(c) Standard BMR for the
　　age and sex of the
　　subject　　= 40 Cal/m² BSA/hour

- -

Oxygen consumption in 6 minutes = 1470 ml
Oxygen consumption in 1 hour = 14.70 liters
When 1 liter of O_2 is consumed, 4.8 Calories are released.
∴ Calories released from consumption
　　of 14.7 liter of O_2 = 4.8 × 14.70 = 70.56

$$BMR = \frac{Calories\ consumed/hr}{Body\ surface\ area} = \frac{70.56}{1.6} = 44$$

Standard BMR for the subject = 40 cal/m² BSA/ hour

∴ Calculated BMR is in excess by 4 calories/m² BSA/hour

$$Percentage\ excess = \frac{4}{40} \times 100 = 10\%$$

Thus, the BMR of the subject is = + 10%
(Normal range = ± 15%).

Q.16 Calculate the cardiac index of the individual from his data given below.

Data
(a) Cardiac output　　　　= 5.20 liters/min
(b) Body surface area (BSA) = 1.65 m²

- -

(Cardiac index is the cardiac output per m² BSA per minute)

$$Cardiac\ index = \frac{Cardiac\ output/min}{BSA} = \frac{5.20}{1.65} = 3.15$$

Cardiac index = 3.15 liters/min.

Q.17 Calculate the heart rate from the ECG provided.

There are two methods to calculate the heart rate from an ECG.

1. Divide 1500 by the number of smallest squares between any two successive R waves: Assume there are 18 smallest squares between two R waves:
   Then the heart rate will be 1500/18 = 82/min.
2. Divide 60 by the time interval, in seconds, between two successive R waves:
   Assume there are 21 smallest squares between two R waves:
   21 smallest squares　　= 0.84 sec
   (each smallest square　= 0.04 sec)
   ∴ Heart rate　　　　　= 60/0.84
   　　　　　　　　　　　= 71/min.

Q.18 Calculate the stroke volume and cardiac output from the data given below.

Data
(a) Oxygen content of mixed
　　venous blood　　　　= 14.8 ml/100 ml
(b) Oxygen content of systemic
　　arterial blood　　　　= 19.5 ml/100 ml

(c) Heart rate = 70/min

(Mixed venous blood is collected from the right ventricle or pulmonary artery via a catheter. Systemic arterial blood can be taken from any artery)

(d) Oxygen consumption per minute = 245 ml

- -

(The cardiac output is calculated by applying Fick principle).

Cardiac output

$$= \frac{Oxygen\ consumption}{Arteriovenous\ oxygen\ difference} \cdot 100$$

$$= \frac{245}{19.5 - 14.8} \cdot 100 = \frac{245}{4.7} \cdot 100 = 5200\ ml$$

Stroke volume

$$= \frac{Cardiac\ output/min}{Heart\ rate} = \frac{5200}{70\ ml} = 74\ ml$$

Comments

In the example cited above, every 100 ml blood that flow through the lungs per minute pick up 4.7 ml of oxygen. Therefore, to pick up 245 ml of oxygen, 5200 ml blood must flow through the lungs per minute. This is an example of Fick principle. Normally, the output of the two ventricles is identical, except at the start of exercise when the output of the right ventricle is higher (due to increased venous return) for a few seconds until the output becomes similar on the two sides.

Q. 19 Calculate the effective filtration pressure from the data given below.

Data

(a) Glomerular capillary
hydrostatic pressure = 55 mm Hg

(b) Glomerular capillary
blood osmotic pressure = 30 mm Hg

(c) Bowman's
capsular fluid pressure = 15 mm Hg

(d) Bowman's capsular
fluid osmotic pressure = 0 mm Hg.

- -

The glomerular capillary hydrostatic pressure is about 55 mm Hg when the mean systemic arterial pressure is 100 mm Hg.

Thus, the effective filtration
pressure = 55 − (30 + 15) = 10 mm Hg

Comments

The effective filtration pressure is the function of two variables: the hydrostatic pressure gradient driving fluid out of the glomerular capillaries and into Bowman's capsule, and the colloid osmotic pressure gradient bringing fluid into the glomerular capillaries. The colloid osmotic pressure of capsular fluid is near zero because it normally contains little protein—only a few milligrams of albumin which is reabsorbed in the proximal tubules.

Q. 20 Calculate the glomerular filtration rate (GFR) from the data provided below.

Data

(a) Concentration of inulin
in plasma (P) = 0.24 mg/ml

(b) Concentration of inulin
in urine (U) = 34 mg/ml

(c) Rate of urine formation (V) = 0.9 ml/min

- -

Plasma inulin clearance =

$$\frac{Concentration\ of\ inulin\ in\ urine \cdot Volume\ of\ urine/min}{Concentration\ of\ inulin\ in\ plasma}$$

$$= \frac{U_{IN} \cdot V}{P_{IN}} = \frac{34 \cdot 0.9}{0.24} = 127\ ml/min$$

Comments

The major determinant of GFR is the hydrostatic pressure within the glomerular capillaries. In addition, the renal blood flow (RBF) through the glomeruli has a great effect on GFR; when the rate of RBF increases, the GFR increases.

The term clearance refers to the volume of plasma from which a substance X is completely removed or "cleared" per unit time, i.e., the ml of plasma that "contained" the substance X that is present in one minute's urine. It is a theoretical volume rather than a volume that can be collected and directly measured. Its value can be calculated from measurable quantities. For example, inulin is only filtered and measures GFR, while p-aminohippuric acid (PAH; see below) is both filtered and secreted into the proximal tubules, and measures renal blood flow (RBF).

Q. 21   Calculate the renal blood flow (RBF) from the data given below.

Data
(a) Concentration of PAH
      in urine (U_{PAH})   = 14 mg/ml
(b) Concentration of PAH
      in plasma (P_{PAH})   = 0.03 mg/ml
(c) Rate of urine flow (V)   = 1.5 ml/min
(d) Hematocrit (Hct)   = 43%

- - - - - - - - - - - - - - - - - - - -

Plasma clearance of PAH

$$= \frac{U_{PAH} \cdot V}{P_{PAH}} = \frac{14 \cdot 1.5}{0.03} = 700 \, ml/min$$

This plasma clearance of PAH is the effective renal plasma flow (ERPF).

The ERPF can be converted into actual renal plasma flow (RPF):

$$Actual \, RPF = \frac{ERPF}{Extraction \, ratio} = \frac{700}{0.9} = 770 \, ml/min$$

(About 90% of PAH in the arterial blood is removed during a single passage through the kidneys, i.e., its extraction ratio is 0.9)
Hematocrit = 43% (given data)
∴ Renal blood flow =

$$\frac{100}{100 - Hct} \cdot RPF = \frac{100}{100 - 43} \cdot 770 = \frac{100}{57} \cdot 770 = 1350$$

The renal blood flow is 1350 ml per minute.

Q. 22   Calculate the urea clearance from the given data.

Data
(a) Concentration of urea
      in urine (U)   = 20 mg/ml
(b) Concentration of urea
      in blood (B)   = 38 mg/100 ml
(c) Rate of urine flow (V)   = 1.5 ml/min

- -

Since the urine flow is less than 2.0 ml/min, the formula of "standard" urea clearance is

$$\frac{U \cdot \sqrt{V}}{B} \times 100$$

$$Urea \, clearance = \frac{20 \cdot \sqrt{1.5}}{38} \cdot 100$$

$$= \frac{20 \cdot 1.22}{38} \cdot 100 = 64 \, ml/min$$

Comments
It has been shown empirically that with rapid flow of urine (2 ml per minute or more), the excretion of urea is maximum—hence called "maximum" urea clearance. The formula for maximum clearance is UV/P. The value for maximum clearance is 65–100 ml per minute, while the normal value for standard clearance is 40-65 ml per minute.

Q. 23   Calculate the safe periods in the two women from the data provided.

Data
Woman A: Menstrual cycles regular, duration of a cycle is 29 days.
Woman B: Menstrual cycles irregular, duration of cycles varies between 26 and 33 days.

- -

Woman A: *Menstrual cycle:* 29 days
               Ovulation: 15th day of the cycle (14

days before the onset of next cycle). *Safe period:* Extends up to 11th day, and continues from 19th day onwards to the end of the cycle.

Woman B: *Menstrual cycle:* 26 days to 33 days (To calculate the safe period in women with irregular menstrual cycles during the pre-ovulatory phase, 18 is subtracted from the shortest recorded cycle. During the luteal phase, 11 is subtracted from the longest recorded cycle).

Safe period: 26 – 18 = 8, and
33 – 11 = 22.

Therefore, in this woman, the safe period extends up to 8th day of any cycle, and continues from day 22 onward till the end of the cycle.

(The first day of the menstrual cycle is the day when the menstrual bleeding starts).

Appendix

UNITS AND MEASURES EMPLOYED IN PHYSIOLOGY

The international system of units (SI Units-system International d' Unites)

Examples of Basic SI Units		
Physical quantity	Name of SI unit	Symbol of SI unit
length	meter	m
mass	kilogram	kg
amount of substance	mole	mol
energy	joule	J
pressure	pascal	Pa
time	second	s (or, sec)
electric current	ampere	A
thermodynamic temperature	kelvin	K
luminous intensity	candela	cd

Decimal Multiples and Submultiples of the SI Units

These are formed by the use of prefixes. The Greek prefixes (deca, hecto, kilo, myria) denote multiplication. The Latin prefixes (deci, centi, milli) denote division. [The METER (Fr, MÉTRÉ), the unit of length is the ten-millionth part of a line drawn from the pole to the equator].

Multiple	Prefix	Symbol	Sub multiple	Prefix	Symbol
10^1	deca	da	10^{-1}	deci	d
10^2	hecto	h	10^{-2}	centi	c
10^3	kilo	k	10^{-3}	milli	m
10^6	mega	M	10^{-6}	micro	μ
10^9	giga	G	10^{-9}	nano	n
10^{12}	tera	T	10^{-12}	pico	p
10^{15}	peta	P	10^{-15}	femto	f
10^{18}	exa	E	10^{-18}	atto	a

Unit of volume. The SI unit of volume is the *cubic meter* (m^3). But because of its inconvenience the *liter (l)* and *deciliter (dl)* are used as the units of volume for most applications in physiology and biochemistry. The equivalents of *metric, United States,* and *English (Imperial)* measures are also shown.

$1\ m^3$ = 1000 liters

1 fl oz = 29.57 ml

1 liter = 1.76 pints

1 liter = 1.06 US liq quart

1 US = 0.83 English gallon (Imperial) gallon

$1\ m^3$ = 275 bus (bushel)

• 1 dl = 100 ml
• 1 inch = 16.39 cm^3
• 1 ml = 0.0352 oz
• 1 mm^3 (1 c mm) = 1 μl (microliter)
• 1 pint = 568 ml = 20 fl oz
• 1 m^3 = 1.31 yd^3
• 1 US = 32 fl oz = 0.95 1 liq quart
• 1 gallon = 4.55 liters
• 1 bus = 0.0364 m^3

Unit of amount of substance. The 'Molar' (e.g., mol/l; μmol/l) is used for substances of defined chemical composition. It replaces the equivalent concentration (mEq/l) which is not part of the SI system for measurements of sodium, potassium, chloride and bicarbonate (the numerical value of these four measurements is unchanged because these ions are univalent).

Unit of weight (mass concentration). The SI unit is the *kilogram* (kg)

1 kg = 1000 g (grams)

1 kg = 2.20 pounds (lb; avoirdupois) = 2.68 pounds (apothecaries')

1 lb = 453.6 g = 16 oz • 1 oz = 28.35 g • 1 grain = 65mg

1 tonne = 1000 kg = 0.984 ton = 2204 lb

1 ton = 1016 kg = 1.02 tonne = 2244 lb

Unit of length. The SI unit is the *meter (m)*

1 Angstrom unit (Å) = 10^{-10} m = 0.1 nm • [1 micrometer (μm) = 10^{-6} m (micron, μ, is obsolete, and in its place, the unit μm is used)].

1 in (inch) = 2.54 cm

•1 cm   = 0.394 in
•1 yd (yard) = 0.9144 m
1 meter = 39.37 in •1 meter   = 1.09144 yd
•1 meter   = 3.28 ft (feet)
1 km = 0.621 mile •1 mile   = 1.609 km
•1 mile   = 1760 yd
1 nautical mile = 1.852 km = 1.14 mile = 6080 ft
Knot = Nautical miles per hour

Unit of Area. The SI unit of area is the *square meter* *(m²)*

$1 \, cm^2 = 0.155 \, inch^2$ •$1 \, in^2 = 6.452 \, cm^2$
•$1 \, ft^2 = 929 \, cm^2$
$1 \, m^2 = 10.8 \, ft^2$ •$1 \, m^2 = 1.20 \, yd^2$
•$1 yd^2 = 0.836 \, m^2$
$1 \, acre = 4840 \, yd^2 = 4047 \, m^2 = 0.4047 \, ha$ (hectare)
1 hectare = 2.471 acres •1 sq mile
$= 2.59 \, km^2 = 640$ acres

Unit of pressure. The SI unit of pressure is the *pascal* *(Pa)*. This is the pressure exerted by 1 Newton force on an area of a square meter ($1 \, Pa = 1 \, N \, m^{-2}$).
1 cm water = 98.1 Pa
•1 mm Hg = 1 torr = 133.3 Pa = 0.1333 kPa
1 kPa = 7.60 mm Hg = 10.1 cm H_2O
• $1 \, lb/in^2 = 6.894$ kPa
1 millibar (mb) = 0.1 kPa
• 1 dyne/cm = 10^{-4} kPa
• 1 normal atmosphere = 1 bar
= 760 mm Hg = 101.3 kPa

Temperature. The SI temperature scale is the kelvin scale (K) but it is inconvenient to use in medicine. The *Celsius* (formerly centrigrade) scale (°C) has been retained.
• To convert Celsius degrees to Fahrenheit, multiply with 9/5 and add 32.
• To convert Fahrenheit degrees to Celsius, substract 32 and multiply by 5/9.

°C –40 –10 0 10 20 30 35 37 40 45 100
°F –40 14 32 50 68 86 95 98.6 104 113 212

LABORATORY VALUES OF CLINICAL IMPORTANCE

The following laboratory values are some of those which have frequent clinical relevance. Values in SI units are shown in brackets after the values in traditional units.

BODY FLUIDS AND OTHER MASS DATA

Body fluid, total volume: 50% (in obese) to 70% (lean) of body weight
• Intracellular : 30-40% of body weight
• Extracellular : 20-30% of body weight
(Of about 40 liters of water in a 70 kg man, 14 liters are in ECF (3.5 liters in vascular, and 10.5 liters in interstitial fluid compartments) and 26 liters in ICF).

Blood (total volume)
Males   : 70 ml/kg body weight
Females : 65 ml/kg body weight (7.5-8% b.w)

Plasma volume
Males   : 39 ml/kg body weight
Females : 40 ml/kg body weight

RBC volume
Males   : 30 ml/kg body weight
Females : 25 ml/kg body weight

BLOOD—Reference intervals

Arterial gases
$PaCO_2$: 35-45 mm Hg
PaO_2 : 80-100 mm Hg at sea level

Arterial oxygen saturation (at rest)
Sea level : 97%
5000 ft   : 90%
15000 ft   : 75%
(Adult blood contains 0.3 ml O_2 in physical solution and about 19 ml/dl in chemical combination with hemoglobin).

Carbon dioxide content, plasma (sea level): 50-70 volumes/dl [21-28 mmol/liter].

Carboxyhemoglobin
• Nonsmokers : 0–2.3%
• Smokers   : 2.1–4.2%

Bleeding time
Duke method (finger, ear lobe) : < 5 minutes
Ivy method (5-mm wound)   : < 9 minutes
Simplate   : < 7 minutes

Coagulation time
Capillary blood   : 2–5 min
Venous blood (Lee and White) : 5–15 min

Erythrocyte sedimentation rate (ESR), mm 1st hour:
> Westergren:
>> Males : 0–15
>> Females : 0–20
> Wintrobe:
>> Males : 0–9
>> Females : 0–20 (Increases with age)

Fragility of red cells: Hemolysis begins at 0.45% NaCl; complete at 0.35% NaCl solution.

Hematocrit (Hct; packed cell volume, (PCV)
> Men   : 40-52%
> Women : 37-47%
> [(SI: Men : 0.4-0.52 l/l, Women: 0.37-0.47 l/l)]

Mean corpuscular (cell) volume (MCV): 75-94 µm^3 [75-94 fl]

Mean corpuscular hemoglobin (MCH): 27-32 pg

Mean corpuscular hemoglobin concentration (MCHC):
> 30-36% [SI: 30-36 g/l]

Osmolality (serum): 275-295 mosm/kg water

Red cell count:
> Males   : 4.5-6.5 million/mm^3
>> [SI: 4.5-6.5 × 10^{12}/l]
> Females : 4.0-5.5 million/mm^3
>> [SI : 4.0-5.5 × 10^{12}/l]
> *Hemoglobin*
> Males   : 13.5-18 g/dl
> Females : 11.5-16 g/dl

White cell count (WCC): 4000-11000/mm^3
[SI: 4.0 - 11.0 × 10^9/l]

Neutrophils	40-75% WCC	[2.0-7.5 × 10^9/l]
Eosinophils	1-6% WCC	[0.04-0.44 × 10^9/l]
Lymphocytes	20-45% WCC	[1.3-3.5 × 10^9/l]
Basophils	0.0-1.0% WCC	[0.0-0.10 × 10^9/l]
Monocytes	2-10% WCC	[0.2-0.8 × 10^9/l]

Platelet count: 150,000-400,000/mm^3 [SI:150.0-400.0 × 10^9/l]
> Life span: 8-10 days

CARDIOVASCULAR SYSTEM

Cardiac output (Fick): 4.5-6 liters/min
(cardiac index: 2.5-3.6 liters/min/m^{2}BSA

Capillary pressure (systemic):
- Arterial end : 32 mm Hg
- Venous end : 12 mm Hg
- Mean   : 20 mm Hg

Pulmonary capillaries (mean):
> 8 mm Hg (osmotic pressure of blood: 25 mm Hg; no tissue fluid formed).

Maximum glucose reabsorptive capacity (Tm$_G$):
> Males: 300-450 mg/min
> Females: 250-350 mg/min

Osmolality: On normal diet and fluid intake: Range: 500-850 mosm/kg water. Achievable range (normal kidney): Dilution 40-80 mosm/kg water. Concentration: at least 3-4 times plasma osmolality.

BIOCHEMISTRY—Reference values (S: serum; P: plasma)

[Values in SI units are given in brackets after the values in traditional units]

Aminotransferases (S)

Aspartate-aminotransferase (AST, SGOT): 10-14 Karmen units/ml; 6-18 IU/l [100-300 µmol/l]

Alanine-aminotransferase (ALT, SGPT): 10-40 Karmen units/ml; 3-26 IU/l [50-430 µmol/l]

Amylase (S): 60-180 Somogyi units/dl [13-53 nmol/l]

Ammonia (whole blood): 80-110 µg/dl [45-65 µmol/l]

Bicarbonate (S or P): 24-30 mEq/l [24-30 mmol/l]

Bilirubin (total, S or P): 0.3-1 mg/dl [5-17 µmol/l] (About half is direct)

Calcium, total (S): 8.5-10.5 mg/dl [2.12-2.62 mmol/l] (varies with protein concentration)

Chloride (S): 350-375 mg/dl; 95-105 mEq/l [95-105 mmol/l]

Cholesterol (S): 140-300 mg/dl [3.6-7.8 mmol/l]

Fibrinogen (P): 150-400 mg/dl [1.5-4 g/l]

Glucose, normal, fasting (P): 80-90 mg/dl [4.4-4.9 mmol/l] Upper limit: 110 mg/dl [6 mmol/l]

2-hour postprandial (or after drinking 75 g glucose (50 g in children under 14)

> Normal: 140 mg/dl [7.8 mmol/l] No value exceeds renal threshold of 180 mg/dl [9.9 mmol/l]

Impaired glucose tolerance: 140-200 mg/dl [7.8-11.1 mmol/l]

Diabetes mellitus: > 200 mg/dl [> 11.1 mmol/l on more than one occasion] •Two fasting levels > 145 mg/dl confirm the diagnosis of diabetes mellitus.

Immunoglobulins (S):
   IgA: 90-350 mg/dl • IgD: 0-8 mg/dl
   IgE: < 0.025 mg/dl • IgG: 800-1500 mg/dl
   IgM: 45-150 mg/dl (SI units in g/l)

Magnesium (S or P): 2-3 mg/dl [0.75-1.05 mmol/l]

Non-protein nitrogen (NPN) (S): 20-30 mg/dl [14-21 mmol/l]

Osmolality (P): 285-295 mosm/kg of serum water

Phosphate (as inorganic P) (P): 2.5-4.5 mg/dl [0.8-1.45 mmol/l]

Phosphatase, acid, serum: 0.2-1.8 IU [3-30 nmol/l]

Phosphatase, alkaline, serum: 21-91 IU at 37°C [0.4-1.5 μmol/l]

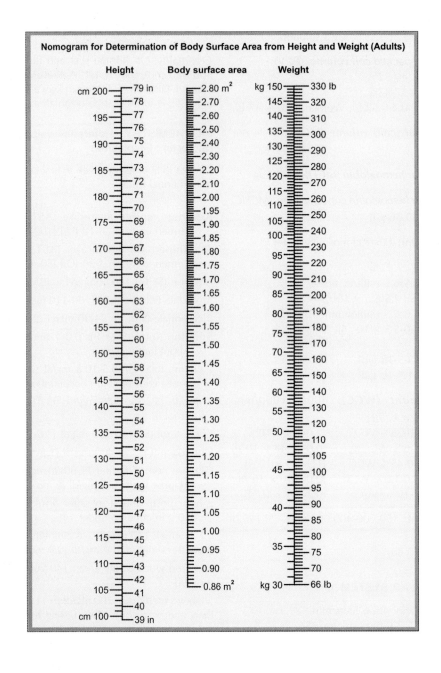

Nomogram for Determination of Body Surface Area from Height and Weight (Adults)

Potassium (S): 14-20 mg/dl [3.5-5.0 mmol/l]

Proteins, total, serum: 5.5-8.0 g/dl [55-80 g/l]

Protein fractions
 Albumin: 3.5-5 g/dl
 Globulin: 2-3.5 g/dl
 Alpha$_1$: 0.2-0.4 g/dl
 Alpha$_2$: 0.5-0.9 g/dl
 Beta: 0.6-1.1 g/dl
 Gamma: 0.7-1.7 g/dl

SGOT, SGPT: See Aminotransferases

Sodium (S): 310-340 mg/dl (136-145 mEq/l) [135-145 mmol/l]

Triglycerides, as triolin (S): 25-150 mg/dl [0.28-1.69 mmol/l]

Thyroid binding globulin (TBG) (P): 7-17 mg/l

Thyroxine (T$_4$) (P): 70-140 nmol/l

Thyroxine (free) plasma: 9-22 pmol/l

Triiodothyronine (T$_3$), plasma: 1.2-3.0 nmol/l

Urea (urea nitrogen) (S): 10-20 mg/dl [3.6-7.1 mmol/l]

Uric acid (urate) (S or P): 2-7 mg/dl [0.15- 0.48 mmol/l] (slightly less in females)

Xylose (B): 5-50 mg/dl [0.33-3.33 mmol/l]

Zinc (S): 50-150 µg/dl [7.65-22.95 µmol/l].